Diagnosis and Treatment of Tinnitus

Diagnosis and Treatment of Tinnitus

Editor: Kimi Brown

AMERICAN
MEDICAL PUBLISHERS
www.americanmedicalpublishers.com

AMERICAN
MEDICAL PUBLISHERS
www.americanmedicalpublishers.com

Cataloging-in-Publication Data

Diagnosis and treatment of tinnitus / edited by Kimi Brown.
p. cm.
Includes bibliographical references and index.
ISBN 979-8-88740-515-5
1. Tinnitus. 2. Tinnitus--Diagnosis. 3. Tinnitus--Treatment. 4. Hearing disorders. I. Brown, Kimi.
RF293.8 .D53 2023
617.8--dc23

American Medical Publishers,
41 Flatbush Avenue,
1st Floor, New York,
NY 11217, USA

ISBN 979-8-88740-515-5 (Hardback)

Contents

Preface

Tinnitus is a hearing disorder which involves hearing noises that are actually not caused by sounds coming from the outside world. A number of underlying causes generated at any level of the auditory system may result in this disorder. Factors such as emotional stress, traumatic brain injury, excessive earwax, and exposure to loud noise can severely affect hearing. Tinnitus is categorized into three types which are named as subjective tinnitus, objective tinnitus, and pulsatile tinnitus. The disorder is typically subjective, which means that the noises a person hears are not identifiable by physicians or hearing technicians using current technology. In certain cases, tinnitus can be detected by an individual using a stethoscope. This condition is called objective tinnitus. Pulsatile tinnitus is described as experiencing sound that beats in time with the pulse. Tinnitus can be cured through talk therapy, sound therapy, or hearing aids. Through this book, the readers would gain knowledge that would broaden their perspective about tinnitus. A number of researches and case studies from all over the globe have been included herein on the diagnosis and treatment of this disease. It is a collective contribution of a renowned group of international experts.

The researches compiled throughout the book are authentic and of high quality, combining several disciplines and from very diverse regions from around the world. Drawing on the contributions of many researchers from diverse countries, the book's objective is to provide the readers with the latest achievements in the area of research. This book will surely be a source of knowledge to all interested and researching the field.

In the end, I would like to express my deep sense of gratitude to all the authors for meeting the set deadlines in completing and submitting their research chapters. I would also like to thank the publisher for the support offered to us throughout the course of the book. Finally, I extend my sincere thanks to my family for being a constant source of inspiration and encouragement.

Editor

1

Neuroanatomical Alterations in Tinnitus Assessed with Magnetic Resonance Imaging

Thomas W. Allan[1†], Julien Besle[1†], Dave R. M. Langers[2,3], Jeff Davies[2,3], Deborah A. Hall[2,3], Alan R. Palmer[1] and Peyman Adjamian[1]*

[1] Medical Research Council Institute of Hearing Research, The University of Nottingham, Nottingham, UK, [2] Nottingham Hearing Biomedical Research Unit, National Institute for Health Research (NIHR), Nottingham, UK, [3] Otology and Hearing Group, Division of Clinical Neuroscience, School of Medicine, The University of Nottingham, Nottingham, UK

***Correspondence:**
Peyman Adjamian
peyman.adjamian@nottingham.ac.uk

† These authors have contributed equally to this work.

Previous studies of anatomical changes associated with tinnitus have provided inconsistent results, with some showing significant cortical and subcortical changes, while others have found effects due to hearing loss, but not tinnitus. In this study, we examined changes in brain anatomy associated with tinnitus using anatomical scans from 128 participants with tinnitus and hearing loss, tinnitus with clinically normal hearing, and non-tinnitus controls with clinically normal hearing. The groups were matched for hearing loss, age and gender. We employed voxel- and surface-based morphometry (SBM) to investigate gray and white matter volume and thickness within regions-of-interest (ROI) that were based on the results of previous studies. The largest overall effects were found for age, gender, and hearing loss. With regard to tinnitus, analysis of ROI revealed numerous small increases and decreases in gray matter and thickness between tinnitus and non-tinnitus controls, in both cortical and subcortical structures. For whole brain analysis, the main tinnitus-related significant clusters were found outside sensory auditory structures. These include a decrease in cortical thickness for the tinnitus group compared to controls in the left superior frontal gyrus (SFG), and a decrease in cortical volume with hearing loss in left Heschl's gyrus (HG). For masked analysis, we found a decrease in gray matter volume in the right Heschle's gyrus for the tinnitus group compared to the controls. We found no changes in the subcallosal region as reported in some previous studies. Overall, while some of the morphological differences observed in this study are similar to previously published findings, others are entirely different or even contradict previous results. We highlight other discrepancies among previous results and the increasing need for a more precise subtyping of the condition.

Keywords: tinnitus, brain anatomy, auditory cortex, voxel-based morphometry, surface-based morphometry

INTRODUCTION

Tinnitus, the perception of a phantom sound in the absence of an external source, is experienced chronically by approximately 5–15% of the population (Baguley et al., 2013). The onset of tinnitus is typically associated with aging or exposure to loud noise, cumulative or sudden, such that hair cell damage occurs with subsequent hearing impairment. Tinnitus can cause significant distress, causing problems such as depression, anxiety and sleep disorders (Henry et al., 2005).

The exact cause of tinnitus and its associated pathophysiology remains unknown. Although tinnitus is commonly initiated by damage to the peripheral auditory system, it is believed that the sound percept is generated and maintained in the brain. This has been confirmed by surgical interventions where the auditory nerve is bisected yet the perception of the tinnitus sound remains (House and Brackmann, 1981). Current consensus is that the initial cause of many forms of tinnitus is strongly related to cochlear damage and the resulting hearing loss, which may cause changes to neural coding properties (Seki and Eggermont, 2003).

Recently, both functional and structural imaging have been used to investigate changes in the brain associated with tinnitus. Functional studies based on changes in regional cerebral blood flow (using positron emission tomography; PET) have found regions of the brain associated with the perception of the tinnitus sound (Mirz et al., 1999, 2000a,b; Reyes et al., 2002). However, PET has limitations due to the required administration of radioactive tracer restricting longitudinal studies. Functional magnetic resonance imaging (fMRI) has also been used to measure changes in brain activity in people with tinnitus. This method has high spatial resolution, but significant acoustic noise is generated by the scanner during the imaging process that may have a confounding effect on the results (Melcher et al., 2000; Lanting et al., 2008, 2009). Moreover, fMRI is able to detect persistent changes in neural baseline activity that can be associated with chronic tinnitus. Magneto- and electroencephalography (MEG, EEG) have been used to examine differences in power spectra and to localize regions of the brain associated with tinnitus. However, these methods suffer from poor spatial resolution and results are contradictory (for review see Adjamian et al., 2009). All functional imaging methods have confounding issues that relate to task performance, and how well the participant is able to describe the changes they are experiencing.

Anatomical brain changes are believed to arise from plasticity and reorganization of the brain. Analysis of high resolution MRI anatomical data of the brain, thus complements functional imaging. Various studies have shown that functional changes are directly linked to structural changes in tinnitus (Mühlau et al., 2006; Schneider et al., 2009; Husain et al., 2011; Leaver et al., 2011, 2012; Mahoney et al., 2011; Aldhafeeri et al., 2012; Schecklmann et al., 2012; Boyen et al., 2013; Melcher et al., 2013). Adjamian et al. (2014) recently provided a comprehensive review of this literature.

Changes in structure, gray and white matter volumes and brain shape are indicative of differences in prolonged neuronal activity and connectivity between brain regions (Pfefferbaum et al., 1994; Good et al., 2001; Draganski et al., 2004; Maguire et al., 2006). We have previously reviewed several approaches to structural analysis that have been growing in popularity in recent years, including: voxel-based morphometry (VBM), surface-based morphometry (SBM), deformation-based morphometry (DBM), tensor-based morphometry (TBM) and diffusion tensor imaging (DTI) (Adjamian et al., 2014). VBM allows assessment using statistical metrics of voxel-wise changes in the gray matter volume of the neocortex between populations, or in any given population relative to a clinical measure. However, VBM has been criticized for being sensitive to image registration procedures that can yield spurious results (Bookstein, 2001). On the other hand, using the surface of the brain, SBM highlights the cortical folding of the brain and avoids the registration problems, to some extent, by investigating differences in the area, thickness of tissue or the curvature of the cortex between subjects (Winkler et al., 2010).

Current evidence regarding the tinnitus-related structural changes in the brain has produced a range of contradictory and varied results. Mühlau et al. (2006) were the first to show structural changes related to tinnitus using whole brain and region-of-interest (ROI) voxel-wise VBM analyses. This study showed a reduction in gray matter in subcallosal areas, such as the nucleus accumbens (NAc), and an increase in the medial geniculate nucleus (MGN). However, other studies have failed to replicate these results using largely similar methods (e.g., Landgrebe et al., 2009; Husain et al., 2011; Melcher et al., 2013). In line with Mühlau et al. (2006) findings, Rauschecker et al. (2010) suggested a gating model in which tinnitus results from a failure to inhibit noise, allowing unpleasant noise signals to reach the auditory cortex (AC). This model is based upon evidence from human neuroimaging and animal studies and involves cortical and subcortical regions consisting of the amygdala, the NAc, the ventromedial prefrontal cortex (vmPFC), and the reticular nucleus of the thalamus (Leaver et al., 2011, 2012; Seydell-Greenwald et al., 2014). This limbic corticostriatal pathway has been shown to play an important role in the suppression of unpleasant sounds. Consequently, abnormalities within these areas of the brain may lead to the perception of a tinnitus sound and the negative emotions associated with chronic tinnitus. As this model predicts tinnitus-related changes in the activity of specific structures, it can be evaluated using MRI-based morphological analysis techniques.

In a recent article, we identified various factors which may underlie the reported inconsistent findings (Adjamian et al., 2014). These include the heterogeneity of tinnitus characteristics such as its etiology, duration and lateralization. Moreover, in most studies, important parameters that may independently affect brain anatomy have not been adequately controlled for, such as age and hearing loss (Lee et al., 2007; Crippa et al., 2010). Another important factor may be the small size of participant groups, often due to recruitment difficulties, with sometimes as few as 11 tinnitus participants. Small sample sizes result in low statistical power, such that effects from one or two participants can dramatically change the overall outcomes. In addition to the low statistical power, many studies employ thresholds uncorrected for multiple comparisons, which increases the chance of false positives. Another possible reason for the inconsistent findings might be the masks used to specify ROIs in the analysis. Six groups have used the same masks as defined in Mühlau et al. (2006), but with varying results (Mühlau et al., 2006; Landgrebe et al., 2009; Husain et al., 2011; Leaver et al., 2011; Boyen et al., 2013; Melcher et al., 2013). Others have focused upon whole-brain analysis (Schecklmann et al., 2012, 2013), specific ROIs such as Heschl's gyri (Schneider et al., 2009) and the inferior/superior/middle frontal gyri (Aldhafeeri et al., 2012), large ROIs such as the temporal lobe, upper brain stem and bilateral orbito-frontal cortices (Mahoney et al., 2011), or a range of brain regions such as the thalamus, caudate, putamen and globus pallidus (Leaver et al., 2012). This range of foci means that it is difficult to distinguish a consistent pattern across studies.

Given the previous inconsistent findings, we aimed to address some of these methodological issues using MRI data collected from a large cohort of tinnitus participants and matched controls at partner research centers in Nottingham. We tested the hypothesis that tinnitus is accompanied by changes in gray and white matter compared to non-tinnitus controls. More specifically, we aimed to detect structural changes using VBM and SBM, whilst controlling for variables such as tinnitus severity, hearing loss, and age. Based on the gating mechanism proposed by Rauschecker et al. (2010), we hypothesize that these changes in brain anatomy will be located in the MGN, the vmPFC, and the NAc. We use various ROI masks based on previous studies, including those by Mühlau et al. (2006) and Leaver et al. (2011) to examine areas beyond the subcallosal region. Finally, given that tinnitus is an ongoing sensation that has been shown to affect resting state activity (Husain and Schmidt, 2014), we also investigated anatomical changes in the areas constituting the default mode network (DMN), which is linked to resting-state activity (Greicius et al., 2003).

MATERIALS AND METHODS

Subject Recruitment

One hundred twenty eight participants (73 tinnitus and 55 controls) were recruited as part of other functional imaging studies at the Medical Research Council (MRC) Institute of Hearing Research (IHR; $n = 61$) and the National Institute for Health Research (NIHR) Nottingham Hearing Biomedical Research Unit (BRU; $n = 67$). The IHR cohort had been recruited as part of MEG studies to investigate oscillatory and evoked responses in tinnitus (Adjamian et al., 2012; Sereda et al., 2013). The BRU cohort was recruited for a study examining hearing aid benefits for tinnitus with functional MRI (Davies et al., 2014). The IHR study was approved by the National Health Service (NHS) East Midlands Nottingham local research ethics Committee 2, and sponsored by the MRC. The BRU study was approved by the North Nottinghamshire Research Ethics Committee, and sponsored by the NHS Nottingham University Hospital Trust.

Audiograms comprising frequencies from 0.25 to 12 kHz were acquired for each subject. Clinically normal hearing was based on the average of the pure-tone hearing threshold levels 250, 500, 1000, 2000 and 4000 Hz <20 dB Hearing Loss (HL; British Society of Audiology, 2011). Participants with tinnitus completed either the Tinnitus Handicap Inventory (THI; Newman et al., 1996; $N = 30$, the IHR cohort) or Tinnitus Handicap Questionnaire (THQ; Kuk et al., 1990; $N = 43$, the BRU cohort) to assess its severity. Because these questionnaire scores have the same range (0–100) and show high convergent validity (Fackrell et al., 2014), we applied a simple stratification to combine both sets of scores so that all tinnitus participants had a tinnitus severity score that fell within one of five categories: grade one, 0–16 (low); grade two, 17–36 (mild); grade three, 37–56 (moderate); grade four, 57–76 (severe); or, grade five, 77–100 (catastrophic). These boundaries were informed by a UK THI grading (McCombe et al., 2001).

Group Classifications

Three separate groups of participants were defined for statistical analysis. The aim of these groups is to isolate particular features so that we could maximize the statistical power to detect various potential effects.

Group 1—All Subjects

The first group consisted of all participants in the study, divided into two subgroups of tinnitus participants and non-tinnitus controls. This comparison maximized the statistical power available to detect possible changes related to tinnitus.

Group 2—Severe Tinnitus vs. Matched Controls

The second group consisted of participants with severe or catastrophic tinnitus and controls individually matched for age, gender and hearing loss. This comparison was made to assess the effect of highly intrusive tinnitus compared to a matched sample.

Group 3—Tinnitus With Clinically Normal Hearing vs. Matched Controls

The final group consisted of tinnitus participants with clinically normal hearing, again matched individually for age and gender to controls with clinically normal hearing. This comparison isolated the effect of tinnitus from the effect of hearing loss.

Information and number of participants pertaining to each of the subgroups are listed in **Table 1** and their mean audiograms are shown in **Figures 1A–C**. There were no significant differences in age, gender or hearing loss between the tinnitus participants and control participants in any of the three groups.

Data Acquisition

Subjects were scanned either on a 3-T or 1.5-T Philips scanner by means of a high resolution magnetization-prepared rapid gradient-echo (MPRAGE) acquisition (resolution = $1 \times 1 \times 1$ mm^3, repetition time (TR) = 8 s, echo time (TE) = 3.74 ms, field of view (FOV) = $256 \times 256 \times 160$ mm^3). One hundred twenty one participants were scanned on the 3 T scanner, and 7 (4 tinnitus and 3 non-tinnitus controls) on the 1.5 T, because, the 3 T scanner was unavailable.

VBM Data Processing

The data processing was performed using Statistical Parametric Mapping (SPM8[1]). Each participant's anatomical image was

[1]http://www.fil.ion.ucl.ac.uk/spm/software/spm8/

TABLE 1 | Demographic information and hearing status for each of the three groupings.

Group	Subgroup	*N*	Age (years)				Gender		PTA (dB HL)
			Mean	Std	Min	Max	Male	Female	Mean (both ears)
1 (All)	Tinnitus	73	58.38	12.41	24	80	43	30	28.62
	Controls	55	56.91	16.39	19	76	30	25	24.19
2 (Severe Tinnitus vs. matched Controls)	Tinnitus	16	55.06	15.53	24	80	8	8	21.51
	Controls	16	53.69	14.85	25	72	8	8	20.91
3 (Tinnitus with clinically normal hearing vs. matched controls)	Tinnitus	15	47.60	16.66	24	80	6	9	8.22
	Controls	15	50.20	17.25	20	71	6	9	8.62

segmented into gray matter, white matter, cerebrospinal fluid (CSF) and other tissues. For each group (described above), Diffeomorphic Anatomical Registration Through Exponentiated Lie algebra (DARTEL: Ashburner, 2007) was used to create a white matter and gray matter template using segmented images of participants from all of the groups to improve the registration to a common space. That is, each group had its own gray and white matter template to which both the tinnitus participants and controls were realigned. Whilst aligning the individual images to the template, the volume of white and gray matter was preserved (i.e., modulated images were computed).

The data were then resampled to 2-mm isotropic resolution, aligned with Montreal Neurological Institute (MNI) space and subsequently smoothed with an isotropic 10-mm full-width at half-maximum (FWHM) kernel. Finally, these images were set at

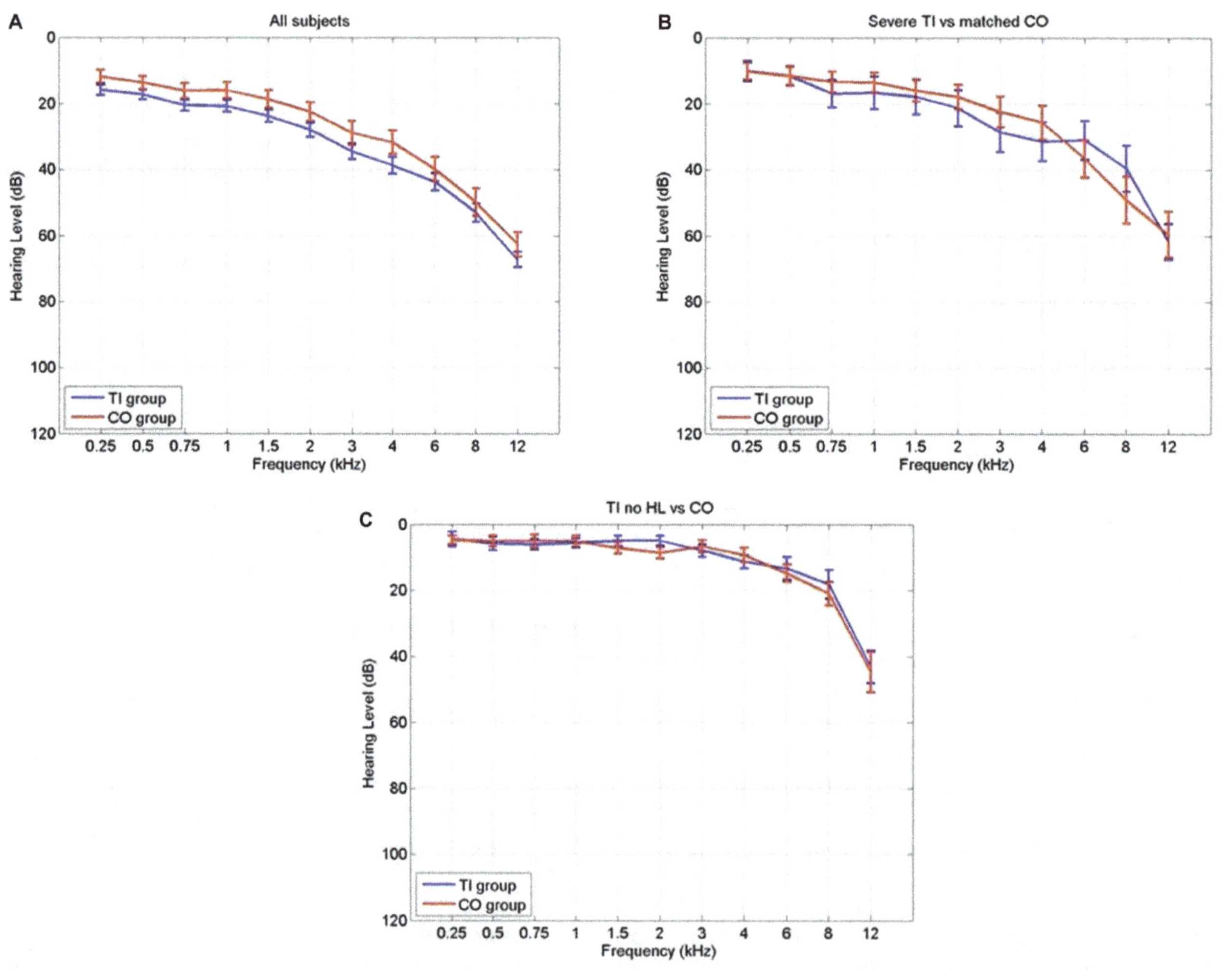

FIGURE 1 | The audiograms for each comparison group for the tinnitus participants (blue) and the controls (red) in (A) all subjects, (B) severe tinnitus and matched controls and (C) tinnitus with no hearing loss and matched controls.

TABLE 2 | The definitions of the masks used and how they were defined.

Mask	Brodmann areas	WFUpickatlas	MNI coordinates (*x, y, z*)	Volume (bilateral, cm^3)
Cochlear nucleus (CN)	–	–	±10, −38, −45	1.30
Superior olivary complex (SOC)	–	–	±13, −35, −41	1.30
Inferior colliculus (IC)	–	–	±6 , −33, −11	1.30
Medial geniculate nucleus (MGN)	–	–	±17, −24, −2	4.11
Heschl gyrus (HG)	41	–	–	13.45*
Auditory cortex (AC)	22, 41 and 42	–	–	74.74*
Superior temporal gyrus (STG)	–	Superior temporal gyrus	–	83.97
Nucleus accumbens (Na$_C$)	–	Nucleus accumbens left and right	–	4.25
Ventromedial prefrontal cortex (vmPFC)	10, 11, 12, 13, 14, 25 and 32	–	–	77.19
Default mode network (DMN)	–	Posterior cingulate, medial frontal gyrus and middle temporal gyrus	–	120.90

**Indicates volume after 2 mm dilation;—Indicates no information available.*

a threshold of 5% to compensate for edge voxels and the blurring effect caused by smoothing the data.

Statistical maps were produced using linear regression through an ANCOVA model with a group factor (tinnitus or control) and additional covariates for tinnitus severity grading (1–5); controls were all assigned a value equal to the average of the tinnitus subgroup in order for this regressor to be orthogonal to the group factor), left and right ear pure tone averages (PTA) over the tested frequencies to 8 kHz, age, and gender. The group factor and all four covariates were tested for statistical significance. In addition, for each subject, the whole brain gray matter and white matter volumes were used as an additional covariate in the respective ANCOVA models to compensate for whole brain volume differences between subjects. In an alternative model, the raw THI/THQ scores were used as a covariate instead of the tinnitus severity grade, but the results were equivalent and are therefore not shown here. All the statistical maps were family-wise error (FWE) corrected for multiple comparisons using Gaussian Field theory with a confidence threshold of 0.05. The statistical analysis was run on the whole brain as well as restricted to each of the masks defined below.

FreeSurfer Data Processing

Cortical surface reconstruction was performed using the standard FreeSurfer v 5.3.0[2] pipeline run on a Linux CentOS 6 platform. In brief, this includes removal of non-brain tissues, automated Talairach transformation, segmentation of the subcortical white matter and deep gray matter volumetric structures, intensity normalization, tessellation of the gray and white matter boundary, automated topological correction and surface deformation. The technical details are fully described in prior publications (Dale et al., 1999; Fischl et al., 1999a,b; Fischl and Dale, 2000).

Measures of each subject's cortical thickness, area and volume were computed. Each subject's cortical surfaces were morphed onto the standard inflated brain and the thickness, area and volume values were smoothed with a 10-mm FWHM Gaussian kernel. The same ANCOVA model as in the VBM analysis, with one group factor and four covariates, was fitted to each measure (one difference with the VBM analysis however is that we did not use mean/total thickness/area/volume as an additional covariate). Monte-Carlo simulations were run to correct for multiple comparisons at the cluster level (Hayasaka and Nichols, 2003), as implemented in Freesurfer (Hagler et al., 2006). For the simulations, the voxelwise (uncorrected) threshold was set to $p = 0.01$ and the clusterwise (corrected) threshold was set to $p = 0.05$. Statistical analysis was conducted on the whole surface as well as in each of the masks, defined below.

Masks

To complement the whole-brain analyses, 10 masks were defined to assess changes in particular regions of the brain that might be attributable to the tinnitus percept. These masks were chosen based on the regions specified by the gating mechanism proposed by Rauschecker et al. (2010), and those used by Mühlau et al. (2006) that had shown tinnitus-related changes in brain volume.

Detailed definition of each mask is given in **Table 2**. The masks based on Rauschecker's gating mechanism are shown in **Figure 2**. The WFUpickatlas in SPM8 was used to define the masks. The AC mask (Brodmann areas 22, 41 and 42) was dilated by 2 mm in all directions to accommodate small registration errors and individual variability issues. The NAc mask was defined from the WFUpickatlas, and the vmPFC consisted of Brodmann areas 10, 11, 12, 13, 14, 25 and 32. Heschl's gyrus (HG; Brodmann area 41) was also dilated by 2 mm to account for small misregistration effects. The DMN comprised the posterior cingulate cortex (pCC), medial frontal gyrus (mFC) and middle temporal gyrus (MTG). The superior temporal gyrus (STG) was selected as it relates to normal auditory functioning, but does not include all areas of the AC that lie on the supratemporal plane. The masks for the AC, HG and STG had overlapping regions. The vmPFC and DMN also showed overlap.

Four subcortical masks were defined using coordinates based on Mühlau's study, to determine if their results could be replicated with our larger cohort of participants. These masks are shown in **Figure 3**. Bilateral 5-mm radius spheres were defined for the Cochlear nucleus (CN), the Superior olivary complex (SOC), and the Inferior colliculus (IC). In addition to these, bilateral 8 mm radius spheres were defined in the MGN.

[2]http://surfer.nmr.mgh.harvard.edu/

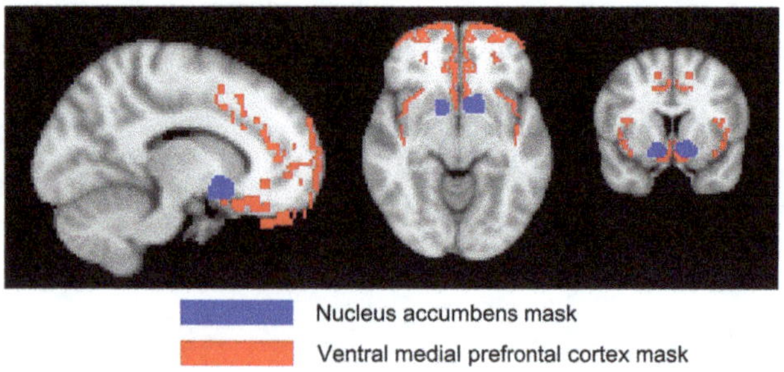

FIGURE 2 | The Rauschecker model brain regions [nucleus accumbens (NAc) and ventromedial prefrontal cortex (vmPFC)] that have been defined as a mask for further analysis.

All of the masks were used for the VBM analysis. Five of these masks were used for the SBM analysis (AC, DMN, HG, vmPFC and STG) as the other masks targeted subcortical structures. To create the surface masks, the volumetric masks were projected onto the standard inflated brain and manually corrected to remove non-contiguous vertices due to projection errors (corresponding to voxels contiguous in volumetric space but belonging to non-contiguous gyri).

ROI Analysis

For all of the masks and groups, ROI analyses were performed to compute the magnitude of differences between the tinnitus participants and controls. The various measures of interest (i.e., gray and white matter volume for VBM; surface thickness, area, and volume for SBM) were averaged (gray and white matter volume, surface cortical thickness) or summed (surface area and volume) across the voxels or vertices in a mask, and statistically compared between subgroups using t-tests. In Freesurfer, surface area/volume measures were normalized by the total surface area/volume of each hemisphere and all individual measures were averaged between the left and right surface masks.

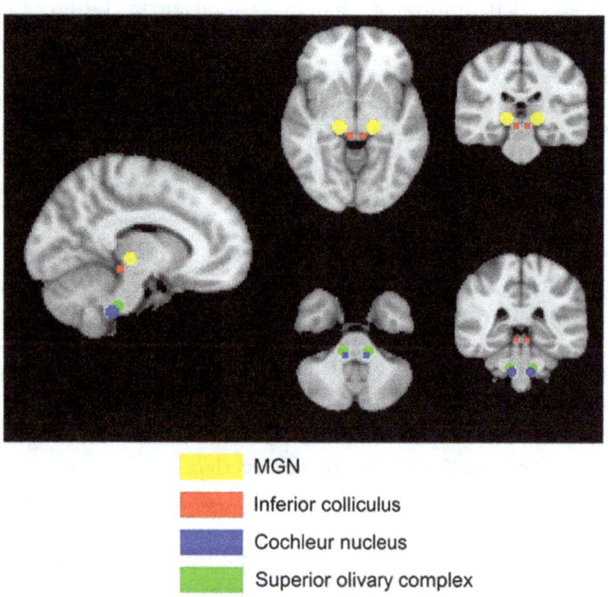

FIGURE 3 | The Mulhau masks that have previously shown anatomical changes relating to tinnitus.

RESULTS

Correlation Analysis

Pearson correlation coefficients were calculated between hearing loss PTA, age and tinnitus severity data to assess whether any covariates were interdependent.

The correlation between age and hearing loss across all subjects was significant ($r = 0.41$, p = 10–6; **Figure 4**). The correlations between tinnitus severity and hearing loss ($r = 0.08$, $p = 0.36$) or tinnitus severity and age ($r = -0.00$, $p = 0.98$) did not reach significance.

Morphometry

Overall, we found a number of clusters of significant effects in various masks and for different contrasts, varying in size. A summary of the significant effects of interest (Tinnitus vs. Controls and Tinnitus severity) is given in **Table 3** and they are described in detail in the following sections and shown in **Figures 6–11**. Full details of all findings, including significant effects of other covariates, are presented in the Supplementary Material Tables SI1–SI5.

Grouping 1—All subjects

Whole-head voxel/vertexwise analysis

In both the VBM and SBM analyses, by far the largest effects (in terms of extent of the significant clusters) were for the age and gender covariates. Regarding tinnitus, tinnitus severity, and hearing loss, only a few small clusters were found and only when using SBM.

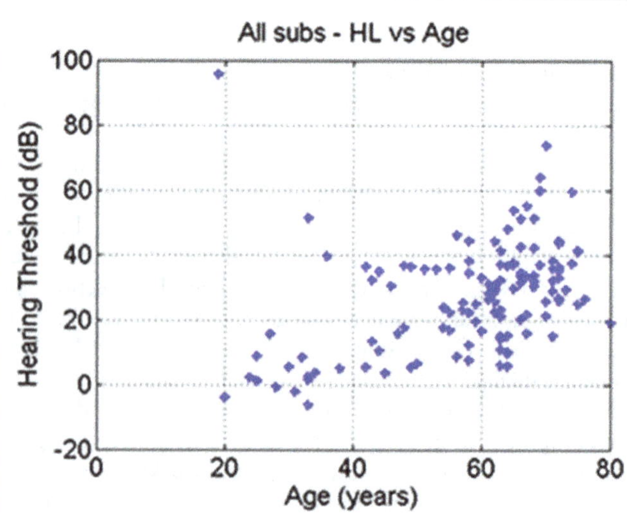

FIGURE 4 | The age of each subject plotted against their hearing threshold.

TABLE 3 | Summary of results.

VBM		
	Gray matter	**White matter**
Grouping 1. (All TI vs. All controls)	Reduction for TI vs. CO in right HG (0.008 cm^3) and with increasing TI severityin right DMN (0.056 cm^3). ROI analysis: increase in SOC for TI vs. CO (5.5%)	Reduction in TI vs. CO in right MGN (0.50 cm^3)
Grouping 2. (Severe TI vs. Matched controls)	No Differences	Reduction in TI vs. CO in right MGN (0.19 cm^3)
Grouping 3. (TI with Clinically normal hearing vs. matched controls)	No Differences	Increase in TI vs. CO in left HG (0.008 cm^3); Increase with TI severity in left CN (0.008 cm^3)

SBM			
	Thickness	**Area**	**Volume**
Grouping 1. (All TI vs. All controls)	Decrease for TI vs. CO in left AC/STG (4.51 cm^2), left superior frontal gyrus (5.04 cm^2), right STS (1.69 cm^2) and right HG (0.33 cm^2). Increase with TI severity in right middle Temporal gyrus (2.61 cm^2), and right rostro medial Frontal gyrus (2.02 cm^2). ROI analysis: 2.1% decrease for TI vs. CO in AC	Decrease with TI severity in right precuneus (12.5 cm^2) ROI analysis: increase for TI vs. CO in vmPFC (1.31%) and decrease in AC (−2.1%)	Decrease for TI vs. CO in right HG (0.27 cm^2) and with TI severity in right precuneus (8.35 cm^2) ROI analysis: decrease for TI vs. CO in Auditory cortex (−3.9%), HG (−4.5%) and STG (−2.4%)
Grouping 2. (Severe TI vs. Matched controls)	Decrease for TI vs. CO in left AC (0.85 cm^2).	No Differences	No Differences
Grouping 3. (TI with Clinically normal hearing vs. matched controls)	Decrease for TI vs. CO in AC/STG (1.17 cm^2) and right rostro-middle frontal gyrus (1.71 cm^2). Increase with tinnitus severity in left midtemporal gyrus (3.18 cm^2)	Decrease with TI severity in left HG/AC (3.18 cm^2), right superior parietal gyrus (5.80 cm^2) and right posterior cingulate (6.37 cm^2)	Decrease with TI severity in left HG/AC (2.50 cm^2)

*Results of VBM voxelwise analysis and SBM vertexwise analysis are reported as volume and surface area of significant clusters. ROI analysis results are reported in % change relative to the average/total ROI value averaged across TI and CO groups (TI, Tinnitus; CO, Control; MTG, Middle Temporal Gyrus; STS, Superior Temporal Sulcus. Other abbreviations as in **Table 1**).*

Whole brain VBM analysis (see Tables SI1,SI2) revealed many significant clusters in various parts of the brain, corresponding mainly to an increase in gray matter volume with age (totalling 10,234 voxels or 81.9 cm^3), and to a lesser extent a decrease in white matter volume with age (totalling 34.7 cm^3) and larger gray matter volume for males vs. female (totalling 13.9 cm^3). The largest of these clusters was an increase in gray matter volume with age in a 20 cm^3 volume near the boundaries of the ventricles (**Figure 5**). This cluster contains very little actual gray matter, being predominantly white matter and CSF. So the voxel grayscale is likely contaminated. As the ventricles are known to expand during the ageing process due to cortical atrophy, there is a likely explanation for this finding and so it is not discussed further. Other significant clusters were small in extent (<1 cm^3) and there were no significant effects of tinnitus, tinnitus severity or hearing loss.

In the whole brain SBM analysis (see Tables SI3–SI5), various clusters showed a decrease of cortical thickness, area and/or volume with age (total areas of the clusters were 558.5, 224.2 and 610.0 cm^2 respectively). There was an increase in cortical area and/or volume for males compared to females (total cluster areas were 1205.1 and 836.3 cm^2 respectively). Additionally, there were clusters of decreased cortical thickness for males in the left hemisphere (total area 7.9 cm^2). There were smaller significant clusters for tinnitus, tinnitus severity and hearing loss. These included a decrease in cortical thickness for the tinnitus group compared to controls in a 5.0 cm^2 area in the left superior frontal gyrus (SFG; **Figure 6A**), a decrease in cortical area and volume with tinnitus severity in an area of the right precuneus (over 12.5

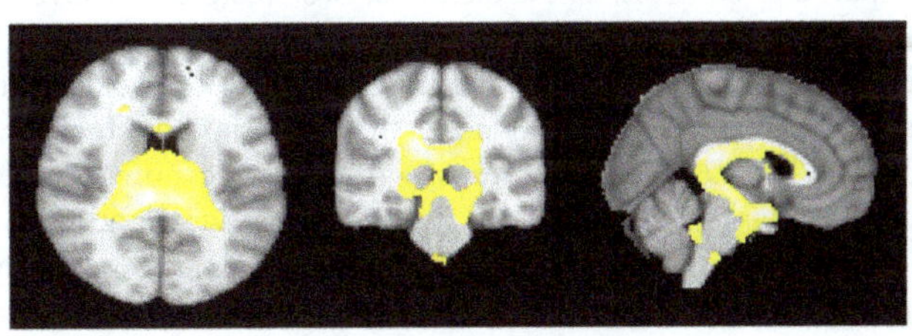

FIGURE 5 | The areas showing that as age increases there is a significant increase in gray matter volume at the cerebrospinal fluid (CSF) boundaries for the regression group of all subjects using age as the regressor of interest.

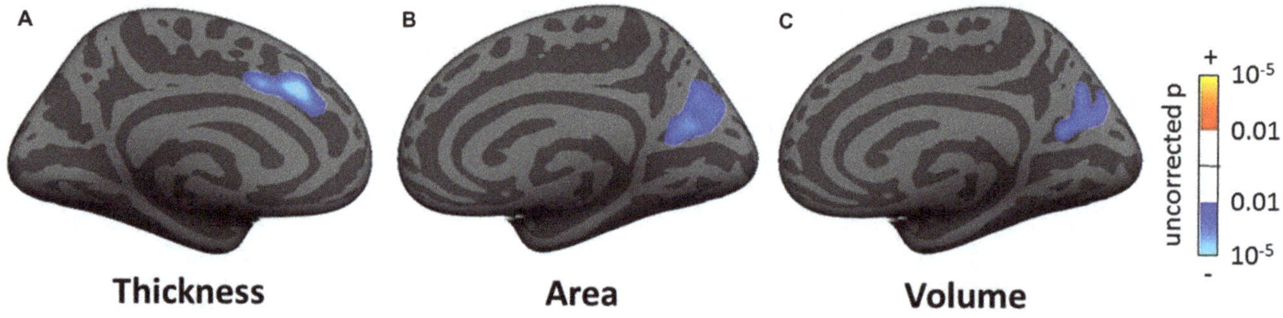

FIGURE 6 | Clusters showing a significant effect ($p < 0.05$ family wise error (FWE)-corrected) of tinnitus in the superior frontal gyrus (SFG; A) and of tinnitus severity in the pre-cuneus (B,C) in the whole-brain surface-based morphometry (SBM) analysis. Blue areas correspond to a negative effect (decrease in thickness for the tinnitus group vs. the control group and decrease in area and volume for increasing tinnitus severity).

and 8.4 cm^2 respectively; **Figures 6B,C**), a decrease in cortical volume with hearing loss in left HG (over 4.8 cm^2; not shown) and a decrease in cortical area and volume with hearing loss in the right fusiform gyrus (over 6.2 and 5.3 cm^2 respectively; not shown).

Masked voxel/vertexwise analysis

When restricting the VBM and SBM analyses to the various masks, the majority of clusters of significance were again found for the effects of age and gender and these effects were generally in the same direction as in the whole-head analysis. These clusters will not be detailed here (see Tables SI1–SI5). There were additional clusters of significance for tinnitus, tinnitus severity and hearing loss, which will be summarized below.

For the VBM masked analyses, we found a decrease in gray matter volume in the right HG (1 voxel or 0.008 cm^3; not shown) and in white matter volume for the tinnitus group compared to the control group in the right MGN (63 voxels or 0.50 cm^3; **Figure 7A**), a decrease in gray matter volume in the right DMN (0.056 cm^3) with increasing tinnitus severity (not shown). There were also two clusters of decreasing white matter volume with hearing loss in the left HG (found using AC, HG and STG masks) and left vmPFC. We also found one cluster of increasing white matter volume with hearing loss in the left NAc (all clusters <0.6 cm^3; not shown).

For the SBM masked analyses, we found several clusters of decreased cortical thickness or volume for the tinnitus group compared to controls. These included, two clusters of decreased thickness in the left AC (total cluster area 4.51 cm^2, **Figure 8A**, found using both the AC and STG masks), one cluster of decreased thickness in the bank of the right superior temporal sulcus (STS; 1.69 cm^2, **Figure 8B**, found using both the AC and STG masks), one cluster of decreased thickness and one of decreased volume in right HG (0.33 and 0.27 cm^2 respectively, **Figures 8C,D**) and one cluster of decreased thickness in the left SFG, identical to the one found in the whole brain analysis (**Figure 6A**). There were also two clusters of increasing cortical thickness with increasing tinnitus severity: one in the right MTG (2.61 cm^2, **Figure 8E**) and one in the right rostro-medial frontal gyrus (2.02 cm^2, **Figure 8F**).

ROI analysis

In the ROI analysis, we averaged the various measures across all voxels/vertices of each mask bilaterally and compared them between the tinnitus and control groups. This analysis showed additional significant effects, some of which were similar to the voxel/vertexwise effects. The only significant effect for the VBM ROI analysis was a 5.5% increase in gray matter volume for the tinnitus group in the SOC. For the SBM ROI analysis, we found a 2.1% decrease in cortical thickness in AC (similar to the vertex-wise effect shown in **Figures 8A,B**), a 1.3% increase in cortical area in vmPFC (similar to the vertexwise effect shown in **Figure 8F**) and decreases in cortical volume in AC, HG and STG (3.9%, 4.5% and 2.4% respectively). All effect sizes for the ROI analysis are reported in Tables SI6–SI10 and significant ones are summarized in **Table 3**).

Grouping 2—Severe Tinnitus vs. Matched Controls

Most significant clusters for this subgroup analysis were for the effect of age and gender and were in a direction similar to the ones described in the whole-head analysis with all subjects (grouping 1). These effects will not be described in detail here (see Tables SI1–SI5). There were a few significant clusters

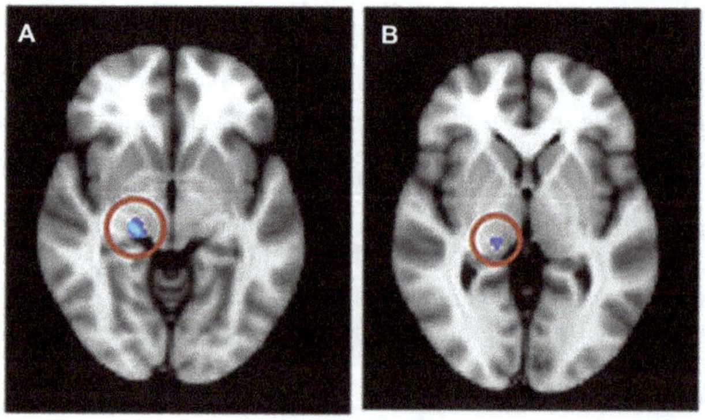

FIGURE 7 | Significant voxels (circled) found in the medial geniculate nucleus (MGN) for a reduction in white matter for tinnitus participants compared to controls for (A) regression group 1, all subjects and (B) regression group 2, severe tinnitus matched to controls.

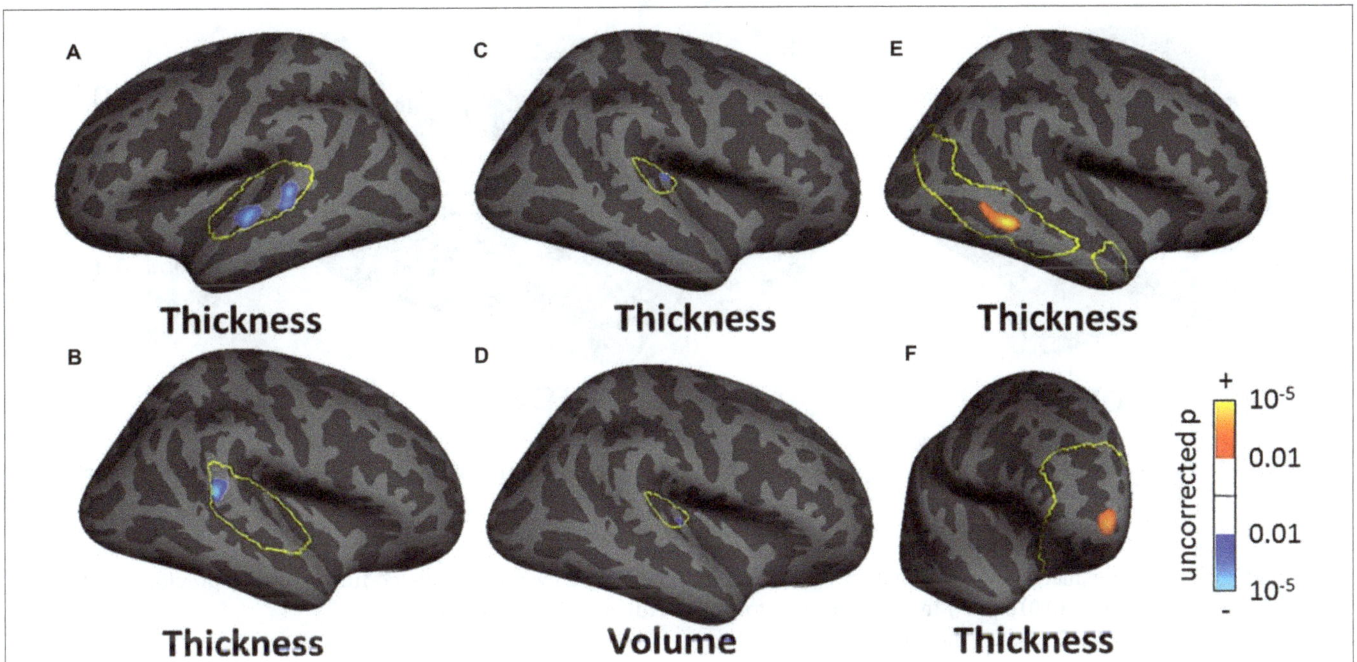

FIGURE 8 | Clusters showing a significant effect ($p < 0.05$ FWE-corrected) of tinnitus in left AC (A) right superior temporal sulcus (STS; B) right Heschl's gyrus (HG) (C,D) and of tinnitus severity in right middle temporal gyrus (MTG) and PFC (E,F) in the masked SBM analysis. The yellow outlines depict the masks used to restrict the vertexwise analysis (auditory cortex, AC for **A,B** HG for **C,D** default mode network (DMN) for **E**; PFC for **F**). Blue areas correspond to a negative effect (decrease in thickness or volume for the tinnitus group vs. the control group) and the red areas to a positive effect (increasing thickness for increasing tinnitus severity).

showing an effect of tinnitus, tinnitus severity or hearing loss (described in the following section), and none in the whole-head analysis.

The masked voxelwise VBM analysis showed a 0.19 cm^3 cluster of decreased white matter volume in the right MGN for the severe tinnitus subgroup compared to matched controls (**Figure 7B**; similar to the effect described above for all subjects and **Figure 7A**) and two clusters of decreasing gray matter volume with increasing hearing loss in the left IC (0.02 cm^3; not shown) and the MGN bilaterally (1.22 cm^3; not shown). The masked vertexwise SBM analysis showed a cluster of decreased cortical thickness for the severe tinnitus subgroup compared to matched controls at the junction of HG and the STG in the left hemisphere (0.85 cm^2; **Figure 9**). There was also a cluster of increasing cortical thickness with increasing hearing loss in the right inferior parietal gyrus (1.47 cm^2, not shown).

The ROI-averaged analysis showed no significant effect of tinnitus for either the VBM or SBM analyses.

Grouping 3—Tinnitus With Clinically Normal Hearing vs. Matched Controls

As for grouping 2, most significant clusters were for the effect of age or gender. There were however a number of clusters of significance for the effect of tinnitus, tinnitus severity and hearing loss, including a few in the whole-head analyses.

The whole-brain SBM analysis showed two clusters of decreasing cortical area with increasing tinnitus severity in the right superior parietal gyrus and pCC (total areas of clusters 12.17 cm^2, **Figure 10**) and one cluster of increasing cortical volume with hearing loss in the right inferior parietal gyrus (4.55 cm^2, not shown).

The masked VBM analysis showed a few small clusters of significance: one voxel in left HG and another in left CN showing an increase in white matter volume for the normal-hearing tinnitus group compared to matched controls, a 0.12 cm^3 cluster

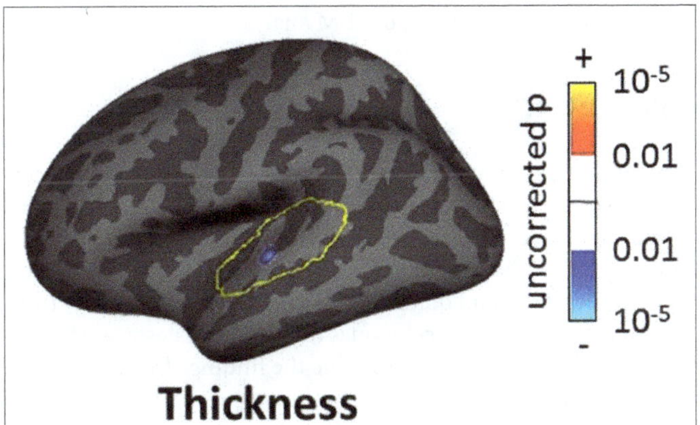

FIGURE 9 | Cluster showing a significant effect ($p < 0.05$ FWE-corrected) of tinnitus in left AC in the masked SBM analysis for the severe tinnitus grouping. The yellow outlines depict the AC masks used to restrict the vertexwise analysis. The blue area corresponds to a negative effect (decrease in thickness for the severe tinnitus group vs. matched controls).

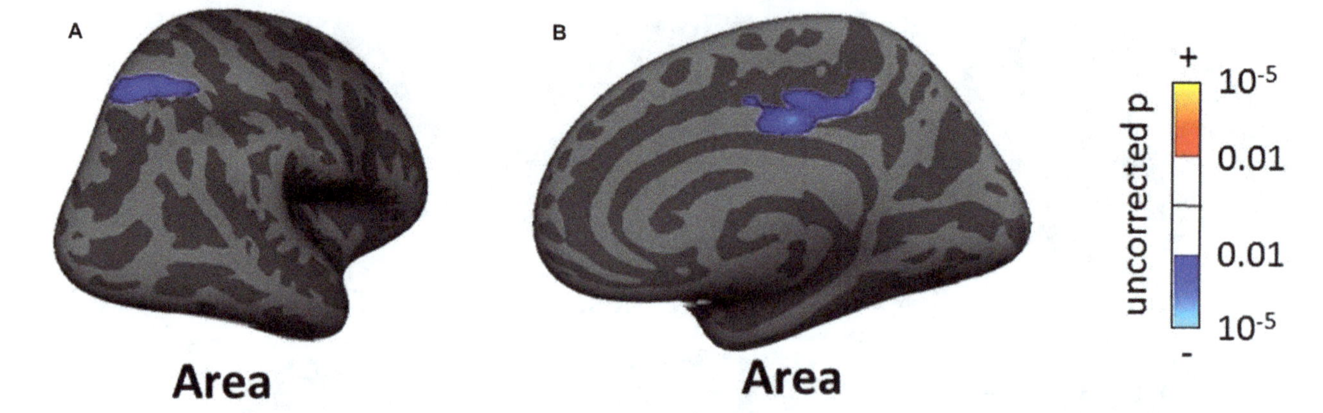

FIGURE 10 | Clusters showing a significant effect (p < 0.05 FWE-corrected) of tinnitus severity in right superior parietal gyrus (A) and right posterior cingulate cortex (B) in the whole-brain SBM analyses. Blue areas correspond to a negative effect (decrease in cortical area with increasing tinnitus severity).

in IC bilaterally showing increasing gray matter volume with hearing loss and two voxels (0.016 cm^3) in the right AC (found using both the AC and STG masks) showing increasing white matter volume with hearing loss (not shown).

The masked SBM analysis showed several clusters of significance for the effect of tinnitus and tinnitus severity: two clusters of decreased cortical thickness for the normal-hearing tinnitus group vs. matched controls in the left STG (1.17 cm^2, **Figure 11A**, found both using the STG and AC masks) and in the right rostro-middle frontal gyrus (1.71 cm^2, **Figure 11B**), one cluster of decreasing cortical area/volume with increasing tinnitus severity in left HG (3.18 cm^2, **Figures 11C,D** found using the AC, HG and STG masks) and one cluster of increasing cortical thickness with increasing tinnitus severity in the left MTG (3.18 cm^2, **Figure 11E**). There was also one cluster of increasing cortical thickness with hearing loss in the right rostro-middle frontal gyrus (1.81 cm^2, not shown).

The ROI-averaged analysis showed no significant effect of tinnitus for either the VBM or SBM analyses.

DISCUSSION

Structural analysis of neuroanatomy offers a unique approach to unraveling the mystery of tinnitus. Different morphological techniques have unique strengths and limitations and results can vary depending on specific algorithms used to register or segment the brain and quantify changes in tissue type. Our study applied a range of these techniques to the same dataset—bringing novel insights into just how variable the findings from structural analysis of the brain can be.

While the large cohort of participants allowed us to control confounding effects of hearing loss and age, these two variables were correlated and so their independent effects cannot be isolated with any degree of precision. Controlling hearing loss and tinnitus severity, we found moderate changes in brain anatomy associated with tinnitus. Important and somewhat disappointing, many of these significant changes were different and some even contradicted findings from previous studies (see Adjamian et al., 2014).

Tinnitus-related Changes—Comparison With Previous Findings

The results of both our VBM and SBM analyses reveal differences between tinnitus and non-tinnitus participants in both cortical and subcortical auditory structures, but only when the analysis was focused on these regions (masked voxel/vertexwise analyses or ROI analysis). Furthermore, as shown in **Table 4**, there was a limited overlap between the location and direction of our effects and those of previously published VBM and SBM studies.

At the subcortical level, our VBM analysis showed an increase in gray matter concentration in the SOC and a reduction in white matter probability in the MGN (**Figure 7A**) for tinnitus participants. None of these effects have been reported before, although there are conflicting reports of changes in gray matter concentration in the medial geniculate body (MGB), with Mühlau et al. (2006) reporting an increase, and Mahoney et al. (2011) a decrease in tinnitus compared to controls. At the cortical level, we found small decreases in gray matter probability and/or thickness in right HG using both the VBM and SBM analyses (**Figures 8C,D**), as well as slightly larger decreases in cortical thickness in left AC (outside HG, **Figure 8A**). This is fairly consistent with previous SBM studies which reported a decrease in cortical thickness in right HG and STG bilaterally (Aldhafeeri et al., 2012) and a decrease in cortical volume in HG (Schneider et al., 2009). It should be borne in mind however that not all SBM studies have found this effect (see Leaver et al., 2012) and that VBM studies have tended to find increases rather than decreases in gray matter concentration in HG or STG in participants with tinnitus (Husain et al., 2011; Mahoney et al., 2011; Boyen et al., 2013).

The only two significant clusters of change related to tinnitus that we found in our whole-brain analysis were located outside sensory auditory structures: we found a decrease in cortical thickness for tinnitus participants in the left SFG and a decrease in cortical volume with tinnitus severity in the right precuneus

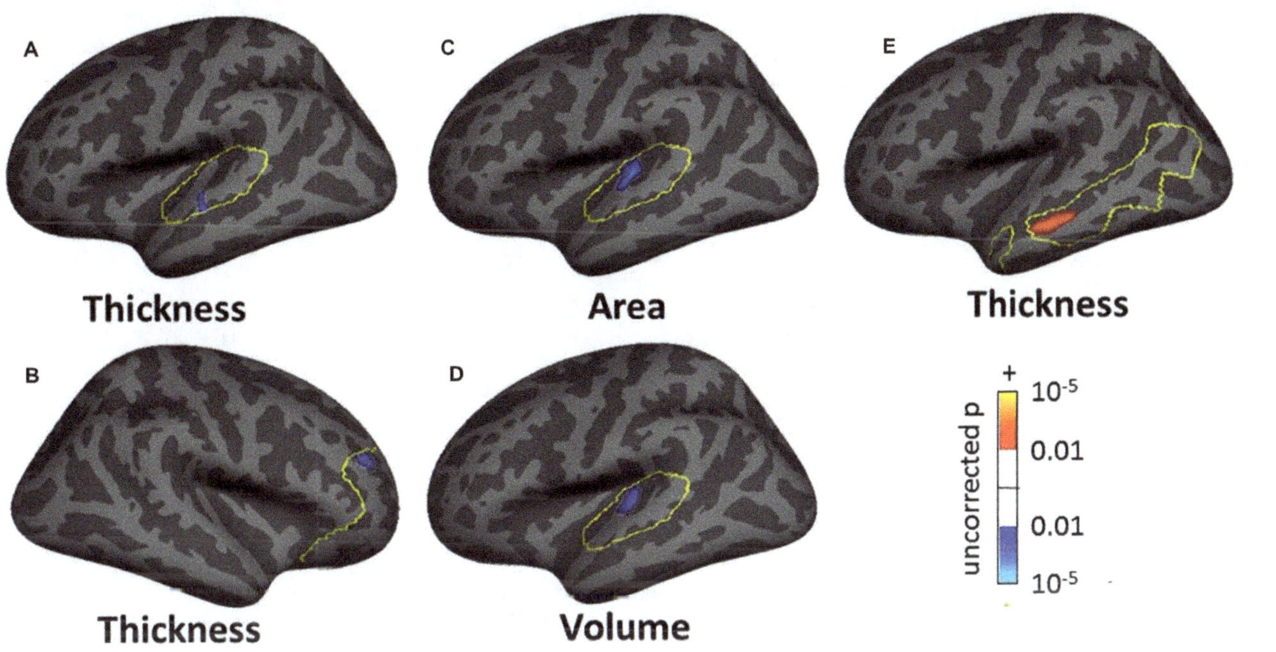

FIGURE 11 | Clusters showing a significant effect (p < 0.05 FWE-corrected) of tinnitus in left AC (A) and right rostromedial frontal cortex (B) of tinnitus severity in left HG (C,D) and left MTG (E) in the masked SBM analyses. The yellow outlines depict the masks used to restrict the vertexwise analysis (AC for **A,C,D**; PFC for **B**; DMN for **E**). Blue areas correspond to a negative effect (decrease in thickness for the normal-hearing tinnitus group vs. matched controls in **(A,B)** decrease in area and volume with increasing tinnitus severity in **(C,D)** and the red areas to a positive effect (increasing thickness for increasing tinnitus severity in **(E)**.

(**Figure 6**). Whereas the effect in precuneus has not been reported before, the location of the effect in the SFG is very similar to that of the gray matter (thickness) reduction reported by Leaver et al. (2012) in dorsomedial PFC using both VBM and SBM, although theirs was on the right side. Aldhafeeri et al. (2012) also reported a general decrease in cortical thickness in the right PFC using SBM. In contrast, Husain et al. (2011) reported an increase in gray matter concentration in tinnitus participants using VBM.

When restricting the analysis to ROIs, we found a few additional effects of tinnitus in non-auditory structures (e.g., increase in cortical thickness with tinnitus severity in MTG in DMN mask). One area of particular interest is the vmPFC: in separate VBM or SBM studies, Mühlau et al. (2006), Leaver et al. (2011) and Leaver et al. (2012) found a decrease in gray matter concentration in tinnitus participants in the subcallosal region, which is included in the vmPFC. On the other hand, at least three other studies have failed to replicate these effects (Landgrebe et al., 2009; Husain et al., 2011; Melcher et al., 2013) even though some of them were specifically designed to do so. Here we find an effect that clearly contradicts previous studies, since our SBM analysis shows a general increase in cortical area in vmPFC for the tinnitus group (ROI analysis) as well as a more focused increase in cortical thickness with tinnitus severity in the right rostro medial frontal gyrus (in the vmPFC-masked vertexwise analysis, **Figure 8F**).

Finally, we note that many significant effects of tinnitus reported in earlier studies (in cingulate cortex, hippocampus, insula, supramarginal gyrus, occipito-parietal cortex; Landgrebe et al., 2009; Leaver et al., 2011; Mahoney et al., 2011; Aldhafeeri et al., 2012; Boyen et al., 2013; Husain and Schmidt, 2014) were not replicated here. Therefore, even though we did find effects that replicated previous studies, the overall picture is one of non-replicability and contradiction.

In this study, we used both VBM and SBM analysis techniques to assess gray/white matter concentration, and thickness, area, and volume of the gray matter, respectively. One might expect that any regions found in the gray matter VBM analysis would also appear in the SBM analysis (at least for the cortical volume measurement), since we applied these to the exact same data. However, we observed a proportionally larger and a higher number of significant clusters in SBM than VBM, with differing locations. There are several differences in the exact details of the VBM and SBM procedures that could explain these discrepancies. First, the nature of the measurement is different: VBM as implemented in SPM measures the probability that a certain voxel belongs to white or gray matter and this is modulated by the amplitude of the deformation necessary to register individual brains onto a common template. On the other hand, SBM as implemented in Freesurfer measures actual geometric properties of the cortical sheet (thickness, area and volume) at each vertex of each subject (modulated by the deformation fields for area and volume). Second, the registration procedure is different: SPM uses non-linear registration in volumetric space, whereas FreeSurfer uses spherical registration in surface space. Whereas in Freesurfer, deformation fields are necessarily limited to the cortical sheet, in SPM, they can occur in

TABLE 4 | Summary of main results of previous tinnitus VBM and SBM studies compared to present results (table adapted from Adjamian et al., 2014).

	Group differences		Modulations	
Brain structure	**Decreases**	**Increases**	**HL**	**TIN**
Auditory gray matter				
Superior olivary complex	K			
Inferior colliculus	B	–	–	-
Medial geniculate body	FK	A	–	-
Heschl's gyrus (A1)	***CG***K***K***	I	***CG***K	I
Superior temporal gyrus (A2)	***GK***	DF	DI	H***H***
Non-auditory gray matter				
vmPFC/subcallosal gyrus	AE***G***H***H***	***(K)***	IJK	***K***
dmPFC	***G***H***H (K)***	D	DIJ	**-**
Nucleus accumbens	–	–	K	-
Anterior cingulate	***G***	D	D	-
Posterior cingulate	***G***	–	J	-
Hippocampus	BI	–	I	-
Insula	–	–	–	H***H***
Supramarginal gyrus	H	–	I	H***H***
Occipito-parietal cortex	–	I	I	-
Orbito-frontal cortex	F	–	–	-
Superior frontal gyrus	***(K)***	–	–	-
Middle frontal gyrus	—	***(K)***	–	-
Middle temporal gyrus	–	I***K***	–	-
Precuneus	–	–	–	***K***
Fusiform gyrus	–	–	***K***	-

Present results are denoted by the letter K and are from grouping 1 only. Regular font letters denote VBM analyses and bold/italics letters SBM analyses. A = Mühlau et al. (2006); B = Landgrebe et al. (2009); C = Schneider et al. (2009); D = Husain et al. (2011); E = Leaver et al. (2011); F = Mahoney et al. (2011); G = Aldhafeeri et al. (2012); H = Leaver et al. (2012); I = Boyen et al. (2013); J = (Melcher et al. (2013); HL, Hearing loss; TIN, Tinnitus severity; vmPFC, ventromedial pre-frontal cortex; dmPFC, dorsomedial prefrontal Cortex.

any direction in volume space. As a result, errors due to imperfect registration will be different in the two techniques. Finally, even though we used almost identical statistical models, there were at least two important differences: we did not correct for total/average brain thickness/area/volume in the SBM analysis and we used different types of FWE correction. The latter could explain why significant cluster sizes are proportionally larger in the SBM analysis: in the VBM analysis, the cluster size corresponds to the voxelwise-corrected p-value whereas in the SBM analysis, it corresponded to the uncorrected p-value (and is therefore larger). It is also likely that the cluster-based FWE correction used in Freesurfer is more sensitive to large clusters of relatively low significance, which could explain why more clusters were found overall in the SBM analysis.

Reasons for Variability Between Studies

Tinnitus is a heterogeneous disorder, typically based on only a single criterion: the perception of a phantom sound. As yet there is no universally agreed separation of tinnitus patients into subgroups based on clinical and etiological factors. Tinnitus etiology, severity, hearing loss, comorbid medical conditions, age of onset, duration and laterality, among others, are factors which can effect brain morphology (Adjamian et al., 2014). Indeed, age and hearing loss seriously confound the interpretation of many results in this field. It is likely that the differences between participants across different studies, exaggerated by the lack of meaningful definitions of tinnitus subgroups, explain the reasons for diversity in findings.

A recent European-funded Cooperation in Science and Technology program (COST Action) for a Tinnitus research Network (TINNET[3]) aims to identify subtypes of tinnitus, and their neural correlates and thus develop an innovative hypothesis-driven treatment approaches. Until such time, future studies should attempt to collect as much information from participants as possible and attempt to recruit participants that are clinically and characteristically homogeneous as far as possible. Studies should ideally administer tinnitus questionnaires, depression questionnaires, measure audiograms at least up to 12 kHz, ascertain the duration, lateralization and cause of their tinnitus and basic demographic information. Participants should be matched on these characteristics as far as possible. Many of these variables were measured in the studies from which the data for the current analysis were obtained.

CONCLUSION

Given the results of the present study, and in the context of previous discrepant findings, we conclude that it is not yet possible with any confidence to associate tinnitus with anatomical changes in specific parts of the brain. This is likely due to the heterogeneity of tinnitus characteristics, and the lack meaningful subtyping. Exploratory analyses might propose a subtyping classification which could then generate hypotheses for future testing. However, the

[3]http://tinnet.tinnitusresearch.net/

more stringent the eligibility criteria for inclusion, the more challenging it will be to recruit sufficient number of participants in each subgroup for valid statistical inference.

AUTHOR CONTRIBUTIONS

PA and DRML conceived the study, wrote the discussion. PA and JD collected the data. TWA and JB analyzed the data and wrote the article. ARP and DAH supervised and provided guidance.

ACKNOWLEDGMENTS

This work was supported by the Medical Research Council (Grant No. U135097129).

REFERENCES

Adjamian, P., Hall, D. A., Palmer, A. R., Allan, T. W., and Langers, D. R. M. (2014). Neuroanatomical abnormalities in chronic tinnitus in the human brain. *Neurosci. Biobehav. Rev.* 45C, 119–133. doi: 10.1016/j.neubiorev.2014.05.013

Adjamian, P., Sereda, M., and Hall, D. A. (2009). The mechanisms of tinnitus: perspectives from human functional neuroimaging. *Hear. Res.* 253, 15–31. doi: 10.1016/j.heares.2009.04.001

Adjamian, P., Sereda, M., Zobay, O., Hall, D. A., and Palmer, A. R. (2012). Neuromagnetic indicators of tinnitus and tinnitus masking in patients with and without hearing loss. *J. Assoc. Res. Otolaryngol.* 13, 715–731. doi: 10.1007/s10162-012-0340-5

Aldhafeeri, F. M., Mackenzie, I., Kay, T., Alghamdi, J., and Sluming, V. (2012). Neuroanatomical correlates of tinnitus revealed by cortical thickness analysis and diffusion tensor imaging. *Neuroradiology* 54, 883–892. doi: 10.1007/s00234-012-1044-6

Ashburner, J. (2007). A fast diffeomorphic image registration algorithm. *Neuroimage* 38, 95–113. doi: 10.1016/j.neuroimage.2007.07.007

Baguley, D., McFerran, D., and Hall, D. (2013). Tinnitus. *Lancet* 382, 1600–1607. doi: 10.1016/S0140-6736(13)60142-7

Bookstein, F. L. (2001). "Voxel-based morphometry" should not be used with imperfectly registered images. *Neuroimage* 14, 1454–1462. doi: 10.1006/nimg.2001.0770

Boyen, K., Langers, D. R. M., de Kleine, E., and van Dijk, P. (2013). Gray matter in the brain: differences associated with tinnitus and hearing loss. *Hear. Res.* 295, 67–78. doi: 10.1016/j.heares.2012.02.010

British Society of Audiology. (2011). Recommended procedure; pure-tone air-conduction and bone-conduction threshold audiometry with and without masking. Available online at: http://www.thebsa.org.uk/wp-content/uploads/2014/04/BSA_RP_PTA_FINAL_24Sept11_MinorAmend06Feb12.pdf.

Crippa, A., Lanting, C. P., van Dijk, P., and Roerdink, J. B. (2010). A diffusion tensor imaging study on the auditory system and tinnitus. *Open Neuroimag. J.* 4, 16–25. doi: 10.2174/1874440001004010016

Dale, A. M., Fischl, B., and Sereno, M. I. (1999). Cortical surface-based analysis. I. Segmentation and surface reconstruction. *Neuroimage* 9, 179–194. doi: 10.1006/nimg.1998.0395

Davies, J., Gander, P. E., Andrews, M., and Hall, D. A. (2014). Auditory network connectivity in tinnitus patients: a resting-state fMRI study. *Int. J. Audiol.* 53, 192–198. doi: 10.3109/14992027.2013.846482

Draganski, B., Gaser, C., Busch, V., Schuierer, G., Bogdahn, U., and May, A. (2004). Neuroplasticity: changes in grey matter induced by training. *Nature* 427, 311–312. doi: 10.1038/427311a

Fackrell, K., Hall, D. A., Barry, J. G., and Hoare, D. J. (2014). "Tools for tinnitus measurement: development and validity of questionnaires to assess handicap and treatment effects," in *Tinnitus: Causes, Treatment and Short and Long-Term Health Effects*, eds F. Signorelli and F. Turjman (New York, NY: Nova Science Publishers), 13–60.

Fischl, B., and Dale, A. M. (2000). Measuring the thickness of the human cerebral cortex from magnetic resonance images. *Proc. Natl. Acad. Sci. U S A* 97, 11050–11055. doi: 10.1073/pnas.200033797

Fischl, B., Sereno, M. I., and Dale, A. M. (1999a). Cortical surface-based analysis. II: inflation, flattening and a surface-based coordinate system. *Neuroimage* 9, 195–207. doi: 10.1006/nimg.1998.0396

Fischl, B., Sereno, M. I., Tootell, R. B., and Dale, A. M. (1999b). High-resolution intersubject averaging and a coordinate system for the cortical surface. *Hum. Brain Mapp.* 8, 272–284. doi: 10.1002/(SICI)1097-0193(1999)8:4<272::AID-HBM10 >3.0.CO;2-4

Good, C. D., Johnsrude, I. S., Ashburner, J., Henson, R. N., Friston, K. J., and Frackowiak, R. S. (2001). A voxel-based morphometric study of ageing in 465 normal adult human brains. *Neuroimage* 14, 21–36. doi: 10.1006/nimg.2001.0786

Greicius, M. D., Krasnow, B., Reiss, A. L., and Menon, V. (2003). Functional connectivity in the resting brain: a network analysis of the default mode hypothesis. *Proc. Natl. Acad. Sci. U S A* 100, 253–258. doi: 10.1073/pnas.0135058100

Hagler, D. J. Jr., Saygin, A. P., and Sereno, M. I. (2006). Smoothing and cluster thresholding for cortical surface-based group analysis of fMRI data. *Neuroimage* 33, 1093–1103. doi: 10.1016/j.neuroimage.2006.07.036

Hayasaka, S., and Nichols, T. E. (2003). Validating cluster size inference: random field and permutation methods. *Neuroimage* 20, 2343–2356. doi: 10.1016/j.neuroimage.2003.08.003

Henry, J. A., Dennis, K. C., and Schechter, M. A. (2005). General review of tinnitus: prevalence, mechanisms, effects and management. *J. Speech Lang. Hear. Res.* 48, 1204–1235. doi: 10.1044/1092-4388(2005/084)

House, J. W., and Brackmann, D. E. (1981). Tinnitus: surgical treatment. *Ciba Found. Symp.* 85, 204–216. doi: 10.1002/9780470720677.ch12

Husain, F. T., Medina, R. E., Davis, C. W., Szymko-Bennett, Y., Simonyan, K., Pajor, N. M., et al. (2011). Neuroanatomical changes due to hearing loss and chronic tinnitus: a combined VBM and DTI study. *Brain Res.* 1369, 74–88. doi: 10.1016/j.brainres.2010.10.095

Husain, F. T., and Schmidt, S. A. (2014). Using resting state functional connectivity to unravel networks of tinnitus. *Hear. Res.* 307, 153–162. doi: 10.1016/j.heares.2013.07.010

Kuk, F. K., Tyler, R. S., Russell, D., and Jordan, H. (1990). The psychometric properties of a tinnitus handicap questionnaire. *Ear Hear.* 11, 434–445. doi: 10.1097/00003446-199012000-00005

Landgrebe, M., Langguth, B., Rosengarth, K., Braun, S., Koch, A., Kleinjung, T., et al. (2009). Structural brain changes in tinnitus: grey matter decrease in auditory and non-auditory brain areas. *Neuroimage* 46, 213–218. doi: 10.1016/j.neuroimage.2009.01.069

Lanting, C. P., De Kleine, E., Bartels, H., and Van Dijk, P. (2008). Functional imaging of unilateral tinnitus using fMRI. *Acta Otolaryngol.* 128, 415–421. doi: 10.1080/00016480701793743

Lanting, C. P., de Kleine, E., and van Dijk, P. (2009). Neural activity underlying tinnitus generation: results from PET and fMRI. *Hear. Res.* 255, 1–13. doi: 10.1016/j.heares.2009.06.009

Leaver, A. M., Renier, L., Chevillet, M. A., Morgan, S., Kim, H. J., and Rauschecker, J. P. (2011). Dysregulation of limbic and auditory networks in tinnitus. *Neuron* 69, 33–43. doi: 10.1016/j.neuron.2010.12.002

Leaver, A. M., Seydell-Greenwald, A., Turesky, T. K., Morgan, S., Kim, H. J., and Rauschecker, J. P. (2012). Cortico-limbic morphology separates tinnitus from tinnitus distress. *Front. Syst. Neurosci.* 6:21. doi: 10.3389/fnsys.2012.00021

Lee, Y. J., Bae, S. J., Lee, S. H., Lee, J. J., Lee, K. Y., Kim, M. N., et al. (2007). Evaluation of white matter structures in patients with tinnitus using diffusion tensor imaging. *J. Clin. Neurosci.* 14, 515–519. doi: 10.1016/j.jocn.2006.10.002

Maguire, E. A., Woollett, K., and Spiers, H. J. (2006). London taxi drivers and bus drivers: a structural MRI and neuropsychological analysis. *Hippocampus* 16, 1091–1101. doi: 10.1002/hipo.20233

Mahoney, C. J., Rohrer, J. D., Goll, J. C., Fox, N. C., Rossor, M. N., and Warren, J. D. (2011). Structural neuroanatomy of tinnitus and hyperacusis in semantic dementia. *J. Neurol. Neurosurg. Psychiatry* 82, 1274–1278. doi: 10.1136/jnnp.2010.235473

McCombe, A., Baguley, D., Coles, R., McKenna, L., McKinney, C., Windle-Taylor, P., et al. (2001). Guidelines for the grading of tinnitus severity: the results of a working group commissioned by the British association of otolaryngologists, head and neck surgeons, 1999. *Clin. Otolaryngol. Allied Sci.* 26, 388–393. doi: 10.1046/j.1365-2273.2001.00490.x

Melcher, J. R., Knudson, I. M., and Levine, R. A. (2013). Subcallosal brain structure: correlation with hearing threshold at supra-clinical frequencies (>8 kHz), but not with tinnitus. *Hear. Res.* 295, 79–86. doi: 10.1016/j.heares.2012.03.013

Melcher, J. R., Sigalovsky, I. S., and Guinan, J. J. Jr., Levine, R. A. (2000). Lateralized tinnitus studied with functional magnetic resonance imaging: abnormal inferior colliculus activation. *J. Neurophysiol.* 83, 1058–1072.

Mirz, F., Gjedde, A., Ishizu, K., and Pedersen, C. B. (2000a). Cortical networks subserving the perception of tinnitus—a PET study. *Acta Otolaryngol. Suppl.* 543, 241–243. doi: 10.1080/000164800454503

Mirz, F., Gjedde, A., Sødkilde-Jrgensen, H., and Pedersen, C. B. (2000b). Functional brain imaging of tinnitus-like perception induced by aversive auditory stimuli. *Neuroreport* 11, 633–637. doi: 10.1097/00001756-200002280-00039

Mirz, F., Gjedde, A., Stodkilde-Jorgensen, H., and Pedersen, C. B. (1999). "Neuroanatomical correlates of tinnitus," in *Proceedings of the Sixth International Tinnitus Seminar*, ed J. Hazell (London: Tinnitus and Hyperacusis Centre), 323–327.

Mühlau, M., Rauschecker, J. P., Oestreicher, E., Gaser, C., Röttinger, M., Wohlschläger, A. M., et al. (2006). Structural brain changes in tinnitus. *Cereb. Cortex* 16, 1283–1288. doi: 10.1093/cercor/bhj070

Newman, C. W., Jacobson, G. P., and Spitzer, J. B. (1996). Development of the Tinnitus Handicap inventory. *Arch Otolaryngol. Head Neck Surg.* 122, 143–148. doi: 10.1001/archotol.1996.01890140029007

Pfefferbaum, A., Mathalon, D. H., Sullivan, E. V., Rawles, J. M., Zipursky, R. B., and Lim, K. O. (1994). A quantitative magnetic resonance imaging study of changes in brain morphology from infancy to late adulthood. *Arch. Neurol.* 51, 874–887. doi: 10.1001/archneur.1994.00540210046012

Rauschecker, J. P., Leaver, A. M., and Mühlau, M. (2010). Tuning out the noise: limbic-auditory interactions in tinnitus. *Neuron* 66, 819–826. doi: 10.1016/j.neuron.2010.04.032

Reyes, S. A., Salvi, R. J., Burkard, R. F., Coad, M. L., Wack, D. S., Galantowicz, P. J., et al. (2002). Brain imaging of the effects of lidocaine on tinnitus. *Hear. Res.* 171, 43–50. doi: 10.1016/s0378-5955(02)00346-5

Schecklmann, M., Lehner, A., Poeppl, T. B., Kreuzer, P. M., Hajak, G., Landgrebe, M., et al. (2012). Cluster analysis for identifying sub-types of tinnitus: a positron emission tomography and voxel-based morphometry study. *Brain Res.* 1485, 3–9. doi: 10.1016/j.brainres.2012.05.013

Schecklmann, M., Lehner, A., Poeppl, T. B., Kreuzer, P. M., Rupprecht, R., Rackl, J., et al. (2013). Auditory cortex is implicated in tinnitus distress: a voxel-based morphometry study. *Brain Struct. Funct.* 218, 1061–1070. doi: 10.1007/s00429-013-0520-z

Schneider, P., Andermann, M., Wengenroth, M., Goebel, R., Flor, H., Rupp, A., et al. (2009). Reduced volume of Heschl's gyrus in tinnitus. *Neuroimage* 45, 927–939. doi: 10.1016/j.neuroimage.2008.12.045

Seki, S., and Eggermont, J. J. (2003). Changes in spontaneous firing rate and neural synchrony in cat primary auditory cortex after localized tone-induced hearing loss. *Hear. Res.* 180, 28–38. doi: 10.1016/s0378-5955(03)00074-1

Sereda, M., Adjamian, P., Edmondson-Jones, M., Palmer, A. R., and Hall, D. A. (2013). Auditory evoked magnetic fields in individuals with tinnitus. *Hear. Res.* 302, 50–59. doi: 10.1016/j.heares.2013.04.006

Seydell-Greenwald, A., Raven, E. P., Leaver, A. M., Turesky, T. K., and Rauschecker, J. P. (2014). Diffusion imaging of auditory and auditory-limbic connectivity in tinnitus: preliminary evidence and methodological challenges. *Neural Plast.* 2014:145943. doi: 10.1155/2014/145943

Winkler, A. M., Kochunov, P., Blangero, J., Almasy, L., Zilles, K., Fox, P. T., et al. (2010). Cortical thickness or grey matter volume? The importance of selecting the phenotype for imaging genetics studies. *Neuroimage* 53, 1135–1146. doi: 10.1016/j.neuroimage.2009.12.028

2

Alexithymia is Associated with Tinnitus Severity

Jan Wielopolski[1], Tobias Kleinjung[2], Melanie Koch[2], Nicole Peter[2], Martin Meyer[3], Michael Rufer[4] and Steffi Weidt[4]*

[1] Department of Psychiatry and Psychotherapy, University Hospital Zurich, University of Zurich, Zurich, Switzerland, [2] Department of Otorhinolaryngology, University Hospital Zurich, University of Zurich, Zurich, Switzerland, [3] Neuroplasticity and Learning in the Healthy Aging Brain, University of Zurich, Zurich, Switzerland, [4] Department of Psychiatry, Psychotherapy and Psychosomatics, Psychiatric Hospital, University of Zurich, Zurich, Switzerland

***Correspondence:**
Jan Wielopolski
jan.wielopolski@usz.ch

Objective: Alexithymia is considered to be a personality trait with a tendency to express psychological distress in somatic rather than emotional form and, therefore, may play a vital role in somatization. Although, such a propensity can be found in patients suffering from tinnitus, the relationship between alexithymic characteristics and the subjective experience of tinnitus severity remains yet unclear. Our aim was to evaluate which alexithymic characteristics are linked to the subjective experience of tinnitus symptomatology.

Methods: We evaluated tinnitus severity (Tinnitus Handicap Inventory, THI), alexithymia (20-item Toronto Alexithymia Scale, TAS-20), and depression (Beck Depression Inventory, BDI) in 207 outpatients with tinnitus. Correlation analyses and multiple regression analyses were calculated in order to investigate the relationship between alexithymic characteristics, tinnitus severity, and depression.

Results: Highly significant positive correlations were found between THI total score and TAS-20 total score as well as BDI score. Regarding the TAS-20 subscales, multiple regression analyses showed that only the TAS-20 subscale "difficulty in identifying feelings" (DIF) and the BDI significantly predicted the subjective experience of tinnitus severity. Regarding the THI subscales, only higher scores of the THI subscale "functional" demonstrated an independent moderate association with higher scores for DIF.

Conclusion: We found an independent association between the subjective experience of tinnitus severity and alexithymic characteristics, particularly with regard to limitations in the fields of mental, social, and physical functioning because of tinnitus and the difficulty of identifying feelings facet of alexithymia. These findings are conducive to a better understanding of affect regulation that may be important for the psychological adaptation of patients suffering from tinnitus.

Keywords: tinnitus, alexithymia, Tinnitus Handicap Inventory, Toronto Alexithymia Scale, depressive symptoms

INTRODUCTION

Tinnitus is defined as the auditory perception of sound without any corresponding external sound stimulation and occurs in 10–19% of persons in industrialized societies, of which one in five will require medical attention (1–3). It is not completely understood why some persons adapt to their tinnitus symptoms and why others do not (4, 5), but many authors suggest that psychological factors have a notable influence on the subjective experience of tinnitus (6, 7). Langguth et al. proved the importance of anxiety and depression as indicators of experiencing of tinnitus severity by using the Tinnitus Handicap Inventory (THI) (8, 9). Furthermore, a substantial association has been described between tinnitus severity and depression as well as a positive effect of antidepressive treatment on tinnitus severity (10). Moreover, Hiller et al. demonstrated that tinnitus occurred more often in patients with somatization or hypochondriacal disorder and stated that tinnitus may be a somatoform symptom with a possible comorbidity of these different conditions (11). Numerous studies support these suggestions by illustrating similar patterns of subjective loudness and of pitch of tinnitus in patients with great annoyance and in those without annoyance of tinnitus (12–14). A further well-described aspect is the association between tinnitus and reduced quality of life assessed by a standard test procedure (15–17) as well as the association between the greater emotional distress due to tinnitus and the attention that is paid to tinnitus (14).

One condition that may complicate the adaption to emotional distress and lead to a maladaptive coping behavior is alexithymia, which was introduced by Nemiah and Sifneos about 40 years ago based on the clinical observations on patients with psychosomatic disorders (18, 19). Alexithymia is a multifacet personality trait characterized by a reduced ability in identifying and describing one's feelings, a reduced ability in distinguishing own feelings from bodily sensations, an externally oriented style of thinking, and a restricted imaginal process (20). Alexithymia is associated with increased individual distress (21), reduced health-related quality of life (22), and reduced empathic brain responses (23). Alexithymic people are prone to express psychological distress in somatic rather than emotional form (24), which is considered a triggering factor for psychiatric and behavioral problems such as somatization (24, 25). Congruously, it was found that alexithymia was more prevalent in people with somatoform disorders than in healthy controls (26). These findings are supported by other studies where important factors of alexithymia like difficulties in identifying and describing feelings were related to a greater amount of severe dizziness symptoms (27). Although originally associated with psychosomatic diseases, many studies also already demonstrated a higher prevalence of alexithymia in different psychiatric disorders like panic disorder (28), eating disorders (29, 30), alcohol dependence (31), posttraumatic stress disorders (32), and personality disorders (33, 34) as well as in somatic diseases like inflammatory bowel disease (35), recurrent severe asthma (36), or essential hypertension (37).

Despite numerous publications on alexithymia and somatic symptoms, there are hardly any studies that deal with the associations among alexithymia and tinnitus. As far as we know, only one study exists and has not revealed any correlation between alexithymia and tinnitus severity in a community sample of elderly people aged between 70 and 85 years (38).

However, due to the assumption of the somatoform symptom quality of tinnitus and the mentioned finding that alexithymic characteristics are more prevalent in somatic symptom reporting, our aim was to investigate the relationship between alexithymia and the subjective experience of tinnitus severity in individuals with tinnitus. Furthermore, we wanted to examine which alexithymic characteristics are linked to the subjective experience of tinnitus symptomatology, because they might play an important role for the psychological adaptation of patients suffering from tinnitus.

MATERIALS AND METHODS

Participants

The study was authorized by the ethics committee of the canton of Zurich. Two hundred eighty patients referred to the tinnitus outpatient service at University Hospital Zurich and seen between December 2012 and May 2014 were asked to participate in the study (16). The patients' medical histories were assessed prior to data recording and all subjects suffering from acute or chronic somatic diseases that could be causing the symptomatology were excluded as well as subjects with chronic psychiatric diseases. All participants gave their written electronic consent before starting to answer the questionnaires online. In case of participants' questions or uncertainties, a trained medical student provided help in completing the questionnaires. The final sample comprised 207 patients who filled out the questionnaires completely, spoke fluent German, and reported to have had tinnitus for at least 1 month in order to exclude people with temporary symptoms and focus on people with post-acute and chronic tinnitus.

Measures

To evaluate tinnitus severity, the validated German version of the THI was used, which represents the most standardized tinnitus handicap measuring tool in the literature with excellent internal consistency (Cronbach's alpha = 0.93) (39, 40). The THI is a self-reported measure consisting of 25 questions grouped into three subscales: functional (11 questions measuring the functional aspects of tinnitus such as mental, social, and physical functioning), emotional (9 questions reflecting affective responses to tinnitus), and catastrophic (5 questions representing catastrophic responses to tinnitus, which include depression and sleep disturbance) (41, 42). Every of the 25 items can be scored with 0 ("no"), 2 ("sometimes"), or 4 ("yes") points. The total score can be calculated in a range from 0 to 100 and can be subdivided into different grades of subjective experience of tinnitus severity: light (0–16), mild (18–36), moderate (38–56), severe (58–76), and catastrophic handicap (78–100) (43). Furthermore, scores can be calculated for the three subscales: functional (maximum score = 44), emotional (maximum score = 36), and catastrophic (maximum score = 20) (44).

In order to assess alexithymia, the 20-item Toronto Alexithymia Scale (TAS-20) (German version) was administered to the participants (45, 46). The TAS-20, the most commonly used measure of alexithymia, is a valid and reliable 20-item self-report questionnaire with a total score from 0 to 100 and consists of three subscales, measuring the difficulty in identifying feelings (DIF), the difficulty in describing feelings (DDF), and the externally oriented thinking (EOT) (45, 47). There is evidence that the TAS-20 is a reliable and valid measure of alexithymia in normal and clinical adult samples (Cronbach's alpha = 0.81) (48).

The severity of depression was assessed by the German version of the Beck Depression Inventory (BDI) that consists of 21 items including clinical symptoms of depression with a total score from 0 to 63, with higher scores reflecting higher levels of depression. A total score of 0–10 corresponds with no or minimal depression, of 11–17 with a mild or moderate depression, of 18–63 with a clinical relevant depression. The German version of the questionnaire has shown good psychometric properties (49, 50).

Statistical Analysis

Descriptive statistics for different measures were calculated for all participants. Data were checked for normal distribution before further statistical analysis. Associations between THI total scores and TAS-20 total scores with subscale scores as well as BDI total scores, and age were tested by using Pearson correlations (two-sided). Afterward, stepwise multiple regression analyses were performed in order to investigate the independent relationship between scores of the TAS-20 with subscales and THI. All statistical calculations were performed using the statistical software package SPSS™/Version 22.0 for Windows (SPSS Inc., Chicago, IL, USA). The significance level was set at $p \leq 0.05$.

RESULTS

Seventy-three out of the 207 patients who completed our questionnaires were females (35.3%). Mean age was 46.7 years (SD = 13.9). The average duration of tinnitus was 66.1 months (SD = 92.5). Mean scores on subjective tinnitus severity, alexithymia, and depression ($n = 207$) are presented in **Table 1**.

Patients showed, on average, moderate levels of tinnitus severity with a mean THI total score of 44.4 (SD = 23.3). In detail, 26 patients (12.6%) of the sample reported a slight handicap, 60 patients (29.0%) reported a mild handicap, 58 patients (28.0%) reported a moderate handicap, 45 patients (21.7%) reported a severe handicap, and 18 patients (8.7%) reported a catastrophic handicap. These findings are similar to results from other studies (51, 52).

The mean value of the TAS-20 total score in our sample was 44.0 (SD = 10.8), which is slightly higher as compared to the mean score of 39.9 (SD = 8.4) in a representative reference sample of the German population ($n = 306$) (53). Using the TAS-20 cut-off score ≥ 61 (54, 55), 19 patients (9.2%) could be classified as alexithymic, which is consistent with prevalence rates of alexithymia in the German general population (56).

In terms of depression severity, patients showed a mean BDI sum-score of 9.3 (SD = 6.9), which indicates none or minimal depression (57). According to the BDI manual, 133 patients (64.3%) were classified as not depressed, 50 patients (24.2%) were classified as mildly to moderately depressed, and 24 patients (11.6%) were classified as clinically relevant depressed.

Table 2 gives an overview of the Pearson correlations between THI total scores and TAS-20 total scores with subscale scores as well as BDI total scores and age. Highly significant correlations were found between THI total score and BDI score as well as TAS-20 total score and two subscales, measuring the DIF and the DDF (all $p < 0.01$; see **Table 2**). The third TAS-20 subscale, measuring EOT, and also age did not correlate with THI total score.

A stepwise multiple regression analysis including all TAS-20 subscales and the BDI score was performed in order to asses for independent relationships between these variables and THI total score (as dependent variable). It was found that only BDI (Beta = 0.64, adjusted $R^2 = 0.49$, $p < 0.01$) and the DIF-subscale (Beta = 0.12, adjusted $R^2 = 0.50$, $p < 0.05$) significantly predicted subjective level of tinnitus severity measured by THI.

In order to further estimate the association between tinnitus severity and DIF, a second stepwise multiple regression analysis was calculated with the THI subscales as independent variables and the TAS-20 DIF subscale as dependent variable. The THI total score was not used in conjunction with the THI subscales to exclude redundancy of the data analyses. According to these findings, only higher scores of the THI subscale "functional" demonstrated an independent association with higher scores for difficulty identifying feelings (Beta = 0.45, adjusted $R^2 = 0.20$, $p < 0.01$).

DISCUSSION

Our findings establish the existence of a moderate relationship between the subjective experience of tinnitus severity and alexithymic deficits in emotion regulation. More specifically, we found a positive correlation between the functional subscale of the THI, which reflects limitations tinnitus causes in the mental, occupational, social, and physical areas, and the TAS-20 dimension for difficulty identifying feelings. To the best of our

TABLE 1 | Mean scores on the Tinnitus Handicap Inventory (THI) with subscales, the Toronto Alexithymia Scale (TAS-20) with subscales, and the Beck Depression Inventory (BDI); $n = 207$.

Variable	Mean	SD
THI total	44.4	23.3
THI functional	20.6	11.5
THI emotional	13.4	8.5
THI catastrophic	10.4	4.9
TAS-20 total	44.0	10.8
TAS-20 difficulty in identifying feelings	14.1	5.4
TAS-20 difficulty in describing feelings	11.0	3.5
TAS-20 externally oriented thinking	18.9	4.4
BDI	9.3	6.9

TABLE 2 | Pearson correlation coefficients between Tinnitus Handicap Inventory (THI), the Toronto Alexithymia Scale (TAS-20) with subscales, the Beck Depression Inventory (BDI), and age; $n = 207$, $^{**}p < 0.01$.

	TAS-20 total	TAS-20 difficulty in identifying feelings	TAS-20 difficulty in describing feelings	TAS-20 externally oriented thinking	BDI	Age
THI total	0.33**	0.46**	0.28**	0.02	0.70**	−0.09
THI functional	0.33**	0.45**	0.28**	0.04	0.68**	−0.07
THI emotional	0.29**	0.42**	0.26**	−0.02	0.64**	−0.12
THI catastrophic	0.30**	0.41**	0.26**	0.03	0.64**	−0.05

knowledge, only one previous study has evaluated the association between tinnitus and alexithymia, but in a community sample of elderly people. In contrast to our findings, Salonen et al. did not find any correlation between TAS-20 scores and tinnitus severity (38). The discrepancy to our results may be explained by the fact that Salonen et al. did not use a standardized instrument to measure tinnitus severity, which was only classified by indicating one of the three groups: no tinnitus, tinnitus without annoyance, and tinnitus with annoyance (38).

Some limitations should be taken into consideration when discussing the results. First, data were collected by self-report questionnaires even though alexithymic patients may have difficulty in adequately assessing their emotional deficits (58). Second, the cross-sectional design of our study precluded any causal interpretation of the relationship between tinnitus severity and alexithymia. We are also quite aware of the fact that the significant association between DIF and THI total score was small in terms of the overall variance explained. Thus, DIF may play a role in the subjective experience of tinnitus severity, but this is not completely confirmed by the actual study. Furthermore, the relation between tinnitus severity and depressive symptoms, which was reported similarly in other studies (43, 59) might be ascribed to a content overlap between the used self-report questionnaires (52). Also further studies are needed to understand the relationship between alexithymic characteristics and the experience of tinnitus severity, which are focused on patients with chronic tinnitus, i.e., tinnitus symptoms for at least 6 months, in order to avoid including patients who are still under posttraumatic distress.

Despite the mentioned limitations our findings suggest that people with difficulties in identifying feelings may tend to experience greater limitations in social, daily, and reading activities involving concentration, auditory acuity, attention, and rest due to tinnitus (as measured by the functional subscale of THI), which is in accordance with De Gucht and Heiser (26). They reported similar outcomes in their review of the empirical literature on somatization and alexithymia: DIF demonstrated the strongest association with the number of symptoms reported, even stronger than the association with general alexithymia. Our results were also consistent with previous investigation that showed that the difficulties identifying feelings factor of the TAS-20 was particularly effective in predicting somatization (60).

Taken together, the disturbances in DIF and the subjective experience of tinnitus severity should be considered in future studies for more precise understanding of this association, preferably with the additional application of observer rated or interview-based methods for measuring alexithymia as the Toronto Structured Interview for Alexithymia (61, 62). Our results benefit a better understanding of emotion regulation difficulties in patients suffering from tinnitus. Furthermore, if replicated, they may have important clinical implications: because people with difficulties in identifying feelings are characterized by using escape-avoidance strategies, individualized psychotherapeutic interventions might potentially benefit these patients. Further research may also point to the fact that not just alexithymic characteristics can predict the experience of tinnitus severity, but a more general impairment in awareness and regulation of mental states (63–65), for example, an impaired self-reflection as found in different psychiatric disorders (66).

ETHICS STATEMENT

The study was authorized by the ethics committee of the canton of Zurich, Switzerland. All participants gave their written (electronic) informed consent in accordance with the Declaration of Helsinki.

AUTHOR CONTRIBUTIONS

JW managed data collection, analyzed and interpreted the collected data, and wrote the first draft for the article. TK initiated the collaborative project, conceptualized and designed the project, collected and monitored data collection, and revised the article. MK, NP, and MM collected data, monitored data collection, and interpreted data, and critically revised the draft paper. MR contributed to the concept and design, interpreted data, and critically revised the draft paper. SW initiated the collaborative project, conceptualized and designed the project, designed data collection tools, collected and monitored data collection, interpreted the data, and revised the article. All authors read and approved the final manuscript.

REFERENCES

Henry JA, Schechter MA, Loovis CL, Zaugg TL, Kaelin C, Montero M. Clinical management of tinnitus using a "progressive intervention" approach. *J Rehabil Res Dev* (2005) 42(4 Suppl 2):95–116. doi:10.1682/JRRD.2005.01.0005

Michikawa T, Nishiwaki Y, Kikuchi Y, Saito H, Mizutari K, Okamoto M, et al. Prevalence and factors associated with tinnitus: a community-based study of Japanese elders. *J Epidemiol* (2010) 20(4):271–6. doi:10.2188/jea. JE20090121

Probst T, Pryss RC, Langguth B, Spiliopoulou M, Landgrebe M, Vesala M, et al. Outpatient tinnitus clinic, self-help web platform, or mobile application to recruit tinnitus study samples? *Front Aging Neurosci* (2017) 9:113. doi:10.3389/fnagi.2017.00113

Scott B, Lindberg P. Psychological profile and somatic complaints between help-seeking and non-help-seeking tinnitus subjects. *Psychosomatics* (2000) 41(4):347–52. doi:10.1176/appi.psy.41.4.347

Durai M, Searchfield G. Anxiety and depression, personality traits relevant to tinnitus: a scoping review. *Int J Audiol* (2016) 55(11):605–15. doi:10.1080/14992027.2016.1198966

Langguth B, Landgrebe M, Kleinjung T, Sand GP, Hajak G. Tinnitus and depression. *World J Biol Psychiatry* (2011) 12(7):489–500. doi:10.3109/15622975.2011.575178

Milerova J, Anders M, Dvorak T, Sand PG, Koniger S, Langguth B. The influence of psychological factors on tinnitus severity. *Gen Hosp Psychiatry* (2013) 35(4):412–6. doi:10.1016/j.genhosppsych.2013.02.008

Langguth B, Kleinjung T, Fischer B, Hajak G, Eichhammer P, Sand PG. Tinnitus severity, depression, and the big five personality traits. *Prog Brain Res* (2007) 166:221–5. doi:10.1016/S0079-6123(07)66020-8

Pinto PC, Marcelos CM, Mezzasalma MA, Osterne FJ, de Melo Tavares de Lima MA, Nardi AE. Tinnitus and its association with psychiatric disorders: systematic review. *J Laryngol Otol* (2014) 128(8):660–4. doi:10.1017/S0022215114001030

Folmer RL, Griest SE, Meikle MB, Martin WH. Tinnitus severity, loudness, and depression. *Otolaryngol Head Neck Surg* (1999) 121(1):48–51. doi:10.1016/S0194-5998(99)70123-3

Hiller W, Janca A, Burke KC. Association between tinnitus and somatoform disorders. *J Psychosom Res* (1997) 43(6):613–24. doi:10.1016/S0022-3999(97)00188-8

Dobie RA, Sakai CS, Sullivan MD, Katon WJ, Russo J. Antidepressant treatment of tinnitus patients: report of a randomized clinical trial and clinical prediction of benefit. *Am J Otol* (1993) 14(1):18–23.

Figueiredo RR, Rates MA, Azevedo AA, Oliveira PM, Navarro PB. Correlation analysis of hearing thresholds, validated questionnaires and psychoacoustic measurements in tinnitus patients. *Braz J Otorhinolaryngol* (2010) 76(4):522–6. doi:10.1590/S1808-86942010000400018

Newman CW, Wharton JA, Jacobson GP. Self-focused and somatic attention in patients with tinnitus. *J Am Acad Audiol* (1997) 8(3):143–9.

Nondahl DM, Cruickshanks KJ, Dalton DS, Klein BE, Klein R, Schubert CR, et al. The impact of tinnitus on quality of life in older adults. *J Am Acad Audiol* (2007) 18(3):257–66. doi:10.3766/jaaa.18.3.7

Weidt S, Delsignore A, Meyer M, Rufer M, Peter N, Drabe N, et al. Which tinnitus-related characteristics affect current health-related quality of life and depression? A cross-sectional cohort study. *Psychiatry Res* (2016) 237:114–21. doi:10.1016/j.psychres.2016.01.065

Krog NH, Engdahl B, Tambs K. The association between tinnitus and mental health in a general population sample: results from the HUNT Study. *J Psychosom Res* (2010) 69(3):289–98. doi:10.1016/j.jpsychores.2010. 03.008

Nemiah JC, Sifneos PE. Psychosomatic illness: a problem in communication. *Psychother Psychosom* (1970) 18(1):154–60. doi:10.1159/000286074

Sifneos PE. The prevalence of 'alexithymic' characteristics in psychosomatic patients. *Psychother Psychosom* (1973) 22(2):255–62. doi:10.1159/000286529

Taylor GJ, Bagby RM. The alexithymia personality dimension In: Widige TA, editor. *The Oxford Handbook of Personality Disorders*. New York, NY: Oxford University Press (2012) p. 648–73.

Humphreys TP, Wood LM, Parker JD. Alexithymia and satisfaction in intimate relationships. *Pers Individ Dif* (2009) 46(1):43–7. doi:10.1016/j.paid. 2008.09.002

Leenen K, Rufer M, Moergeli H, Grabe H-J, Jenewein J, Nuñez DG, et al. Alexithyme Patientenmerkmale und Lebensqualität-Eine Querschnittsstudie an 79 ambulanten Patienten mit Angststörungen. *Z Psychiatr Psychol Psychother* (2015) 61:17–26. doi:10.1024/1661-4747/a000136

Bird G, Silani G, Brindley R, White S, Frith U, Singer T. Empathic brain responses in insula are modulated by levels of alexithymia but not autism. *Brain* (2010) 133(Pt 5):1515–25. doi:10.1093/brain/awq060

Lundh LG, Simonsson-Sarnecki M. Alexithymia, emotion, and somatic complaints. *J Pers* (2001) 69(3):483–510. doi:10.1111/1467-6494.00153

Taylor GJ, Bagby RM, Parker JDA. *Disorders of Affect Regulation: Alexithymia in Medical and Psychiatric Illness*. Cambridge; New York: Cambridge University Press (1997). xxii,359 p.

De Gucht V, Heiser W. Alexithymia and somatisation: quantitative review of the literature. *J Psychosom Res* (2003) 54(5):425–34. doi:10.1016/S0022-3999(02)00467-1

von Rimscha S, Moergeli H, Weidt S, Straumann D, Hegemann S, Rufer M. Alexithymia and health-related quality of life in patients with dizzi- ness. *Psychopathology* (2013) 46(6):377–83. doi:10.1159/000345357

Parker JD, Taylor GJ, Bagby RM, Acklin MW. Alexithymia in panic disorder and simple phobia: a comparative study. *Am J Psychiatry* (1993) 150(7):1105–7. doi:10.1176/ajp.150.7.1105

Corcos M, Guilbaud O, Speranza M, Paterniti S, Loas G, Stephan P, et al. Alexithymia and depression in eating disorders. *Psychiatry Res* (2000) 93(3):263–6. doi:10.1016/S0165-1781(00)00109-8

Taylor GJ, Parker JD, Bagby RM, Bourke MP. Relationships between alexithymia and psychological characteristics associated with eating disorders. *J Psychosom Res* (1996) 41(6):561–8. doi:10.1016/S0022-3999(96) 00224-3

Loas G, Otmani O, Lecercle C, Jouvent R. Relationships between the emotional and cognitive components of alexithymia and dependency in alcoholics. *Psychiatry Res* (2000) 96(1):63–74. doi:10.1016/S0165-1781(00) 00189-X

Zeitlin SB, McNally RJ, Cassiday KL. Alexithymia in victims of sexual assault: an effect of repeated traumatization? *Am J Psychiatry* (1993) 150(4):661–3. doi:10.1176/ajp.150.4.661

Joyce AS, Fujiwara E, Cristall M, Ruddy C, Ogrodniczuk JS. Clinical correlates of alexithymia among patients with personality disorder. *Psychother Res* (2013) 23(6):690–704. doi:10.1080/10503307.2013.803628

Nicolo G, Semerari A, Lysaker PH, Dimaggio G, Conti L, D'Angerio S, et al. Alexithymia in personality disorders: correlations with symptoms and interpersonal functioning. *Psychiatry Res* (2011) 190(1):37–42. doi:10.1016/j. psychres.2010.07.046

Porcelli P, Zaka S, Leoci C, Centonze S, Taylor GJ. Alexithymia in inflammatory bowel disease. A case-control study. *Psychother Psychosom* (1995) 64(1):49–53. doi:10.1159/000288990

Serrano J, Plaza V, Sureda B, de Pablo J, Picado C, Bardagi S, et al. Alexithymia: a relevant psychological variable in near-fatal asthma. *Eur Respir J* (2006) 28(2):296–302. doi:10.1183/09031936.06.00008105

Jula A, Salminen JK, Saarijarvi S. Alexithymia: a facet of essential hypertension. *Hypertension* (1999) 33(4):1057–61. doi:10.1161/01.HYP.33.4.1057

Salonen J, Johansson R, Joukamaa M. Alexithymia, depression and tinnitus in elderly people. *Gen Hosp Psychiatry* (2007) 29(5):431–5. doi:10.1016/j. genhosppsych.2007.05.002

Kleinjung T, Fischer B, Langguth B, Sand PG, Hajak G, Dvorakova J, et al. Validation of the German-version Tinnitus Handicap Inventory (THI). *Psychiat Prax* (2007) 34:S140–2. doi:10.1055/s-2006-940218

Newman CW, Jacobson GP, Spitzer JB. Development of the Tinnitus Handicap Inventory. *Arch Otolaryngol Head Neck Surg* (1996) 122(2):143–8. doi:10.1001/archotol.1996.01890140029007

Newman CW, Sandridge SA, Jacobson GP. Psychometric adequacy of the Tinnitus Handicap Inventory (THI) for evaluating treatment outcome. *J Am Acad Audiol* (1998) 9(2):153–60.

Wrzosek M, Szymiec E, Klemens W, Kotylo P, Schlee W, Modrzynska M, et al. Polish translation and validation of the Tinnitus Handicap Inventory and the Tinnitus Functional Index. *Front Psychol* (2016) 7:1871. doi:10.3389/fpsyg.2016.01871

Zeman F, Koller M, Langguth B, Landgrebe M, Tinnitus Research Initiative Database Study Group. Which tinnitus-related aspects are relevant for quality of life and depression: results from a large international multicentre sample. *Health Qual Life Outcomes* (2014) 12:7. doi:10.1186/1477-7525-12-7

Rejali D, Sivakumar A, Balaji N. *Ginkgo biloba* does not benefit patients with tinnitus: a randomized placebo-controlled double-blind trial and meta-analysis of randomized trials. *Clin Otolaryngol Allied Sci* (2004) 29(3): 226–31. doi:10.1111/j.1365-2273.2004.00814.x

Bach M, Bach D, de Zwaan M, Serim M, Bohmer F. [Validation of the German version of the 20-item Toronto Alexithymia Scale in normal persons and psychiatric patients]. *Psychother Psychosom Med Psychol* (1996) 46(1):23–8.

Bagby RM, Parker JD, Taylor GJ. The twenty-item Toronto Alexithymia Scale – I. Item selection and cross-validation of the factor structure. *J Psychosom Res* (1994) 38(1):23–32. doi:10.1016/0022-3999(94)90005-1

Taylor GJ, Bagby RM, Parker JD. The 20-Item Toronto Alexithymia Scale. IV. Reliability and factorial validity in different languages and cultures. *J Psychosom Res* (2003) 55(3):277–83. doi:10.1016/S0022-3999(02)00601-3 Popp K, Schafer R, Schneider C, Brahler E, Decker O, Hardt J, et al. [Factor structure and reliability of the Toronto Alexithymia Scale (TAS-20) in the German population]. *Psychother Psychosom Med Psychol* (2008) 58(5):208–14. doi:10.1055/s-2007-986196

Beck AT, Ward CH, Mendelson M, Mock J, Erbaugh J. An inventory for measuring depression. *Arch Gen Psychiatry* (1961) 4:561–71. doi:10.1001/archpsyc.1961.01710120031004

Hautzinger M. [The Beck Depression Inventory in clinical practice]. *Nervenarzt* (1991) 62(11):689–96.

Andersson G, Freijd A, Baguley DM, Idrizbegovic E. Tinnitus distress, anxiety, depression, and hearing problems among cochlear implant patients with tinnitus. *J Am Acad Audiol* (2009) 20(5):315–9. doi:10.3766/jaaa.20.5.5

Ooms E, Meganck R, Vanheule S, Vinck B, Watelet JB, Dhooge I. Tinnitus severity and the relation to depressive symptoms: a critical study. *Otolaryngol Head Neck Surg* (2011) 145(2):276–81. doi:10.1177/0194599811403381

Koch AS, Kleiman A, Wegener I, Zur B, Imbierowicz K, Geiser F, et al. Factorial structure of the 20-item Toronto Alexithymia Scale in a large sample of somatoform patients. *Psychiatry Res* (2015) 225(3):355–63. doi:10.1016/j.psychres.2014.12.013

Parker JD, Michael Bagby R, Taylor GJ, Endler NS, Schmitz P. Factorial validity of the 20-item Toronto Alexithymia Scale. *Eur J Personality* (1993) 7(4):221–32. doi:10.1002/per.2410070403

Parker JD, Taylor GJ, Bagby RM. Alexithymia and the recognition of facial expressions of emotion. *Psychother Psychosom* (1993) 59(3–4):197–202. doi:10.1159/000288664

Franz M, Popp K, Schaefer R, Sitte W, Schneider C, Hardt J, et al. Alexithymia in the German general population. *Soc Psychiatry Psychiatr Epidemiol* (2008) 43(1):54–62. doi:10.1007/s00127-007-0265-1

Beck AT, Steer RA, Carbin MG. Psychometric properties of the Beck Depression Inventory: twenty-five years of evaluation. *Clin Psychol Rev* (1988) 8(1):77–100. doi:10.1016/0272-7358(88)90050-5

Lumley MA, Neely LC, Burger AJ. The assessment of alexithymia in medical settings: implications for understanding and treating health problems. *J Pers Assess* (2007) 89(3):230–46. doi:10.1080/00223890701629698

Crocetti A, Forti S, Ambrosetti U, Bo LD. Questionnaires to evaluate anxiety and depressive levels in tinnitus patients. *Otolaryngol Head Neck Surg* (2009) 140(3):403–5. doi:10.1016/j.otohns.2008.11.036

Grabe HJ, Spitzer C, Freyberger HJ. Alexithymia and personality in relation to dimensions of psychopathology. *Am J Psychiatry* (2004) 161(7):1299–301. doi:10.1176/appi.ajp.161.7.1299

Bagby RM, Taylor GJ, Parker JD, Dickens SE. The development of the Toronto Structured Interview for Alexithymia: item selection, factor structure, reliability and concurrent validity. *Psychother Psychosom* (2006) 75(1):25–39. doi:10.1159/000089224

Grabe HJ, Lobel S, Dittrich D, Bagby RM, Taylor GJ, Quilty LC, et al. The German version of the toronto structured interview for alexithymia: factor structure, reliability, and concurrent validity in a psychiatric patient sample. *Compr Psychiatry* (2009) 50(5):424–30. doi:10.1016/j.comppsych.2008.11.008

Lysaker PH, Gumley A, Luedtke B, Buck KD, Ringer JM, Olesek K, et al. Social cognition and metacognition in schizophrenia: evidence of their independence and linkage with outcomes. *Acta Psychiatr Scand* (2013) 127(3): 239–47. doi:10.1111/acps.12012

Semerari A, Carcione A, Dimaggio G, Falcone M, Nicolo G, Procacci M, et al. How to evaluate metacognitive functioning in psychotherapy? The metacognition assessment scale and its applications. *Clin Psychol Psychot* (2003) 10(4):238–61. doi:10.1002/cpp.362

Velotti P, Garofalo C, Petrocchi C, Cavallo F, Popolo R, Dimaggio G. Alexithymia, emotion dysregulation, impulsivity and aggression: a multiple mediation model. *Psychiatry Res* (2016) 237:296–303. doi:10.1016/j.psychres.2016.01.025

Dimaggio G, Vanheule S, Lysaker PH, Carcione A, Nicolo G. Impaired self-reflection in psychiatric disorders among adults: a proposal for the existence of a network of semi independent functions. *Conscious Cogn* (2009) 18(3):653–64. doi:10.1016/j.concog.2009.06.003

3

Clinical Validation of a New Tinnitus Assessment Technology

Sylvie Hébert[1,2]* *and Philippe Fournier*[1,2†]

[1] *Faculty of Medicine, School of Speech Pathology and Audiology, Université de Montréal, Montréal, QC, Canada,*
[2] *BRAMS – International Laboratory for Research on Brain, Music, and Sound, Université de Montréal, Montréal, QC, Canada*

Correspondence:
Sylvie Hébert
sylvie.hebert@umontreal.ca

Current clinical assessment of tinnitus relies mainly on self-report. Psychoacoustic assessment of tinnitus pitch and loudness are recommended but methods yield variable results. Herein, we investigated the proposition that a previously validated fixed laboratory-based method (Touchscreen) and a newly developed clinically relevant portable prototype (Stand-alone) yield comparable results in the assessment of psychoacoustic tinnitus pitch and loudness. Participants with tinnitus [*N* = 15, 7 with normal hearing and 8 with hearing loss (HL)] and participants simulating tinnitus (simulators, *N* = 15) were instructed to rate the likeness of pure tones (250—16 kHz) to their tinnitus pitch and match their loudness using both methods presented in a counterbalanced order. Results indicate that simulators rated their "tinnitus" at lower frequencies and at louder levels (~10 dB) compared to tinnitus participants. Tinnitus subgroups (with vs. without HL) differed in their predominant tinnitus pitch (i.e., lower in the tinnitus with HL subgroups), but not in their loudness matching in decibel SL. Loudness at the predominant pitch was identified as a factor yielding significant sensitivity and specificity in discriminating between the two groups of participants. Importantly, despite differences in the devices' physical presentations, likeness and loudness ratings were globally consistent between the two methods and, moreover, highly reproducible from one method to the other in both groups. All in all, both methods yielded robust tinnitus data in less than 12 min, with the Stand-alone having the advantage of not being dependent of learning effects, being user-friendly, and being adapted to the audiogram of each patient to further reduce testing time.

Keywords: tinnitus, psychoacoustic test tool, loudness, pitch, hearing loss

INTRODUCTION

Tinnitus is a common health condition that affects from 11.9 to 30.3% of the general population and its prevalence increases with increasing age (1, 2). Tinnitus can interfere with daily life and is associated with significant psychological distress, anxiety, and other health-related issues (1). Individuals with tinnitus seeking clinical services are at a clear disadvantage compared to others because there are no established guidelines for the clinical assessment and intervention for tinnitus. At the basis of clinical service is assessment, which confirms diagnosis, as well as determines and monitors intervention, and yet, current clinical assessments of tinnitus mostly rely on patients' self-report.

Tinnitus can be characterized by its psychoacoustic properties (pitch and loudness), which pertain to the auditory domain, and by its associated distress, which pertains to the psychological domain. Some clinical settings assess psychoacoustic measurements of pitch and loudness. Classical forced-choice paradigm and the method of adjustment are the preferred methods used (3). However, the procedure is passive, with clinicians controlling the stimulus parameters presented to the patient (3). These techniques are usually mastered by highly skilled clinicians and yet do not provide stable measurements of the tinnitus percept within a session or between sessions over time (3). This lack of reliability compromises tinnitus assessments such that clinical trials often have to rely on visual analog scales or tinnitus questionnaires as main treatment outcomes (4, 5). These outcomes, however, are highly unsatisfactory because some therapeutic interventions (e.g., transcranial magnetic stimulation of the auditory cortex, deep brain stimulation, noise-notched music) are targeted primarily at decreasing the psychoacoustic loudness of tinnitus, which in turn would supposedly decrease the associated psychological distress. However, the precise relationship between loudness and distress is unknown and usually statistical correlations are not very high (6). Therefore, the best tinnitus assessment should include reliable measures of both of these aspects.

Recently, an active method allowing the patient to control parameters using a Touchscreen has shown good test–retest reliability for tinnitus predominant pitch and loudness matching over several months (6, 7). Moreover, psychoacoustic tinnitus loudness matches were higher for simulators than for participants with tinnitus and was a better predictor for specificity (e.g., correctly detecting simulators) than predominant pitch (4). A similar method specifically designed for clinical settings could be very useful for health-care professionals to assess the progression of the tinnitus over several months in individual patients and assess treatment' efficacy with confidence. High levels of sensitivity and specificity of the method are interesting features that would be valuable in medicolegal cases of tinnitus. For these purposes, a new Stand-alone prototype (hereafter, Stand-alone) was developed from the first laboratory device (hereafter, Touchscreen), in order to capture the main tinnitus characteristics—likeness and loudness ratings—but in a format that is more suited for clinical purposes.

The aim of the present study was, therefore, to compare performance of the two methods, including participants simulating having tinnitus. As previously reported, the tinnitus likeness and most importantly the loudness should be significantly different between tinnitus participants and simulators for both methods. Likewise, loudness should be a better predictor of tinnitus presence compared to tinnitus predominant pitch, again for both methods.

As time efficiency is a major issue for clinicians, testing time for the two devices was assessed and compared. We predicted that the modification made to the Stand-alone device should provide a more efficient testing time than the Touchscreen method for patients with hearing loss (HL). Finally, the effect of presenting two pure tones instead of the standard three pure tones was assessed, as it could also potentially reduce testing time.

A second objective was to compare two tinnitus subtypes. In particular, tinnitus with and without HL has been shown to engage two different types of brain structures (8, 9). In addition, differences in tinnitus spectrum have been noted across studies between tinnitus patients with and without HL mostly in the very high frequency region (6, 10). From a clinical standpoint, these two groups are also very different in term of assessment and therapeutic approach. For instance, hearing assessment for tinnitus patients with HL is usually longer than for patients without HL, and thus, any saved time in the assessment of tinnitus would be a valuable asset for a clinical device. In that respect, tinnitus subgroups were further examined on the basis of this criterion.

MATERIALS AND METHODS

Participants

Two groups of participants who had not participated in our previous studies using the Touchscreen method were recruited through word of mouth or advertisements in local newspapers. Tinnitus participants had to have chronic bilateral tinnitus, not have complete deafness in one or both ears, and be in good health. Health was further verified by questions on possible diseases (e.g., neurological disease), conditions (e.g., uncontrolled hypertension), and medication. This group consisted of 15 adults (9M, 6F) with a mean age of 45 years (min: 23; max: 69). Simulator participants had to have had a previous experience of transient tinnitus (less than a day) more than 3 months before the experiment so that they could rely on this past experience to fake tinnitus. Most participants reported having previous experience of transient tinnitus after loud sound exposure such as a music concert, a very frequent phenomenon (10). This group consisted of 15 adults (7M, 8F) with a mean age of 32 years (min: 21; max: 62). They were instructed to simulate this sound perception with the intention of convincing the experimenter that they had tinnitus. None of the participants reported otologic condition other than HL and none of the participants were smokers.

Tinnitus Subtypes

The normal hearing (NH) Tinnitus subgroup ($N = 7$) had hearing thresholds ≤25 dB hearing loss (HL) at all frequencies from 250 to 8 kHz in both ears. The HL tinnitus subgroup ($N = 8$) had hearing thresholds >25 dB HL at least at one frequency between 250 and 8 kHz in either ear.

Hearing Assessment

An otoscopy was performed in order to rule out earwax compaction and outer ear pathology. Standard hearing detection thresholds were assessed in each ear monaurally from 0.25 to 8 kHz in half-octave steps by a clinical audiologist using the standard modified Hughson–Westlake up–down procedure (5) with an AC-40 clinical audiometer and ER-3A insert earphones in a sound-proof booth (ANSI S3.6-2004 standard norms). Very-high frequency thresholds (9–16 kHz) were also assessed monaurally in each ear using Sennheiser HDA-200 supra-aural headphones.

Tinnitus Matching Method

Tinnitus assessment was run with both the Touchscreen and the Stand-alone in each participant in a counterbalanced order. Both methods used 3-s pure tones ranging from 0.25 to 16 kHz presented three times in a pseudorandom order such that no two identical frequencies were presented in a row. Participants were first asked to rate the likeness of the tone to their tinnitus pitch on a Likert-type scale in which 0 = "does not match my tinnitus at all" and 10 = "perfectly matches my tinnitus." During the same trial, they had to match the loudness of the tone—that is, the sound level at which that specific frequency contributed to their tinnitus—by moving a visual gauge (Touchscreen) or a potentiometer (Stand-alone) that increased and decreased the sound level by 1 dB steps. Participants were allowed to play each pure tone as many times as needed for both methods. The sound was presented binaurally using closed DT 770 Pro/250 dynamic headphones (Beyerdynamic, Heilbronn, Germany) for the Touchscreen method and HDA-300 Sennheiser (Sennheiser electronic GmbH & Co. KG, Germany) headphones for the Stand-alone device. The main difference between the two methods (see **Figure 1**) is that the Stand-alone uses standard buttons for playing sounds and rating likeness and a potentiometer for loudness matching. The design of the Stand-alone maximizes ergonomics and comfort to improve its use by older patients.

In addition, in order to make the method more time-efficient, especially for participants with some degree of HL, an additional step was implemented in the Stand-alone method. The audiogram of each participant was taken into account such that (1) frequencies for which a threshold could not be found (i.e., higher than the limits of the audiometer) were not presented and (2) levels of the frequencies presented were always beyond threshold. This information was added to the device just before the task began.

Calibration

Headphones were calibrated before each session with a SoundPro SE/DL sound level meter using a QE-4170 microphone model (Quest Technologies, Oconomowoc, WI, USA) and an EC-9A 2cc ear coupler (Quest Electronics, Oconomowoc, WI, USA).

Procedure

All participants were first assessed with the hearing evaluation. Then, they were tested with one of the two matching methods (Touchscreen or Stand-alone) in a counterbalanced order. They were next tested with the other method, both taking place in the same sound attenuated room. Participants were asked to provide repeatable tinnitus matching responses to the best of their ability. Simulators were instructed to use their past experience of tinnitus to convince the experimenter that they had tinnitus but were not instructed to use any particular method to provide consistent responses during matching. The time required to perform the tinnitus-matching task for each device was assessed using a conventional chronometer. The experimenter started the chronometer as soon as the participant press the « play » button for the first time, that is, after the instruction was given for each device individually. The study was approved by the ethics committee of Université de Montréal and was conducted with the understanding and written consent of each participant.

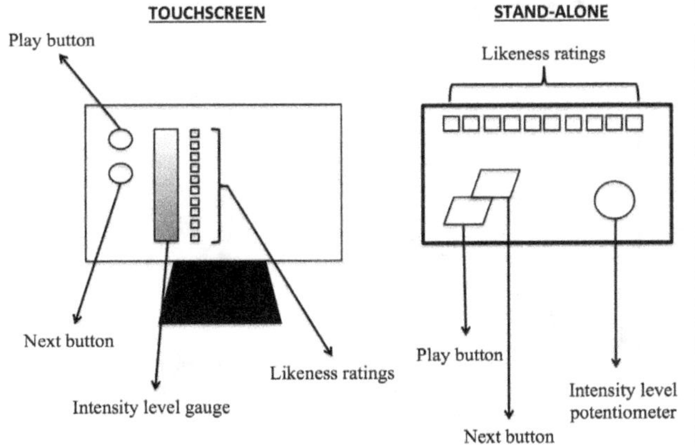

FIGURE 1 | **Schematization of the Touchscreen and the Stand-alone devices used in the experiment.**

Analyses

In all analyses below, the two groups (Tinnitus vs. Simulators) were first compared, and in a second step, the Tinnitus subgroups (NH vs. HL) were compared. Hearing thresholds were analyzed with a 2 × (2 × 16) ANOVA with Group (first, Tinnitus vs. Simulators; second, Tinnitus NH vs. HL) as a between-subject factors and ear (right, left) and frequency (250–16 kHz) as within-subject factors. Similar analyses were run on likeness ratings and loudness matching but with Methods (Touchscreen vs. Stand-alone) rather than ear as a within-subject factor. Product-to-moment Pearson correlations and paired-sample *T*-tests were run on these data to compare the two methods. The first and second predominant pitches and their corresponding loudness were extracted from the tinnitus spectrum of each participant and compared between groups and subgroups as described above.

Sensitivity and specificity analyses were run for each method (Touchscreen, Stand-alone) using logistic regressions taking group as the dependent factor putting the first predominant pitch and its corresponding loudness match as independent predictors.

To investigate potential learning effects in using devices, testing time was analyzed using a 2 × (2 × 2) ANOVA with Group [(1) Tinnitus vs. Simulators; (2) Tinnitus NH vs. HL] as between-subject factors and order of presentation (Touchscreen first vs. Stand-alone first) and Method (Touchscreen vs. Stand-alone) as within-subject factors. Finally, comparisons were made between using all three instances of pure tones and the first two instances only.

RESULTS

Hearing Thresholds

Hearing thresholds of all 16 frequencies did not differ across ears (all *ps* >0.05) except at 12.5 kHz ($p = 0.001$) and, therefore, were averaged. When considering two groups (Tinnitus, Simulators), the two-way interaction between frequency and group was significant, $F(15, 420) = 3.32, p < 0.001$. Thresholds for the Tinnitus group were higher from 3 to 14 kHz, all *ps* <0.05 and only marginally higher at 16 kHz, $p = 0.07$. When considering only the tinnitus subgroups NH vs. HL, the same pattern emerged, $F(15, 195) = 23.59, p < 0.001$. Thresholds for the HL subgroup were higher from 2 to 16 kHz, all *ps* <0.04. **Figure 2** displays the best thresholds for the three groups for Tinnitus and Simulator group (**Figure 2A**) and Tinnitus subgroups NH and HL (**Figure 2B**).

Tinnitus Pitch Matching

On likeness ratings, there was no significant main effect of Methods or any interaction involving this factor (all *ps* >0.05), suggesting that the two methods work similarly (see **Table 1**). Paired-sample *T*-tests revealed only one significant difference at 9 kHz with a seven mean difference in the ratings between the two methods (see **Table 1**). Overall, correlations between the two methods were very high (mean $r = 0.74$, min: 0.53, max: 0.95). **Figure 2A** shows the likeness ratings for the Tinnitus and Simulator groups with merged Methods. There was a two-way interaction between Group and Frequency, $F(15, 420) = 1.70$, $p < 0.05$. Simulators' ratings were higher compared to Tinnitus' for frequencies 250–3 kHz irrespective of Methods, all *ps* <0.05.

For the Tinnitus subgroups, there was no effect of Methods or interaction involving this factor (all *ps* >0.05). **Figure 2B** shows the likeness ratings for the two subgroups NH and HL tinnitus. There was a significant interaction between frequency and subgroups, $F(15, 195) = 5.16$, $p < 0.001$. Ratings were higher for frequencies 14 and 16 kHz for the NH subgroup ($p < 0.001$) and marginally significant for the 12.5 kHz ($p = 0.05$). None of the other frequency differed (all *ps* >0.14). There was also a main effect of subgroup, $F(1, 13) = 7.02$, $p = 0.02$, with NH tinnitus subgroup rating their tinnitus with higher scores than the HL subgroup (means of 4 and 3, respectively).

When considering the first and the second predominant pitch, that is, the frequencies with the first and the second highest ratings in each individual participant, the Tinnitus group did not differ from the Simulator group (see **Table 2**). Interestingly, the Tinnitus subgroups differed from one another in terms of the first predominant pitch, with a higher predominant pitch for the NH subgroup compared to the HL subgroup (see **Table 2**).

Tinnitus Loudness Matching

On loudness ratings, there was no main effect of Methods or any interaction between Methods and Groups (all *ps* >0.10), again suggesting that both methods work similarly. However, there was a two-way interaction between Methods and Frequency, $F(15, 420) = 2.43$, $p = 0.002$: loudness matches with the Touchscreen were significantly lower for 2, 3, and 4 kHz and higher for 9 kHz (see **Table 1**). Overall, correlations between the two methods were again very high (mean $r = 0.65$, min: 0.26, max: 0.88). The expected group effect was significant $F(1, 28) = 7.32$, $p = 0.011$, with higher loudness matches for the Simulator compared to the Tinnitus group (mean of 17.7 and 6.1 dB SL, respectively) (see **Figure 3**). For the Tinnitus subgroups, there was no effect of Methods or interaction involving this factor (all *ps* >0.05). There was no main effect or interaction involving subgroups (means were: 7.97 and 4.41 dB SL for the NH and HL tinnitus, respectively).

When considering the loudness associated with the first and the second predominant pitches, the Tinnitus and Simulator groups differed significantly (see **Table 2**). The two Tinnitus subgroups did not differ on loudness for the two predominant frequencies.

Testing Time

Figure 4 displays testing times for the two methods according to order of presentation. Analyses revealed learning effects depending on the method used, as supported by a significant interaction between Method and Order of presentation, $F(1, 26) = 28.02$, $p < 0.001$: for the Stand-alone method, the order of presentation did not matter (testing times of 9 min 22 s, n.s.) whereas when the Touchscreen method was presented first, it took significantly

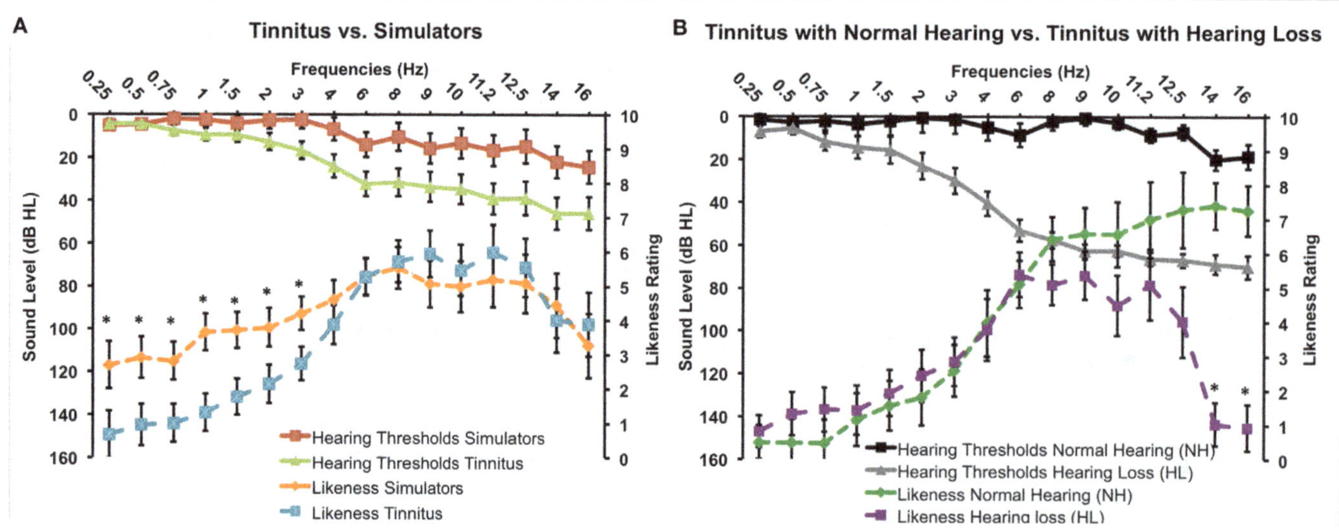

FIGURE 2 | **Best hearing thresholds and tinnitus likeness ratings for the Tinnitus and Simulator groups (A) and the two Tinnitus subgroups with normal hearing and with hearing loss (B) (SEM).**

TABLE 1 | Mean differences and product-to-moment Pearson correlations between the two methods (Touchscreen vs. Stand-alone) and the two groups (Simulators and Tinnitus groups merged) for likeness ratings and loudness matching at each frequency.

	Likeness ratings				Loudness matching			
Frequency (kHz)	**Mean difference**	***p*-Value**	***r***	***p*-Value**	**Mean difference (dB)**	***p*-Value**	***r***	***p*-Value**
0.25	0.1	0.70	0.95	<0.001	−0.4	0.76	0.88	<0.001
0.5	0.2	0.59	0.76	<0.001	−0.4	0.88	0.78	<0.001
0.75	−0.2	0.33	0.85	<0.001	−2.3	0.49	0.70	<0.001
1	0.3	0.33	0.79	<0.001	−1.9	0.56	0.71	<0.001
1.5	−0.4	0.27	0.66	<0.001	−5.0	0.15	0.67	<0.001
2	−0.3	0.43	0.66	<0.001	**−8.4**	**0.05**	0.56	0.001
3	−0.4	0.21	0.64	<0.001	**−14.0**	**<0.001**	0.74	<0.001
4	−0.4	0.37	0.62	<0.001	**−7.5**	**0.05**	0.69	<0.001
6	−0.3	0.46	0.53	0.003	−5.3	0.07	0.68	<0.001
8	0.2	0.64	0.65	<0.001	5.9	0.07	0.65	<0.001
9	**0.7**	**0.04**	0.81	<0.001	**9.9**	**0.01**	0.56	0.001
10	0.1	0.87	0.81	<0.001	4.4	0.11	0.73	<0.001
11.2	0.1	0.71	0.87	<0.001	1.0	0.72	0.61	<0.001
12.5	0.4	0.37	0.76	<0.001	−7.7	0.07	0.44	0.014
14	**1.0**	**0.04**	0.76	<0.001	1.6	0.55	0.67	<0.001
16	0.9	0.09	0.76	<0.001	0.0	1.00	0.26	0.164
Grand mean	0.1		0.74		−1.9		0.65	

Significant differences between the two methods are in bold.

TABLE 2 | Comparisons between the first and second predominant pitches of the tinnitus spectrum (in kHz) and their corresponding loudness (in dB SL) for the two methods.

	Tinnitus	**Simulators**	***p*-Value**	**Tinnitus with normal hearing**	**Tinnitus with hearing loss**	***p*-Value**
Touchscreen						
First predominant pitch (kHz)	11.37	8.98	n.s.	14.64	8.5	**=0.001**
Second predominant pitch (kHz)	9.06	9.86	n.s.	11.03	8.84	n.s.
Loudness predominant pitch (SL)	−1.9	20	**=0.015**	−10	5.2	n.s.
Loudness second predominant pitch (SL)	6.1	22	**=0.046**	6.3	5.9	n.s.
Stand-alone						
First predominant pitch (kHz)	11.09	8.39	n.s.	14	8.55	**=0.02**
Second predominant pitch (kHz)	10.01	7.06	n.s.	12.21	8.08	**=0.04**
Loudness predominant pitch (SL)	10.8	24.92	**=0.02**	5.75	15.2	n.s.
Loudness second predominant pitch (SL)	9.18	27.48	**=0.002**	5.7	12.23	n.s.

Significant differences between the two methods are in bold.
n.s., not significant.

more time than when it was presented after the Stand-alone method (12 min 44 s vs. 8 min 32 s, $p = 0.009$). There was also a main effect of Method, with overall testing time shorter for the Stand-alone compared to the Touchscreen, $F(1, 26) = 10{,}37$, $p = 0.003$ (testing time Stand-alone = 10 min 46 s; range = 4 min 30 s to 20 min 01 s; testing time Touchscreen = 9 min 21 s; range: 5 min 23 s and 16 min 48 s). Finally, there was also a main effect of group, with the Simulator group being faster than the Tinnitus group, $F(1, 26) = 7.24$, $p = 0.011$ (8 min 23 s vs. 11 min 36 s for the two groups, respectively).

Analyses were also run to examine testing time differences between methods for the tinnitus subtypes (with or without HL) with the implemented audiogram. The two-way interaction between Method (Touchscreen, Stand-alone) and subgroup (without, with HL) with order of presentation as a co-variable was significant, $F(1, 12) = 7.03$, $p = 0.021$. For the subgroup without HL, testing time did not differ between methods (11 min 5 s vs. 10 min 41 s for the Touchscreen and Stand-alone, respectively, $p = 0.75$) whereas for the subgroup HL, testing time was—marginally—shorter with the Stand-alone (13 min 48 s vs. 10 min 54 s for the Touchscreen and Stand-alone, respectively, $p = 0.052$). All but one tinnitus participant with HL took less time with the Stand-alone device (see **Figure 5**).

Two vs. Three Instances Presentation

The impact of presenting the two first vs. three instances of each frequency on the likeness ratings and loudness matching was also examined (see **Table 3**). Only two significant differences were found, one at 9 kHz for the likeness ratings (mean difference = 0.27) and one at 12.5 kHz for the loudness matches (mean difference = 3.4 dB SL). The analysis between the Tinnitus and Simulator groups was rerun on likeness and loudness matches. Similar results were obtained: for pitch matching, the frequency by groups interaction was marginally significant $F(15, 420) = 1.62$, $p = 0.066$ and *post hoc* tests revealed significant differences in ratings between the two groups for the frequencies 0.25–3 kHz, with higher ratings for the Simulators. For the loudness matching, the Frequency by Methods interaction was significant $F(15, 420) = 2.51$, $p = 0.001$, similar to the three instances results. The main group effect was also significant $F(1, 28) = 7.14$, $p = 0.012$,

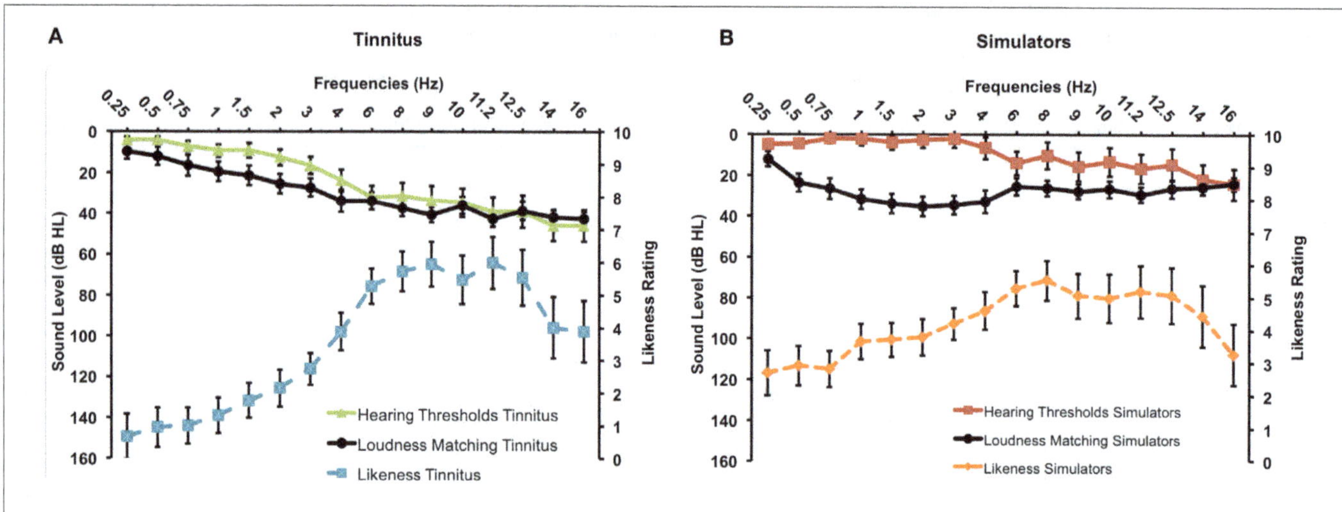

FIGURE 3 | **Tinnitus spectrum (likeness ratings and loudness matches) for the Tinnitus (A) and the Simulator (B) groups (SEM).**

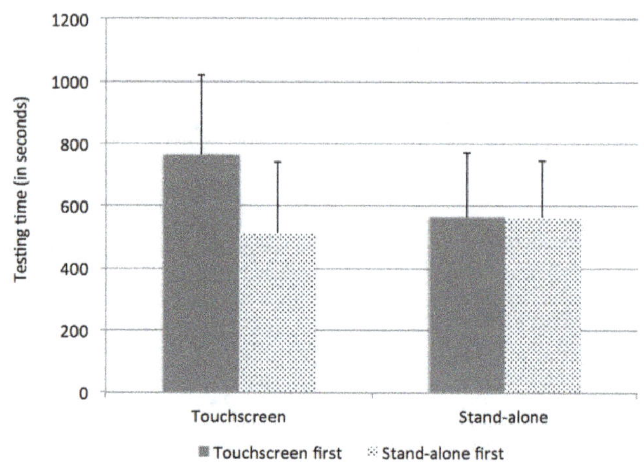

FIGURE 4 | **Testing time (SD) for the two methods and the two groups according to the order of presentation (Touchscreen or Stand-alone first).**

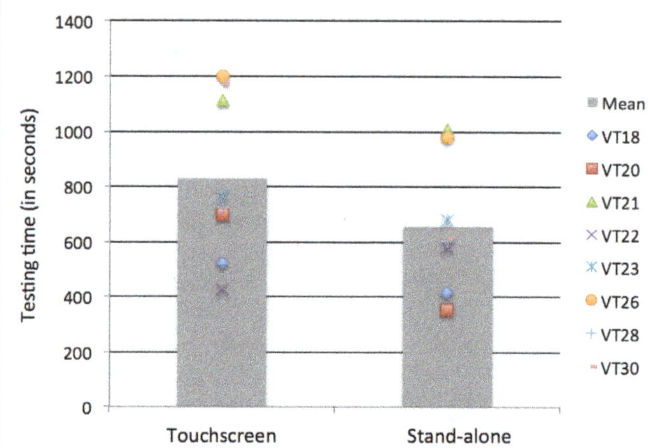

FIGURE 5 | **Testing time for the subgroup Tinnitus with hearing loss using the Touchscreen or Stand-alone device.** Individual data are shown.

with Simulators having higher loudness matches (mean: 18 dB SL) than the Tinnitus participants (mean: 6.8 dB SL).

Predominant Pitch vs. Loudness as Predictors of Having Tinnitus

The logistic regression model taking tinnitus predominant pitch and loudness (in dB SL) at the tinnitus predominant pitch as predictor variables for the likelihood of having tinnitus was significant for the Touchscreen, $\chi^2(2) = 6.855, p = 0.032$. The model explained 27.2% (Nagelkerke R^2) of the variance and correctly classified 70.0% of cases, with 73.3% sensitivity (i.e., correctly classifying tinnitus participants in the Tinnitus group) and 67.7% specificity (i.e., correctly classifying Simulators in the Simulator group). This model only included loudness as a significant predictor ($p = 0.062$), and not pitch ($p = 0.90$): lower loudness values were associated with greater likelihood of having tinnitus. A very similar pattern was found for the Stand-alone, $\chi^2(2) = 7.261$, $p = 0.026$. The model explained 28.7% (Nagelkerke R^2) of the variance and correctly classified 73.3% of cases, with 73.3% sensitivity and 73.3% specificity. Likewise, the model only included loudness as a significant predictor ($p = 0.064$), and not pitch ($p = 0.48$): lower loudness values were associated with greater likelihood of having tinnitus. Running the same analyses taking only the first two instances rather than three yielded basically the same pattern of results.

DISCUSSION

The two methods examined here performed very similarly for participants with tinnitus as well as for participants simulating having tinnitus. Indeed, both methods produced replicable tinnitus spectrum, with similar likeness frequency ratings and very

TABLE 3 | Mean differences and product-to-moment Pearson correlations between two methods instances (three vs. two) for likeness ratings and loudness matching at each frequency for merged Methods.

	Likeness ratings				Loudness matching			
Frequency (kHz)	Mean difference	*p*-Value	*r*	*p*-Value	Mean difference (dB)	*p*-Value	*r*	*p*-Value
0.25	0.02	0.61	0.99	<0.001	−0.37	0.44	0.98	<0.001
0.5	0.05	0.41	0.99	<0.001	−0.30	0.59	0.99	<0.001
0.75	0.06	0.28	0.99	<0.001	0.002	1.0	0.99	<0.001
1	−0.07	0.12	0.99	<0.001	−0.11	0.80	0.99	<0.001
1.5	−0.09	0.45	0.96	<0.001	−0.76	0.47	0.96	<0.001
2	0.07	0.40	0.98	<0.001	1.24	0.06	0.98	<0.001
3	0.04	0.75	0.94	<0.001	−0.67	0.56	0.96	<0.001
4	0.11	0.30	0.96	<0.001	−1.73	0.25	0.94	<0.001
6	0.04	0.74	0.94	<0.001	1.03	0.17	0.98	<0.001
8	0.11	0.24	0.98	<0.001	−0.39	0.71	0.94	<0.001
9	**0.27**	**0.004**	0.98	<0.001	0.76	0.14	0.99	<0.001
10	0.08	0.40	0.98	<0.001	−1.40	0.15	0.96	<0.001
11.2	-0.01	0.97	0.99	<0.001	−0.17	0.77	0.99	<0.001
12.5	0.07	0.46	0.99	<0.001	**−3.42**	0.04	0.88	<0.001
14	0.04	0.56	0.99	<0.001	−0.67	0.10	0.99	<0.001
16	0.05	0.61	0.99	<0.001	−1.18	0.29	0.89	<0.001
Grand mean	0.05		0.98		−0.51		0.96	

Significant mean differences between the two methods are in bold.

few differences in loudness matches. Both methods had highly correlated likeness ratings and loudness matches. Our study confirms that tinnitus spectrum, including frequency and loudness, can be quickly, yet robustly measured in the laboratory as well as in the clinic. Time efficiency is a major issue for clinicians and much research efforts are dedicated to the development of automated tests that are reliable and can be run while recruiting minimal clinician's participation (11–14). Studies have endeavored to reduce test time in almost every domain of audiology including electrophysiology (13), conventional audiometry (12), speech audiometry (15), hearing screening (11), and ototoxicity monitoring (14). Our test fits perfectly in this movement by offering a testing time less than 12 min to get robust tinnitus data. While the participant is performing the task, clinicians' expertise can be used for other purposes, such as writing reports, planning therapy, or consulting colleagues. Considering time efficiency, the Stand-alone device seems to be a better choice than the Touchscreen device for several reasons. First, the Stand-alone device has shown similar testing time independently of the order of presentation, which suggest that this device is so "user-friendly" and so easy to use, that pre-training is not necessary to improve time efficiency. In addition, the implementation of the audiogram of each patient reduces further the testing time and that is not dependent on learning effects such that it can be used confidently to measure therapeutic success or evolution of patients. This new feature might also be of particular interest to clinicians currently using the « conventional » pitch and loudness matching procedure with the audiometer. Indeed, the conventional method requires high skills from clinicians who need to consider, before each sound presentation, the frequency, the presentation level, and the degree of HL while focusing on the feedback provided by the patient during the tinnitus evaluation. These downfalls are potentially avoided with the proposed patient-directed methods. In addition, and despite the small number of participants tested in this study, the test offers good sensitivity and specificity (70% and above), lending itself for medicolegal purposes.

Presenting two pure tones instead of the standard three pure tones yielded essentially the same results. These results suggest that it could be possible to reduce testing time even more by using only two instances instead of three. This would mean that a tinnitus evaluation of pitch and loudness matching could be obtained in about 6–7 min instead of 9–10 min. Since the comparison between three and two instances was made from the same data, however, the current analysis should be taken cautiously: significant differences would mean that the third instance has a value that would be remote from the mean of the two first instances. A within-subject study design comparing two different testing sessions, one using three instances and the other one using two instances is needed before concluding on the validity of reducing the instances of presentation to two. Until further research is carried out, we believe that, for a test under 10 min, the safest solution for now would be to keep three instances.

As reported previously (6), Simulators rated lower frequencies as more similar to their tinnitus than Tinnitus participants, and overall they "matched" their tinnitus about 10 dB louder than the Tinnitus group. When considering the first and second predominant pitches of the tinnitus spectrum, only loudness matches differed between Tinnitus and Simulator participants.

Regarding tinnitus subgroups, both methods again produced comparable results, but given our small sample size, these results are tentative. Tinnitus participants with NH and HL differed mainly on the predominant pitch of their tinnitus, with—unsurprisingly—a lower predominant pitch for tinnitus participants with HL compared to those with NH. Combined with previous studies from other laboratories that have reported similar findings on likeness ratings (15–18), our study strengthens the evidence that tinnitus spectrum is mirroring the HL. Overall, the tinnitus spectrums of both tinnitus subgroups were almost identical with the exception of two very high frequencies: 14 and 16 kHz. Such differences have been noted previously, sometimes as a decline when looking at heterogeneous tinnitus groups with a wide range of HL (10) or as an increase in ratings when looking at tinnitus groups with NH (7). In the present study, hearing thresholds at those high frequencies were too elevated in the HL subgroup to be tested efficiently with either method. Considering that both subgroups (NH or HL) displayed very similar ratings for all frequencies with the exception of those two, it can be presumed that they are probably part of the tinnitus spectrum for the HL group as well, but it was not possible to assess them successfully. These results also suggest that simulators are different in their low-frequency likeness ratings from both tinnitus subgroups, either with or without HL. In addition, our study brings new information about tinnitus subgroups, in that they did not differ from one another in their loudness ratings when expressed in decibel above thresholds (dB SL). Loudness matching, an original asset of our methods compared to previous studies, is particularly important given loudness—not frequency—is the most important predictor of the presence of tinnitus. Therefore, our findings suggest that the effect of recruitment on tinnitus loudness matching did not affect significantly the results obtained by the HL subgroups. Yet, the mean loudness matching for the NH group was slightly higher (~8 dB SL) than for the HL group (~4 dB SL), which could be attributed to loudness recruitment. Most importantly, both loudness measures were lower than the Simulator group (~18 dB SL), yielding again confidence that the methods can be used with tinnitus patients displaying different types of HL. From the current data, if loudness recruitment does have an effect on tinnitus loudness matching, this aspect seems to be clinically irrelevant. Further studies with larger groups should help answering this question.

AUTHOR CONTRIBUTIONS

SH and PF designed the study and analyzed the data. SH wrote the manuscript and both authors finalized and approved the manuscript.

ACKNOWLEDGMENTS

We thank Nathanaël Lécaudé for programming the Touchscreen device and Julie Roy and Anaïs Mihoubi for their help in testing participants. This study was sponsored by MENODYS Inc., which is developing a medical technology related to the research described in this paper. The study was executed by both authors following a contractual agreement with Université de Montréal. Neither author has equity interest in MENODYS.

REFERENCES

Shargorodsky J, Curhan GC, Farwell WR. Prevalence and characteristics of tinnitus among US adults. *Am J Med* (2010) 123(8):711–8. doi:10.1016/j.amjmed.2010.02.015

McCormack A, Edmondson-Jones M, Somerset S, Hall D. A systematic review of the reporting of tinnitus prevalence and severity. *Hear Res* (2016) 337:70–9. doi:10.1016/j.heares.2016.05.009

Henry JA, Zaugg TL, Schechter MA. Clinical guide for audiologic tinnitus management I: assessment. *Am J Audiol* (2005) 14(1):21–48. doi:10.1044/1059-0889(2005/005)

Hall DA, Haider H, Kikidis D, Mielczarek M, Mazurek B, Szczepek AJ, et al. Toward a global consensus on outcome measures for clinical trials in tinnitus: report from the First International Meeting of the COMiT Initiative, November 14, 2014, Amsterdam, The Netherlands. *Trends Hear* (2015) 19. doi:10.1177/2331216515580272

Langguth B, Goodey R, Azevedo A, Bjorne A, Cacace A, Crocetti A, et al. Consensus for tinnitus patient assessment and treatment outcome measurement: Tinnitus Research Initiative meeting, Regensburg, July 2006. *Prog Brain Res* (2007) 166:525–36. doi:10.1016/S0079-6123(07)66050-6

Basile CÉ, Fournier P, Hutchins S, Hébert S. Psychoacoustic assessment to improve tinnitus diagnosis. *PLoS One* (2013) 8(12):e82995. doi:10.1371/journal.pone.0082995

Fournier P, Hébert S. Gap detection deficits in humans with tinnitus as assessed with the acoustic startle paradigm: does tinnitus fill in the gap? *Hear Res* (2013) 295:16–23. doi:10.1016/j.heares.2012.05.011

De Ridder D, Vanneste S, Freeman W. The Bayesian brain: phantom percepts resolve sensory uncertainty. *Neurosci Biobehav Rev* (2014) 44:4–15. doi:10.1016/j.neubiorev.2012.04.001

Vanneste S, De Ridder D. Deafferentation-based pathophysiological differences in phantom sound: tinnitus with and without hearing loss. *Neuroimage* (2016) 129:80–94. doi:10.1016/j.neuroimage.2015.12.002

Degeest S, Corthals P, Vinck B, Keppler H. Prevalence and characteristics of tinnitus after leisure noise exposure in young adults. *Noise Health* (2014) 16(68):26–33. doi:10.4103/1463-1741.127850

Hagerman B. Efficiency of speech audiometry and other tests. *Br J Audiol* (1993) 27(6):423–5. doi:10.3109/03005369309076719

Driscoll C, Kei J, McPherson B. Outcomes of transient evoked otoacoustic emission testing in 6-year-old school children: a comparison with pure tone screening and tympanometry. *Int J Pediatr Otorhinolaryngol* (2001) 57(1):67–76. doi:10.1016/S0165-5876(00)00445-6

Mahomed-Asmail F, Swanepoel de W, Eikelboom RH. Diagnostic hearing assessment in schools: validity and time efficiency of automated audiometry. *J Am Acad Audiol* (2016) 27(1):42–8. doi:10.3766/jaaa.15041

Vander Werff KR. Accuracy and time efficiency of two ASSR analysis methods using clinical test protocols. *J Am Acad Audiol* (2009) 20(7):433–52. doi:10.3766/jaaa.20.7.5

Moffat G, Adjout K, Gallego S, Thai-Van H, Collet L, Noreña AJ. Effects of hearing aid fitting on the perceptual characteristics of tinnitus. *Hear Res* (2009) 254(1–2):82–91. doi:10.1016/j.heares.2009.04.016

Roberts LE, Moffat G, Baumann M, Ward LM, Bosnyak DJ. Residual inhibition functions overlap tinnitus spectra and the region of auditory threshold shift. *J Assoc Res Otolaryngol* (2008) 9(4):417–35. doi:10.1007/s10162-008-0136-9

Norena A, Micheyl C, Chéry-Croze S, Collet L. Psychoacoustic characterization of the tinnitus spectrum: implications for the underlying mechanisms of tinnitus. *Audiol Neurootol* (2002) 7(6):358–69. doi:10.1159/000066156

Heijneman KM, de Kleine E, Wiersinga-Post E, van Dijk P. Can the tinnitus spectrum identify tinnitus subgroups? *Noise Health* (2013) 15(63):101–6. doi:10.4103/1463-1741.110290

4

Assessing Auditory Processing Deficits in Tinnitus and Hearing Impaired Patients with the Auditory Behavior Questionnaire

Isabel Diges[1], *Francisco Simón*[2] *and Pedro Cobo*[2*]

[1] ACURE-Tinnitus and Hyperacusis Clinic, Madrid, Spain,

[2] Institute of Physical and Information Technologies, Consejo Superior de Investigaciones Científicas (CSIC), Madrid, Spain

Correspondence:
Pedro Cobo
pedro.cobo@csic.es

Background and Purpose: Auditory processing disorders (APD), tinnitus and hearing loss (HL) are typical issues reported by patients in audiologic clinics. These auditory impairments can be concomitant or mutually excluding. APD are not necessarily accompanied by significant HL, whereas many adults exhibit peripheral HL and typical cognitive deficits often associated with APD. Since HL, tinnitus and APD affects to several parts of the ascending auditory pathway from the periphery to the auditory cortex, there could be some interrelationship between them. For instance, tinnitus has been reported to degrade the auditory localization capacity. Tinnitus is believed to be triggered by deafferentation of normal peripheral input to the central auditory system. This peripheral deficit can be accompanied by HL or not, since a type of permanent cochlear damage (thus deafferentation) without an elevation of hearing thresholds might persist. Therefore, a combined study of APD, tinnitus and HL on the same cohort of patients can be audiologically relevant and worthy.

Methods: Statistical analysis is applied to a cohort of 305 patients attending an audiology clinic in Madrid (Spain). This group of patients is first categorized in four subgroups, namely, HLTG (with tinnitus and HL), NHLTG (with tinnitus and without HL), HLNTG (with HL but no tinnitus), and NHLNTG (neither tinnitus nor HL). The statistical variables include Age, Average Auditory Threshold (ATT), for assessing HL, Tinnitus Handicap Inventory (THI), for measuring tinnitus, and a new 25-item Auditory Behavior Questionnaire (ABQ), for scoring APD. Factor analysis is applied to arrange these items into 4 subscales. The internal consistency reliability of this ABQ is confirmed by calculating Cronbach's coefficients α. The test-retest reliability is assessed by the intraclass correlation coefficients, *ICC*. Statistical techniques applied to the data set include descriptive analysis of variables and Spearman rank correlations (ρ) between them.

Results: Overall reliability of ABQ is confirmed by an α value of 0.89 and by an *ICC* of 0.91. Regarding the internal consistency reliability, the four subscales prove a fairly good consistency with α coefficients above 0.7. Average values of statistical variables show significantly lower age of patients with tinnitus and no HL, which can provide a cue of noise overexposure of this segment of population. These younger patients show also decreased ABQ and similar THI in comparison with patients in the other subgroups. A strong correlation ($\rho = 0.63$) was found between AAT and Age for the HLNTG subgroup. For the HLTG subgroup, a moderate correlation ($\rho = 0.44$) was found between ABQ and THI.

Conclusion: The utilized questionnaire (ABQ), together with AAT and THI, can help to study comorbid hearing impairments in patients regularly attending an audiological clinic.

Keywords: auditory processing disorder, tinnitus, hearing loss, questionnaires

INTRODUCTION

The auditory system transmits sounds from the environment to the auditory cortex where they are processed to produce a perception. The sound signal, a vibroacoustic wave, is transduced into an electrical train of pulses at the synapses between the hair cells of the Corti organ and the auditory nerve. This interface is a powerful device able to transmit signals from the periphery to the auditory pathway spanning 12 decades in amplitude (120 dB) and 3 decades in frequency (20–20 kHz) (Knipper et al., 2013). This mechano-electrical transduction of sound waves into a train of electrical spikes is completed within 1–4 ms with standard deviation of roughly 0.8 ms, which is even lesser than the corresponding constant time of mammalian visual cells (Kopp-Scheinpflug and Tempel, 2015). Auditory signals are thus reliably transmitted along large diameter axons and across highly specialized synapses through the afferent auditory pathway.

Acoustic signals (coded as electrical spike trains) spread from the auditory nerve to the higher central auditory system through the brainstem, an intricate network of neurons with soma grouped into the ascending auditory nuclei. The auditory brainstem involves many sophisticated auditory processing including frequency analysis, sound localization, temporal integration and discrimination, binaural cues for spatial analysis, multisensorial processing, and others. Processing mechanisms for higher order patterns of sound are carried out in the primary auditory cortex (Griffiths, 2002). Any abnormal deviation of this rather sophisticated sound transduction, coding, and processing system arises auditory impairments, including hearing loss (HL), tinnitus and auditory processing disorders (APD).

Peripheral deficits afford HL or hypoacusis. The prevalence of HL has, due to aging of the population, doubled over the past 30 years (Knipper et al., 2013). HL is usually measured as an elevation of hearing thresholds expressed in dB. However, recent studies have revealed a type of permanent cochlear damage, without an elevation of hearing thresholds (Weisz et al., 2006; Schaette and McAlpine, 2011). This subtle damage should be linked to a permanent and progressive degeneration of auditory fibers that occurs in association with damage of the inner hair cell synapse (Knipper et al., 2013).

Tinnitus is the medical term for the auditory perception of sounds in the absence of any external source. As an auditory phantom perception, it seems to be the correlate of maladaptive attempts of the brain to reorganize due to distorted sensory input (Kleinjung et al., 2009). This notion is confirmed by the finding that HL is the most important risk factor for developing tinnitus and that most people with sudden unilateral deafness experience tinnitus. In general, there is increasing evidence that tinnitus is related to alterations of neuronal functioning in the central auditory system which compensates for diminished input by upregulating its responsiveness in sub-cortical and cortical networks (Eggermont, 2012). This auditory percept presents in a great variety: a rustling, whistling, ringing, murmuring or humming sound (neural sounds) which can come in high or low tones, be loud or soft and be continuous or interrupted. Tinnitus is an uncomfortable symptom affecting severely the quality of life of adults (Holm et al., 2005). This sound sensation may cause many audiological, cognitive and neurological issues ranging from hearing and attention deficits to anxiety, annoyance, irritability, disturbed sleep patterns, and depression (Zeng et al., 2011; Zhang, 2013). Tinnitus as such is not an abnormal sensation. Most people will experience tinnitus after a couple of minutes in a silent anechoic room. Tinnitus that occurs every day for more than 5 min is reported by 10–15% of the population, and for 1–2% it affects their quality of life considerably (Van de Heyning et al., 2007; Hall et al., 2015).

APD refers to difficulties in the auditory mechanisms underlying the following abilities of the auditory system: sound localization and lateralization, auditory discrimination, auditory pattern recognition, temporal aspect of audition, and auditory performance in competing, or with degraded, acoustic signals (ASHA-American Speech-Language-Hearing Association, 2005). Therefore, it is a disorder associated with the impaired capability of the auditory system to process complex sound signals, especially in degraded or noisy scenarios (Griffiths, 2002). It may be associated with difficulties in listening, speech understanding, language development, and learning (Jerger and Musiek, 2000). The prevalence of APD is 2–7% for school-aged children (with a ratio of 2:1 in boys with respect to girls), and 10–20% in the elderly (Skarzynski et al., 2015). APD is not necessarily accompanied by a significant increase in the pure tone hearing thresholds, especially in young people. Furthermore, increased audiometric thresholds cannot fully account for the difficulty that elderly listeners experience in processing speech in noise (George et al., 2007). These concomitant problems make the diagnosis of APD more difficult. In normal hearing patients, APD can be diagnosed using screening tests including competing words, competing sentences, dichotic listening, speech understanding in noise, filtered speech, and phonemic synthesis (Skarzynski et al., 2015; Weihing et al., 2015). More recently, speech-evoked auditory brainstem responses (Kopp-Scheinpflug and Tempel, 2015; Rocha-Muniz et al., 2016) and mismatch negativity (MMN)

(Rocha-Muniz et al., 2015) have been proposed to objectively detect APD.

Since HL, tinnitus and APD are associated with pathologies (or alterations) at different locations on the ascending auditory pathway, it can be hypothesized that these might be interrelated. The main goal of this work is to present a correlational analysis to assess associations between HL, tinnitus and APD in a sample of patients exhibiting these hearing disorders. Furthermore, a new measure for assessing APD, the Auditory Behavior Questionnaire is introduced.

MATERIALS AND METHODS

Participants

The study sample consists of a cohort of 305 patients, 174 men (age = 44 ± 14 years) and 131 women (47 ± 14 years), attending an audiologic clinic in Madrid (Spain) between 2011 and 2014.

Firstly we performed *post-hoc* comparisons in the basis of HL obtaining two groups: NHLG composed of subjects with normal hearing, and HLG formed with subjects with hearing loss. The threshold for being included in these groups was calculated as the average of the tonal audiometric thresholds (AAT) for 0.25, 0.5, 1, 2, 4, and 8 kHz frequency bands (George et al., 2007; Savastano, 2008):

$$AAT = \frac{1}{6}\sum_{n=1}^{6} HL\left(f_n\right) \quad (1)$$

where f_n are the octave band frequencies between 250 Hz and 8 kHz. Individuals with average threshold under (over) 25 dB were included in the NHLG (HLG). According with this criterion, 195 patients were found to fit into the HLG and 110 into the NHLG.

Then, subjects were classified as suffering of tinnitus (182 patients) or not (123 patients). All tinnitus sufferers were asked to fill in the THI questionnaire (Spanish version proposed and validated by Herraiz et al., 2001). From the 182 tinnitus sufferers, 53 belonged to the NHLG and the other 129 were included in the HLG. From the 123 non tinnitus patients, 57 belonged to the NHLG and the other 66 were included in the HLG. The categorizing of patients is summarized in **Table 1**.

Measures

All patients referring hypoacusis, tinnitus, hyperacusis, APD, acoustic distortion, aural pressure, acoustic trauma, or otalgy were selected for this study. All of them were subjected to audiological and ENT explorations. Audiological exploration was carried out into an audiological cabin, using a two-channel clinic audiometer AC40 from Interacoustics, including tonal audiometry, logoaudiometry, discomfort threshold, and distortion products otoacoustic emissions (DPOAEs). ENT exploration consisted of otoscopy, rhinoscopy, and faringoscopy. Besides AAT and THI, all patients were asked to fill in the Auditory Behavior Questionnaire described in the following Section.

TABLE 1 | Categorizing of patients.

Normal Hearing Group (NHLG)		Hearing Loss Group (HLG)	
110		195	
Tinnitus (NHLTG)	Non tinnitus (NHLNTG)	Tinnitus (HLTG)	Non tinnitus (HLNTG)
53	57	129	66

The Auditory Behavior Questionnaire

A large number of validated questionnaires have been proposed for quantifying tinnitus distress, disability or handicap. The patient responses to these questionnaires are summed resulting in a final score, which is then used to rate their tinnitus severity. A percentage of tinnitus patients also report listening difficulties typically related with the auditory processing disorder. Although, some of these questionnaires include auditory perceptual difficulties (e.g., the Tinnitus Functional Index, Meikle et al., 2012; Henry et al., 2016) as one of the assessed subscales, none of them was designed to deal with the auditory processing issues undergone by tinnitus patients. In this work a new 25-item questionnaire, the Auditory Behavior Questionnaire (ABQ), is used to assess the auditory processing difficulties associated to hearing impaired subjects. This questionnaire can be useful to complement current measures of auditory processing deficits, like speech-in-noise tests, in tinnitus sufferers (Gilles et al., 2016).

In a first stage, the questionnaire was based on 114 items, including questions about the auditory functions that could be altered as a consequence of the APD. A pre-test pilot study helped to choose the correct extension of the questions, the resistance or rejection degree to some of them and the time needed for completion. This pilot study was led by a consulting panel, consisting of three ENT specialists with substantial experience with hearing impaired patients, one audiologist with direct experience with APD, and one psychologist expert in development of questionnaires.

In a second stage, the 114 initial items were reduced to 25 final items. The main criteria for choosing the 25 final items from these initial 114 were the descriptive analysis and the repetition frequency of each one. The opinion of patients was also taken into account, asking them to rank the items with which they felt more identified. The final 25 items were those that got a greater punctuation from patients. All items were related with the altered processing functions reported by the ASHA-American Speech-Language-Hearing Association (2005), as well as with the alteration of cognitive functions as attention, memory and auditory comprehension. Furthermore, a 25-item questionnaire should facilitate the inter-comparison with a well-established 25-item questionnaire for tinnitus, the THI. The original version in Spanish of the ABQ questionnaire is shown in Figure S1. For understanding purposes to non-Spanish readers, an English adaptation of the items (non-tested and non-validated) is provided in Figure S2. Factor analysis was applied for reliably grouping these items into 4 subscales.

Scoring of the ABQ

Likewise as with THI, each patient response of the ABQ is rated as 0 (no), 2 (sometimes), or 4 (yes). Therefore, the total score of the ABQ, the sum of the individual responses, ranges between 0 and 100. Auditory processing handicap is then rated as slight (ABQ≤28), moderate (29≤ABQ≤58) or severe (ABQ≥59).

Statistical Analyses

Firstly, a factor analysis is applied for categorizing the 25 items into 4 subscales. Then, the internal consistency of each subscale and the full questionnaire is assessed by the Cronbach's alpha coefficient (α). α values greater than 0.7 are considered to provide acceptable internal consistency (Müller et al., 2016). Test-retest allowed checking the reliability of the questionnaire over the time by the intraclass correlation coefficient, *ICC*.

Age, ABQ score, AAT score (as calculated by Equation 1), and THI score (Spanish version) will be the statistical variables for this analysis. A descriptive analysis will be carried out for each of the subgroups defined in **Table 1**.

Finally, Spearman rank correlation analysis will be applied to paired variables for each subgroup. Spearman rank correlation will be used to identify and test the strength of relationships between these variables. Positive Spearman correlation coefficients (ρ) between x and y variables denote that both variables increase monotonically, and vice-versa, a negative correlation coefficient indicates that when x increases y decreases monotonically. The correlation between the variables is considered to be very weak for $|\rho| \leq 0.2$, weak for $0.2 < |\rho| \leq 0.4$, moderate for $0.4 < |\rho| \leq 0.6$, strong for $0.6 < |\rho| \leq 0.8$ and very strong for $|\rho| > 0.8$. Omitting algebraic signs, when comparing different questionnaires for the same construct, $\rho \geq 0.4$ denotes that both measure the same construct (convergent validity), whilst $\rho < 0.4$ signifies that both measure different aspects (discriminant validity) (Müller et al., 2016).

Data sets will be analyzed with MATLAB and R, with significance level $p \leq 0.05$.

RESULTS

Factor Analysis

The 25 questions were aimed to identify those aspects of the auditory processing that can produce some kind of disablement related to the auditory processing capabilities, such as the attentional and memory capacity or selective attention, the auditory discrimination capability, the time aspects required for the correct comprehension of the sound message, the comprehension and integration of information, including discrimination and multisensory integration, the ability to structure thoughts and to coordinate auditory process with non-verbal auditory information, and the ability to assess space orientation features. A factor analysis was carried out to identify the underlying subscales.

Table 2 summarizes the correlation values between the ABQ items, arranged in a way that stands out the similarities. It can be seen that there are a subset of items with higher correlation values, thus a pattern can be envisaged that allows discerning three or four significant groups of items. A scree plot, **Figure 1**, shows that there are 5 eigenvalues greater than 1. On the other hand, a parallel analysis suggests 3 as the number of factors to be retained in the analysis. A comparison between models with 3, 4, and 5 factors evidenced that the 5-factor model provided latent factors with only 2 items that, in turn, were closely related to items from other factors. In addition, some parameters (as the Root Mean Square Error of Approximation, RMSEA) proved a poor performance of the 3-factor model. Therefore, the 4-factor model based on principal axis factoring with oblique rotation was selected. This model gave a $\chi^2 = 283.25$, with 206 degrees of freedom, and a RMSEA = 0.061, what seems adequate to our case (Hutchinson and Olmos, 1998).

Table 3 summarizes the loadings of the items as a function of the factors. The 4 subscales resulting from this analysis have then been defined as:

- Auditory Discrimination (AD): consists of 8 items and is expected to assess attention, memory, auditory discrimination, and the time aspects required for the correct comprehension of the sound message.
- Multisensorial Integration (MI): consists of 9 items supposed to evaluate comprehension and integration of information, as well as discrimination and multisensorial integration.
- Concentration Capacity (CC): consists of 5 items expected to pick up the selective attention and difficulties to concentrate in sound environments.
- Understanding Capacity (UC): consists of 3 items that would allow measuring the ability to understand speech in noisy and reverberant environments.

The resulting model is shown in **Figure 2**. The English version of the final questionnaire (originally in Spanish), defined according to this model, is shown in Figure S2. Notice that this English version consists of a translation by the authors and has not been rigorously tested nor validated (Müller et al., 2016). Users interested in using this version should request permission to use to the first author (idiges8@gmail.com).

Reliability

Table 4 summarizes the results of the reliability tests. Third column shows the results for the internal consistency reliability tests that turns out to have an α above 0.75 for all the subscales, except for "Concentration Capacity" ($\alpha = 0.69$) which is yet acceptable.

Fourth column of **Table 4** shows the values of the *ICC* resulting of applying the test-retest to 35 patients. As it can be seen test-retest reliability evidences a good consistency for all the subscales.

Descriptive Analysis of Variables

Some relevant statistical parameters of the variables (Age, ABQ, AAT, and THI) for each subgroup are summarized in **Table 5** and **Figures 3–6**.

A significant difference in age was found between the median of patients with or without HL, with a confidence level of 95%, regardless they suffer from tinnitus or not, **Figure 3**. The median ages of patients in NHLTG and NHLNTG are 11 and 15.5 years lower than HLTG and HLNTG, respectively. Both NHLTG and

TABLE 2 | Correlation values between the questionnaire items ordered to show compact groups of values.

	1	2	7	5	9	6	12	10	11	3	4	14	16	18	19	17	20	21	22	23	8	13	24	15	25
1	–																								
2	0.67	–																							
7	0.25	0.32	–																						
5	0.32	0.46	0.34	–																					
9	0.36	0.49	0.35	0.62	–																				
6	0.37	0.47	0.36	0.52	0.48	–																			
12	0.33	0.52	0.36	0.51	0.56	0.61	–																		
10	0.03	0.23	0.26	0.20	0.21	0.18	0.22	–																	
11	0.38	0.54	0.39	0.49	0.43	0.49	0.54	0.26	–																
3	0.34	0.55	0.29	0.41	0.31	0.40	0.39	0.25	0.53	–															
4	0.35	0.59	0.27	0.43	0.38	0.43	0.45	0.31	0.55	0.83	–														
14	0.25	0.42	0.28	0.36	0.38	0.38	0.45	0.24	0.38	0.39	0.40	–													
16	0.18	0.39	0.25	0.39	0.38	0.36	0.45	0.24	0.42	0.46	0.50	0.44	–												
18	0.12	0.19	0.30	0.15	0.23	0.13	0.18	0.14	0.17	0.19	0.12	0.07	0.14	–											
19	0.04	0.11	0.13	0.18	0.12	0.07	0.18	0.08	0.11	0.15	0.15	0.08	0.06	0.38	–										
17	0.05	0.13	0.25	0.04	0.08	0.20	0.24	0.12	0.12	0.17	0.13	0.11	0.09	0.35	0.26	–									
20	0.09	0.18	0.29	0.24	0.17	0.19	0.25	0.11	0.18	0.24	0.19	0.16	0.19	0.28	0.35	0.28	–								
21	0.03	0.09	0.16	0.14	0.13	0.15	0.15	0.10	0.14	0.18	0.19	0.11	0.21	0.33	0.30	0.33	0.40	–							
22	0.06	0.12	0.27	0.17	0.17	0.19	0.26	0.15	0.11	0.14	0.20	0.16	0.15	0.27	0.36	0.32	0.40	0.46	–						
23	0.10	0.07	0.28	0.10	0.15	0.11	0.12	0.21	0.17	0.10	0.06	0.12	0.04	0.34	0.26	0.28	0.21	0.20	0.29	–					
8	0.20	0.25	0.37	0.18	0.18	0.09	0.15	0.23	0.28	0.24	0.19	0.17	0.17	0.31	0.19	0.17	0.15	0.16	0.18	0.39	–				
13	0.20	0.21	0.31	0.17	0.18	0.17	0.20	0.20	0.20	0.17	0.19	0.20	0.17	0.23	0.18	0.25	0.18	0.14	0.21	0.41	0.53	–			
24	0.14	0.24	0.31	0.27	0.23	0.16	0.25	0.20	0.20	0.20	0.20	0.30	0.17	0.19	0.28	0.16	0.35	0.19	0.24	0.31	0.18	0.25	–		
15	0.19	0.18	0.28	0.11	0.16	0.22	0.20	0.11	0.22	0.26	0.24	0.23	0.29	0.32	0.21	0.30	0.32	0.39	0.22	0.24	0.28	0.24	0.22	–	
25	0.07	0.20	0.25	0.13	0.13	0.22	0.15	0.17	0.19	0.24	0.24	0.19	0.24	0.27	0.15	0.19	0.19	0.24	0.20	0.26	0.29	0.17	0.23	0.40	–

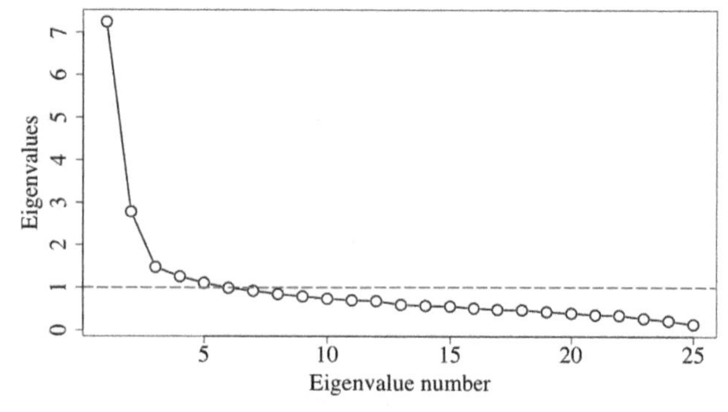

FIGURE 1 | Scree plot of the test correlation matrix.

TABLE 3 | Loadings of the items for the resulting factors.

ID	AD	MI	CC	UC
9	0.86			
12	0.85			
5	0.8			
6	0.75			
2	0.57			0.27
11	0.51			0.24
1	0.46			
14	0.45			
21		0.77		
20		0.65		
22		0.65		
19		0.54		
17		0.48		
18		0.41	0.25	
15		0.41		
24		0.27		
25		0.24	0.23	
8			0.89	
13			0.71	
23			0.59	
7	0.34		0.35	
10			0.23	
4				0.82
3				0.81
16	0.34			0.34

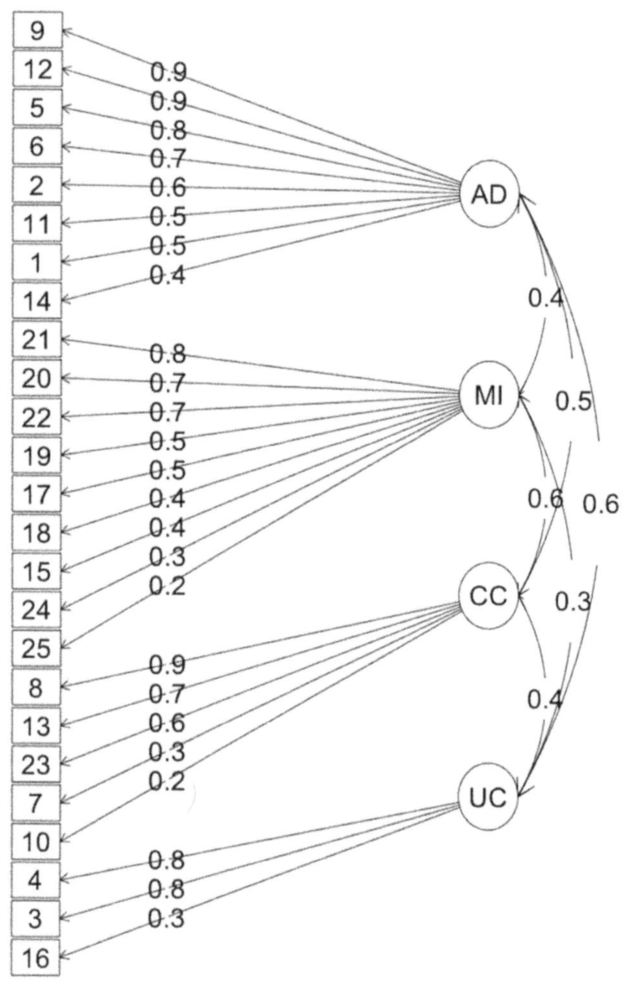

FIGURE 2 | Diagram of the resulting model from the factor analysis.

TABLE 4 | Initial and test-retest Cronbach's alpha for each subscale of the ABQ.

Subscale	No. of Items	$\alpha_{initial}(N = 310)$	$ICC_{test\text{-}retest}(N = 35)$
Overall	25	0.89	0.91
AD	8	0.87	0.77
MI	9	0.78	0.88
CC	5	0.69	0.83
UC	3	0.81	0.75

NHLNTG also have a smaller variability as compared to the HLTG and HLNTG. Thus, in average, patients without HL are younger than patients with HL.

Regarding the ABQ, and considering the median values for all the subgroups, patients exhibit a moderate processing disorder ($29<ABQ\leq58$) in the HLNTG (thus, with HL and without tinnitus), and a slight processing disorder ($ABQ<28$) in the HLTG, NHLTG, and NHLNTG. The skewness of the ABQ for the different subgroups is much greater for the NHLTG than for the rest of the subgroups, so that the relative amount of cases with high ABQ scores for this subgroup is greater than in the other subgroups. Furthermore, AAT distribution is more asymmetric than the rest of variables. Also, AAT and THI values of patients in the different subgroups do not show significant differences, **Figures 5, 6**.

Rank Correlations

Table 6 summarizes the Spearman rank correlation coefficients between paired statistical variables. As it can be seen, AAT

TABLE 5 | Descriptive analysis for the variables of the four subgroups.

	Age				ABQ				AAT		THI	
	HLTG	**HLNTG**	**NHLTG**	**NHLNTG**	**HLTG**	**HLNTG**	**NHLTG**	**NHLNTG**	**HLTG**	**HLNTG**	**HLTG**	**NHLTG**
N	129	66	53	57	129	66	53	57	129	66	129	53
Median	49	52.5	38	37	28	35	14	28	40	40	44	44
SD	12.7	15.6	9.2	11.0	19.6	19.5	13.8	16.7	22.1	22.0	25.4	22.1
Skewness	0.081	−0.23	0.49	0.013	0.44	0.17	1.032	0.451	1.29	1.087	0.11	−0.11

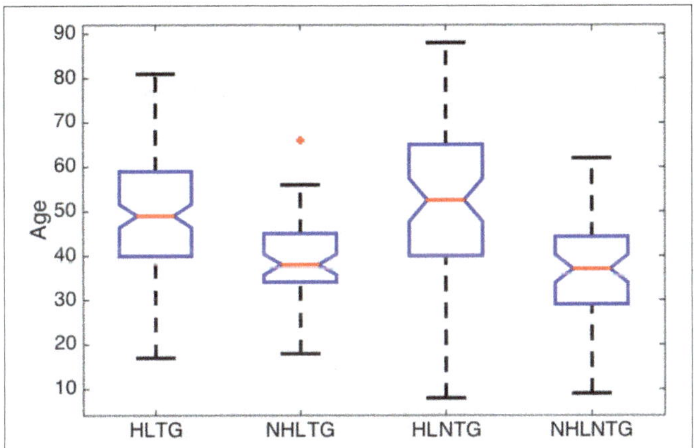

FIGURE 3 | Boxplot of descriptive analysis of age by subgroups.

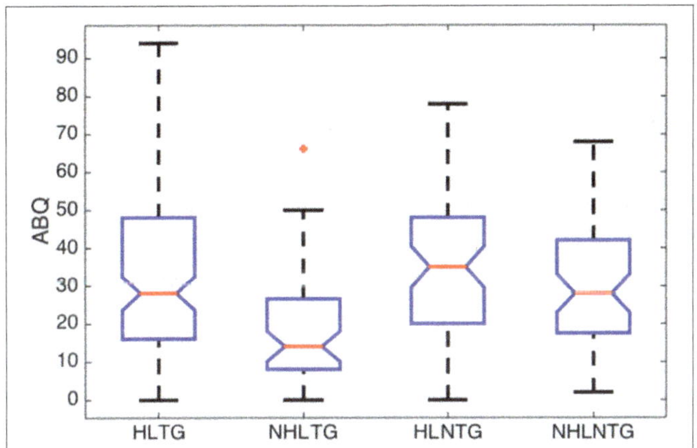

FIGURE 4 | Boxplot of descriptive analysis of ABQ by subgroups.

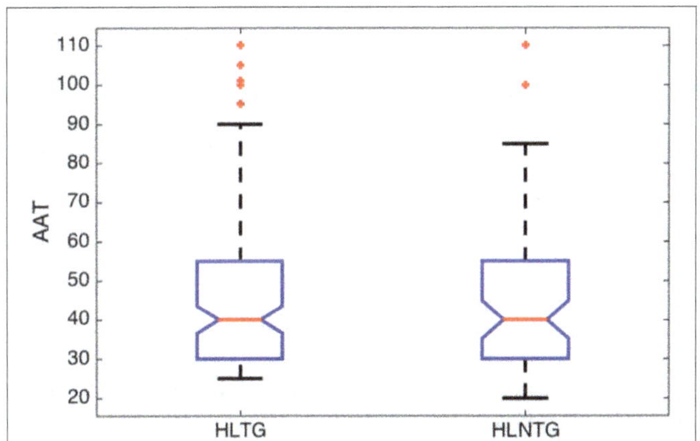

FIGURE 5 | Boxplot of descriptive analysis of AAT by subgroups.

exhibits a strong monotonic increasing relationship with age for patients in the HLNTG subgroup, and a weak relationship in the HLTG subgroup. Thus, HL seems to increase strongly with age for patients without tinnitus, and weakly for patients with tinnitus. ABQ shows a weak monotonically decreasing relationship with age for patients in the NHLTG subgroup. Furthermore, the relationship between ABQ and THI is moderate for the HLTG subgroup, and weak for the NHLTG subgroup. Hence, ABQ increases moderately or weakly with THI in patients without or with HL, respectively. The interrelationship of ABQ with AAT is weak for both HLTG and HLNTG subgroups. All the other paired variables reveal a very weak interrelationship ($|\rho| < 0.2$).

Table 7 shows the expected inter-relationships between the analyzed hearing impairments as well as their variation with age. The usually reported increasing HL with age is confirmed in our results of **Table 6**. Furthermore, the rank correlation coefficient is almost double for patients without tinnitus (HLNTG) in comparison to patients with tinnitus (HLTG). For illustrating better some of these inter-relationships, **Figures 7**, **8** show the scatter plots of AAT vs. Age, for the HLTG and HLNTG subgroups, and ABQ vs. THI, for the HLTG and NHLTG subgroups, respectively.

DISCUSSION

The descriptive analysis of the statistical variables has provided remarkable results. Firstly, it was found that the average age of patients without HL is significantly lower that the corresponding average age of patients with HL, see **Figure 3**. This is consistent with the fact that younger people begins to experience auditory troubles even though HL has not been developed yet. Many authors attribute these troubles to noise overexposure (Emmerich et al., 2002; Gilles et al., 2016). According to Liberman and Liberman (2015), diffuse loss of internal hair cells (IHC), or the auditory nerve fibers they innervate, has to exceed 80–90% before auditory thresholds increase significantly. Secondly, for patients with tinnitus, the average ABQ score is significantly lower (half) without HL than

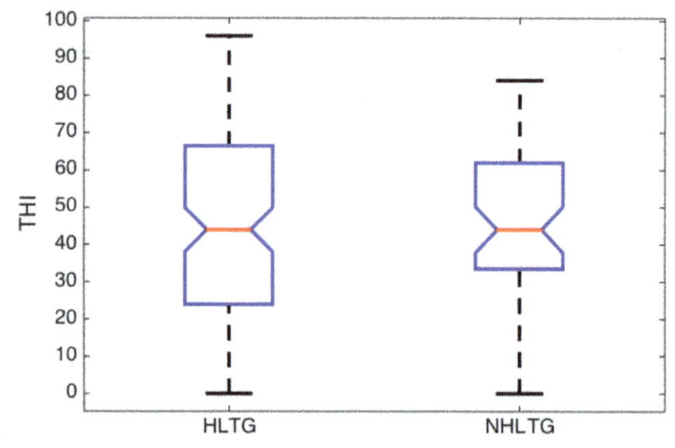

FIGURE 6 | Boxplot of descriptive analysis of THI by subgroups.

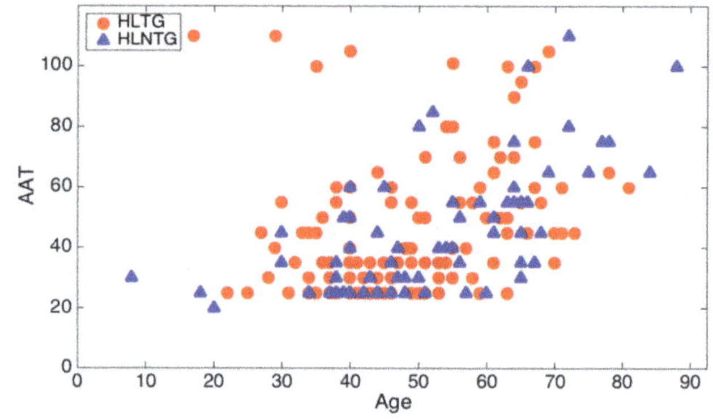

FIGURE 7 | Scatter plot of AAT vs. age for the HLTG and HLNTG subgroups.

TABLE 6 | Spearman rank correlation coefficients between variables for each subgroup.

	Age	ABQ	AAT	THI
ABQ	0.13 (HLTG)			
	0.13 (HLNTG)			
	−0.31 (NHLTG)	1		
	0.06 (NHLNTG)			
AAT	0.34 (HLTG)	0.31 (HLTG)	1	
	0.63 (HLNTG)	0.21 (HLNTG)		
THI	−0.06 (HLTG)	0.44 (HLTG)	−0.02 (HLTG)	1
	−0.17 (NHLTG)	0.34 (NHLTG)		

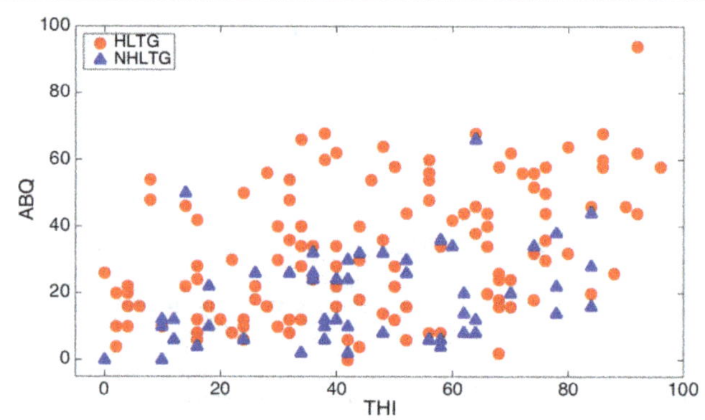

FIGURE 8 | Scatter plot of ABQ vs. THI for the HLTG and NHLTG subgroups.

TABLE 7 | Expected inter-relationship between Age, HL, Tinnitus, and APD.

	Age	APD	HL	Tinnitus
APD	⇑		⇑	⇑
HL	⇑	≈		≈
Tinnitus	⇑	≈	⇑	

with HL (see **Table 5**). In other words, HL seems to weaken the auditory processing capabilities of subjects with tinnitus. Hyvärinen et al. (2016) found that tinnitus may degrade auditory localization ability, although this effect can also be due to the associated levels of HL. And thirdly, we have not found differences between the average THI score in patients with or without HL (see **Figure 6**). In principle, this could contradict the finding that subjective discomfort seems to be higher in tinnitus patients with HL than in those without HL (Ganz Sanchez et al., 2005; Savastano, 2008). Nevertheless, if we take into consideration that, in our patients cohort, the average age of subjects in the NHLTG subgroup is 11 years lower than those in the HLTG subgroup, this result reinforce the idea that tinnitus in young people can be triggered by damage in the IHC-auditory nerve synapses (Liberman and Liberman, 2015).

The prevalence of APD is expected to increase with age (Skarzynski et al., 2015). Our results provided a weak monotonic increasing dependence of ABQ with age for subjects with HL (HLTG and HLNTG), see **Table 6**. For patients with normal hearing, this dependence is decreasing for patients with tinnitus (NHLTG) and practically plane for patients without tinnitus (NHLNTG). Thus, the expected increasing dependence of ABQ with age is not confirmed in patients with normal hearing.

APD is also expected to increase with HL (George et al., 2007). However, our results provided a weak correlation of ABQ with AAT, regardless the patients are suffering of tinnitus or not, see **Table 6**.

The increasing interdependency between APD and tinnitus has been reported by some authors. Newman et al. (1994) investigated the relationship between psychoacoustic judgements, speech understanding ability and self-perceived handicap in tinnitus and hearing impaired subjects. Hyvärinen et al. (2016) reported that tinnitus may degrade auditory localization ability, although this effect is, for the most part, due to the associated levels of HL. Gilles et al. (2016) showed that young people with noise induced tinnitus, but normal hearing thresholds, proved impaired speech-in-noise performance. Jain and Sahoo (2014) found that tinnitus has an effect on certain aspects of auditory processing like temporal resolution, speech perception in noise and frequency discrimination in individuals with normal hearing. Our results confirm a monotonically increasing inter-relationship between ABQ and THI, moderate for patients with concomitant HL (HLTG), and weak for patients with normal hearing (NHLTG).

We have not found significant correlation of THI score with age, which does not contradict the generalized idea that the incidence of tinnitus increases with aging, since THI measures negative reactions of tinnitus, not its prevalence.

Most patients of tinnitus have a related HL, attributable to aging, noise exposure, or chronic otitis media (Holm et al., 2005). Although, HL is an important risk factor for tinnitus, this can occur independently from broad increase of hearing thresholds. Normal hearing thresholds can also be accompanied by impaired function of efferent fibers that project from the brainstem to the cochlea (Schaette and McAlpine, 2011). We have not found a significant correlation factor between THI and AAT, see **Table 6**. Therefore, our results do not support the generalized belief that tinnitus increases with HL. Again, this result reinforces the model of tinnitus triggered by cochlear synaptopathy, which can occur due to noise overexposure (Liberman and Liberman, 2015; Gilles et al., 2016).

The subjective discomfort has been reported to be higher in tinnitus patients with HL than in those without HL (Ganz Sanchez et al., 2005; Savastano, 2008). However, we have found the same average THI in patients with HL (HLTG) and normal hearing (NHLTG), see **Table 5**.

Limitations

Since audiological assessment of subjects was obtained at a single point of time, the study presented here is cross-sectional in itself. Thus, although the results have been interpreted as an estimation of co-occurring hearing impairments in a cohort, they should not be given a prospective significance. The current study, as applied in this work, has been used to analyse comorbidities between hearing impairments, but cannot discriminate between causes and effects. It is also worth mentioning that the above discussed results and interpretations have the known limitations of behavior science studies. Namely, correlational analysis is able to assess the direction and strength of inter-relationships between paired variables but does not provide causal links between them (Stangor, 2011). Thus, the correlational analysis applied in this work has demonstrated that some of the variables are associated, as discussed above, but this relationship could be due to another external variable. Furthermore, although factor analysis results suggest the existence of four latent variables, the need of using oblique rotation, together with the value of the loadings of some of the items, suggests the existence of interactions between them that would require further in-depth studies. It should be considered that the analysis reported here was based on descriptive analysis which has not controlled for the effects of other explanatory and confounding variables such as age, sex, AAT, THI, or type of work experience, and environmental (noise levels) or biological factors. Also, we are currently collecting relevant data, firstly, to carry out statistical diagnostic on ABQ in predicting HL, and secondly, to allow control for other variables in the statistical analysis.

CONCLUSIONS

An inter-relationship study between hearing loss, tinnitus and auditory processing disorder in 305 patients attending an audiological clinic has been carried out in this work. Such audiological disorders have been measured by the average auditory threshold, tinnitus handicap inventory and auditory behavior questionnaire, respectively. The results of this study have confirmed the expected monotonically increasing dependency of auditory behavior questionnaire score and average auditory threshold with age, as well as auditory behavior questionnaire score with average auditory threshold and tinnitus handicap inventory score. However our results, unlike those previously reported by others, show that tinnitus handicap inventory score does not increase with either age or average auditory threshold.

ETHICS STATEMENT

The study presented in this manuscript contains a post-analysis of tests and questionnaires from a dataset that did not require approval from a medical ethical board. All the patients attending an audiological clinic (ACURE) were subjected to standard audiological tests and asked to fill the questionnaires. Thus, the analyses we include in this manuscript resulted from a post-processing of these data, paying special attention to keep all patients de-identified. Anyway, the study would be approved by an ethical committee if it had been submitted.

AUTHOR CONTRIBUTIONS

ID designed the ABQ. FS and PC analyzed the data. PC and FS drafted the initial and final versions of the manuscript.

REFERENCES

ASHA-American Speech-Language-Hearing Association (2005). *(Central) Auditory Processing Disorders.* Technical Report.

Eggermont, J. J. (2012). *The Neuroscience of Tinnitus.* London: Oxford University Press.

Emmerich, E., Richter, F., Hagner, H., Giessler, F., Gehrlein, S., and Dieroff, H.-G. (2002). Effects of discotheque music on audiometric results and central acoustic evoked neuromagnetic responses. *Int. Tinnitus J.* 8, 13–19.

Ganz Sanchez, T., Torres de Madeiros, I. R., Dias levy, C. P., Oiticica Ramalho, J. R., and Ferreira Bento, R. (2005). Tinnitus in normally hearing patients: clinical aspects and repercussions. *Rev. Bras. Otorrinolaringol.* 71, 427–431. doi: 10.1590/S0034-72992005000400005

George, E. L. J., Zekveld, A. A., Kramer, S. E., Goverts, S. T., Festen, J. M., and Houtgast, T. (2007). Auditory and nonauditory factos affecting speech reception in noise by older listeners. *J. Acoust. Soc. Am.* 121, 2362–2375. doi: 10.1121/1.2642072

Gilles, A., Schlee, W., Rabau, S., Wouters, K., Fransen, E., and Van de Heyning, P. (2016). Decreased speech-in-noise understanding in young adults with tinnitus.

Frontiers Neurosci. 10:288. doi: 10.3389/fnins.2016.00288

Griffiths, T. D. (2002). Central auditory processing disorders. *Curr. Opin. Neurol.* 15, 31–33. doi: 10.1097/00019052-200202000-00006

Hall, D. A., Haider, H., Kikidis, D., Mielczarek, M., Mazurek, B., Szczepek, A. J., et al. (2015). Toward a global consensus on outcome measures for clinical trials in tinnitus: report from the First International Meeting of the COMiT Initiative, November 14, 2014, Amsterdam, The Netherlands. *Trends Hear.* 19:2331216515580272. doi: 10.1177/2331216515580272

Henry, J. A., Griest, S., Thielman, E., McMillan, G., Kaelin, C., and Carlson, K. F. (2016). Tinnitus Functional Index: development, validation, outcomes research, and clinical application. *Hear. Res.* 334, 58–64. doi: 10.1016/j.heares.2015.06.004

Herraiz, C., Hernández Calvín, F. J., Plaza, G., et al. (2001). Evaluación de la incapacidad en los pacientes con acufenos. *Acta Otorrinolaringol. Esp.* 52, 142–145. doi: 10.1016/S0001-6519(01)78247-7

Holm, A. F., Staal, M. J., Mooij, J. J. A., and Albers, F. W. J. (2005). Neurostimulation as a new treatment for severe tinnitus: a pilot study. *Otol. Neurotol.* 26, 425–428. doi: 10.1097/01.mao.0000169784.15083.61

Hutchinson, S. R., and Olmos, A. (1998). Behavior of descriptive fit indexes in confirmatory factor analysis using ordered categorical data. *Struct. Equ. Model.* 5, 344–364. doi: 10.1080/10705519809540111

Hyvärinen, P., Mendonça, C., Santala, O., Pulkki, V., and Aarnisalo, A. A. (2016). Auditory localization by subjects with unilateral tinnitus. *J. Acoust. Soc. Am.* 139, 2280–2289. doi: 10.1121/1.4946897

Jain, C., and Sahoo, J. P. (2014). The effect of tinnitus on some psychoacoustical abilities in individuals with normal hearing sensitivity. *Int. Tinnitus J.* 19, 28–35. doi: 10.5935/0946-5448.20140004

Jerger, J., and Musiek, F. (2000). Report of the consensus conference on the diagnosis of Auditory Processing Disorders in school-aged children. *J. Am. Acad. Audiol.* 11, 467–474.

Kleinjung, T., Steffens, T., Struz, J., and Langguth, B. (2009). Curing tinnitus with a Cochlear Implant in a patient with unilateral sudden deafness: a case report. *Cases J.* 2-7462, 1–3. doi: 10.1186/1757-1626-2-7462

Knipper, M., Van Dijk, P., Nunes, I., Rüttiger, L., and Zimmermann, U. (2013). Advances in the neurobiology of hearing disorders: recent developments regarding the basis of tinnitus and hyperacusis. *Progr. Neurobiol.* 111, 17–33. doi: 10.1016/j.pneurobio.2013.08.002

Kopp-Scheinpflug, C., and Tempel, B. L. (2015). Decreased temporal precision of neuronal signalling as a candidate mechanism of auditory processing disorder. *Hear Res.* 330, 213–220. doi: 10.1016/j.heares.2015.06.014

Liberman, L. D., and Liberman, M. C. (2015). Dynamics of cochlear synaptopathy after acoustic overexposure. *J. Assoc. Res. Otolaryn.* 16, 205–219. doi: 10.1007/s10162-015-0510-3

Meikle, M. B., Henry, J. A., Griest, S. E., Stewart, B. J., Abrams, H. B., McArdle, R., et al. (2012). The Tinnitus Functional Index: development of a new clinical measure for chronic, intrusive tinnitus. *Ear Hear.* 32, 153–176. doi: 10.1097/AUD.0b013e31822f67c0

Müller, K., Edvall, N. K., Idrizbegovic, E., Huhn, R., Cima, R., Persson, V., et al. (2016). Validation of online versions of tinnitus questionnaires translated into Swedish. *Front. Aging Neurosci.* 8:272. doi: 10.3389/fnagi.2016.00272

Newman, C. W., Wharton, J. A., Shivapuja, B. G., and Jacobson, G. P. (1994). Relationships among psychoacoustic judgements, speech understanding ability and self-received handicap in tinnitus subjects. *Audiology* 33, 47–60. doi: 10.3109/00206099409072954

Rocha-Muniz, C. N., Befi-Lopes, D. M., and Schochat, E. (2015). Mismatch negativity in children with specific language impairment and auditory processing disorder. *Braz. J. Otorhinolaryngol.* 81, 408–415. doi: 10.1016/j.bjorl.2014.08.022

Rocha-Muniz, C. N., Filippini, R., Neves-Lobo, I. F., Rabelo, C. M., Morais, A. A., Murphy, C. F. B., et al. (2016). Can speech-evoked Auditory Brainstem Response become a useful tool in clinical practice? *CoDAS* 28, 77–80. doi: 10.1590/2317-1782/20162014231

Savastano, M. (2008). Tinnitus with or without hearing loss: are its characteristics different? *Eur. Arch Otorhinolaryngol.* 265, 1295–1300. doi: 10.1007/s00405-008-0630-z

Schaette, R., and McAlpine, D. (2011). Tinnitus with a normal audiogram: physiological evidence for hidden hearing loss and computational model. *J. Neurosci.* 31, 13452–13457. doi: 10.1523/JNEUROSCI.2156-11.2011

Skarzynski, P. H., Wlodarczyk, A. W., Kochanek, K., Pilka, A., Jedrzejczak, W. W., Olszewski, L., et al. (2015). Central auditory processing disorder (CAPD) tests in a school-age hearing screening programme – analysis of 76,429 children. *Ann. Agric. Environ. Med.* 22, 90–95. doi: 10.5604/12321966.1141375

Stangor, C. (2011). *Research Methods for the Behavioral Sciences.* Wadsworth: Cengage Learning.

Van de Heyning, P., Meeus, O., Blaivie, C., Vermeire, K., Boudewyns, A., and De Ridder, D. (2007). Tinnitus: a multidisciplinary clinical approach. *B-ENT*, 3, 3–10.

Weihing, J., Guenette, L., Chermak, G., Brown, M., Ceruti, J., Fitzgerald, K., et al. (2015). Characteristics of pediatric performance of tests battery commonly used in the diagnosis of central auditory processing disorder. *J. Am. Acad. Audiol.* 26, 652–659. doi: 10.3766/jaaa.14108

Weisz, N., Hartmann, T., Dohrmann, K., Schlee, W., and Nore-a, A. (2006). High-frequency tinnitus without hearing loss does not mean absence of deafferentation. *Hear Res.* 222, 108–114. doi: 10.1016/j.heares.2006.09.003

Zeng, F. G., Tang, Q., Dimitrijevic, A., Starr, A., Larki, J., and Blevins, N. H. (2011). Tinnitus suppression by low-rate electric stimulation and its electrophysiological mechanisms. *Hear. Res.* 277, 61–66. doi: 10.1016/j.heares.2011.03.010

Zhang, J. (2013). Auditory cortex stimulation to suppress tinnitus: mechanisms and strategies. *Hear. Res.* 295, 38–57. doi: 10.1016/j.heares.2012.05.007

5

Paired Associative Stimulation of the Temporal Cortex: Effects on the Auditory Steady-State Response

Sarah Engel, Robert Daniel Heinrich Markewitz, Berthold Langguth and Martin Schecklmann*

Department of Psychiatry and Psychotherapy, University of Regensburg, Regensburg, Germany

Correspondence:
Sarah Engel
sarah@engelvita.de

Background: Paired associative stimulation (PAS) is the repeated combination of a sensory stimulus with transcranial magnetic stimulation (TMS) in close temporal association. Recently, a study demonstrated that PAS of an auditory stimulus together with TMS of the temporal cortex is capable of changing the amplitude of auditory evoked potentials (AEP).

Objective: This study examined the influence of tone duration and habituation in temporal cortex PAS as elicited by 40 and 20 Hz amplitude modulated auditory steady-state responses (aSSR).

Methods: Eighteen subjects participated in two experiments, including two PAS protocols each, which consisted of 200 auditory stimuli (4 kHz) paired with temporal cortex TMS with an interstimulus interval (ISI) of 45 ms between tone onset and TMS pulse, delivered at 0.1 Hz. Experiment 1 compared auditory stimuli with different lengths [PAS (23 ms) vs. PAS (400 ms)]. Experiment 2 investigated verum vs. sham PAS. aSSR for the paired tone (4 kHz) and a control tone (1 kHz) were measured pre- and post-interventional—using 40 Hz aSSR in experiment 1 and both 20 and 40 Hz aSSR in experiment 2.

Results: A statistically significant, sham-controlled decrease in amplitude was observed for the 20 Hz aSSR using the 4 kHz PAS carrier frequency in experiment 2.

Conclusion: Frequency-specific effects for the 20 Hz aSSR confirm the feasibility of auditory PAS and highlight the secondary auditory cortex as its target site, introducing new possible treatment protocols for patients suffering from tinnitus. The amplitude decrease can be explained by principles of spike timing-dependent plasticity and the superposition model of aSSR.

Keywords: paired associative stimulation, auditory steady-state response, temporal cortex, tinnitus, spike-timing dependent plasticity

INTRODUCTION

Transcranial magnetic stimulation (TMS) is a non-invasive stimulation technique which uses a coil placed on the scalp to apply magnetic stimulation to possible target areas of the cortex (1). A series of TMS pulses is called repetitive TMS (rTMS), which can induce changes of excitability *via* processes similar to long term potentiation (LTP) and long term depression (LTD) (2). Paired associative stimulation (PAS) is the pairing of external sensory stimuli with TMS pulses applied to the corresponding cortical region of the peripheral stimulus capable of inducing changes in neuroplasticity (3). Based on the concept of spike timing-dependent plasticity (STDP), the effects of PAS depend strongly on the order of the cortical processing of the peripheral stimulus and the TMS pulse. If cortical neurons are stimulated post-synaptically with TMS before they are excited pre-synaptically by the sensory stimulus, synaptic connectivity is reduced *via* LTD-like effects (3). If this order is reversed, LTP-like effects are expected (3). A recent pilot study revealed that the principles of PAS apply not only to the motor cortex (4) and the primary somatosensory cortex (5) but to the human secondary auditory cortex as well (6).

Tones of a specific carrier frequency can have sinusoidally modulated sound levels. These amplitude modulated tones (AM) are used to evoke auditory steady-state responses (aSSR) in the auditory cortex (7). They are recorded in the electroencephalogram as sinusoidal waves of the same frequency as the frequency of the amplitude modulation of the tone (8). So far there is no complete understanding of the mechanism underlying the aSSR. In theory, depending on the modulation frequency different parts of the auditory cortex can be activated and the generated neural responses are thought to correspond with those of transient auditory evoked potentials (AEP) (7). For example, 40-Hz AM aSSR have a modulated sound level with a period of 25 ms. Therefore, the 40-Hz AM aSSR most likely correlates with the Pa-component, a middle latency AEP with a latency of about 25 ms (9–12). There is a lot of evidence that the source of the 40 Hz aSSR is localized in the Heschl's gyrus, which is considered to be the primary auditory cortex (13–15), which is also be presumed to be the origin of the Pa-component (16). Equivalent to the 40 Hz AM tone, a 20-Hz aSSR may reflect the P1-component, a late AEP with a latency of 50 ms generated in the secondary auditory cortex (16).

A pilot study showed that PAS of the auditory cortex is capable to induce timing- and tone-specific inhibitory effects as indicated by amplitude decreases of long-latency AEP (6). PAS (45 ms) showed greater decreases than PAS (10 ms) [PAS protocol with an interstimulus interval (ISI) of 45 ms between tone onset and TMS pulse vs. a PAS protocol with an ISI of 10 ms] (6). Schecklmann et al. assumed that the auditory evoked signal reaches the secondary auditory cortex, which has been stimulated with TMS, after about 50 ms (6). Thus, the more pronounced amplitude reduction after PAS (45 ms) was interpreted as a consequence of the shorter interval between pre- and postsynaptic excitation as compared to PAS (10 ms) (6). The effects seemed also to be frequency specific, as the amplitude decrease was more pronounced for the 4 kHz tone which had been used for the PAS intervention in contrast to a 1 kHz control tone (6). No significant effects on the AEP were observed after 0.1 or 1 Hz rTMS without acoustic stimulation that were used as control conditions (6). In this pilot study, the paired tone had a duration of 400 ms which represents a relatively long duration as PAS of the somatosensory or motor system uses electric stimuli in the range of microseconds (3). Thus, the long duration might have contributed to the inhibitory effect. One further limitation of the pilot study was the lack of a control condition that consisted of auditory stimulation in combination with sham stimulation (6). Therefore, habituation effects induced by numerous repetitions of the presented tones could not be ruled out as a potential confounder, even if the timing-specific effects (same number of presented acoustic stimuli) argued against pure habituation effects as an explanation for the observed amplitude decreases (6). Furthermore, only effects on the secondary auditory cortex were evaluated by assessing late AEP (6).

The aims of the present work were to control for effects of the duration of the paired auditory stimulus and for unspecific effects such as habituation. For this purpose, we conducted two experiments contrasting long- and short PAS tones (experiment 1) and verum (using a defined stimulation intensity) and sham stimulation (experiment 2) for the PAS stimulation. Effects were measured *via* aSSR using 40 Hz amplitude (experiment 1) and both 40 and 20 Hz amplitude modulation (experiment 2). Therefore, effects on the primary (40 Hz AM aSSR) and on the secondary (20 Hz aSSR) auditory cortex can be evaluated.

We hypothesized that PAS of the temporal cortex can induce changes in neuroplasticity. According to the model of STDP the chosen ISI of 45 ms between tone onset and the TMS pulse will lead to an increase in amplitude of the 40 Hz AM aSSR representing the primary auditory cortex and to a decrease in amplitude of the 20 Hz AM aSSR representing the secondary auditory cortex (16).

MATERIALS AND METHODS

Subjects and Recruitment

Eighteen students from the University of Regensburg participated in the study. We recruited all subjects by word of mouth. All volunteers received a monetary compensation and had no relevant neurological or medical disorders. Seventeen subjects completed a multiple choice vocabulary test ("Mehrfach-Wortschatz-Intelligenztest", third edition, MWT-B) (17). Participant 18 was excluded from this test as she was not a German native speaker. Hearing function was assessed by pure tone audiometry testing seven frequencies between 125 Hz and 8 kHz (Midimate 622D, Madsen Electronics, GN Otometry, Denmark). All participants had a hearing threshold below 30 dB HL for all tested frequencies. All subjects gave written informed consent after being informed about contraindications, side effects (3), and study procedure. The study was approved by the Ethics Committee of the University of Regensburg and performed in accordance with the last revision of the Declaration of Helsinki.

General Study Procedure

All participants completed four different sessions of PAS, two within each experiments. We (Sarah Engel and Robert Daniel Heinrich Markewitz) conducted the experiments in a quiet room of the Department of Psychiatry and Psychotherapy of the University of Regensburg at the Bezirksklinikum Regensburg. One of us operated the TMS stimulator, while the other one overviewed the stimulus presenting computer program. Within experiment 1 and 2, we presented the different PAS-conditions in a randomized order 1 week apart with a 6-month interval between experiments 1 and 2. We measured aSSR before and after each PAS-condition (see **Figure 1**).

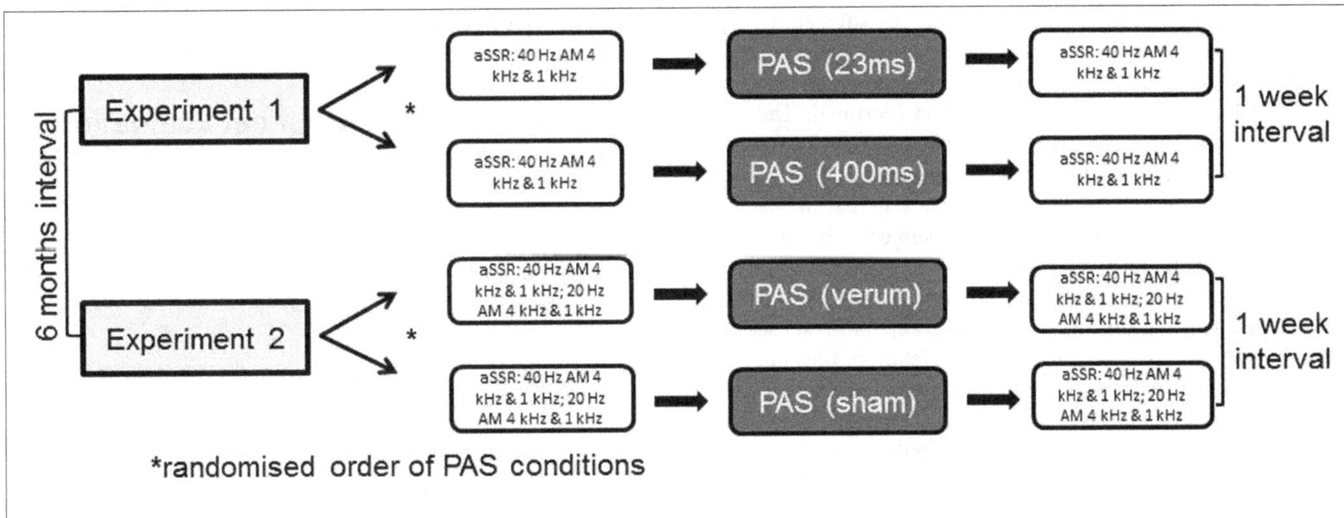

FIGURE 1 | General study procedure.

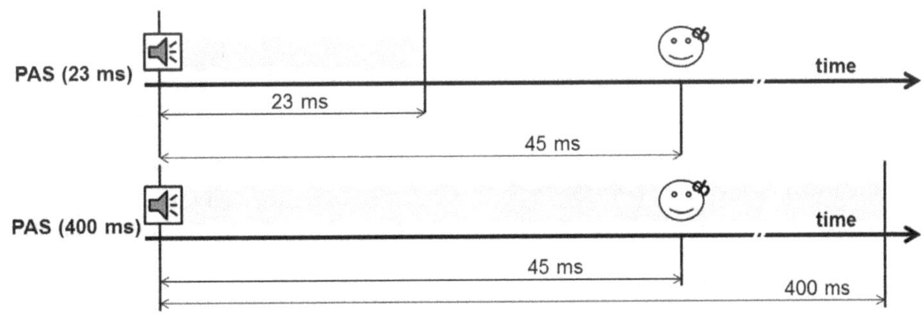

FIGURE 2 | Design experiment 1.

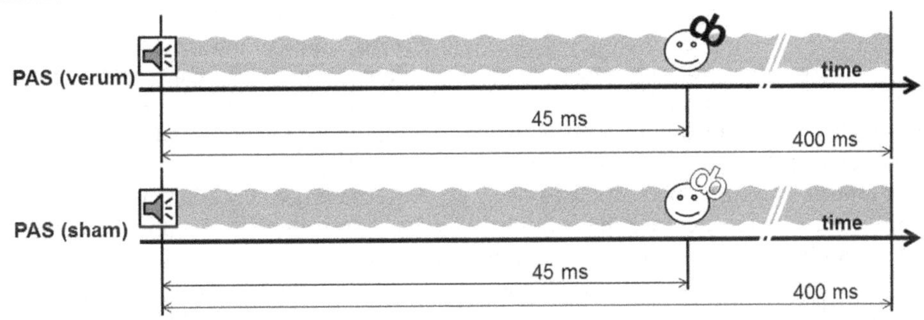

FIGURE 3 | Design experiment 2.

In the first session of each experiment, we determined the stimulation intensity [110% resting motor threshold (RMT)] for each subject following the protocol of Schecklmann and colleagues (6, 18).

For each experiment, we evaluated the sensation levels for the tones used during the experiments using Adobe audition 3.0 (Adobe Systems, DE, USA). We presented all tones binaurally through inserted earphones (E-A-RLINK, Foam Eartips for Insert Earphones, 3M, E-A-R, Etymotic Research, Inc.) at 60 dB sensation level.

PAS Protocols

All PAS protocols lasted around 33 min and consisted of 200 stimulus pairs of an auditory stimulus of 4 kHz and a TMS pulse with an ISI of 45 ms presented with a stimulation frequency of 0.1 Hz. We used an ISI of 45 ms as the pilot study showed the largest effects for this condition (6).

During experiment 1, we performed two different PAS protocols, using a 400-ms tone and a 23-ms tone [PAS (23 ms) vs. PAS (400 ms)] (see **Figures 2** and **3**). The shortest tone length enabling a pure tone percept was 23 ms as evaluated by subjective judgment and fourier analysis as implemented in Adobe Audition.

Experiment 2 included a sham and a verum PAS protocol, using a 400-ms tone [PAS (sham) vs. PAS (verum)]. The PAS (verum) protocol was the same protocol as the PAS (400 ms) protocol used in experiment 1. In the sham condition, the water-cooled figure of eight coil was reverted in a way that the back of the coil was directed to the head of the subject. The magnetic field is decreased to one-sixth on this side of the coil as indicated by own measurements [compare technique in van Doren et al. (19)]. This sham condition guaranteed comparable sensations with respect to the click sound and the vibration of the coil.

We placed the coil over the left auditory cortex following the protocol of the pilot study (6) by using a standard procedure based on EEG coordinates (20). The TMS pulses were presented with a water-cooled figure of eight coil (MAGPRO, Medtronic, USA, outer diameter: 90 mm; water-cooled double coil). The computer software Presentation (Neurobehavioral Systems, Inc., USA) triggered the TMS pulse and presented the auditory stimuli. To ensure the exact timing of the ISI (45 ms), we measured the acoustic stimuli from the insert earplugs with a sound-level meter linked to one channel of the EEG amplifier and the TMS artifact which is induced by stimulation of the electrode cap.

aSSR Recording and Measurement

We recorded aSSR with an EEG cap (Braincap Fast'n Easy 64 Ch for TMS, Standard Layout, Easycap, Germany), reduced impedances below 10 kΩ. We sampled EEG data with a frequency of 500 Hz (BrainAmp MR plus, Germany). We used AM tones of 800 ms duration (rise- and fall time: 75 ms) with a carrier frequency of 4 kHz (paired tone) or 1 kHz (control tone), presented in a randomized order with a variable ISI (2,800–3,200 ms). For recording EEG, we used BrainVision (Brain Products GmbH, Germany).

Experiment 1

In experiment 1, we compared two PAS protocols, one using a 23-ms tone of 4 kHz [PAS (23 ms)] and the other one using a 400 ms tone of 4 kHz [PAS (400 ms)]. As read-out parameter we used 40 Hz AM aSSR, measured as described above, in order to evaluate the effects on the primary auditory cortex. We used two different carrier frequencies: a 4-kHz tone, correlating with the 4 kHz we used during the PAS intervention (paired tone), and a 1-kHz tone (control tone). The aSSR measurments before and after the PAS intervention lasted about 7.5 min each.

Experiment 2

In experiment 2, we compared a verum condition (actual stimulation of the auditory cortex) with a sham condition [PAS (verum) vs. PAS (sham)]. As in experiment 1, we also used a 400-ms tone with a carrier frequency of 4 kHz for the PAS intervention. In order to evaluate the effects on the primary and secondary cortex, we measured 20 and 40 Hz AM aSSR before and after the intervention with two different carrier frequencies, 4 (paired tone) and 1 kHz (control tone). Accordingly, four acoustic stimuli were presented (40 Hz AM aSSR of 4 kHz carrier frequency, 40 Hz AM aSSR of 1 kHz carrier frequency, 20 Hz AM aSSR of a 4 kHz carrier frequency, and 20 Hz AM aSSR of 1 kHz carrier frequency). Measurements of the aSSR lasted about 15 min each.

Data Analysis and Statistical Evaluation

We transferred all recorded EEG data to EEGLAB (21), created epochs of 4.5 s (from 2 s before till 2.5 s after tone onset), and processed the EEG data using a high (0.1 Hz) and a low (90 Hz) pass filter. After visual inspection, we excluded segments containing muscle artifacts, electrodes with signal loss, and segments with strong background noise. Further artifacts were rejected using independent component analysis.

After a subsequent visual inspection for any remaining artifacts, we interpolated the EEG data and re-referenced it to an average reference. The electrode FCz, which was used as a reference electrode during measurements, was reconstructed. EEG channels which were omitted before due to artifacts were then reconstructed using surrounding electrodes for interpolation purposes.

For the analysis of the 20-Hz aSSR, we filtered the data with 18–22 Hz, while a filter of 38–42 Hz was used for analysis of the 40-Hz aSSR.

After manually inspecting all segments of each participant for artifacts, we identified 59 as the minimum number of segments, i.e., the measurement with the smallest number of remaining segments counted 59 segments. Therefore, we used the first 59 trials of each participant and of each condition for further calculations.

Then we transferred the EEG data to FieldTrip (21). We calculated and rectified the mean voltage of all trials. Thereafter, we performed a baseline correction for the interval of 300 ms before the tone onset. We inspected the averaged and rectified trials for plausibility using topographies and trajectories. We decided to use time-locked data (averaging of the single segments) and evoked activity as the principle of STDP is related to an exact and constant timing of two stimuli.

For further statistical analysis and based on plausibility checks, we chose a time of interest of 500–800 ms to avoid interference with long-latency AEP. Our region of interest was in the fronto-parietal area (F1, Fz, F2, FC1, FCz, FC2, C1, Cz, C2). We extracted the data from these electrodes and imported it into SPSS 18.0.0 (SPSS, USA).

We computed 2 × 2 analyses of variance with two within-subjects factors "time" (pre vs. post) and "PAS-condition" (experiment 1: short vs. long tone; experiment 2: sham vs. verum condition), for both tones (1 kHz control tone and 4 kHz paired tone) and both types of AM tones in experiment 2 (20 Hz AM and 40 Hz AM). We used a two tailed paired Student's t-test for *post hoc* analysis for statistically significant interaction effects. We performed corrections for multiple comparisons using Bonferroni correction.

RESULTS

All participants had a mean age of 21.28 years [±2.37 standard deviation (SD)] with an age range from 19 to 28 years. All participants were right handed, 10 were female. The mean hearing level (dB HL) was 13.318 ± 2.572 SD with a range (dB HL) of 8.890–17.78. There was no significant difference between the

RMT for experiment 1 and 2 ($T = -0.414$; $df = 1;17$; $p = 0.684$). Experiment 1 and 2 were completed by all 18 participants without any reports of side effects.

Explanation of Plausibility

For all subjects, we could identify the typical topography of both the 20- and the 40-Hz aSSRs as a positive maximum in the fronto-central region for the sensitive interval of 500–800 ms including the electrodes: F1, Fz, F2, FC1, FCz, FC2, C1, Cz, C2.

Effects of PAS Adjusted for Multiple Comparisons (Bonferroni)

Experiment 1 showed no significant effects for the 1 kHz tone (all *F*-values < 5.375; all *p*-values > 0.066) and no significant effect for the 4 kHz tone (all *F*-values < 2.232; all *p*- values > 0.306).

Looking at the results of experiment 2, we found a significant result for the 20 Hz AM 4 kHz paired tone for the main effect PAS condition ($F = 8.816$; $df = 1;17$; $p = 0.018$) as well as for the interaction "time by PAS condition" ($F = 6.11$; $df = 1;17$; $p = 0.048$) (see **Figure 4**), but not for the time main effect ($F = 0.167$; $df = 1;17$; $p = 1.376$). The *post hoc* paired Student's *t*-test showed a significant decrease in the amplitude from pre to post stimulation for the verum condition ($t = 3.505$; $df = 1;17$; $p = 0.012$) but no significant decrease in amplitude of the verum condition in contrast to the sham condition after the stimulation ($t = 2.120$; $df = 1;17$; $p = 0.196$). For the sham condition there were no differences between the pre- and post-measurement ($t = 0.253$; $df = 1;17$; $p = 1.606$). Before stimulation verum and sham differed not significant ($t = -1.374$; $df = 1;17$; $p = 0.374$). Therefore, a significant decrease of the 20 Hz AM 4 kHz tone—which was paired in the PAS—could be observed for the verum condition with no changes for the sham condition. There were no significant effects for the 40 Hz AM 4 kHz tone (all *F*-values < 1.521, all *p*-values > 0.468). All effects for both 40 and 20 Hz AM tones with the carrier frequency of 1 kHz were not significant (all *F*-values < 2.188; all *p*-values > 0.314).

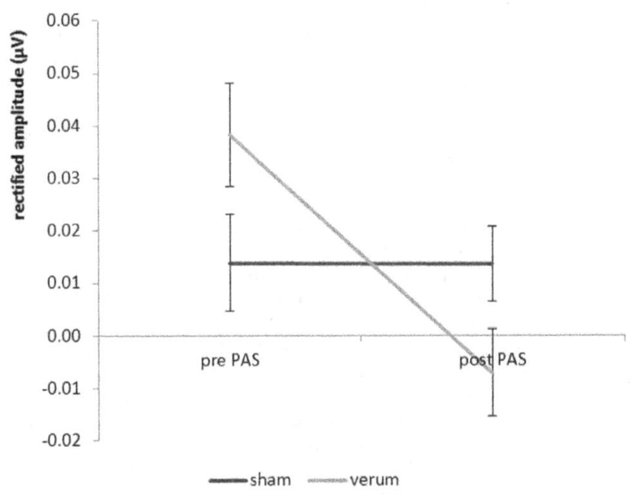

FIGURE 4 | Results for the 20 Hz AM 4 kHz paired tone in experiment 2 (± standard deviation).

DISCUSSION

The main finding of our experiments was a significant interaction effect showing a sham-controlled PAS induced decrease of the 20 Hz aSSR amplitude. This effect was frequency specific as it occurred only for the 4 kHz tone (carrier frequency which was used for pairing in the PAS) but not for the 1 kHz control tone. We could not find any statistically significant results for the 40 Hz aSSR, neither for the 1 kHz nor for the 4 kHz carrier frequency, including experiment 1 (short tone vs. long tone) and 2 (verum vs. sham condition). The significant frequency-specific interaction effect may support the notion that PAS with combined auditory and TMS induces an inhibitory mechanism by inducing STDP. A pure habituation effect can be excluded as auditory stimulation combined with sham TMS (experiment 2) did not induce a significant amplitude reduction of the aSSR. The observed frequency specificity is in line with the results of the pilot study (6), where inhibitory effects were also observed primarily for the frequency of the tone that was paired with TMS in the PAS protocol. The frequency specificity is a further argument for the assumption that combined auditory stimulation and TMS is critical for the observed inhibitory effects.

The reduction of the 20 Hz aSSR after PAS fits well with superposition theory which explains the generation of aSSR (9–12). Based on the theory of STDP (2, 3) the PAS protocol with an ISI of 45 ms should lead to LTD-like effects for external stimuli which arrive in the stimulated cortical area later than 45 ms after auditory stimulation. Under the assumption that the 20 Hz aSSR is generated by superposition of the P1/P50 (which has a latency of 50 ms), effects of a PAS (45 ms) protocol should lead to amplitude decrease which was the case in the present study.

There were no significant effects for the 40 Hz aSSR neither in experiment 1 nor in experiment 2. As shown in the plausibility check, we were able to evoke the 40 Hz aSSR, but the PAS protocols did not induce any changes of the amplitude of the 40 Hz aSSR. 40 Hz aSSR are presumably generated by the primary auditory cortex (12), whereas the 20 Hz aSSR are most likely generated in the secondary cortex (16). Therefore, the significant decrease in amplitude of the 20 Hz aSSR as compared to no significant change in amplitude for the 40 Hz aSSR might be explained by the different anatomical origins of the 20- and the 40-Hz aSSR as described above. While the primary auditory cortex occupies most of the Heschl's gyrus deep in the Sylvian fissure (22), the secondary auditory cortex (22), lies next to the primary auditory cortex on the external surface of the cortex. Due to its superficial location the secondary auditory cortex can be better reached with TMS than the primary auditory cortex. The individual stimulation intensity for the PAS intervention was determined as 110% of the RMT and, therefore, depended on the anatomy of the motor cortex, which lies as part of the precentral gyrus on the outer surface of the cortex as well (22). As such, we assumed that a 10% increase of the RMT will also be able to reach the auditory cortex. However, whether the stimulation intensity is high enough to have a direct effect on the primary auditory cortex is questionable. Since effects on the secondary auditory cortex could be observed, but none on the primary auditory cortex, we can assume that the intensity level of 110% of the RMT, we used during the intervention, may not be high enough to induce direct changes in neuroplasticity in the primary auditory cortex. For further experiments, we should take into account that the intensity of the electromagnetic field is inversely proportional to the distance from the TMS-coil (3).

Notably, we cannot exclude that TMS effects propagate from the secondary to the primary auditory cortex (23). However, such transsynaptically propagated effects on the primary auditory cortex would be too late to induce any STDP like effects in the investigated PAS protocols. Because we did not see any statistically significant results for the 40 Hz aSSRs neither in experiment 1 nor in experiment 2, we cannot draw any conclusions about the influence of different tone lengths of the paired tone. Further experiments using 20 Hz aSSR as read-out parameter will be needed to investigate the relevance of the tone length of the paired tone. Moreover, further experiments investigating the impact of different PAS intervals would be useful to confirm STDP as the underlying mechanism for the observed results.

Further experiments will also be necessary for additional evaluation of tonotopical effects of PAS on aSSR (e.g., using different frequencies as different stimulation conditions for the tones paired with the TMS-pulse during the intervention). Only then can an assessment of the potential of PAS as a tool both for research purposes and treatment of medical conditions be undertaken. For instance, PAS could be applied therapeutically to attenuate tinnitus symptoms. Pathogenesis of tinnitus, a phantom perception of sound (24), is thought to originate from abnormal neural activity (24, 25) and a decrease of functional inhibiting pathways (26). Our study contributes to the findings of the previous study (6) that depending on timing PAS is capable of inhibiting neural activities in the auditory cortex. Therefore, PAS of the auditory cortex could be used to reduce abnormal neural activity and to compensate the missing inhibiting pathways found in patients with tinnitus. If PAS proves to have a strictly tonotopical effect on aSSR it might even offer an individualized therapy option for people with tonal tinnitus, who could be treated with an inhibitory PAS intervention using their individual tinnitus pitch as a paired tone, other than rTMS which has shown moderate effects lasting from weeks to several months (27, 28). The potential therapeutic value of PAS in this context remains speculative.

ETHICS STATEMENT

This study was carried out in accordance with the recommendations of the last revision of the Declaration of Helsinki with written informed consent from all subjects. All subjects gave written informed consent in accordance with the Declaration of Helsinki. The protocol was approved by the Ethics Committee of the University of Regensburg.

AUTHOR CONTRIBUTIONS

All authors conceived and designed the research, as well as interpreted the results of the experiments. SE and RM performed the experiments. SE drafted the manuscript and prepared figures. MS and BL edited and revised the manuscript. All authors approved the final version of the manuscript.

ACKNOWLEDGMENTS

The authors would like to thank all participants and Dr. Larry Roberts for special advice on auditory steady-state responses.

REFERENCES

Hunter DJ. Gene-environment interactions in human diseases. *Nat Rev Genet* (2005) 6:287–98. doi:10.1038/nrg1578

Hallett M. Transcranial magnetic stimulation: a primer. *Neuron* (2007) 55(2):187–99. doi:10.1016/j.neuron.2007.06.026

Pascual-Leone A, Valls-Sole J, Wassermann EM, Hallett M. Responses to rapid-rate transcranial magnetic stimulation of the human motor cortex. *Brain* (1994) 117(Pt 4):847–58. doi:10.1093/brain/117.4.847

Siebner HR, Ziemann U. *Das TMS-Buch: Handbuch der transkraniellen Magnetstimulation.* Heidelberg: Springer Medizin (2007).

Stefan K, Kunesch E, Cohen LG, Benecke R, Classen J. Induction of plasticity in the human motor cortex by paired associative stimulation. *Brain* (2000) 123(Pt 3):572–84. doi:10.1093/brain/123.3.572

Wolters A, Sandbrink F, Schlottmann A, Kunesch E, Stefan K, Cohen LG, et al. A temporally asymmetric Hebbian rule governing plasticity in the human motor cortex. *J Neurophysiol* (2003) 89(5):2339–45. doi:10.1152/jn.00900.2002

Schecklmann M, Volberg G, Frank G, Hadersdorfer J, Steffens T, Weisz N, et al. Paired associative stimulation of the auditory system: a proof-of-princi- ple study. *PLoS One* (2011) 6(11):e27088. doi:10.1371/journal.pone.0027088

Santarelli R, Maurizi M, Conti G, Ottaviani F, Paludetti G, Pettorossi VE. Generation of human auditory steady-state responses (SSRs). II: addition of responses to individual stimuli. *Hear Res* (1995) 83(1–2):9–18. doi:10.1016/0378-5955(94)00185-S

Müller N, Schlee W, Hartmann T, Lorenz I, Weisz N. Top-down modulation of the auditory steady-state response in a task-switch paradigm. *Front Hum Neurosci* (2009) 3:1. doi:10.3389/neuro.09.001.2009

Plourde G, Stapells DR, Picton TW. The human auditory steady-state evoked potentials. *Acta Otolaryngol Suppl* (1991) 491:153–9; discussion 160. doi:10.3109/00016489109136793

Gutschalk A, Mase R, Roth R, Ille N, Rupp A, Hahnel S, et al. Deconvolution of 40 Hz steady-state fields reveals two overlapping source activities of the human auditory cortex. *Clin Neurophysiol* (1999) 110(5):856–68. doi:10.1016/ S1388-2457(99)00019-X

Suzuki T, Kobayashi K, Umegaki Y. Effect of natural sleep on auditory steady state responses in adult subjects with normal hearing. *Audiology* (1994) 33(5):274–9. doi:10.3109/00206099409071887

Presacco A, Bohorquez J, Yavuz E, Ozdamar O. Auditory steady-state responses to 40-Hz click trains: relationship to middle latency, gamma band and beta band responses studied with deconvolution. *Clin Neurophysiol* (2010) 121(9):1540–50. doi:10.1016/j.clinph.2010.03.020

Brugge JF, Nourski KV, Oya H, Reale RA, Kawasaki H, Steinschneider M, et al. Coding of repetitive transients by auditory cortex on Heschl's gyrus. *J Neurophysiol* (2009) 102(4):2358–74. doi:10.1152/jn.91346.2008

Godey B, Schwartz D, de Graaf JB, Chauvel P, Liegeois-Chauvel C. Neuromagnetic source localization of auditory evoked fi lds and intracerebral evoked potentials: a comparison of data in the same patients. *Clin Neurophysiol* (2001) 112(10):1850–9. doi:10.1016/S1388-2457(01)00636-8

Bidet-Caulet A, Fischer C, Besle J, Aguera P, Giard M, Bertrand O. Effects of selective attention on the electrophysiological representation of concurrent sounds in the human auditory cortex. *J Neurosci* (2007) 27(35):9252–61. doi:10.1523/JNEUROSCI.1402-07.2007

Eckert J, Lang N, Maurer K. *Praxis der evozierten Potentiale: SEP, AEP, MEP, VEP; mit 60 Tabellen.* 2nd ed. Darmstadt: Steinkopff (2005).

Lehrl S. *Manual zum MWT-B.* 5th ed. Balingen: Spitta-Verl (2005).

Pridmore S, Fernandes Filho JA, Nahas Z, Liberatos C, George MS. Motor threshold in transcranial magnetic stimulation: a comparison of a neurophysiological method and a visualization of movement method. *J ECT* (1998) 14(1):25–7. doi:10.1097/00124509-199803000-00004

van Doren J, Langguth B, Schecklmann M. Electroencephalographic effects of transcranial random noise stimulation in the auditory cortex. *Brain Stimul* (2014) 7:807–12. doi:10.1016/j.brs.2014.08.007

Langguth B, Zowe M, Landgrebe M, Sand P, Kleinjung T, Binder H, et al. Transcranial magnetic stimulation for the treatment of tinnitus: a new coil positioning method and first results. *Brain Topogr* (2006) 18(4):241–7. doi:10.1007/s10548-006-0002-1

Delorme A, Makeig S. EEGLAB: an open source toolbox for analysis of single-trial EEG dynamics including independent component analysis. *J Neurosci Methods* (2004) 134(1):9–21. doi:10.1016/j.jneumeth.2003.10.009

Benninghoff A, Drenckhahn D. *Taschenbuch Anatomie.* 1st ed. München: Elsevier, Urban & Fischer (2008).

Gueguin M, Le Bouquin-Jeannes R, Faucon G, Chauvel P, Liegeois-Chauvel C. Evidence of functional connectivity between auditory cortical areas revealed by amplitude modulation sound processing. *Cereb Cortex* (2006) 17(2):304–13. doi:10.1093/cercor/bhj148

Møller AR, Langguth B, de Ridder D, Kleinjung T. *Textbook of Tinnitus.* New York, NY: Springer New York (2011).

Norena AJ, Eggermont JJ. Changes in spontaneous neural activity immediately after an acoustic trauma: implications for neural correlates of tinnitus. *Hear Res* (2003) 183(1–2):137–53. doi:10.1016/S0378-5955(03)00225-9

Roberts LE, Moff t G, Baumann M, Ward LM, Bosnyak DJ. Residual inhibition functions overlap tinnitus spectra and the region of auditory threshold shift. *J Assoc Res Otolaryngol* (2008) 9(4):417–35. doi:10.1007/s10162-008-0136-9

Langguth B, de Ridder D. Chapter 36 – Tinnitus: therapeutic use of superficial brain stimulation. In: Lozano AM, Hallett M, editors. *Handbook of Clinical Neurology: Brain Stimulation.* Elsevier (2013). p. 441–67. Available from: http://www.sciencedirect.com/science/article/pii/B978044453497200036X

Langguth B, Schecklmann M, Lehner A, Landgrebe M, Poeppl TB, Kreuzer PM, et al. Neuroimaging and neuromodulation: complementary approaches for identifying the neuronal correlates of tinnitus. *Front Syst Neurosci* (2012) 6:15. doi:10.3389/fnsys.2012.00015

6

A State-of-the-Art Review: Personalization of Tinnitus Sound Therapy

Grant D. Searchfield, Mithila Durai and Tania Linford*

Section of Audiology, Eisdell Moore Centre, The University of Auckland, Auckland, New Zealand

***Correspondence:**
Grant D. Searchfield
g.searchfield@auckland.ac.nz

Background: There are several established, and an increasing number of putative, therapies using sound to treat tinnitus. There appear to be few guidelines for sound therapy selection and application.

Aim: To review current approaches to personalizing sound therapy for tinnitus.

Methods: A "state-of-the-art" review (Grant and Booth, 2009) was undertaken to answer the question: how do current sound-based therapies for tinnitus adjust for tinnitus heterogeneity? Scopus, Google Scholar, Embase and PubMed were searched for the 10-year period 2006–2016. The search strategy used the following key words: "tinnitus" AND "sound" AND "therapy" AND "guidelines" OR "personalized" OR "customized" OR "individual" OR "questionnaire" OR "selection." The results of the review were cataloged and organized into themes.

Results: In total 165 articles were reviewed in full, 83 contained sufficient details to contribute to answering the study question. The key themes identified were hearing compensation, pitched-match therapy, maskability, reaction to sound and psychosocial factors. Although many therapies mentioned customization, few could be classified as being personalized. Several psychoacoustic and questionnaire-based methods for assisting treatment selection were identified.

Conclusions: Assessment methods are available to assist clinicians to personalize sound-therapy and empower patients to be active in therapy decision-making. Most current therapies are modified using only one characteristic of the individual and/or their tinnitus.

Keywords: tinnitus, treatment, therapy, review, person-centered

INTRODUCTION

State-of-the-art reviews are a specific form of review that focus on current issues and new perspectives, often in areas with a need of further research (Grant and Booth, 2009). The last 10 years has seen the emergence of many new tinnitus therapies using sound (Hoare et al., 2013a, 2014b). Although the heterogeneity of tinnitus is widely acknowledged by clinicians, many common sound-based tinnitus treatments are applied with limited assessment of individual differences (Hoare et al., 2014b). The ambiguity underlying tinnitus mechanisms and the rapid development of commercial interests in digital sound technology for tinnitus treatment have resulted in an increase in treatment options but few selection guidelines (Searchfield, 2016). There appears to be little information as to how to choose between treatments and how to apply them based on individual differences. In this state-of-the-art review we focus on how sound-based therapies are modified for individual characteristics and needs.

Research into the benefits of sound as a tinnitus therapy medium has not been systematic (Mckenna and Irwin, 2008; Hobson et al., 2012). There have been concerns as to whether the claims made regarding the effectiveness of sound therapy are correct (Mckenna and Irwin, 2008). We believe that some of the ambiguity surrounding sound therapy arises by applying the title "sound therapy" as a blanket term to the use of (any) sound that may have a positive effect on tinnitus. There are numerous mechanisms by which sounds could interfere with tinnitus (Norena, 2015). Tinnitus may be masked by sound interfering with encoding (e.g., energetic masking, Vernon, 1977) or pattern recognition (e.g., informational masking, Kidd et al., 1998, 2002). Sounds may desynchronize neural ensembles suspected in tinnitus generation (Eggermont and Tass, 2015). Sounds with positive emotional associations can affect mood and arousal (Handscomb, 2006; Tang et al., 2009). Hearing aids may mask tinnitus and have psychosocial benefits by improving communication (Shekhawat et al., 2013b; Searchfield, 2015). Long-term alleviation of tinnitus may occur through habituation (Jastreboff, 2000), inhibition (Teismann et al., 2011), gain reduction (Norena, 2015) or possible elevations in individual signal detection thresholds (Welch and Dawes, 2008). Attention, cognition and context of perception also appear to be important factors that manipulate long-term adaptation to tinnitus (Searchfield et al., 2012; Searchfield, 2014; Andersson et al., 2016).

Across the health sciences the personalized medicine movement has created a shift in focus from a "one size fits all" model to one that tailors diagnosis and treatment to the individual (Tutton, 2012; Schleidgen et al., 2013). At the same time health services are beginning to shift from evidence-based medicine to evidence-informed individualized care (Miles and Loughlin, 2011). Personalized medicine tends to incorporate traditional assessment methods, genotyping and genomic evaluation to explain and predict risk and treatment outcomes (Ginsburg and Willard, 2009). There is a search for biomarkers and endophenotypes in tinnitus (Sand et al., 2007). The current absence of clear genetic and blood-based biomarkers for tinnitus does not preclude personalization of treatments. The view of personalized medicine should be broadened away from just genetic markers (Anon, 2012). Tinnitus has both psychoacoustic (sound) (Tyler, 2000) and psychological (emotion, reaction) markers (Meikle et al., 2012). The context of tinnitus experience is also likely to affect its perception (Andersson et al., 2016) so that tinnitus is the result of psychosocial, psychoacoustic and individual psychological factors (Searchfield, 2014). In addition to modifying treatments based on assessment outcomes there are good arguments for applying principles of person-centered care to tinnitus therapy. In person-centered care patients are encouraged to be active participants in their treatment through the creation of a power-balanced, therapeutic relationship with their health professionals (Michie et al., 2003). Patients who participate in their own care report greater satisfaction, better adherence and health outcomes (Grenness et al., 2014). Research in the treatment of various health conditions such as chronic pain, balance disorders, and diabetes shows that self-efficacy beliefs also play an important role in treatment outcomes and management of the condition (Smith and Fagelson, 2011). Tinnitus self-efficacy is the confidence that individuals have in their capabilities to perform the treatment courses of action needed to manage their tinnitus successfully (Smith and Fagelson, 2011).

Person-centered needs-based care in rehabilitative audiology is not a new concept (Grenness et al., 2014). Most audiologists will be familiar with needs-based assessment for hearing aid selection (Dillon et al., 1987); similar principles could be applied in tinnitus therapy. Such an approach requires clinicians to take into account the needs of individual tinnitus patients, and provide custom-tailored therapeutic approaches. Our purpose in reviewing the literature was to identify the current state-of-the-art in personalizing sound-based therapies.

METHODS

A state-of-art review (Grant and Booth, 2009) was undertaken in December 2016 with cataloging of results in January and February 2017. All studies irrespective of quality were included as long as they addressed the topic and the research occurred in the last 10 years. There were no other inclusion/exclusion criteria. The research question for the current scoping review was: how do current sound-based therapies for tinnitus adjust for tinnitus heterogeneity? Sound-based therapies were defined as those that included the use of sound (either with or without counseling), but not psychological therapies used without sound or based on the scope of practice of psychologists (e.g., Cognitive Behavioral Therapy). From the included studies, all data were charted; themes and key issues were identified.

To identify relevant studies, the search was carried out using the databases Scopus, Google Scholar, Embase and PubMed for the 10-year period 2006–2016. The search strategy used the following key words: "tinnitus" AND "sound" AND "therapy" AND "guidelines" OR "personalized" OR "customized" OR "individual" OR "questionnaire" OR "selection." The search on Google scholar was terminated when two full pages of consecutive results contained no entries of relevance to the study question. After initial consideration of title relevance to the study by one author (GDS), 199 articles were shortlisted. After reading the abstracts, 150 articles were read in full independently by two authors (GDS and MD). The reference lists of these 150 articles were searched for additional pertinent articles. This returned a further 15 articles for which the text was read in full, of those 165 articles for which full text was reviewed 83 studies described personalization (customization, individual adjustment) methods sufficiently to extract meaningful data. Two authors (GDS and MD) achieved a consensus on classification of content with the third author (TL) verifying categorization.

Studies were charted according to the method used to personalize therapy. The application of psychoacoustical and/or psychosocial assessment tools to treatment selection and management was cataloged along with the method used to customize the treatment for individual characteristics. A therapy might employ multiple types of customization and tools, in which case cross-referencing was used. In addition, evidence for person-centered care was recorded (including: getting to know patient or client as a person, sharing of power and responsibility, informed of treatment choice, accessibility and flexibility of service provider, coordination and integration, environment that is conducive to person-centered care).

RESULTS

Five themes were identified from the literature surveyed as categorical answers to the question: "how do current sound-based therapies for tinnitus adjust for tinnitus heterogeneity?" The themes were "hearing compensation" (adjustment to audiometry) "pitch matched" (adjustment using the predominant tinnitus pitch) "maskability" (adjustment to a desired level of masking) "reaction to sound" (selection based on the emotional or relaxing characteristics of sound) and "psychosocial factors" (use of psychological and/or environmental factors to select therapy). The therapy themes, the treatments using the approach, and the assessment used, are cataloged in **Table 1**.

Hearing Compensation

Treatments that modified their response on the basis of hearing sensitivity were hearing aids and sound stimulation compensating for reduced audibility (**Table 1**). Hearing aids were used to correct for loss of audibility of sounds that accompanied hearing loss. When the primary focus of hearing aid fitting was to improve hearing for speech an emphasis was placed on amplifying sound in a frequency specific manner to improve intelligibility (McNeill et al., 2012; Shekhawat et al., 2013b). When tinnitus was the primary focus a secondary goal for amplification was raising the audibility of environmental sounds (Shekhawat et al., 2013a). The basis for modification was the individuals hearing thresholds obtained using pure-tone audiometry. The amount of amplification was determined using a prescription based on the audiogram (Shekhawat et al., 2013a). Hearing aids were considered to reduce hearing handicap, reduce the levels of attention paid to tinnitus, and compensate for deafferentation, and possibly improve cognition (Searchfield, 2006, 2015; Shekhawat et al., 2013b; Sereda et al., 2015; Zarenoe et al., 2017). McNeill et al. (2012) identified those most likely to achieve benefit from hearing aids as having good low frequency hearing and tinnitus pitch within the amplification range of the hearing aids (McNeill et al., 2012). Jalilvand et al. (2015) suggested that hearing aids might be more successful in management of tinnitus from blast injuries than sound generators (Jalilvand et al., 2015). Frequency lowering processing was suggested as an alternative strategy to conventional amplification (Peltier et al., 2012). Several studies suggested sound therapy device selection based on the audiogram (from hearing aids, combination instruments and cochlear implants) (Folmer and Carroll, 2006; Mazurek et al., 2006; Tyler et al., 2015; Searchfield, 2016). Searchfield (2016) recommended normal hearing would be fitted with sound generators; high frequency hearing loss with hearing aids; hearing loss encompassing low frequencies with combination instruments; severe-profound hearing loss with cochlear implants.

Hearing loss will affect the perception of therapeutic sounds in addition to reducing the audibility of speech and environmental sounds. To address this several sound therapies adjusted the spectrum of music (Davis et al., 2007; Wazen et al., 2011; Peltier et al., 2012; Vanneste et al., 2013; Henin et al., 2016; Li et al., 2016), fractal tones (Herzfeld et al., 2014) or noise (Uriz et al., 2013) for the presence of hearing loss. The intent from threshold-adjusted sounds was to make the sound audible across a broad frequency range rather than stimulating the frequencies with best thresholds (Davis, 2006; Távora-Vieira et al., 2011). In some cases too severe a hearing loss was an exclusion factor for therapy (Davis et al., 2007). One study suggested that adjusting music levels for hearing threshold was of no benefit to tinnitus suppression (Vanneste et al., 2013).

Pitch-Based Therapy

Several therapies used the pitch or spectrum of tinnitus as the basis for stimulation. Sound stimuli were individualized to span a frequency range centered on the dominant tinnitus pitch (**Table 1**). The sounds used and intended mechanisms of effect varied greatly: some therapies attempt to change the synchronized firing of neural assemblies near tinnitus pitch using tonal stimulation (Hanley and Davis, 2008; Reavis et al., 2010, 2012; Eggermont and Tass, 2015; Hauptmann et al., 2015, 2016; Hoare et al., 2015; Williams et al., 2015); others changed the phase of sounds presented at tinnitus pitch (Herraiz et al., 2007; Vermeire et al., 2007; Choy et al., 2010; Meeus et al., 2010; Fioretti et al., 2011; Heijneman et al., 2012) and another paired tonal stimulation with vagus nerve stimulation (De Ridder et al., 2015). Tinnitus pitch was used as the basis for selecting band-pass noise (Serquera et al., 2015) notched music (Courtenay et al., 2010; Teismann et al., 2011; Györi, 2016) or noise (Lugli et al., 2009) for lateral inhibition (Courtenay et al., 2010) and one method provided extra stimulation at tinnitus pitch (Mahboubi et al., 2012) while another used tinnitus pitch-matched sound embedded in nature sounds as a therapy (Bessman et al., 2009). Another form of pitch-based therapy employed participants undertaking active training tasks in discrimination (Herraiz et al., 2007; Roberts and Bosnyak, 2011; Hoare et al., 2013b, 2014b; Wise et al., 2016) or categorization tasks (Jepsen et al., 2010). The intended mechanism of effect for these training tasks is reorganization of tonotopic maps, but their main effect may be in modifying attention to tinnitus (Hoare et al., 2010). Several studies used more complex replicas (avatars) of tinnitus for passive stimulation (Viirre, 2010) and stimulation only while asleep (Pedemonte et al., 2010). Auditory training in a game format used the individual's tinnitus avatar as a distractor (Wise et al., 2016).

The variability in tinnitus pitch matching is a critical concern issue for pitch-based treatments (Hoare et al., 2014a; Serquera et al., 2015). Variability in pitch match that is more than one octave between consecutive sessions may preclude some therapies (Hoare et al., 2014a). Pitch matching is

TABLE 1 | Therapy themes and references.

Therapy theme	Treatments	Assessment
Hearing compensation	**Hearing aids** Folmer and Carroll, 2006; Searchfield et al., 2010; McNeill et al., 2012; Peltier et al., 2012; Oz et al., 2013; Shekhawat et al., 2013b; Jalilvand et al., 2015; Searchfield, 2015; Sereda et al., 2016 **Threshold adjusted sound** Davis, 2006; Davis et al., 2007; Wazen et al., 2011; Peltier et al., 2012; Vanneste et al., 2013; Parra, 2015; Henin et al., 2016; Li et al., 2016 **Cochlear implant** Tyler et al., 2015	**Pure Tone Audiogram** Davis, 2006; Folmer and Carroll, 2006; Davis et al., 2007; Searchfield et al., 2010; Wazen et al., 2011; McNeill et al., 2012; Peltier et al., 2012; Oz et al., 2013; Shekhawat et al., 2013b; Vanneste et al., 2013; Jalilvand et al., 2015; Parra, 2015; Searchfield, 2015; Tyler et al., 2015; Henin et al., 2016; Li et al., 2016; Sereda et al., 2016
Pitched-matched	**Notched sound** Lugli et al., 2009; Courtenay et al., 2010; Teismann et al., 2011; Györi, 2016 **Band-pass noise** Serquera et al., 2015 **Tonal stimulation** Hanley and Davis, 2008; Reavis et al., 2010, 2012; De Ridder et al., 2015; Eggermont and Tass, 2015; Hauptmann et al., 2015, 2016; Hoare et al., 2015; Williams et al., 2015 **Auditory training** Herraiz et al., 2007; Hoare et al., 2010, 2014b; Jepsen et al., 2010; Roberts and Bosnyak, 2011; Spiegel et al., 2015; Wise et al., 2015, 2016 **Phase shifting** Herraiz et al., 2007; Vermeire et al., 2007; Choy et al., 2010; Meeus et al., 2010; Fioretti et al., 2011; Heijneman et al., 2012 **Hearing aids** Schaette et al., 2010; McNeill et al., 2012; Searchfield, 2016 **Replica tinnitus** Viirre, 2010; Drexler et al., 2016 **Emphasis tinnitus pitch** Bessman et al., 2009; Mahboubi et al., 2012	**Pitch matching** Herraiz et al., 2007; Vermeire et al., 2007; Hanley and Davis, 2008; Bessman et al., 2009; Lugli et al., 2009; Choy et al., 2010; Courtenay et al., 2010; Meeus et al., 2010; Reavis et al., 2010, 2012; Schaette et al., 2010; Fioretti et al., 2011; Roberts and Bosnyak, 2011; Teismann et al., 2011; Heijneman et al., 2012; Mahboubi et al., 2012; McNeill et al., 2012; Hoare et al., 2014a, 2015; Hutter et al., 2014; Eggermont and Tass, 2015; Hauptmann et al., 2015, 2016; Serquera et al., 2015; Spiegel et al., 2015; Williams et al., 2015; Györi, 2016 **Tinnitus Avatar** Viirre, 2010; Spiegel et al., 2015; Wise et al., 2015, 2016; Drexler et al., 2016
Maskability	**Partial masking** Tyler et al., 2007, 2012; Suzuki et al., 2016 **Mixing point masking** Henry et al., 2006; Huang et al., 2006; Jastreboff and Jastreboff, 2006; Jastreboff, 2007, 2011, 2015; Kim et al., 2014; Ostermann et al., 2016 **Hearing aids** McNeill et al., 2012; Searchfield, 2016 **Spatial** Oishi et al., 2013; Searchfield et al., 2016	**Patient report** Jastreboff and Jastreboff, 2006; Jastreboff, 2007, 2011, 2015; Tyler et al., 2007, 2012; McNeill et al., 2012; Oishi et al., 2013; Kim et al., 2014; Ostermann et al., 2016; Searchfield, 2016; Suzuki et al., 2016 **Calculation** Huang et al., 2006 **Localization** Searchfield et al., 2016
Reaction to sound	**Nature sounds / sound type** Handscomb, 2006; Ito et al., 2009; Piskosz, 2012; Herzfeld et al., 2014; Durai et al., 2015; Henry et al., 2015; Barozzi et al., 2016 **Music** Hann et al., 2008 Hann et al., 2008 **Notched music** Lugli et al., 2009; Courtenay et al., 2010; Teismann et al., 2011; Györi, 2016 **Filtered music** Davis, 2006; Davis et al., 2007; Hutter et al., 2014; Li et al., 2016 **Discomfort to sound** Bartnik and Skarzynski, 2006; Jastreboff and Jastreboff, 2006; Jastreboff, 2007, 2011, 2015; Durai et al., 2015	**Patient report** Davis, 2006; Handscomb, 2006; Davis et al., 2007; Hann et al., 2008; Ito et al., 2009; Lugli et al., 2009; Courtenay et al., 2010; Teismann et al., 2011; Piskosz, 2012; Herzfeld et al., 2014; Hutter et al., 2014; Durai et al., 2015; Henry et al., 2015; Barozzi et al., 2016; Györi, 2016; Li et al., 2016 **Categorization of report** Bartnik and Skarzynski, 2006; Jastreboff and Jastreboff, 2006; Jastreboff, 2007, 2011, 2015
Psychosocial factors	**Hearing aids** Searchfield, 2006; Hoare et al., 2012; Sereda et al., 2015	**COSIT** Searchfield, 2006, 2015

(Continued)

TABLE 1 | Continued

Therapy theme	Treatments	Assessment
	Partial masking Tyler et al., 2007; Anwar, 2013; Sereda et al., 2016 **Adaptation** Durai et al., 2015 **Mixing point masking** Mazurek et al., 2006; Herraiz et al., 2007; Ariizumi et al., 2010 **Selection** Tyler et al., 2006; Newman, 2008 #19; Newman et al., 2008; Tyler, 2012	**STOP** Newman et al., 2008 **TAQ** Tyler et al., 2006, 2007 **Demographics and clinical history** Mazurek et al., 2006; Herraiz et al., 2007; Hoare et al., 2012; Tyler, 2012; Sereda et al., 2015 **Motivation** Ariizumi et al., 2010 Ariizumi et al., 2010 **Personality** Tyler et al., 2006; Durai et al., 2015

The references were categorized to the major theme of the research or review. There were occasions where references were cross-referenced to different themes or treatment categories. Assessment was broadly classified into categories; there was variation between studies in how specific features were measured (e.g., different forms of pitch matching). TAQ, Tinnitus Activities Questionnaire; STOP, Sound Therapy Option Profile; COSIT, Client Oriented Scale of Improvement in Tinnitus.

not considered very useful in methods based on counseling and broad noise therapy (Baguley et al., 2013). However, tinnitus pitch within the effective range of sound therapy device may be a prognostic factor for treatment success (Schaette et al., 2010; McNeill et al., 2012; Searchfield, 2016). Momentary analysis may have a role in guiding treatments in which the feature measured (e.g., pitch) guides treatment sound selection. Incorporating such assessments into daily routine in a non-threatening manner or even game (Wise et al., 2016) may mitigate the potential negative effects of momentary analysis in priming individuals to focus on their tinnitus.

Maskability

We used a psychoacoustic definition of masking: when the perception of tinnitus is affected by the presence of another sound. The level of sound used in theory has been one of the more contentious issues in audiology-based tinnitus therapy (Jastreboff, 2007; Tyler et al., 2012). Masking can be used to totally or partially reduce the audibility of tinnitus by covering it with another sound. Tinnitus Retraining Therapy (TRT) advocates a masking level in which the sound mixes with, but does not cover, the tinnitus (Henry et al., 2006; Huang et al., 2006; Jastreboff and Jastreboff, 2006; Jastreboff, 2007, 2011, 2015; Kim et al., 2014; Ostermann et al., 2016) while others suggest use of the minimum level resulting in relief (Tyler et al., 2007, 2012; Suzuki et al., 2016). Most therapies set their target level based on patients' reports of tinnitus audibility and sound being comfortable, although Huang et al. (2006) reported that the mixing level could be predicted on the basis of the MML (Huang et al., 2006). Kim et al. (2014) reported TRT with broadband noise to have a higher success rate than mixed or narrowband noise (Kim et al., 2014). TRT and masking is typically practiced using sound presentation to both ears; Oishi et al. suggested that monaural presentation can be successful (Oishi et al., 2013) and Searchfield et al. (2016) showed the potential for binaural sound presentation using interaural cues and Head Related Transfer Function to achieve spatial as well as spectral masking.

Reaction to Sound

In order for sound therapy to be effective it must be comfortable to the user. Under this theme we cataloged therapies that considered individual's sensitivity to, or, reaction to sounds. A key factor in allocating participants to the treatment categories used in TRT was known discomfort to sound (Jastreboff and Jastreboff, 2006; Jastreboff, 2007, 2011, 2015). Personality may be a predictive factor in determining if a participant is sound responsive or sound sensitive (Durai et al., 2015). A positive individual response to therapeutic sounds will increase the individual's ability to achieve treatment goals as well as compliance to treatment. The strong emotional response to music has seen its use as a therapeutic tool (Hann et al., 2008). Music has been adopted as the sound manipulated in the Neuromonics Tinnitus Treatment (Davis et al., 2007; Li et al., 2016) and notched music therapies (Lugli et al., 2009; Courtenay et al., 2010; Teismann et al., 2011; Györi, 2016). Fractal tones also have music-like relaxation properties (Herzfeld et al., 2014). Advances in hearing aid technology allow relaxing music or nature sounds to be directly streamed from a patient's smart phone to their hearing aids (Piskosz, 2012). Studies to date suggest that modulated sounds (Henry et al., 2015) or nature sounds (Barozzi et al., 2016) achieve tinnitus benefits similar to broadband noise stimulation.

Psychosocial

We defined psychosocial factors in sound therapy as social moderators and individual thoughts and behaviors that determine the treatment approach. In an evaluation of tinnitus management in NHS audiology departments in the UK by Hoare et al. (2012) identified a wide range of factors that influenced clinicians management strategies (in order of high-low reporting): level of hearing loss, evidence of stress or anxiety, state of mind, severity, willingness to try treatment, sleep disturbance, health, understanding, lifestyle preferences, coping ability, hyperacusis, age, and depression. Although these results were not described in terms of sound-therapy specific decision-making, three of the top four treatments reported were sound-based or could use sound (hearing aids, sound generator,

TABLE 2 | Examples of tinnitus assessments that can be chosen to help guide sound therapy selection.

Assessment tool	Suggested use
TFI (Meikle et al., 2012) TPFQ (Tyler et al., 2014)	Intake and outcome questionnaires developed to be sensitive to treatment effects. Determine effect of tinnitus on individual and areas of life most affected by tinnitus. Assist in priority setting
Audiometry (Sereda et al., 2011)	Identify degree of hearing loss accompanying tinnitus, as basis for modifying audibility of sound therapy
HHI (A or E) (Zarenoe et al., 2017)	Assists in determining if hearing aids should be trialed based on effect of hearing
Psychoacoustic matching (Henry et al., 2013; Hoare et al., 2014a)	Identify tinnitus characteristics on which to base sound stimulation. Essential for pitch-based therapies, helpful in predicting hearing aid success
HADS (Zigmond and Snaith, 1983)	Measure of anxiety and depression, assists in identifying need for referral and focus of therapy (e.g., CBT vs. sound therapies)
MPQ (Tellegen, 1982; Durai and Searchfield, 2016)	Personality typing helps identify sound sensitive patients and tendency for chronic tinnitus
NIH Cognitive Toolbox (Heaton et al., 2014)	Assess cognition (attention, memory) have influence therapy selection and settings (e.g., sow processing for hearing aids)
TAQ (Tyler et al., 2006, 2007)	Identify activities requiring therapy focus
STOP (Newman et al., 2008)	Assists selection of sound therapy types
SETMQ (Smith and Fagelson, 2011)	Identify areas where patients are struggling to manage tinnitus
COSIT (Searchfield, 2006)	Identify and prioritize individuals needs and goals

TFI, Tinnitus Functional index; TPFQ, Tinnitus Primary Function Questionnaire; HHI (A or E), Hearing Handicap Inventory (Adults or Elderly); HADS, Hearing Anxiety and Depression Scale; MPQ, Multidimensional Personality Questionnaire; TAQ, Tinnitus Activities Questionnaire; STOP, Sound Therapy Option Profile; SETMQ, Self-Efficacy for Tinnitus Management Questionnaire; COSIT, Client Oriented Scale of Improvement in Tinnitus.

habituation). In a similar population psychosocial factors were used in selecting hearing aids for tinnitus and mild hearing loss (Sereda et al., 2015). Skepticism, length of treatment and attitude can influence treatment success (Herraiz et al., 2007). Willingness to pay may affect client decision-making (Tyler, 2012). Older patients and tinnitus of longer duration may benefit less from sound therapies (Mazurek et al., 2006; Anwar, 2013). Questionnaires have been used in several person-centered tinnitus therapies to guide treatment (**Table 2**). In Tinnitus Activities Treatment (TAT), the Iowa Tinnitus Activities Questionnaire is recommended to identify patient's needs and treatment priorities (Tyler et al., 2007). Searchfield (2006) advocated the use of a tinnitus version of the Client Orientated Scale of Improvement (COSIT) to identify and set goals for treatment. Newman et al. (2008) used the Sound Therapy Option Profile (STOP) to assist in therapy selection and understanding patient attitudes to different treatments and the Self-Efficacy for Tinnitus Management Questionnaire (SETMQ) can be used to assess patient confidence in using different treatments (Smith and Fagelson, 2011; Fagelson and Smith, 2016).

DISCUSSION

Tinnitus is a heterogeneous disorder: tinnitus sound can differ between individuals, it can result from many different types of injury and its effect can vary from a minor annoyance to catastrophic impact on daily life (Stouffer and Tyler, 1990).

The review of the literature identified five sound therapy themes. Some treatments were included across themes. The majority of studies considered tailored or customized therapy to be selection of treatment sound on the basis of either audiometric threshold or tinnitus pitch. There were approaches that used dimensions of tinnitus severity, sound sensitivity and hearing to categorize or subtype groups of sufferers (Jastreboff, 2011). Another approach was a hierarchy or stepped care model in which individually tailored treatments were used if less resource intensive methods were unsuccessful (Myers et al., 2014). Stepped care has been implemented in environments where universal individually focused therapy would be economically unsustainable (Department of Health, 2009; Myers et al., 2014). Unlike single characteristic therapies whole-person approaches involved patients in decision making as to which of several approaches are best suited to them (Tyler et al., 2007; Newman et al., 2008). We believe that a contributing factor to the inconsistent benefit reported with sound therapies (Mckenna and Irwin, 2008; Hobson et al., 2012) is application of a single title "sound therapy" to a very heterogeneous collection of different sound-based approaches. In addition individual needs and reaction to therapy sounds differ (Durai and Searchfield, 2017) we ascribe to the philosophy that individuals are most likely to manage their tinnitus better when the treatment plan is tailored to their needs (Fisher and Boswell, 2016).

Planning Individual Tinnitus Care

The review did not identify any comprehensive guidelines for optimal sound therapy selection. We believe that many of the sound therapies identified could be effective when selected for the right patients at the right time and appropriate context. To do this we suggest careful assessment and then use of an individual care plan. In this review we deliberately focus on sound therapy, but we strongly believe any treatment plan should consider counseling (Tyler et al., 2007; Searchfield et al., 2011), and referral for psychological therapies such as Cognitive Behavioral Therapy (Martinez-Devesa et al., 2006) when appropriate. By determining individual needs and priorities, alongside assessment measures such as pure-tone audiometry and pitch matching, a plan can be developed that we believe reduces the risk for ineffective treatment. An effective individual care plan may also reduce the time required for treatment, reducing stress, anxiety and loss of hope for the sufferer. We believe those factors of the individual's complaint that are likely to be driving other symptoms should be addressed by therapy first (Fisher and Boswell, 2016).

Based on the review, along with our clinical experience, we suggest that the individual care plan use various clinical assessment methods. When patients first attend the clinic their clinical history, a thorough hearing assessment and tinnitus matching should be undertaken (Langguth et al., 2007). A questionnaire assessing aspects of tinnitus effects on quality of life should be used to provide an overview of tinnitus impact, and serve as a baseline for future assessments of outcomes. The Tinnitus Functional Index (Meikle et al., 2012) and Tinnitus Primary Function Questionnaire (Tyler et al., 2014) are two recent questionnaires developed for this purpose. Based on a clinical history an evaluation of anxiety and depression (e.g., the Hospital Anxiety and Depression Scale, Andersson et al., 2003) or cognition [e.g., National Institutes for Health (NIH) Toolbox Cognition Battery, Heaton et al., 2014] may be important. The comorbidity of anxiety and depression with tinnitus is well known (Andersson et al., 2003). The Hospital Anxiety and Depression Scale (HADS) (Zigmond and Snaith, 1983) or similar questionnaire scores can assist decision-making as to the necessity and priorities for psychological therapies. Tinnitus negatively impacts on cognition (Zarenoe et al., 2017). We do not know yet if differences in cognition should influence selection of sound therapy type, however research suggests that slow-acting hearing aid processing strategies may lead to better hearing when users memory is impaired (Lunner et al., 2009). We also recommend the assessment of personality. The use of personality questionnaires such as the Multidimensional Personality Questionnaire (MPQ) subscales (Tellegen, 1982) in clinics may be useful in identifying at-risk individuals for distressing tinnitus. Four key "maladaptive" personality traits are suspected in playing a role in diverting attention and processing resources toward tinnitus and which may subsequently act to prevent adaptation. These include higher levels of stress reaction, lower social closeness, lower self-control and higher alienation (Durai and Searchfield, 2016). If, for example, an individual has high stress reactions and low self-control and reacts negatively to sound psychological-based interventions may be needed before sound therapy.

Hoare et al. (2014b) recommended that clinicians be guided by the patient's point of care, patient motivation and expectations of sound therapy. The acceptability of the intervention both in terms of the sound stimuli to be used and whether patients are willing to use sound extensively or intermittently is important (Hoare et al., 2014b). A step in this direction is counseling patients about the therapies that are available. Information should be provided about the basis of the treatment, evidence for effectiveness, speed of effects, and costs. Aazh et al. (2009) suggest a poster format for this pre-consultation information; clinics websites and marketing material also can provide useful appointment scene setting. A tinnitus needs assessment can assist in the shared decision making process. The Hearing and Tinnitus clinic at the University of Auckland has used the COSIT as a decision making and goal setting tool for over a decade (Searchfield, 2006). The COSIT is a modification of the COSI, a tool frequently used in needs assessment for hearing problems (Dillon et al., 1987). Other questionnaires that may assist needs assessment include the TAQ (Tyler et al., 2007), STOP (Newman et al., 2008) and SETMQ (Smith and Fagelson, 2011). The TAQ determines the areas in which tinnitus creates problems (emotion, sleep, communication and/or concentration). The TAQ can highlight areas of life in which tinnitus is having the most debilitating effect, which can then be used to focus or tailor treatment (Tyler et al., 2007). The STOP is an 11-item tool that takes into account motivation, acceptance, expectations and willingness to use sound therapy devices (Newman et al., 2008). The SETMQ is a 40-item measure that quantifies the patient's confidence in managing tinnitus in five areas: (1) routine management, (2) emotional response, (3) internal thoughts and interaction with others, (4) tinnitus concepts, and (5) use of assistive devices such as hearing aids and maskers (Smith and Fagelson, 2011).

The relative effectiveness of these questionnaires in informing successful treatment has to be determined. However the usefulness and time savings achieved by use of these questionnaires should not be underestimated, as they can be completed by the patient prior to their appointment and can be assessed by the clinician prior to meeting the patient; saving time during the appointment. There is overlap in the questions asked by the questionnaires so not all need be used. It is important that clinicians choose those questionnaires best suited to the treatments they offer and their health care setting and patient population. We suggest that many audiologists will find the open-ended format of the COSIT familiar, and may wish to combine with one or more closed question formats (TAQ, STOP, SETMQ). The outcome of appropriately selected assessments can result in an efficient tinnitus clinic. Unnecessary or inappropriate treatments can be avoided, reducing the risk that patients become disillusioned with the clinician's methods. With patient "buy-in," motivation and compliance to treatments should be high. Understanding and choosing the treatments to use immediately, and as the impact of tinnitus changes, may be empowering to the patient.

Advancing Sound Therapy and Recognizing Its Limitations

The literature review highlighted the diverse basis and application of sound therapy. Researchers and publications need to be clear on what aspect or type of sound therapy is being used. Mckenna and Irwin (2008) wrote a useful critique of sound therapy with the provocative title "Sound therapy: sacred cow or idol worship?" Mckenna and Irwin's (2008) main arguments were that the mechanisms of sound therapy were not necessarily those claimed, effects may be cognitive or psychological rather than purely auditory, and benefits were modest, if any, above counseling alone. Sound therapy is potentially confusing, given the numerous approaches and various potential mechanisms of effect. While more evidence for sound therapies is becoming available there is still a need to prove benefits. The individualized sound therapy approach also needs to be validated relative to single therapy protocols. In order to provide this evidence we may a need to move away from the dominant nomothetic research approach to an idiographic method that embraces individual variance (Fisher and Boswell, 2016). Group comparisons are limited in their ability to identify effective sound therapies when there is heterogeneity. Sound therapy is, in general, a slow-acting therapy that requires long-term use of some form of sound delivery device; so longitudinal data is needed. Research also needs to continue to investigate whether auditory-based therapies can be enhanced, or sped up, by combining with non-invasive brain (Shekhawat et al., 2014; De Ridder et al., 2015) or multisensory (Spiegel et al., 2015) stimulation.

CONCLUSIONS

The basis of sound therapy is the belief that increasing extrinsic sound driven activity of the auditory system reduces tinnitus. This does not mean sound therapy is uniform in its application; instead it covers many dimensions and presumed mechanisms of effect. Current commentary on sound therapy fails to fully recognize this heterogeneity in application. At the same time few sound therapies can truly be considered personalized to make the most of their purported mechanisms. Much of the literature surveyed used the terms "customized" or "tailored" in terms of a single dimension rather than viewing tinnitus as a complex combination of dimensions. Tools exist for personalizing and planning treatments, they should be integrated into patient care, and their usefulness tested.

AUTHOR CONTRIBUTIONS

GS undertook the initial database search, cataloging, and prepared the manuscript and revisions. MD was involved in manuscript preparation and cataloging of results. TL reviewed the cataloging and contributed to the manuscript with a focus on clinical application.

FUNDING

The researchers are supported by the JM Cathie Trust Fund of the Auckland Medical Research Foundation, the American Tinnitus Association, and the Oticon Foundation of NZ.

REFERENCES

Aazh, H., Moore, B. C., and Roberts, P. (2009). Patient-centered tinnitus management tool: a clinical audit. *Am. J. Audiol.* 18, 7–13. doi: 10.1044/1059-0889(2009/08-0037)

Andersson, G., Heesser, H., and McKenna, L. (2016). "Psychological mechanisms and tinnitus," in *Tinnitus Clinical and Research Perspectives*, eds D. Baguley and M. Fagelson (San Diego, CA: Plural Publishing), 63–74.

Andersson, G., Kaldo-Sandstrom, V., Strom, L., and Stromgren, T. (2003). Internet administration of the hospital anxiety and depression scale in a sample of tinnitus patients. *J. Psychosom. Res.* 55, 259–262. doi: 10.1016/S0022-3999(02)00575-5

Anon (2012). What happened to personalized medicine? *Nature Biotechnology* 30:1. doi: 10.1038/nbt.2096

Anwar, M. N. (2013). Mining and analysis of audiology data to find significant factors associated with tinnitus masker. *Springerplus* 2:1. doi: 10.1186/2193-1801-2-595

Ariizumi, Y., Hatanaka, A., and Kitamura, K. (2010). Clinical prognostic factors for tinnitus retraining therapy with a sound generator in tinnitus patients. *J. Med. Dent. Sci.* 57, 45–53. doi: 10.11480/jmds.570106

Baguley, D., McFerran, D., and Hall, D. (2013). Tinnitus. *Lancet* 382, 1600–1607. doi: 10.1016/S0140-6736(13)60142-7

Barozzi, S., Del Bo, L., Crocetti, A., Dyrlund, O., Passoni, S., Zolin, A., et al. (2016). A comparison of nature and technical sounds for tinnitus therapy. *Acta. Acust. United Acust.* 102, 540–546. doi: 10.3813/AAA.918971

Bartnik, G. M., and Skarzynski, H. (2006). "Tinnitus retraining therapy," in *Tinnitus Treatment: Clinical Protocols*, ed R. Tyler (New York, NY: Thieme Medical Publishers, Inc.), 133–145.

Bessman, P., Heider, T., Watten, V. P., and Watten, R. G. (2009). The tinnitus intensive therapy habituation program: a 2-year follow-up pilot study on subjective tinnitus. *Rehabil. Psychol.* 54, 133–137. doi: 10.1037/a0015660

Choy, D., Lipman, R., and Tassi, G. (2010). Worldwide experience with sequential phase-shift sound cancellation treatment of predominant tone tinnitus. *L. Laryngol Otol.* 124, 366–369. doi: 10.1017/S0022215109992167

Courtenay, E. W., Schlaug, G., and Pantev, C. (2010). Listening to filtered music as a treatment option for tinnitus: a review. *Music Percept.* 27, 327–330. doi: 10.1525/mp.2010.27.4.327

Davis, P. (2006). "Music and the acoustic desensitization protocol for tinnitus," in *Tinnitus Treatment*, ed R. S. Tyler (New York, NY: Thieme), 146–160.

Davis, P. B., Paki, B., and Hanley, P. J. (2007). Neuromonics tinnitus treatment: third clinical trial. *Ear. Hear.* 28, 242–259. doi: 10.1097/AUD.0b013e3180312619

Department of Health (2009). Provision of *Services* for *Adults* with *Tinnitus: A Good Practice Guide*. London: Central office of information.

De Ridder, D., Kilgard, M., Engineer, N., and Vanneste, S. (2015). Placebo-controlled vagus nerve stimulation paired with tones in a patient with refractory tinnitus: a case report. *Otol. Neurotol.* 36, 575–580. doi: 10.1097/MAO.0000000000000704

Dillon, H., James, A., and Ginis, J. (1987). Client oriented scale of improvement (COSI) and its relationship to several other measures of benefit and satisfaction provided by hearing aids. *J. Am. Acad. Audiol.* 8, 27–43.

Drexler, D., Lopez-Paullier, M., Rodio, S., Gonzalez, M., Geisinger, D., and Pedemonte, M. (2016). Impact of reduction of tinnitus intensity on patients' quality of life. *Int. J. Audiol.* 55, 11–19. doi: 10.3109/14992027.2015.1072772

Durai, M., Kobayashi, K., and Searchfield, G. (2015). A preliminary examination of the roles of contextual stimuli and personality traits under the adaptation level theory model of tinnitus. *Acta. Acust United Acust.* 101, 543–551. doi: 10.3813/AAA.918851

Durai, M., and Searchfield, G. (2016). Anxiety and depression, personality traits relevant to tinnitus: a scoping review. *Int. J. Audiol.* 55, 605–615. doi: 10.1080/14992027.2016.1198966

Durai, M., and Searchfield, G. D. (2017). A mixed-methods trial of broad band noise and nature sounds for tinnitus therapy: group and individual responses modeled under the adaptation level theory of tinnitus. *Front. Aging. Neurosci.* 9:44. doi: 10.3389/fnagi.2017.00044

Eggermont, J. J., and Tass, P. A. (2015). Maladaptive neural synchrony in tinnitus: origin and restoration. *Front. Neurol.* 6:29. doi: 10.3389/fneur.2015.00029

Fagelson, M. A., and Smith, S. L. (2016). Tinnitus self-efficacy and other tinnitus self-report variables in patients with and without post-traumatic stress disorder. *Ear Hear.* 37, 541–546. doi: 10.1097/AUD.0000000000000290

Fioretti, A., Eibenstein, A., and Fusetti, M. (2011). New trends in tinnitus management. *Open Neurol. J.* 5:12. doi: 10.2174/1874205X01105010012

Fisher, A. J., and Boswell, J. F. (2016). Enhancing the personalization of psychotherapy with dynamic assessment and modeling. *Assessment* 23, 496–506. doi: 10.1177/1073191116638735

Folmer, R. L., and Carroll, J. R. (2006). Long-term effectiveness of ear-level devices for tinnitus. *Otol. Head Neck Surg.* 134, 132–137. doi: 10.1016/j.otohns.2005.09.030

Ginsburg, G. S., and Willard, H. F. (2009). Genomic and personalized medicine: foundations and applications. *Transl. Res.* 154, 277–287. doi: 10.1016/j.trsl.2009.09.005

Grant, M. J., and Booth, A. (2009). A typology of reviews: an analysis of 14 review types and associated methodologies. *Health Info. Libr. J.* 26, 91–108. doi: 10.1111/j.1471-1842.2009.00848.x

Grenness, C., Hickson, L., Laplante-Lévesque, A., and Davidson, B. (2014). Patient-centred care: a review for rehabilitative audiologists. *J. Audiol.* 53, S60–S67. doi: 10.3109/14992027.2013.847286

Györi, A. (2016). "Tailor-made notched music training-a therapy of chronic tinnitus," in *Computer Music Seminar Aachen*. Available online at: https://www.researchgate.net/publication/310046636_Tailor-Made_Notched_Music_Training_-_a_therapy_of_chronic_tinnitus

Handscomb, L. (2006). Use of bedside sound generators by patients with tinnitus-related sleeping difficulty: which sounds are preferred and why? *Acta Otolaryngol.* 126, 59–63. doi: 10.1080/03655230600895275

Hanley, P. J., and Davis, P. B. (2008). Treatment of tinnitus with a customized, dynamic acoustic neural stimulus: underlying principles and clinical efficacy. *Trends Amp.* 12, 210–222. doi: 10.1177/1084713808319942

Hann, D., Searchfield, G. D., Sanders, M., and Wise, K. (2008). Strategies for the selection of music in the short-term management of mild tinnitus. *ANZ. J. Audiol.* 30:129. doi: 10.1375/audi.30.2.129

Hauptmann, C., Ströbel, A., Williams, M., Patel, N., Wurzer, H., von Stackelberg, T., et al. (2015). Acoustic coordinated reset neuromodulation in a real life patient population with chronic tonal tinnitus. *BioMed. Res. Int.* 2015:569052. doi: 10.1155/2015/569052

Hauptmann, C., Wegener, A., Poppe, H., Williams, M., Popelka, G., and Tass, P. A. (2016). Validation of a mobile device for acoustic coordinated reset neuromodulation tinnitus therapy. *J. Am. Acad. Audiol.* 27, 720–731. doi: 10.3766/jaaa.15082

Heaton, R. K., Akshoomoff, N., Tulsky, D., Mungas, D., Weintraub, S., Dikmen, S., et al. (2014). Reliability and validity of composite scores from the NIH toolbox cognition battery in adults. *J. Int. Neuropsychol. Soc.* 20, 588–598. doi: 10.1017/S1355617714000241

Heijneman, K. M., De Kleine, E., and Van Dijk, P. (2012). A randomized double-blind crossover study of phase-shift sound therapy for tinnitus. *Otolaryngol. Head Neck Surg.* 147, 308–315. doi: 10.1177/0194599812442615

Henin, S., Fein, D., Smouha, E., and Parra, L. C. (2016). The effects of compensatory auditory stimulation and high-definition transcranial direct current stimulation (hd-tdcs) on tinnitus perception - a randomized pilot study. *PLoS ONE* 11:e0166208. doi: 10.1371/journal.pone.0166208

Henry, J. A., Frederick, M., Sell, S., Griest, S., and Abrams, H. (2015). Validation of a novel combination hearing aid and tinnitus therapy device. *Ear Hear.* 36, 42–52. doi: 10.1097/AUD.0000000000000093

Henry, J. A., Roberts, L. E., Ellingson, R. M., and Thielman, E. J. (2013). Computer-automated tinnitus assessment: noise-band matching, maskability, and residual inhibition. *J. Am. Acad. Audiol.* 24, 486–504. doi: 10.3766/jaaa.24.6.5

Henry, J. A., Schechter, M. A., Zaugg, T. L., Griest, S., Jastreboff, P. J., Vernon, J. A., et al. (2006). Outcomes of clinical trial: tinnitus masking versus tinnitus retraining therapy. *J. Am. Acad. Audiol.* 17, 104–132. doi: 10.3766/jaaa.17.2.4

Herraiz, C., Hernandez, F. J., Toledano, A., and Aparicio, J. M. (2007). Tinnitus retraining therapy: prognosis factors. *Am. J. Otol.* 28, 225–229. doi: 10.1016/j.amjoto.2006.09.004

Herzfeld, M., Enza, C., and Sweetow, R. (2014). Clinical trial on the effectiveness of widex zen therapy for tinnitus. *Hear. Rev.* 21, 24–29.

Hoare, D. J., Adjamian, P., Sereda, M., and Hall, D. A. (2013a). Recent technological advances in sound-based approaches to tinnitus treatment: a review of efficacy considered against putative physiological mechanisms. *Noise Health* 15, 107. doi: 10.4103/1463-1741.110292

Hoare, D. J., Edmondson-Jones, M., Gander, P. E., and Hall, D. A. (2014a). Agreement and reliability of tinnitus loudness matching and pitch likeness rating. *PLoS ONE* 9:e114553. doi: 10.1371/journal.pone.0114553

Hoare, D. J., Gander, P. E., Collins, L., Smith, S., and Hall, D. A. (2012). Management of tinnitus in english nhs audiology departments: an evaluation of current practice. *J. Eval. Clin. Prac.* 18, 326–334. doi: 10.1111/j.1365-2753.2010.01566.x

Hoare, D. J., Pierzycki, R. H., Thomas, H., McAlpine, D., and Hall, D. A. (2013b). Evaluation of the acoustic coordinated reset (CR ®) neuromodulation therapy for tinnitus: study protocol for a double-blind randomized placebo-controlled trial. *Trials* 14:207. doi: 10.1186/1745-6215-14-207

Hoare, D. J., Searchfield, G. D., El Refaie, A., and Henry, J. A. (2014b). Sound therapy for tinnitus management: practicable options. *J. Am. Acad. Audiol.* 25, 62–75. doi: 10.3766/jaaa.25.1.5

Hoare, D. J., Stacey, P. C., and Hall, D. A. (2010). The efficacy of auditory perceptual training for tinnitus: a systematic review. *Annals. Behav. Med.* 40, 313–324. doi: 10.1007/s12160-010-9213-5

Hoare, D. J., Whitham, D., Henry, J. A., and Shorter, G. W. (2015). Neuromodulation (desynchronisation) for tinnitus in adults. *Cochrane Database Syst. Rev.* 6:CD011760. doi: 10.1002/14651858.CD011760.

Hobson, J., Chisholm, E., and El Refaie, A. (2012). Sound therapy (masking) in the management of tinnitus in adults. *Cochrane Database Syst. Rev.* 11:CD006371. doi: 10.1002/14651858.CD006371.pub3

Huang, C.-Y., Wu, J.-L., Cheng, C.-C., Sher, Y.-J., and Chung, K.-C. (2006). Evaluation of the mixing point in tinnitus sound therapy by a psychoacoustic matching protocol with a digital tinnitus evaluation system. *Orl* 68, 110–114. doi: 10.1159/000091213

Hutter, E., Grapp, M., Argstatter, H., and Bolay, H. V. (2014). Music therapy for chronic tinnitus: variability of tinnitus pitch in the course of therapy. *J. Am. Acad. Audiol.* 25, 335–342. doi: 10.3766/jaaa.25.4.5

Ito, M., Soma, K., and Ando, R. (2009). Association between tinnitus retraining therapy and a tinnitus control instrument. *Auris Nasus Larynx* 36, 536–540. doi: 10.1016/j.anl.2009.01.003

Jalilvand, H., Pourbakht, A., and Haghani, H. (2015). Hearing aid or tinnitus masker: which one is the best treatment for blast-induced tinnitus? The results of a long-term study on 974 patients. *Audiol. Neurotol.* 20, 195–201. doi: 10.1159/000377617

Jastreboff, M. M. (2007). Sound therapies for tinnitus management. *Prog. Brain Res.* 166, 435–440. doi: 10.1016/S0079-6123(07)66042-7

Jastreboff, P. (2015). 25 Years of tinnitus retraining therapy. *HNO* 63, 307–311. doi: 10.1007/s00106-014-2979-1

Jastreboff, P. J. (2000). "Tinnitus habituation therapy (THT) and tinnitus retraining therapy (TRT)," in *Tinnitus Handbook*, ed R. Tyler (San Diego, CA: Singular Publishing Group), 357–376.

Jastreboff, P. J. (2011). "Tinnitus retraining therapy," in *Textbook of Tinnitus*, eds A. R. Møller, B. Langguth, D. DeRidder, and T. Kleinjung (New York, NY: Springer-Verlag), 575–596.

Jastreboff, P., and Jastreboff, M. M. (2006). Tinnitus retraining therapy: a different view on tinnitus. *Orl* 68, 23–30. doi: 10.1159/000090487

Jepsen, K., Sanders, M., Searchfield, G., and Kobayashi, K. (2010). Perceptual training of tinnitus. proceedings of 'tinnitus discovery': Asia-Pacific tinnitus symposium, 11-12 Sept 2009. *NZ. Med. J.* 123, 141–153.

Kidd, G. Jr., Arbogast, T. L., Mason, C. R., and Walsh, M. (2002). Informational masking in listeners with sensorineural hearing loss. *JARO* 3, 107–119. doi: 10.1007/s101620010095

Kidd, G. J., Mason, C. R., Rothla, T. L., and Deliwala, P. S. (1998). Release from masking due to spatial separation of sources in the identification of nonspeech auditory patterns. *J. Acous. Soc. Am.* 104, 422–431. doi: 10.1121/1.423246

Kim, B. J., Chung, S. W., Jung, J. Y., and Suh, M. W. (2014). Effect of different sounds on the treatment outcome of tinnitus retraining therapy. *Clin. Exp. Otorhinolaryn* 7, 87–93. doi: 10.3342/ceo.2014.7.2.87

Langguth, B., Goodey, R., Azevedo, A., Bjorne, A., Cacace, A., Crocetti, A., et al. (2007). Consensus for tinnitus patient assessment and treatment outcome measurement: tinnitus research initiative meeting, regensburg, july 2006. *Prog. Brain Res.* 166, 525–536. doi: 10.1016/S0079-6123(07)66050-6

Li, S.-A., Bao, L., and Chrostowski, M. (2016). Investigating the effects of a personalized, spectrally altered music-based sound therapy on treating tinnitus: a blinded, randomized controlled trial. *Audiol. Neurotol.* 21, 296–304. doi: 10.1159/000450745

Lugli, M., Romani, R., Ponzi, S., Bacciu, S., and Parmigiani, S. (2009). The windowed sound therapy: a new empirical approach for an effective personalized treatment of tinnitus. *Int. Tin. J.* 15, 51–61.

Lunner, T., Rudner, M., and Ronnberg, J. (2009). Cognition and hearing aids. *Scand. J. Psychol.* 50, 395–403. doi: 10.1111/j.1467-9450.2009.00742.x

Mahboubi, H., Ziai, K., and Djalilian, H. R. (2012). Customized web-based sound therapy for tinnitus. *Int. Tin. J.* 17, 26–30.

Martinez-Devesa, P., Waddell, A., and Theodoulou, M. (2006). Cognitive behavioural therapy for tinnitus. *Cochrane Database Syst. Rev.* 1:1. doi: 10.1002/14651858.CD005233.pub3.

Mazurek, B., Fischer, F., Haupt, H., Georgiewa, P., Reisshauer, A., and Klapp, B. F. (2006). A modified version of tinnitus retraining therapy: observing long-term outcome and predictors. *Audiol. Neurotol.* 11, 276–286. doi: 10.1159/000093526

Mckenna, L., and Irwin, R. (2008). Sound therapy for tinnitus–sacred cow or idol worship? an investigation of the evidence. *Audiol. Med.* 6, 16–24. doi: 10.1080/16513860801899389

McNeill, C., Távora-Vieira, D., Alnafjan, F., Searchfield, G. D., and Welch, D. (2012). Tinnitus pitch, masking, and the effectiveness of hearing aids for tinnitus therapy. *Int. J. Audiol.* 51, 914–919. doi: 10.3109/14992027.2012.721934

Meeus, O., Heyndrickx, K., Lambrechts, P., De Ridder, D., and Van de Heyning, P. (2010). Phase-shift treatment for tinnitus of cochlear origin. *Eur. Arch. Otorhinolaryngol.* 267, 881–888. doi: 10.1007/s00405-009-1145-y

Meikle, M. B., Henry, J. A., Griest, S. E., Stewart, B. J., Abrams, H. B., McArdle, R., et al. (2012). The tinnitus functional index: development of a new clinical measure for chronic, intrusive tinnitus. *Ear Hear.* 32, 153–176. doi: 10.1097/AUD.0b013e31822f67c0

Michie, S., Miles, J., and Weinman, J. (2003). Patient-centredness in chronic illness: what is it and does it matter? *Patient Ed. Couns.* 51, 197–206. doi: 10.1016/S0738-3991(02)00194-5

Miles, A., and Loughlin, M. (2011). Models in the balance: evidence-based medicine versus evidence-informed individualized care. *J. Eval. Clin. Prac.* 17, 531–536. doi: 10.1111/j.1365-2753.2011.01713.x

Myers, P. J., Griest, S., Kaelin, C., Legro, M. W., Schmidt, C. J., Zaugg, T., et al. (2014). Development of a progressive audiologic tinnitus management program for veterans with tinnitus. *J. Rehab. Res. Dev.* 51:609. doi: 10.1682/JRRD.2013.08.0189

Newman, C. W., Sandridge, S. A., Meit, S. S., and Cherian, N. (2008). Strategies for managing patients with tinnitus: a clinical pathway model. *Sem. Hear.* 29, 300–309. doi: 10.1055/s-0028-1082035

Norena, A. J. (2015). Revisiting the cochlear and central mechanisms of tinnitus and therapeutic approaches. *Audiol. Neurootol.* 20(Suppl. 1), 53–59. doi: 10.1159/000380749

Oishi, N., Shinden, S., Kanzaki, S., Saito, H., Inoue, Y., and Ogawa, K. (2013). Effects of tinnitus retraining therapy involving monaural noise generators. *Eur. Arch. Oto. Rhino. Laryngol.* 270, 443–448. doi: 10.1007/s00405-012-1951-5

Ostermann, K., Lurquin, P., Horoi, M., Cotton, P., Herve, V., and Thill, M. P. (2016). Somatic tinnitus prevalence and treatment with tinnitus retraining therapy. *B-ENT* 12, 59–65.

Oz, I., Arslan, F., Hizal, E., Erbek, S. H., Eryaman, E., Senkal, O. A., et al. (2013). Effectiveness of the combined hearing and masking devices on the severity and perception of tinnitus: a randomized, controlled, double-blind study. *ORL J. Otorhinolaryngol. Relat. Spec.* 75, 211–220. doi: 10.1159/00034 9979

Parra, P. C. (2015). Tinnitus: mechanisms, measures and sound treatments. *Loquens* 2:24. doi: 10.3989/loquens.2015.024

Pedemonte, M., Drexler, D., Rodio, S., Geisinger, D., Bianco, A., Pol-Fernandes, D., et al. (2010). Tinnitus treatment with sound stimulation during sleep. *Inter. Tin. J.* 16, 37–43.

Peltier, E., Peltier, C., Tahar, S., Alliot-Lugaz, E., and Cazals, Y. (2012). Long-term tinnitus suppression with linear octave frequency transposition hearing AIDS. *PLoS ONE* 7:e51915. doi: 10.1371/journal.pone.0051915

Piskosz, M. (2012). The Role of wireless streaming in tinnitus management. *Hear. Rev.* 12–15.

Reavis, K. M., Chang, J. E., and Zeng, F.-G. (2010). Patterned sound therapy for the treatment of tinnitus. *Hear. J.* 63, 21–22. doi: 10.1097/01.HJ.0000390817.79500.ed

Reavis, K. M., Rothholtz, V. S., Tang, Q., Carroll, J. A., Djalilian, H., and Zeng, F.-G. (2012). Temporary suppression of tinnitus by modulated sounds. *JARO* 13, 561–571. doi: 10.1007/s10162-012-0331-6

Roberts, L. E., and Bosnyak, D. J. (2011). "Auditory training in tinnitus," in *Textbook of Tinnitus*, eds A. R. Møller, B. Langguth, D. DeRidder, and T. Kleinjung (New York, NY: Springer-Verlag), 563–573.

Sand, P., Langguth, B., Kleinjung, T., and Eichhammer, P. (2007). Genetics of chronic tinnitus. *Prog. Brain Res.* 166, 159–168. doi: 10.1016/S0079-6123(07)66014-2

Schaette, R., Konig, O., Hornig, D., Gross, M., and Kempter, R. (2010). Acoustic stimulation treatments against tinnitus could be most effective when tinnitus pitch is within the stimulated frequency range. *Hear. Res.* 269, 95–101. doi: 10.1016/j.heares.2010.06.022

Schleidgen, S., Klingler, C., Bertram, T., Rogowski, W. H., and Marckmann, G. (2013). What is personalized medicine: sharpening a vague term based on a systematic literature review. *BMC Med. Ethics* 14:55. doi: 10.1186/1472-6939-14-55

Searchfield, G. D. (2006). "Hearing aids and tinnitus," in *Tinnitus Protocols*, ed R. Tyler (New York, NY: Thieme), 161–175.

Searchfield, G. D. (2014). Tinnitus what and where: an ecological framework. *Front. Neurol.* 5:271. doi: 10.3389/fneur.2014.00271

Searchfield, G. D. (2015). "Hearing aids for tinnitus," in *Tinnitus: Clinical and Research Perspectives*, eds D. Baguley and M. Fagelson (San Diego, CA: Plural Publishing), 197–212.

Searchfield, G. D. (2016). "Tinnitus sound therapy options," in *The Consumer Handbook on Tinnitus, 2nd Edn.* ed R. Tyler (Sedona, AZ: Auricle Ink Publishers), 179–195.

Searchfield, G. D., Kaur, M., and Martin, W. H. (2010). Hearing aids as an adjunct to counseling: tinnitus patients who choose amplification do better than those that don't. *Int. J. Audiol.* 49, 574–579. doi: 10.3109/14992021003 777267

Searchfield, G. D., Kobayashi, K., Hodgson, S.-A., Hodgson, C., Tevoitdale, H., and Irving, S. (2016). Spatial masking: development and testing of a new tinnitus assistive technology. *Assist Tech* 28, 115–125. doi: 10.1080/10400435.2015.1110214

Searchfield, G. D., Kobayashi, K., and Sanders, M. (2012). An adaptation level theory of tinnitus audibility. *Front. Syst. Neurosci.* 6:46. doi: 10.3389/fnsys.2012.00046

Searchfield, G. D., Magnusson, J., Shakes, G., Biesinger, E., and Kong, O. (2011). "Counseling and psycho-education for tinnitus management," in *Textbook of Tinnitus*, eds A. R. Møller, B. Langguth, D. DeRidder, and T. Kleinjung (New York, NY: Springer-Verlag), 535–556.

Sereda, M., Davies, J., and Hall, D. A. (2016). Pre-market version of a commercially available hearing instrument with a tinnitus sound generator: feasibility of evaluation in a clinical trial. *Int. J. Audiol.* 56, 286–294. doi: 10.1080/14992027.2016.1254822

Sereda, M., Hall, D. A., Bosnyak, D. J., Edmondson-Jones, M., Roberts, L. E., Adjamian, P., et al. (2011). Re-examining the relationship between audiometric profile and tinnitus pitch. *Int. J. Audiol.* 50, 303–312. doi: 10.3109/14992027.2010.551221

Sereda, M., Hoare, D. J., Nicholson, R., Smith, S., and Hall, D. A. (2015). Consensus on hearing aid candidature and fitting for mild hearing loss, with and without tinnitus: delphi review. *Ear Hear.* 36:417. doi: 10.1097/AUD.0000000000000140

Serquera, J., Schlee, W., Pryss, R., Neff, P., and Langguth, B. (2015). "Music technology for tinnitus treatment within tinnet," in *Audio Engineering Society Conference: 58th International Conference: Music Induced Hearing Disorders: Audio Engineering Society* (Aalborg).

Shekhawat, G. S., Searchfield, G. D., Kobayashi, K., and Stinear, C. M. (2013a). Prescription of hearing-aid output for tinnitus relief. *Int. J. Audiol.* 52, 617–625. doi: 10.3109/14992027.2013.799787

Shekhawat, G. S., Searchfield, G. D., and Stinear, C. M. (2013b). Role of hearing aids in tinnitus intervention: a scoping review. *J. Am. Acad. Audiol.* 24, 747–762. doi: 10.3766/jaaa.24.8.11

Shekhawat, G. S., Searchfield, G. D., and Stinear, C. M. (2014). Randomized trial of transcranial direct current stimulation and hearing aids for tinnitus management. *Neurorehabil. Neural Repair* 28, 410–419. doi: 10.1177/1545968313508655

Smith, S. L., and Fagelson, M. (2011). Development of the self-efficacy for tinnitus management questionnaire. *J. Am. Acad. Audiol.* 22, 424–440. doi: 10.3766/jaaa.22.7.4

Spiegel, D. P., Linford, T., Thompson, B., Petoe, M. A., Kobayashi, K., Stinear, C. M., et al. (2015). Multisensory attention training for treatment of tinnitus. *Sci. Rep.* 5:10802. doi: 10.1038/srep10802

Stouffer, J. L., and Tyler, R. S. (1990). Characterization of tinnitus by tinnitus patients. *J. Speech Hear. Dis.* 55, 439–453. doi: 10.1044/jshd.5503.439

Suzuki, B., Suzuki, F. A., Yonamine, F. A., Onishi, F. K., Penido, E. T., and Oliveira, N. (2016). Effectiveness of sound therapy in patients with tinnitus resistant to previous treatments: importance of adjustments. *Brazil J. Otorhinolaryngol.* 82, 297–303. doi: 10.1016/j.bjorl.2015.05.009

Tang, H. Y., Harms, V., Speck, S. M., Vezeau, T., and Jesurum, J. T. (2009). Effects of audio relaxation programs for blood pressure reduction in older adults. *Eur. J. Cardiovasc. Nurs.* 8, 329–336. doi: 10.1016/j.ejcnurse.2009.06.001

Távora-Vieira, D., Eikelboom, R. H., and Miller, S. (2011). Neuromonics tinnitus treatment for patients with significant level of hearing loss: an adaptation of the protocol. *In. J. Audiol.* 50, 881–886. doi: 10.3109/14992027.2011.606286

Teismann, H., Okamoto, H., and Pantev, C. (2011). Short and intense tailor-made notched music training against tinnitus: the tinnitus frequency matters. *PLoS ONE* 6:e24685. doi: 10.1371/journal.pone.0024685

Tellegen, A. (1982). *Brief Manual for the Multidimensional Personality Questionnaire.* Minneapolis: University of Minnesota Minneapolis, 1031–1010.

Tutton, R. (2012). Personalizing medicine: futures present and past. *Soc. Sci. Med.* 75, 1721–1728. doi: 10.1016/j.socscimed.2012.07.031

Tyler, R. (2000). "Psychoacoustical measurement," in *Handbook of Tinnitus*, ed R. Tyler (San Diego, CA: Singular Publications), 149–180.

Tyler, R., Ji, H., Perreau, A., Witt, S., Noble, W., and Coelho, C. (2014). Development and validation of the tinnitus primary function questionnaire. *Am. J. Audiol.* 23, 260–272. doi: 10.1044/2014_AJA-13-0014

Tyler, R. S. (2012). Patient preferences and willingness to pay for tinnitus treatments. *J. Am. Acad. Audiol.* 23, 115–125. doi: 10.3766/jaaa.23.2.6

Tyler, R. S., Coelho, C., and Noble, W. (2006). Tinnitus: standard of care, personality differences, genetic factors. *ORL* 68, 14–22. doi: 10.1159/000090486

Tyler, R. S., Gogel, S. A., and Gehringer, A. K. (2007). Tinnitus activities treatment. *Prog. Brain Res.* 166, 425–434. doi: 10.1016/S0079-6123(07)66041-5

Tyler, R. S., Keiner, A. J., Walker, K., Deshpande, A. K., Witt, S., Killian, M., et al. (2015). A series of case studies of tinnitus suppression with mixed background stimuli in a cochlear implant. *Am. J. Audiol.* 24, 398–410. doi: 10.1044/2015_AJA-15-0005

Tyler, R. S., Noble, W., Coelho, C. B., and Ji, H. (2012). Tinnitus retraining therapy: mixing point and total masking are equally effective. *Ear. Hear.* 33, 588–594. doi: 10.1097/AUD.0b013e31824f2a6e

Uriz, A. J., Agüero, P. D., Tulli, J. C., Moreira, J. C., González, E. L., Moscardi, G., et al. (2013). "A development and implementation of a tinnitus treatment method," in *Journal of Physics: Conference Series,* Vol. 477 (Tucumán: IOP Publishing), 012026.

Vanneste, S., van Dongen, M., De Vree, B., Hiseni, S., van der Velden, E., Strydis, C., et al. (2013). Does enriched acoustic environment in humans abolish chronic tinnitus clinically and electrophysiologically? A double blind placebo controlled study. *Hear. Res.* 296, 141–148. doi: 10.1016/j.heares.2012.10.003

Vermeire, K., Heyndrickx, K., De Ridder, D., and Van de Heyning, P. (2007). Phase-shift tinnitus treatment: an open prospective clinical trial. *B-ENT* 3(Suppl. 7), 65–69.

Vernon, J. (1977). Attempts to relieve tinnitus. *J. Am. Acad. Audiol.* 2, 124–131.

Viirre, E. (2010). Customized Sound Therapy (CST): a therapy for low-level tinnitus. *Hear. J.* 63, 30–34. doi: 10.1097/01.HJ.0000390819.17619.2c

Wazen, J. J., Daugherty, J., Pinsky, K., Newman, C. W., Sandridge, S., Battista, R., et al. (2011). Evaluation of a customized acoustical stimulus system in the treatment of chronic tinnitus. *Otol. Neurotol.* 32, 710–716. doi: 10.1097/MAO.0b013e318217d459

Welch, D., and Dawes, P. J. (2008). Personality and perception of tinnitus. *Ear Hear.* 29, 684–692. doi: 10.1097/AUD.0b013e318177d9ac

Williams, M., Hauptmann, C., and Patel, N. (2015). Acoustic CR neuromodulation therapy for subjective tonal tinnitus: a review of clinical outcomes in an independent audiology practice setting. *Front. Neurol.* 6:54. doi: 10.3389/fneur.2015.00054

Wise, K., Kobayashi, K., and Searchfield, G. (2015). Feasibility study of a game integrating assessment and therapy of tinnitus. *J. Neurosci. Methods* 249, 1–7. doi: 10.1016/j.jneumeth.2015.04.002

Wise, K., Kobayashi, K., Magnusson, J., Welch, D., and Searchfield, G. D. (2016). Randomized controlled trial of a perceptual training game for tinnitus therapy. *Games Heal. J.* 5, 141–149. doi: 10.1089/g4h.2015.0068

Zarenoe, R., Hallgren, M., Andersson, G., and Ledin, T. (2017). Working memory, sleep, and hearing problems in patients with tinnitus and hearing loss fitted with hearing aids. *J. Am. Acad. Audiol.* 28, 141–151. doi: 10.3766/jaaa.16023

Zigmond, A. S., and Snaith, R. P. (1983). The hospital anxiety and depression scale. *Acta. Psychiatr. Scand.* 67, 361–370. doi: 10.1111/j.1600-0447.1983.tb09716.x

7

Acoustic Coordinated Reset Neuromodulation: A Systematic Review of a Novel Therapy for Tinnitus

Marie Wegger[1], Therese Ovesen[1,2] and Dalia Gustaityte Larsen[3]*

[1] *Department of Clinical Medicine, Aarhus University, Aarhus, Denmark,* [2] *Department of Otorhinolaryngology, Holstebro Regional Hospital, Holstebro, Denmark,* [3] *Department of Otorhinolaryngology, Aarhus University Hospital, Aarhus, Denmark*

***Correspondence:**
Marie Wegger
mw1804@gmail.com

Background: There are growing technological advances in the development of sound-based methods for the treatment of tinnitus. Most of these methods intend to affect the speculated underlying neurological causes of tinnitus. Acoustic coordinated reset (CR) neuromodulation is one of them. A novel method that as of yet seems inadequately reviewed.

Purpose: To evaluate the current evidence on acoustic CR neuromodulation as a method for the treatment of tinnitus and to assess whether the method can be implemented in daily clinical practice.

Methods: A systematic literature search was performed in 13 databases in the period from February 1, 2015 to May 1, 2016. Studies regarding acoustic CR neuromodulation as a treatment method for tinnitus were included in the present review.

Results: A total of 8 studies were eligible for being reviewed comprising a total of 329 patients. Overall, the evidence level of the published literature was low. The main findings in the included studies were that acoustic CR neuromodulation was safe and well tolerated and most patients reported reduction of tinnitus symptoms. The neurophysiological basis of the method was claimed to be desynchronization, anti-kindling, and change of abnormal frequency couplings in a widespread tinnitus network comprising both auditory and non/auditory brain areas based on EEG analyses.

Conclusion: The available evidence is insufficient for clinical implementation of acoustic CR neuromodulation. The limited level of evidence suggests that acoustic CR neuromodulation may have positive effects on tinnitus symptoms. Preliminary electroencephalographic data are compatible with the claim that tinnitus reduction after CR treatment is mediated by a desynchronizing effect. However, a proof for this claim is still lacking.

Keywords: acoustic coordinated reset neuromodulation, desynchronizing, anti-kindling, tinnitus, systematic review

INTRODUCTION

Subjective tinnitus (ST) is an auditory phantom phenomenon, where an auditory perception is not related to a physical, external or internal, and sound source (1, 2). Approximately 10–15% of the adult population experience tinnitus (3). Tinnitus occurs in varying degrees and may have different etiologies (2). Up to 85% of tinnitus cases are accompanied by hearing loss related to external noise trauma (4). Other risk factors include longevity, ototoxic medication, otological diseases, head injury, cerebral diseases, and mandibular joint disorders (5, 6).

There are several theories regarding the mechanisms of ST generation such as phantom auditory perception (7), stimulated acoustic emissions (8), the dorsal cochlear nucleus hypothesis (9–11), and increased spontaneous firing rate (SFR) (12, 13). Tinnitus is most frequently related to damage of the peripheral hearing system, thereby leading to a deafferentiation of neurons influencing more central parts of the auditory system. One of the tinnitus generation theories is that cochlear damage results in deafferentiation-induced cortical map reorganization (1). When central auditory neurons are deprived of their normal input, they begin to show responsiveness to the characteristic frequency of neighboring, less affected regions in the tonotopic map (14). Also included among the neuronal changes are increased SFRs, abnormal synaptic connectivity, and synchronization (15).

The varying causes of tinnitus generation have led to development of a wide variety of treatments. Several methods have been studied, although the benefit has not been conclusively demonstrated. The efficacy of cognitive behavioral therapy, however, is well established, and studies have shown a beneficial effect on tinnitus distress.[1] Other methods include medical treatments (e.g., intravenous Lidocaine) and psychological approaches in combination with therapeutic sound, such as tinnitus retraining therapy. Sound therapies alone include the use of music, white noise generators, and hearing aids (16). Potential mechanisms through which sound therapy may act involve masking, habituation, and reversing of cortical reorganization through lateral inhibition.

There are growing technological advances in sound-based approaches of which the majority is designed to target the maladaptive plasticity perceived as the underlying mechanism of ST (16). Acoustic coordinated reset (CR) neuromodulation® is one of them (6, 14).

The concept of CR neuromodulation was initially developed as a treatment method for Parkinson's disease, where pathological neural synchronization was counteracted by desynchronizing, electrical deep brain stimulation. Since the inventors considered the pathological nerve activity of both Parkinson's and ST to be characterized by hyperactivity and pathological synchronization, acoustic CR neuromodulation was introduced as a non-invasive counterpart (14).

Coordinated reset neuromodulation has been examined in several animal (17, 18) and human studies (19). Over the past few years, studies regarding the effects and mechanisms of acoustic CR neuromodulation have also been presented.

Acoustic CR neuromodulation is a patterned stimulation with tones adjusted to the patient's dominant tinnitus frequency, which aims at counteracting pathological neuronal synchronization. Phase reset is proposed to be achieved by a repetitive stimulus delivery of tones with different frequencies gathered around the dominant tinnitus pitch (2).

To facilitate understanding of CR neuromodulation in general, some principles should be addressed (**Figure 1**):

1. CR neuromodulation (**Figure 1**) is based on the phase reset of oscillatory neuronal activity through desynchronization. It is proposed to counteract the deafferentiation-induced upregulated synchrony and connectivity through desynchronizing and anti-kindling effects (20, 21).
2. Neural populations display spike timing-dependent plasticity (STDP), i.e., they continuously regulate the strength of their synaptic connectivity relative to the pre- and postsynaptic firing (spikes). In other words, neural activity and the strength of their connections are related.
3. CR neuromodulation is designed to cause long-lasting anti-kindling effects; desynchronizing stimulation of neuronal populations causes the neurons to unlearn their pathological connectivity. The method attempts to change spike firing timing networks using series of tones and to force firing from a pathological state with abnormally synchronized synapses to a desynchronized state with weaker synapses. It achieves this

[1] Dinces EA. *Tinnitus*. Available from: http://www.uptodate.com/contents/treatment-of-tinnitus?source=machineLearning&search=tinnitus&selectedTitle=2~150&sectionRank=1&anchor=H2#H2

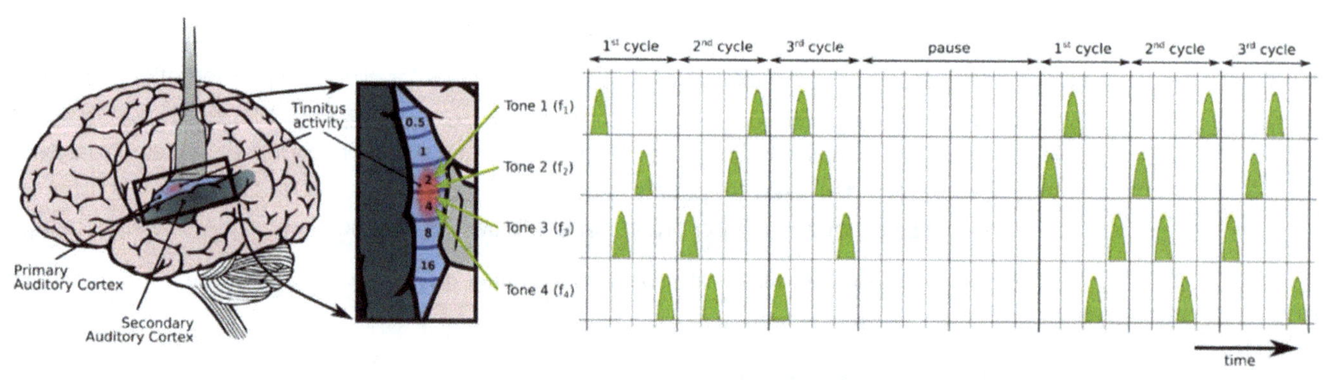

FIGURE 1 | Acoustic coordinated reset neuromodulation: the spatiotemporal organization of stimuli (23). The figure shows how stimuli are comprised by four different tones (triangles) gathered around the dominant tinnitus pitch in a randomized sequence during three cycles, followed by two silent cycles in a 3:2 ON–OFF pattern, to ideally enhance the desynchronizing effect (20, 24). Adapted from Chittka and Brockmann (25), with permission from Tass et al.

through tones played through hearing aid style earphones. The patients are supposed to listen to the tones 4–6 h per day for, e.g., 12 weeks.

4. The phenomenon when such states are present at the same time is known as STDP-induced multistability (2, 22).

The present review provides a systematic overview of studies of acoustic CR neuromodulation as a novel treatment method for ST. The purpose was to establish the current level of evidence available for the intervention and to assess whether the method can be recommended in the clinical setting.

METHODS

Literature search was performed in 13 databases in the period from 1st February to 1st May 2016, using the following search strings: (i) "Tinnitus" AND "acoustic coordinated reset neuromodulation," (ii) Tinnitus AND acoustic coordinated reset neuromodulation, (iii) Tinnitus AND acoustic CR neuromodulation, and (iv) Tinnitus and acoustic coordinated reset (CR) neuromodulation. MeSH terms were not available for either tinnitus or neuromodulation. The highest number of search results was found using search string (ii). None of the other search strings resulted in additional articles. The reference lists of articles identified by this search strategy were reviewed, and one article was considered relevant and selected (26). Trial registers were also searched. A complete list of searched resources is included in **Table 1**.

The present systematic review was intended to follow the PRISMA 2009 guideline. No case control studies could be found, and only one randomized controlled trial (RCT) was available. Therefore, with regards to inclusion and exclusion criteria no restrictions were placed on study design, sample size, or date of release. Study language was restricted to English, German, Danish, Norwegian, or Swedish. Unpublished data were excluded from the review. The intention was to evaluate all studies of patients suffering from subjective tonal tinnitus treated with acoustic CR neuromodulation. Hence, the *a posteriori* inclusion criteria for suitable articles were any original research article concerning tinnitus and acoustic CR neuromodulation, its effect, and/or mechanisms of action. All articles were read by all the three authors.

The following outcomes parameters were identified: visual analog scale (VAS) score (VAS-L: loudness and VAS-A: annoyance), Tinnitus Handicap Inventory, Tinnitus Questionnaire (TQ), Tinnitus Handicap Questionnaire (THQ), The World Health Organization Quality of Life-BREF, tinnitus frequency, spontaneous EEG analysis [including changes regarding connectivity and cross-frequency coupling (CFC) in the tinnitus network], tinnitus pitch change, Tinnitus Functional Index questionnaire, TQ (TBF-12), Global Clinical Improvement-Impression Scale (CGI-I7), and Numeric Rating Scale.

TABLE 1 | Resources searched in following databases.

Resources	No. hits
PubMed	14
Embase	18
Scopus	14
Web of Science	9
SveMed+	0
Cochrane	8
TRIP database	9
ProQuest	22
EBSCOhost	7
Biotechnology research abstract	1
BMJ journal	0
BIBSYS (Oria.no)	1
AMED alternative medicine	0
Others	
http://Clinicaltrials.gov	3
http://Controlled-trials.com	0
http://Clinicaltrialsregister.eu	0

RESULTS

A total of 8 publications were eligible for the review comprising a total of 329 patients in 3 main study populations (**Figure 2**). Details with regard to study population, design, and outcome measures are listed in **Table 2**. Due to the low number of studies, heterogeneous designs, overlap between study populations, and incomparability, each of the studies is commented in the following.

In 2012, Tass et al. published a computational study (27) where they illustrated the simplified neuronal model concept of CR anti-kindling and desynchronizing: an algorithm that was also applicable to the concept of non-invasive acoustic CR neuromodulation. In addition, they pointed to some important features of CR: (1) the pitches of the CR tones should be grouped around the patient-specific tinnitus frequency; (2) CR was effective no matter whether the CR stimulus was confined to the deafferentiated region (most effective) or if both the deafferentiated and non-deafferentiated regions were stimulated; and (3) an optimized spacing of the different CR tone pitches was present, neither too narrow, to ideally stimulate distinct subpopulations, nor too wide, to primarily affect the deafferentiated region. Acoustic CR stimulation requires sufficient hearing ability in the deafferentiated region, which can be achieved by hearing aids. The study suggested that acoustic CR neuromodulation may be a reliable method for the control of synchronization and abnormal interactions in affected neuronal populations.

Subsequently, in a single blind RCT (RESET study) (23), Tass et al. examined the safety and effects of acoustic CR neuromodulation in 63 patients with chronic tonal ST, randomly allocated into 5 different treatment arms (G1–G5). They found the intervention to be safe and well tolerated. Acoustic CR neuromodulation resulted in a significant reduction of tinnitus symptoms, as well as VAS loudness and annoyance, improvement in TQ severity levels, reduction in mean TQ scores, and a reduction of tinnitus frequency. Effects gained in 12 weeks of treatment persisted through a 4-week therapy pause. After a long-term extension period (24 weeks), already gained treatment effects were sustained or improved further. Placebo treatment (G5) did not lead to any significant changes in outcome measures. A comparison between groups revealed that CR therapy was more efficacious

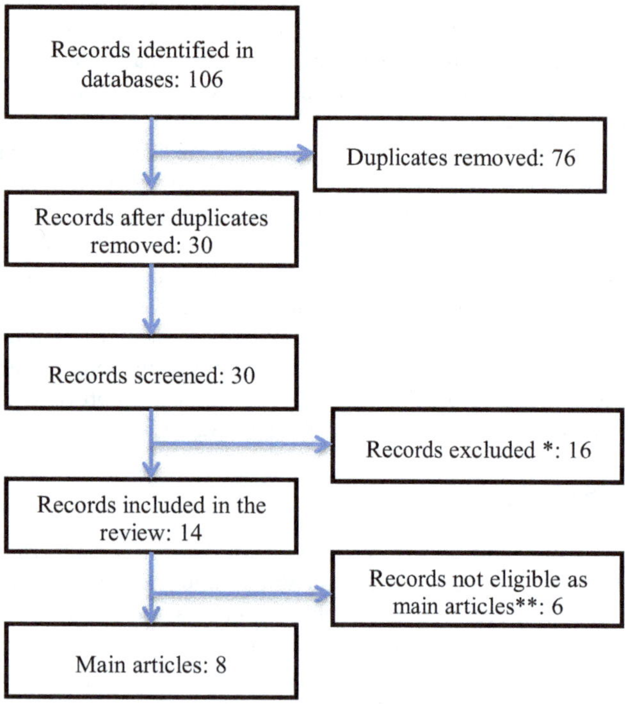

FIGURE 2 | Flowchart of the study selection. *Abstracts, conference–proceedings, reviews, editorials, dissertations and theses, and records not on subject. **Articles assessing endpoints, Hungarian article (language restrictions), not published data, and letters.

when used 4–6 h per day as opposed to 1 h per day. After 12 weeks of therapy, tinnitus associated EEG alterations were reversed. Pathologically elevated δ and γ activity were both decreased in the primary and secondary auditory cortex, as well as in frontal brain areas. Tinnitus-related reduction of α activity was reversed, leading to an enhancement in auditory and prefrontal areas. Thus, CR-induced neuronal changes comprised both auditory and non-auditory brain areas.

Based on existing data from 59 of the 63 patients from the RESET study, Adamchic et al. (28) found a significant correlation between the absolute value of the tinnitus pitch (frequency) change induced by acoustic neuromodulation, and absolute changes of VAS loudness and annoyance scores. The study also found that changes of brain synchrony patters, induced by CR neuromodulation, were associated with pitch change. These changes included the decreases in γ power and increases in α activity in distinctive brain regions, as well as alterations in functional connectivity in the γ frequency band between brain areas of this network. Brain areas found to be associated with these changes involved left temporal cortex, right and left frontal areas, the dorsolateral prefrontal region, and the anterior cingulate cortex. The study discovered that acoustic CR neuromodulation induced tinnitus pitch change, with a simultaneous reduction in tinnitus symptoms and positive changes in oscillatory brain activity.

In another evaluation of the data from the RESET study, Adamchic et al. (29) compared the EEG data from 28 patients with bilateral ST with the spontaneous EEG data from healthy controls. The study showed that acoustic CR neuromodulation shifted the abnormal brain activity associated with tinnitus toward physiological levels. Hence, in a group of "good responders" (TQ improvement >12 points), acoustic CR neuromodulation significantly normalized the patient's brain oscillations and even led to a complete abolishment of pathological power in several brain regions and frequency bands. These changes were significantly correlated with a reduction of tinnitus severity.

In 2013, using the same study population, Silchenko et al. (30) investigated if acoustic CR neuromodulation induced alterations of effective connectivity in the neuronal network underlying tinnitus perception. The effective connectivity in gamma, delta, and alpha frequency bands between brain areas comprising the primary auditory cortex, posterior cingulate cortex, dorsolateral prefrontal areas, and temporal areas were found to be significantly different in ST patients as opposed to healthy controls. When analyzing the types of interactions, they found a significant imbalance of excitation and inhibition in the tinnitus network of brain sources. Acoustic CR therapy significantly altered the strength of these connections so that they approached or even became indistinguishable to the healthy state network structure. Such restoration of effective connectivity was not seen in the group of non-responders.

To further investigate the communicative pathways within the tinnitus network, Adamchic et al. (31) performed a re-analysis of the existing dataset from the RESET study. They found that abnormal CFC[2] in tinnitus patients might coordinate tinnitus-relevant activity and thus provide effective communication between nodes of the tinnitus network. Reduction of tinnitus severity after acoustic CR stimulation led to a partial normalization of abnormal CFC. Treatment-induced tinnitus pitch change significantly modulated changes in CFC.

In 2015, Hauptmann et al. (26) published a prospective, non-randomized, non-controlled, multicenter, and clinical study with 200 chronic tinnitus patients. TQ "Tinnitus-Beeinträchtigungs-Fragebogen TBF12" (TBF-12) and CGI-I7 were used to study the safety and efficacy of acoustic CR neuromodulation. The treatment was found to be well tolerated and with no adverse events. Acoustic CR neuromodulation caused a statistically and clinically significant decrease in TBF-12 scores as well as in CGI-I7 after 12 months of therapy.

The same year, Williams et al. (32), published a clinical case study, where they described the quantitative treatment outcomes of patients undergoing acoustic CR neuromodulation. In line with the abovementioned clinical study, they showed a statistically and clinically significant improvement in tinnitus symptoms after 22–26 weeks of treatment, measured by VAS scores (loudness and annoyance) and THQ.

A protocol for a double-blind RCT study on the evaluation of acoustic CR neuromodulation was suggested by Hoare et al. (34). Although the behavioral results of the study have not been published, they are available on a trial

[2]Cross-frequency coupling (CFC) is a phenomenon proposed to coordinate neural dynamics across spatial and temporal scales (33).

TABLE 2 | Overview of the eight studies included in the review.

Reference, country	Study design	Sample	Outcome measures	Main results
Tass et al. (27), Germany	Computer analysis	None	Coordinated reset (CR) neuromodulation: model presentation illustrating the concept of CR in a simplified neuronal model, considering neurons with spike timing-dependent plasticity transformation of the concept of deep brain stimulation into non-invasive, acoustic CR stimulation	Non-invasive acoustic CR neuromodulation may be a novel therapy for tinnitus
Tass et al. (23), Germany	Prospective, randomized, single blind, placebo-controlled trial: RESET	63	Visual analog scale (VAS) Tinnitus Questionnaire (TQ) Tinnitus frequency Spontaneous EEG	CR neuromodulation caused a significant decrease of tinnitus loudness and symptoms, and reversed tinnitus-related EEG alterations
Adamchic et al. (28), Germany	Part of RESET	59	Tinnitus pitch change versus tinnitus loudness and/or annoyance (VAS score) Changes of brain synchrony induced by CR neuromodulation versus tinnitus pitch change	VAS scores significantly correlated with the absolute value of the CR neuromodulation-induced tinnitus pitch change ($r = 0.92$ baseline to 12 weeks, $p < 0.01$) Significant changes in brain activity were associated with a pronounced tinnitus pitch change
Adamchic et al. (29), Germany	Part of RESET	28	EEG pattern in the tinnitus patients after CR neuromodulation versus EEG pattern in healthy controls EEG in tinnitus patients before and after acoustic CR neuromodulation Relationship between CR neuromodulation-induced changes of different resting EEG parameters and tinnitus symptoms	Tinnitus patients significantly deviated from healthy controls concerning oscillatory brain activity CR neuromodulation significantly normalized patient's brain oscillations in all frequency bands CR neuromodulation-induced normalization of EEG power was significantly associated with reduction of tinnitus severity
Silchenko et al. (30), Germany	Part of RESET	28	Comparison of EEG in tinnitus patients before and after CR neuromodulation Comparison of EEG in tinnitus patients with healthy controls	CR neuromodulation significantly normalized both power and causal interactions within a tinnitus-related network CR neuromodulation specifically counteracted an imbalance of excitation and inhibition in tinnitus patients CR neuromodulation qualitatively changed the spectral response of the tinnitus network by modifying the shape of the averaged transfer function, so that the latter became similar to the control group
Adamchic et al. (31), Germany, USA	Re-analysis of existing dataset from RESET	59	To investigate how the oscillations in the various frequency bands interact	Identification of changes of cross-frequency coupling (CFC) Phase–amplitude CFC increased in tinnitus patients within the auditory cortex and the dorsolateral prefrontal regions between the phase of delta-theta and the amplitude of gamma oscillations Theta phase in the anterior cingulate region modulated gamma in the auditory and dorsolateral prefrontal regions
Hauptmann et al. (26), Germany, UK, USA	Prospective open-label, non-randomized, non-controlled multicenter clinical study	200 23 study centers	TQ (TBF-12) Global Clinical Improvement-Impression Scale (CGI-I7) Numeric Rating Scale (NRS) (0–100)	TBF-12 (total score) showed a mean reduction of 4.1 points (−37.9%) compared to baseline ($p < 0.01$) CGI-I7 revealed that 66.9% of the patients reported an improvement of tinnitus [very much improved (8.7%), much improved (25%), or slightly improved (33.2%)] ($p < 0.01$) Tinnitus-related loudness and annoyance were reduced by 11.1 points (18.9%) and 14.7 points (25.2%), respectively, compared to baseline ($p < 0.01$) on the NRS

(*Continued*)

TABLE 2 | Continued

Reference, country	Study design	Sample	Outcome measures	Main results
Williams et al. (32), UK, Germany	Clinical case study, open-label, non-randomized, non-controlled	66	Tinnitus Handicap Questionnaire (THQ) score	VAS scores were significantly improved: 25.8% mean reduction in tinnitus loudness, 32% mean reduction in tinnitus annoyance ($p < 0.01$ compared to baseline)
			VAS for tinnitus annoyance and loudness	A clinically significant reduction in tinnitus loudness and annoyance was recorded in 59.1 and 72.7% of the patient group, respectively THQ scores were significantly improved by an average of 19.4% ($p < 0.01$) 58.8% of patients experienced a clinically significant reduction in THQ score

outcomes website (https://clinicaltrials.gov/ct2/show/results/NCT01541969?sect=X0125#all). The efficacy of acoustic CR neuromodulation was compared to placebo (tinnitus masking), with crossover of the placebo group to receive the proprietary intervention. The study was completed on February 24, 2016. However, deviations from trial protocol and lack of compliance with the manufacturer's fitting instructions led to doubts about the validity of the results. Hence, results could not be published with evidence, and therefore, it was not included in the present review (35, 36).

DISCUSSION

This review was performed to provide a view over the existing evidence and use of acoustic CR neuromodulation in the treatment of ST. Overall, relatively few publications were found through the search, and the general evidence level was low except for a single RCT. The technique demands assessment of the specific tinnitus frequency and that the patient has (aided) hearing capacity within the given frequency area. A total of 329 patients with chronic tinnitus were included in basically 3 various study populations. Outcome measures were psycho-acoustic tests and EEG. The majority of the included patients reported reduction of tinnitus that was associated with EEG changes toward normalization. The method intends to counteract abnormal synchronization and connectivity through desynchronizing and anti-kindling effects. More specifically, acoustic CR neuromodulation induced pitch change and partially reversed abnormal CFC in a widespread tinnitus network comprising both auditory and non-auditory brain areas. However, several shortcomings of the studies impede generalization of the obtained results and the neurophysiological basis of the method may also be questioned (see below). Thus, the available evidence is insufficient for confident clinical implementation of acoustic CR neuromodulation as a treatment modality for tinnitus at the present moment.

We only identified 8 original reports about acoustic CR neuromodulation based on 3 different populations, i.e., a maximum of 329 patients. Different scopes of the studies, designs, and outcome parameters impede comparison between them as well as use of mutual quality and bias assessment methods. Moreover, many complicated statistical analyses were applied making it difficult to decipher and interpret the results and overall conclusions. Hence, PRISMA guidelines could not be followed in all aspects.

The same authors have generated most of the studies and articles, using the same populations. Independent replication of the positive pilot results is still lacking.

The proof-of-concept study performed by Tass et al. (23) was a RCT—a study design with the greatest evidential value. However, as also pointed out by Rücker and Antes in their reply (37) to Tass et al., the study had several shortcomings: a small number of participants, use of five treatment arms, and most importantly, the lack of direct comparison between the different treatment arms, which is the main idea of RCT studies. Besides baseline to post treatment comparisons within each treatment arm, no direct comparisons between groups were conducted. Tass et al. argued that the study showed quality features not often encountered in tinnitus research (38). A sample size calculation in order to ensure inclusion of sufficient numbers of participants in the different treatment schedules is recommended prior to such studies: the more subgroups, the more participants. A pilot study is also advantageous, for instance, to determine variation of the outcome measures.

In an additional analysis, different treatment arms were *post hoc* pooled and a comparison between an "effective" versus an "ineffective" group was performed. Such pooling results in loss of information and confounders are introduced due to use of different stimuli within the same group, and a false treatment effect may be the result (37, 39). And finally, the applied statistics were rather complex and unusual (e.g., Euclidean distance).

Clinical series or reports, such as the two clinical case studies (26, 32), are associated with a low level of evidence and the main reason is the absence of a control group. A clinical case study, such as the one conducted by Hauptman et al., is meant to consolidate the results from studies with higher level of evidence, e.g., RESET. With an intention to reinforce previously conducted studies, the risk of bias due to the desire for an effect can be comprised. It should also be mentioned that the use of fee-paying participants in the study by Williams et al. might have affected the results due to selection bias. Despite the low level of evidence, both Hauptman and Williams stated that acoustic CR neuromodulation caused a significant decrease of tinnitus. This trend was seen in different outcome measures.

The clinical case studies differ with respect to inclusion criteria, providing heterogeneous study populations. Future studies should be based on precise inclusion criteria to make them more homogenous. This includes consensus regarding the definition of chronic tinnitus, inclusion of both unilateral and bilateral cases, hearing thresholds, etc. Information about confounding factors such as age, psychiatric disorders, medication, and previously received tinnitus therapy should be addressed. Consensus regarding exclusion criteria is important as well. And finally, use of the same reliable and valid outcome measures in different studies is mandatory for comparing results, e.g., VAS and TQ scores (40, 41).

The fundamental challenge in tinnitus research goes far beyond the abovementioned problems with clinical designs and choice of outcome measures because we still know only little about the underlying pathophysiology. As a consequence hereof, the optimal objective parameters are chosen more or less in the dark, whether EEG or other neuroimaging techniques. In an opinion article by Elgoyhen et al. (42), they critically assessed the results of recent neuroimaging studies of ST. The authors concluded that neuroimaging results are highly variable, but interpretation of available data indicates ST to follow auditory deafferentiation leading to lack of sensory information. Elgoyhen et al. suggested that increased activity in auditory pathways could explain the perception of the sound itself, maybe permitted or facilitated by interactions or communication with non-auditory brain areas. The relevance of cortical map reorganization as the cause of tinnitus was questioned, and the authors pointed out that the apparent distortion of the tonotopic map associated with tinnitus may merely be a compensatory response and not the cause of tinnitus. If so, cortical reorganization becomes less relevant to understanding the mechanisms eliciting the perception of phantom sounds and questions the theoretical basis of acoustic CR neuromodulation. In the light of the suggestions by Elgoyhen et al., the obvious questions are: what do the apparent findings in the reviewed reports represent and what is the background for them? Can listening to series of tones be able to interfere with a complex brain disorder involving several brain structures and functions like tinnitus? Regardless of the physiological mechanisms, the RESET study had limitations in design.

Future studies of acoustic CR neuromodulation should comprise RCTs with strict inclusion and exclusion criteria and using several neuroimaging techniques.

CONCLUSION

Acoustic CR neuromodulation has been introduced as a novel treatment for ST. The current evidence level is low, and the assumed underlying physiological mechanisms have been questioned. Therefore, further studies are needed before the method can be recommended as a tinnitus treatment modality.

DEFINITIONS (22)

Phase reset (43) – Phase resetting in neurons is when the dynamical behavior of an oscillation is shifted. This occurs when a stimulus perturbs the phase within an oscillatory cycle and a change in period occurs.

Synchrony – The relation that exists when things occur at the same time, e.g., when neurons fire simultaneously.

Desynchronization – The reverse of or absence of synchrony. Initially synchronized oscillating (fluctuating) systems desynchronize as parameters (existing conditions) changes, or might do so under influence of external stimulation.

Anti-kindling – Unlearning of pathologically strong interactions and/or connectivity of neural networks. The intention is to approach or even regain physiological activity.

Spike timing-dependent plasticity (STDP) (44) – A process by which neurons continuously regulate the strength of their synaptic connections. The neurons adjust the connection strengths based on the relative timing of a particular neuron's firing (or spikes).

Multistability (45) – Multistability is the characteristic of a system that presents two or more mutually exclusive stable states (attractors) for a given set of parameters or conditions. If a system has multiple coexisting attractors and stimulus is sufficiently strong to cause switching among stable states, it may be said to be multistable.

AUTHOR CONTRIBUTIONS

MW: design, data analysis, drafting, acquisition of data final approval, and responsibility for content of manuscript. TO and DL: data analysis, critically revision, final approval, and responsibility for content of manuscript.

REFERENCES

Eggermont JJ, Roberts LE. The neuroscience of tinnitus. *Trends Neurosci* (2004) 27(11):676–82. doi:10.1016/j.tins.2004.08.010

Eggermont JJ, Tass PA. Maladaptive neural synchrony in tinnitus: origin and restoration. *Front Neurol* (2015) 6:29. doi:10.3389/fneur.2015.00029

Hall DA, Láinez MJ, Newman CW, Sanchez TG, Egler M, Tennigkeit F, et al. Treatment options for subjective tinnitus: self reports from a sample of general practitioners and ENT physicians within Europe and the USA. *BMC Health Serv Res* (2011) 11:302. doi:10.1186/1472-6963-11-302

Axelsson A, Prasher D. Tinnitus induced by occupational and leisure noise. *Noise Health* (2000) 2(8):47–54.

Noreña AJ. Revisiting the cochlear and central mechanisms of tinnitus and therapeutic approaches. *Audiol Neurotol* (2015) 20(1):53–9. doi:10.1159/000380749

Baguley D, McFerran D, Hall D. Tinnitus. *Lancet* (2013) 382(9904):1600–7. doi:10.1016/S0140-6736(13)60142-7

Jastreboff PJ. Phantom auditory perception (tinnitus): mechanisms of generation and perception. *Neurosci Res* (1990) 8(4):221–54. doi:10.1016/0168-0102(90)90031-9

Kemp DT. Stimulated acoustic emissions from within the human auditory system. *J Acoust Soc Am* (1978) 64(5):1386–91. doi:10.1121/1.382104

Kaltenbach JA, Zhang J, Finlayson P. Tinnitus as a plastic phenomenon and its possible neural underpinnings in the dorsal cochlear nucleus. *Hear Res* (2005) 206(1–2):200–26. doi:10.1016/j.heares.2005.02.013

Kaltenbach JA. The dorsal cochlear nucleus as a contributor to tinnitus: mechanisms underlying the induction of hyperactivity. *Prog Brain Res* (2007) 166:89–106. doi:10.1016/S0079-6123(07)66009-9

Levine RA. Somatic (craniocervical) tinnitus and the dorsal cochlear nucleus hypothesis. *Am J Otolaryngol* (1999) 20(6):351–62. doi:10.1016/ S0196-0709(99)90074-1

Noreña AJ, Eggermont JJ. Changes in spontaneous neural activity imme- diately after an acoustic trauma: implications for neural correlates of tinnitus. *Hear Res* (2003) 183(1–2):137–53. doi:10.1016/S0378-5955(03) 00225-9

Kaltenbach JA. Summary of evidence pointing to a role of the dorsal cochlear nucleus in the etiology of tinnitus. *Acta Otolaryngol Suppl* (2006) (556):20–6. doi:10.1080/03655230600895309

Hoare D, Sereda M, Adjamian P, Hall D. Recent technological advances in sound-based approaches to tinnitus treatment: a review of efficacy considered against putative physiological mechanisms. *Noise Health* (2013) 15(63):107. doi:10.4103/1463-1741.110292

Eggermont JJ, Roberts LE. The neuroscience of tinnitus: understanding abnormal and normal auditory perception. *Front Syst Neurosci* (2012) 6:53. doi:10.3389/fnsys.2012.00053

Hoare DJ, Searchfield GD, Refaie AE, Henry JA. Sound therapy for tinnitus management: practicable options. *J Am Acad Audiol* (2014) 30(1):62–75. doi:10.3766/jaaa.25.1.5

Tass PA, Silchenko AN, Hauptmann C, Barnikol UB, Speckmann E-J. Long-lasting desynchronization in rat hippocampal slice induced by coordinated reset stimulation. *Phys Rev E Stat Nonlin Soft Matter Phys* (2009) 80(1):11902. doi:10.1103/PhysRevE.80.011902

Tass PA, Qin L, Hauptmann C, Dovero S, Bezard E, Boraud T, et al. Coordinated reset has sustained aftereffects in parkinsonian monkeys. *Ann Neurol* (2012) 72(5):816–20. doi:10.1002/ana.23663

Adamchic I, Hauptmann C, Barnikol UB, Pawelczyk N, Popovych O, Barnikol TT, et al. Coordinated reset neuromodulation for Parkinson's disease: proof- of-concept study. *Mov Disord* (2014) 29(13):1679–84. doi:10.1002/mds.25923

Tass PA. A model of desynchronizing deep brain stimulation with a demand-controlled coordinated reset of neural subpopulations. *Biol Cybern* (2003) 89(2):81–8. doi:10.1007/s00422-003-0425-7

Tass PA, Majtanik M. Long-term anti-kindling effects of desynchronizing brain stimulation: a theoretical study. *Biol Cybern* (2006) 94(1):58–66. doi:10.1007/s00422-005-0028-6

Popovych OV, Tass PA. Control of abnormal synchronization in neurological disorders. *Front Neurol* (2014) 5:268. doi:10.3389/fneur.2014.00268

Tass PA, Adamchic I, Freund HJ, Von Stackelberg T, Hauptmann C. Counteracting tinnitus by acoustic coordinated reset neuromodulation. *Restor Neurol Neurosci* (2012) 30(2):137–59. doi:10.3233/RNN-2012-110218

Lysyansky B, Popovych OV, Tass PA. Desynchronizing anti-resonance effect of m: n ON–OFF coordinated reset stimulation. *J Neural Eng* (2011) 8(3):36019. doi:10.1088/1741-2560/8/3/036019

Chittka L, Brockmann A. Perception space—the final Frontier. *PLoS Biol* (2005) 3(4):e137. doi:10.1371/journal.pbio.0030137

Hauptmann C, Ströbel A, Williams M, Patel N, Wurzer H, von Stackelberg T, et al. Acoustic coordinated reset neuromodulation in a real life patient population with chronic tonal tinnitus. *Biomed Res Int* (2015) 2015:569052. doi:10.1155/2015/569052

Tass PA, Popovych OV. Unlearning tinnitus-related cerebral synchrony with acoustic coordinated reset stimulation: theoretical concept and modelling. *Biol Cybern* (2012) 106(1):27–36. doi:10.1007/s00422-012-0479-5

Adamchic I, Hauptmann C, Tass PA. Changes of oscillatory activity in pitch processing network and related tinnitus relief induced by acoustic CR neuromodulation. *Front Syst Neurosci* (2012) 6:18. doi:10.3389/fnsys.2012.00018

Adamchic I, Toth T, Hauptmann C, Tass PA. Reversing pathologically increased EEG power by acoustic coordinated reset neuromodulation. *Hum Brain Mapp* (2014) 35(5):2099–118. doi:10.1002/hbm.22314

Silchenko AN, Adamchic I, Hauptmann C, Tass PA. Impact of acoustic coordinated reset neuromodulation on effective connectivity in a neural network of phantom sound. *Neuroimage* (2013) 77:133–47. doi:10.1016/j.neuroimage.2013.03.013

Adamchic I, Langguth B, Hauptmann C, Tass PA. Abnormal cross-frequency coupling in the tinnitus network. *Front Neurosci* (2014) 8:284. doi:10.3389/fnins.2014.00284

Williams M, Hauptmann C, Nitesh P. Acoustic CR neuromodulation therapy for subjective tonal tinnitus: a review of clinical outcomes in an independent audiology practice setting. *Front Neurol* (2015) 6:54. doi:10.3389/fneur.2015.00054

Aru J, Aru J, Priesemann V, Wibral M, Lana L, Pipa G, et al. Untangling cross-frequency coupling in neuroscience. *Curr Opin Neurobiol* (2015) 31:51–61. doi:10.1016/j.conb.2014.08.002

Hoare DJ, Pierzycki RH, Thomas H, McAlpine D, Hall DA. Evaluation of the acoustic coordinated reset (CR®) neuromodulation therapy for tinnitus: study protocol for a double-blind randomized placebo-controlled trial. *Trials* (2013) 14(1):207. doi:10.1186/1745-6215-14-207

Hoare DJ, Pierzycki RH, Thomas H, Hall DA. *Evaluation of the CR Neuromodulation Treatment for Tinnitus – Study Results – ClinicalTrials.* (2015). Available from: https://clinicaltrials.gov/ct2/show/results/NCT01541969?sect=X01256#all

Hall DA, Hoare DJ, Pierzycki RH, et al. *59257caf5076ef0653477c-5964fa1512e468b0e8.* (2015). Available from: www.hearing.nihr.ac.uk; http://www.hearing.nihr.ac.uk/research/a-systematic-evaluation-of-the-acoustic-cr-neuromodulation-treatment-for-ti/

Rücker G, Antes G. Reply to Tass et al. on "Counteracting tinnitus by acoustic coordinated reset neuromodulation". *Restor Neurol Neurosci* (2012) 30(2); *Restor Neurol Neurosci* (2013) 31(3):235–7. doi:10.3233/RNN-121123

Tass PA, Adamchic I, Freund H-J, von Stackelberg T, Hauptmann C. Rebuttal to reply by G. Rücker and G. Antes on Tass et al. "Counteracting tinnitus by acoustic coordinated reset neuromodulation". *Restor Neurol Neurosci* (2012) 30(2); *Restor Neurol Neurosci* (2013) 31(3):235–7. doi:10.3233/RNN-121123

Senn S, Julious S. Measurement in clinical trials: a neglected issue for statisticians? *Stat Med* (2009) 28(26):3189–209. doi:10.1002/sim.3603

Adamchic I, Langguth B. Psychometric evaluation of Visual Analog Scale for the assessment of chronic tinnitus. *Am J Audiol* (2012) 21:215–26. doi:10.1044/1059-0889(2012/12-0010)impairment

Adamchic I, Tass PA, Langguth B, Hauptmann C, Koller M, Schecklmann M, et al. Linking the Tinnitus Questionnaire and the subjective Clinical Global Impression: which differences are clinically important? *Health Qual Life Outcomes* (2012) 10(1):79. doi:10.1186/1477-7525-10-79

Elgoyhen AB, Langguth B, De Ridder D, Vanneste S. Tinnitus: perspectives from human neuroimaging. *Nat Rev Neurosci* (2015) 16(10):632–42. doi:10.1038/nrn4003

Krogh-Madsen T, Butera R, Ermentrout GB, Glass L. Chapter 2: Phase resetting neural oscillators: topological theory versus the realworld. In: Schultheiss NW, Prinz AA, Butera RJ, editors. *Phase Response Curves in Neuroscience, Theory, Experience End Analysis*. Vol. 6. New York: Springer New York (2012).

Markram H, Gerstner W, Sjöström PJ. Spike-timing-dependent plasticity: a comprehensive overview. *Front Synaptic Neurosci* (2012) 4:2. doi:10.3389/fnsyn.2012.00002

Kelso JAS. Multistability and metastability: understanding dynamic coordination in the brain. *Philos Trans R Soc Lond B Biol Sci* (2012) 367:906–18. doi:10.1098/rstb.2011.0351

8

Visualization of Global Disease Burden for the Optimization of Patient Management and Treatment

*Winfried Schlee[1], Deborah A. Hall[2,3], Niklas K. Edvall[4], Berthold Langguth[1], Barbara Canlon[4] and Christopher R. Cederroth[4]**

[1] Department for Psychiatry and Psychotherapy, University Hospital Regensburg, Regensburg, Germany, [2] National Institute for Health Research (NIHR) Nottingham Biomedical Research Centre, Nottingham, United Kingdom, [3] Otology and Hearing Group, Division of Clinical Neuroscience, School of Medicine, University of Nottingham, Nottingham, United Kingdom, [4] Experimental Audiology, Department of Physiology and Pharmacology, Karolinska Institutet, Stockholm, Sweden

***Correspondence:**
Christopher R. Cederroth
christopher.cederroth@ki.se

Background: The assessment and treatment of complex disorders is challenged by the multiple domains and instruments used to evaluate clinical outcome. With the large number of assessment tools typically used in complex disorders comes the challenge of obtaining an integrative view of disease status to further evaluate treatment outcome both at the individual level and at the group level. Radar plots appear as an attractive visual tool to display multivariate data on a two-dimensional graphical illustration. Here, we describe the use of radar plots for the visualization of disease characteristics applied in the context of tinnitus, a complex and heterogeneous condition, the treatment of which has shown mixed success.

Methods: Data from two different cohorts, the Swedish Tinnitus Outreach Project (STOP) and the Tinnitus Research Initiative (TRI) database, were used. STOP is a population-based cohort where cross-sectional data from 1,223 non-tinnitus and 933 tinnitus subjects were analyzed. By contrast, the TRI contained data from 571 patients who underwent various treatments and whose Clinical Global Impression (CGI) score was accessible to infer treatment outcome. In the latter, 34,560 permutations were tested to evaluate whether a particular ordering of the instruments could reflect better the treatment outcome measured with the CGI.

Results: Radar plots confirmed that tinnitus subtypes such as occasional and chronic tinnitus from the STOP cohort could be strikingly different, and helped appreciate a gender bias in tinnitus severity. Radar plots with greater surface areas were consistent with greater burden, and enabled a rapid appreciation of the global distress associated with tinnitus in patients categorized according to tinnitus severity. Permutations in the arrangement of instruments allowed to identify a configuration with minimal variance and maximized surface difference between CGI groups from the TRI database, thus affording a means of optimally evaluating the outcomes in individual patients.

Conclusion: We anticipate such a tool to become a starting point for more sophisticated measures in clinical outcomes, applicable not only in the context of tinnitus but also in other complex diseases where the integration of multiple variables is needed for a comprehensive evaluation of treatment response.

Keywords: diagnostic tests, patient management, value-based decision-making, treatment outcome, disease progression, treatment response, subtyping, gender differences

INTRODUCTION

Complex health-care conditions can be characterized by a combination of identified and unidentified etiological factors including genetics, environment, and lifestyle (1). Among them are found Alzheimer's disease, schizophrenia, scleroderma, asthma, Parkinson's disease, multiple sclerosis, and osteoporosis. Phenotypic heterogeneity in the expression of etiological factors adds complexity to clinical assessment and management and can underlie a mixed response to the same management strategy. Indeed, a new area of research has emerged to characterize complex disorders as profiles that possess a defined set of characteristics (2). Identifying important parameters for patient profiling is a challenging task, yet it is an important step toward being able to provide personalized treatment and would support efforts to develop new treatments. However, in many complex health-care conditions, this has been hard to achieve. Tinnitus is one such example, with a wide range of problems experienced by those who suffer from this condition (3, 4). Tinnitus is defined as the phantom perception of sounds in the absence of any external stimulus. Diagnosis primarily relies on self-report, yet because the impact of tinnitus can be so varied from one patient to another, how it is best treated in individuals is still unclear (5). For example, some patients can complain primarily from sleeping problems (6), or from impaired cognitive function (7, 8) or from communication disabilities (9). Tinnitus is a highly unmet clinical need and there are still no singularly effective therapies that reliably reduce tinnitus percept or its symptoms (10–13). Inter-subject variability in the severity of different tinnitus complaints at diagnostic assessment and at outcome assessment of treatment-related response poses challenges for clinical research. Researchers would benefit from being able to build up an overall picture of the different independent components (or domains) of this complex condition, in order to meaningfully capture key discriminative features between individuals or treatment-related differences.

Based on the tinnitus psychological model of Dauman and Tyler that clearly distinguishes the mechanisms of tinnitus from the reactions to tinnitus (14), the use of multiple measurement instruments has been proposed to address the challenges in quantifying the different aspects of tinnitus (15, 16). However, different laboratories deal with these measures in various ways. One option is the presentation of scores for each measurement instrument. The rationale of this approach is that even if most of these measurements correlate with each other, they assess slightly different aspects of an individual's tinnitus (17, 18). A further option is the use of statistical methods (namely Principal Components Analysis) to tease apart independent components of the condition in a data-driven way (19). Tyler and colleagues also suggested focusing only on areas that show an impact (20, 21). However, whereas this approach might be useful in clinical practice where a dominant problematic has been found in an individual patient and justifies a primary focus, this should be avoided when performing clinical trials. Indeed, more than a hundred instruments have been used as primary outcome measures in tinnitus clinical trials, which hampers the synthesis of existing evidence (e.g., with meta-analyses) and the delivering of conclusive guidelines for clinical care (22). In order to avoid the random selection of instruments in tinnitus studies and facilitate the comparison and synthesis of clinical data, an approach has been proposed as part of the COMiT initiative (Core Outcome Measures in Tinnitus), which aims to establish an international standard for outcome measurements in clinical trials of tinnitus (23). This approach still uses multiple measurement instruments, but their selection is informed by first identifying in a consensus-manner which tinnitus-related complaints are judged to be the most important ones from the perspective of assessing whether a treatment has been beneficial or not, and then identifying one measurement instrument to assess each relevant complaint (23). This approach thus seeks to tease apart independent components of the condition in a hypothesis-driven way. Independent of which approach is taken, they all require the presentation of multiple measures simultaneously for an individual or group. A graphical visualization approach would facilitate the rapid interpretation and would be more attractive to clinicians and patients than a numerical presentation style. How best to visualize this multiplicity of data and to integrate the complex data patterns into a single clinical interpretation is a challenge that is shared across all approaches described above and that is relevant for many complex disorders.

Any aggregated visualization of data relating to a complex health-care condition should meet a number of requirements to facilitate clinic usage: (i) it should be possible to display measures with different scales (interval, ordinal, etc.), (ii) it should be possible to display individual and group data, with SDs if relevant, (iii) it should be visually appealing, (iv) it should be easy to interpret, and (v) it should be able to represent pre- and post-intervention data.

Here, we introduce a method for the holistic representation of components of health status relevant to a complex multi-attribute condition based on radar plots. Radar plots allow the representation of multivariate data on a two-dimensional graphical illustration and have been suggested as a useful approach for the visualization of multivariate clinical data (24). By selecting tinnitus as a model, we illustrate the usefulness of using radar plots to give a holistic representation of multiple variables used in the assessment of tinnitus. In a first aim, we assess the performance of the radar plots in conveying an ensemble of clinical data from the Swedish Tinnitus Outreach Project (STOP) cohort. In a second aim, we evaluate the performance of the various instruments working together to provide a meaningful overview of treatment outcome using data from the Tinnitus Research Initiative (TRI) database. We propose that this methodology can be applied to any complex clinical disorder where multiple assessment tools are used, for single subjects or group data, cross-sectional or longitudinal data.

METHODS

Participants

Data are reported from two datasets. The first dataset comes from the STOP recruiting participants with or without tinnitus from the Swedish population[1] and the second dataset comes from the TRI database.[2] STOP is a nationwide population cohort with the aims

[1] http://stop.ki.se.

[2] www.tinnitus-database.de.

of identifying tinnitus biomarkers. Free-willing registration was done on a website and after participants provided their informed consent, they were invited to fill an online survey (25). The project was approved by the local ethics committee "Regionala etikprövningsnämnden" in Stockholm (#2014/1998-31/4). The database project and server are coordinated and located at the Department of Physiology and Pharmacology of the Karolinska Institutet, Sweden. For this study, a first cross-sectional set of data collected until the 11th of October 2016 included 311 occasional and 328 constant tinnitus subjects. A second cross-sectional set of data was extracted on the 5th of December 2016. That dataset included 1,223 non-tinnitus control subjects and added 294 constant tinnitus subjects. The socio-demographics of the current STOP dataset are presented in Table S1 in Supplementary Material.The second dataset comes from the TRI database (26). and includes 571 individuals who participated in any clinical treatment study at the University Hospital Regensburg, Germany and had consented to reuse of their anonymized data to address new research questions (34.5% female, 65.5% male, age distribution: 17–87 years, mean age ± SD: 52.3 ± 12.2 years). Collection of data for the TRI database was approved by the Ethics Committee of the University of Regensburg, Germany (#08/046).

Selection of Outcome Domains and Measurement Instruments

A range of health domains were assessed using investigator-administered tests and patient-reported questionnaires. Collectively, they provide an overall clinical impression of global health burden. All domains and associated instruments have been identified from a review of clinical trials of tinnitus treatments in adults (22).

STOP Cohort

In the STOP cohort, 5 domains of tinnitus and associated comorbidities (psychological distress, tinnitus-related worries and fears, emotional affects, hyperacusis, and quality of life) were measured by 14 separate tinnitus instruments, in which adaptation to Swedish was validated in a previous study (25). In a pilot study, of which two subjects are shown in **Figure 1**, auditory values were included as an additional measure of hearing loss. The Tinnitus Handicap Inventory (THI) (27, 28) was used to measure tinnitus-related psychological distress. Participants rated each of the 25 items on a categorical 3-point scale ("yes" = 4/"sometimes" = 2/"no" = 0). The mean global score reflects the sum of all responses with a maximum score of 100 indicating the greatest impact on everyday function. For the purposes of analysis, the THI global score was used since it is considered a unidimensional measure (29). The THI cutoffs were defined previously (30) and are split in five different categories from slight (0–16), mild (18–36), moderate (38–56), severe (58–76), and catastrophic (78–100). For sake of clarity and the rapid interpretation of severity, we combined light and moderate together as well as severe and catastrophic. In the radar plots, three colors helped classifying severity: green (negligible), orange (light/moderate), and red (severe/catastrophic). Three Numerical Rating Scales were taken from the Tinnitus Sample Case History Questionnaire (26). One measured tinnitus loudness (Lo): "Describe the loudness of your tinnitus using a

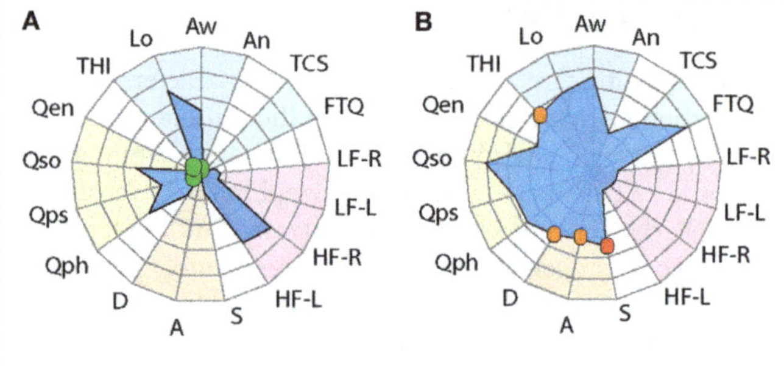

FIGURE 1 | Radar plot profiling for characterizing global health burden in individuals with constant tinnitus. Two tinnitus cases are represented in the radar plots. **(A)** A 72-year-old male subject with high loudness and awareness values displays high-frequency hearing loss but little tinnitus-associated burden. **(B)** A 31-year-old male subject with no hearing loss shows high loudness and awareness scores but with mild/moderate THI scores, moderate depression and anxiety, and severe stress scores. Domains of tinnitus-related burden are grouped in the dark blue region, hearing loss comorbidities in light blue, emotional comorbidities in orange region, and health-related quality of life in yellow. Instruments are labeled as follows: THI, tinnitus-related psychological distress; Lo, tinnitus loudness; Aw, tinnitus awareness; An, tinnitus annoyance; TCS, tinnitus catastrophizing; FTQ, tinnitus fears; LF, low frequency hearing in the left (-L) and right (-R) ears; HF, high-frequency hearing in the left (-L) and right (-R) ears; S, stress; A, anxiety; D, depression scores; Qph, Quality of Life for physical; Qps, psychological, Qso, social; Qen, environment. Color dots illustrate the severity score of those instruments with published severity category boundaries: negligible (green), moderate (orange), and severe (red).

scale from 1 (very faint) to 100 (very loud)." One measured tinnitus awareness (Aw): "What percent of your total awake time, over the last month, have you been aware of your tinnitus?" The third measured tinnitus annoyance (An): "What percent of your total awake time, over the last month, have you been annoyed, distressed, or irritated of your tinnitus?"

The Fear of Tinnitus Questionnaire measures the worries and fears of patients experiencing tinnitus [FTQ; (31)]. There are 17 items that are rated on a true or false scale. A greater score indicates more extreme fear. Catastrophic cognitive misinterpretations of tinnitus sounds were measured by the Tinnitus Catastrophizing Scale [TCS; (31)]. This is an adapted version of the Pain Catastrophizing Scale in which the word "pain" was substituted by the word "tinnitus" (32). There are 13 items, in which participants indicated the extent to which each statement applies to them using a 5-point scale ("always" = 4 to "not at all" = 0). A greater score indicates more extreme perceptions. TCS has a unidimensional structure and the global score was used (31).

Five important comorbidities are anxiety, depression, stress, hearing loss, and hyperacusis. Measurement instruments for each domain are described as follows: anxiety and depression were measured by the Hospital Anxiety and Depression Scale [HADS; (33)]. HADS comprises 7 items on anxiety (A) and 7 items on depression (D), with each item scored from 0 to 3. Higher scores indicate greater severity, with the maximum score being 21. The HADS cutoffs were defined previously by Zigmond and Snaith (33) and are split in three different categories from normal (0–7, shown in green), borderline (8–10, shown in orange), and abnormal (11–21, shown in red). The Perceived Stress Questionnaire assesses chronic and acute relationships with stressful events and activities [PSQ-30; (34)]. Thirty items are answered using a 4-point scale, from "almost always" = 4 to "almost never" = 1. The sum of the answers is substracted by 30 and the resulting value is divided by 90, yielding a score between 0.0 and 1.0. Higher scores indicate more severe perceived stress. There is no consensus about the factor structure of the PSQ-30 (34, 35) and so here we used the global score, not any subscale scores. The PSQ-30 cutoffs were defined previously by Levenstein et al. (34, 35) and are split in three different categories from low stress level (<0.34, shown in green), moderate stress level (0.34–0.46, shown in orange), and high stress level (>0.46, shown in red).

Hyperacusis is defined as sound intensities that others would find normal, but are experienced as intolerably loud by affected individuals. This marked intolerance to everyday environmental sounds happens even at moderate levels, in spite of quite often normal hearing thresholds. We measured the condition using the Hyperacusis Questionnaire [HQ; (36)]. The second part of the questionnaire comprises 14 negatively worded items, which are rated on a 4-point scale ("yes, a lot" = 3 to "no" = 0). The total provides the measure of hypersensitivity to sound with higher scores indicating greater sensitivity. The maximum global score is 42 and a global score greater than 28 indicates clinically significant hyperacusis (shown in red), while a global score equal to or less than 28 indicates a negligible problem (shown in green). Again there is no consensus about the factor structure of the HQ (36, 37) and so here we used the global score, not any subscale scores.

For the two tinnitus cases presented in **Figure 1**, hearing loss was reported separately for both low and high frequencies. Hearing was assessed by fixed frequency Bekesy audiometry using a Madsen Astera 2 audiometer and Sennheiser HDA 200 headphone at standard and high audiometric frequencies. Hearing thresholds reported in dB HL (hearing level) were averaged from 0.125 to 6 kHz for lower frequencies. High-frequency thresholds were averaged for frequencies between 8 and 16 kHz. Thresholds were reported separately for left and right ears.

Four domains of health-related quality of life formed the last set of measures [physical health (Qph), psychological (Qps), social relationships (Qso), and environment (Qen)]. We used the WHOQOL-BREF which is a 26-item questionnaire providing a broad reliable measurement with four validated subscale scores (38). Each item has a range of 1–5 and the four domain scores are scaled in a positive direction with higher scores indicating a more positive quality of life. The items on the quality of life must be reversed before scoring.

TRI Database

For the assessment of tinnitus within cases from the TRI database, the WHOQoL-BREF, THI, and five numeric rating scales (0–10) were used (26). Numeric rating scales refer to tinnitus loudness ("How STRONG or LOUD is your tinnitus at present?" Tlou), tinnitus annoyance ("How ANNOYING is your tinnitus at present?" Tann), ability to ignore tinnitus ("How easy is it for you to IGNORE your tinnitus at present?" Tign), tinnitus unpleasantness ("How UNPLEASANT is your tinnitus at present?" Tunp), and the uncomfortable aspect of tinnitus ("How UNCOMFORTABLE is your tinnitus at present, if everything around you is quiet?" Tunc).

For assessing perceived treatment-related change, an additional measure was the Clinical Global Impression (CGI) scale (39). This is a single question asked at the end of treatment and requires the patient to give an overall rating of his/her current state compared to the pretreatment baseline. The response is scored on a 7-point scale ("very much better" = 1; "much better" = 2; "minimally better" = 3; "no change" = 4; "minimally worse" = 5; "much worse" = 6; "very much worse" = 7).

Designing the Visualization

A radar plot displays multivariate data in two dimensions. The radar plot comprises a sequence of equi-angular spokes (radii), with each spoke representing one of the measures. The data length of a spoke is proportional to the magnitude of the measurement score, from minimum at the center to maximum at the circumference. A line can then be drawn connecting the data values for each spoke. This gives the plot a star-like appearance and a quantifiable surface area. A patient with high scores across multiple measures is represented by a large surface area (high burden) and conversely a patient with low scores is represented by a small surface area. Evaluation of overall burden takes into account the shape of the radar plot and the size of the plot to address in which domains there are greatest burden experienced. When plots contained two average datasets such as for comparisons of gender or treatment, colors such as blue for men and pink for women, or yellow for pretreatment and orange for posttreatment, were used. Several forms of color coding can be used to facilitate the visualization of the data. Observers do not require any specialized knowledge of the measurement instruments to make an overall judgment about the patient profile. Its interpretation is intuitive. Nevertheless, to support the interpretation of those instruments with published severity category boundaries, we represented negligible problem in green, mild/moderate problems in orange, and severe problems in red. This novel feature of the graphical representation helps the observer to rapidly determine individual burden.

For the STOP dataset, five domains were considered including (i) tinnitus severity (assessed by four instruments, blue background), (ii) tinnitus-related fears (assessed with two questionnaires, light blue background), (iii) hyperacusis (measured with one questionnaire, shown in purple), (iv) emotional comorbidities (assessed by two instruments, orange background), and (v) health-related quality of life (assessed with one questionnaire, yellow background). All scores were adjusted to the same minimum–maximum scale of 0–100. For the TCS, FTQ, and HADS, this was done calculating the percentage of the maximum score (total score/maximum score × 100). The PSQ with a maximum score between 0 and 1 was multiplied by 100. The THI and Numerical rating scales all result in a score between 0 and 100 and were left unmodified. Since the WHOQoL-BREF has higher scores with better life quality, we inversed the scale (100 total score) so that the interpretation of the 0–100 scale was consistent across all measurement instruments. The score from the WHOQoL-BREF was translated into a 0–100 score using the method provided in the WHOQoL user manual using the formula: TRANSFORMED SCORE = (SCORE-4) × (100/16). A value of 100 corresponds to greater severity of negative symptoms. Average hearing threshold values were obtained only in the individual examples and were left unmodified as the range from 0 dB HL (normal hearing) to >90 dB HL (profound) covers the full range of expected hearing loss (40). For the TRI dataset, a smaller number of domains were available between baseline and follow-up and thus consisted of (i) health-related quality of life (measured with the WHOQoL-BREF), (ii) the tinnitus-related psychological distress (assessed with the THI), and (iii) the individual aspects of tinnitus assessed by the five numeric rating scales.

Statistical Methods

95% confidence intervals were obtained according to the formula: Z*std/sqrt(n). Group differences were tested by a two-way ANOVA, and multiple comparison tests were mentioned in the legends (Prism version 4.0, GraphPad software). Differences were considered significant if $p < 0.05$.

RESULTS

During a pilot study from the STOP, two tinnitus cases were identified that displayed strikingly different tinnitus-associated burden (**Figure 1**). While both cases displayed relatively high tinnitus loudness and awareness, their radar plot profile indicated a different health burden. Since the THI, the HADS, and the PSQ-30 contain cutoffs for different degrees of severity, these were marked with a color label to grade negligible (green), moderate (orange), or severe (red) scores. A blue surface was used to specify the male gender. A 72-year-old male has a comorbid high-frequency hearing loss, but low scores on tinnitus-related psychological distress (THI), negligible stress (S), anxiety (A), or depression (D) and good quality of life (Qph, Qps, Qso, and Qen) (**Figure 1A**). By contrast, another male, 31 years old, shows good hearing, mild/moderate tinnitus-related psychological distress (THI), moderate stress (S) and anxiety (A), severe depression (D), and poorer quality of life (Qph, Qps, Qso, and Qen) (**Figure 1B**). These two examples capture distinct tinnitus-associated burden across individuals. Based on these findings, we utilized the radar plot as a visualization instrument for assessing cross-sectional data in the STOP cohort.

Cross-sectional Questionnaire-Based Profiling in the STOP Cohort

The two examples provided in **Figure 1** are clearly distinguishable from one another, but how do tinnitus profiles vary in a larger sample? To investigate this question, we analyzed information based on the abovementioned measurement instruments gathered from 639 participants who reported occasional or constant tinnitus in the ongoing STOP study. Since the auditory assessment is still ongoing, these values were not included here. We compared the profiles between occasional and constant tinnitus and took the opportunity to evaluate the differences between men and women (**Figure 2**; **Table 1**). The tinnitus-associated burden denoted by the surface area of each plot appeared greater in constant tinnitus, than in occasional tinnitus (**Figure 2**). Although most scores indicated negligible symptoms in the occasional tinnitus group, scores for the THI and the anxiety subscale of the HADS were mild/moderate in constant tinnitus (**Table 1**). When assessing gender differences for intermittent tinnitus, the overall burden appeared very similar between men and women, with the exception of hyperacusis whereby the plots highlighted a small difference in scores [♀: HQ = 16.60 (15.38–17.82), and ♂: HQ = 12.32 (10.88–13.75), **Figure 2C**]. However, while this difference was statistically significant ($p < 0.0001$), both gender subgroups were below the grading of a clinically meaningful hyperacusis (cutoff = 28). This difference between men and women can be appreciated in the radar plots where an extension of the HQ radii can be seen in women (**Figure 2C**), indicating that the radar plots allow to visually capture subtle changes. For constant tinnitus, many of the tinnitus domains had greater scores in women than in men, including awareness, annoyance, and catastrophic cognitive misinterpretations (**Figure 2F**). Comorbidities were also slightly higher, including hyperacusis and anxiety. Psychological distress (THI) and stress (HADS) were the only instruments showing a shift from the negligible toward the moderate category. Analysis of the data using a two-way ANOVA confirmed that genders differed significantly [$F_{(1, 8,715)} = 193.4$; $p < 0.0001$, **Table 1**]. Again, the visualization of the radar plots merged for men and women enable to observe a greater surface area for women.

Although the radar plots allowed to distinguish contrasting tinnitus-associated burden in constant tinnitus versus occasional as well as subtle differences between genders in both subgroups, we sought to determine whether the radar plots could support the interpretation of those instruments with published severity category boundaries. To do so, an additional set of questionnaire data was collected from 294 subjects with constant tinnitus and added to the previous dataset of 328 for a total of 622 subjects with constant tinnitus. These were classified according to three grades of the THI from slight (range: 0–16, n = 272), mild and moderate (range: 18–56, n = 305), and severe to catastrophic (range: 58–100, n = 45). The HQ, HADS, PSQ-30, and WHOQoL-BREF data from the slight group did not differ from that of non-tinnitus control subjects (n = 1,845, **Table 2**). Consistently, the radar plots showed no clinically meaningful scores for the slight THI group (**Figure 2G**); however, the mild/moderate THI groups displayed an increased in tinnitus-associated burden with stress scores being *moderate* (**Figure 2H**; **Table 2**), whereas the severe/catastrophic THI group showed much larger surface of the radar plots with *severe* stress and *moderate* anxiety levels (**Figure 2I**; **Table 2**). Hyperacusis scores increased significantly from negligible to mild/moderate and from mild/moderate to severe/catastrophic tinnitus groups, but remained below clinically meaningful hyperacusis values (**Table 2**). Overall, the radar plots facilitated the appreciation of greater tinnitus-associated burden in cross-sectional data from the STOP cohort and suggest that this visualization tool may help in evaluating global tinnitus burden.

Evaluation of Treatment Outcome with the TRI Database

We reasoned that these plots could also be informative with respect to treatment-related response. To investigate this question, we analyzed information from the TRI database that contains information from baseline and posttreatment measures collected from 574 individuals based on three sets of questions

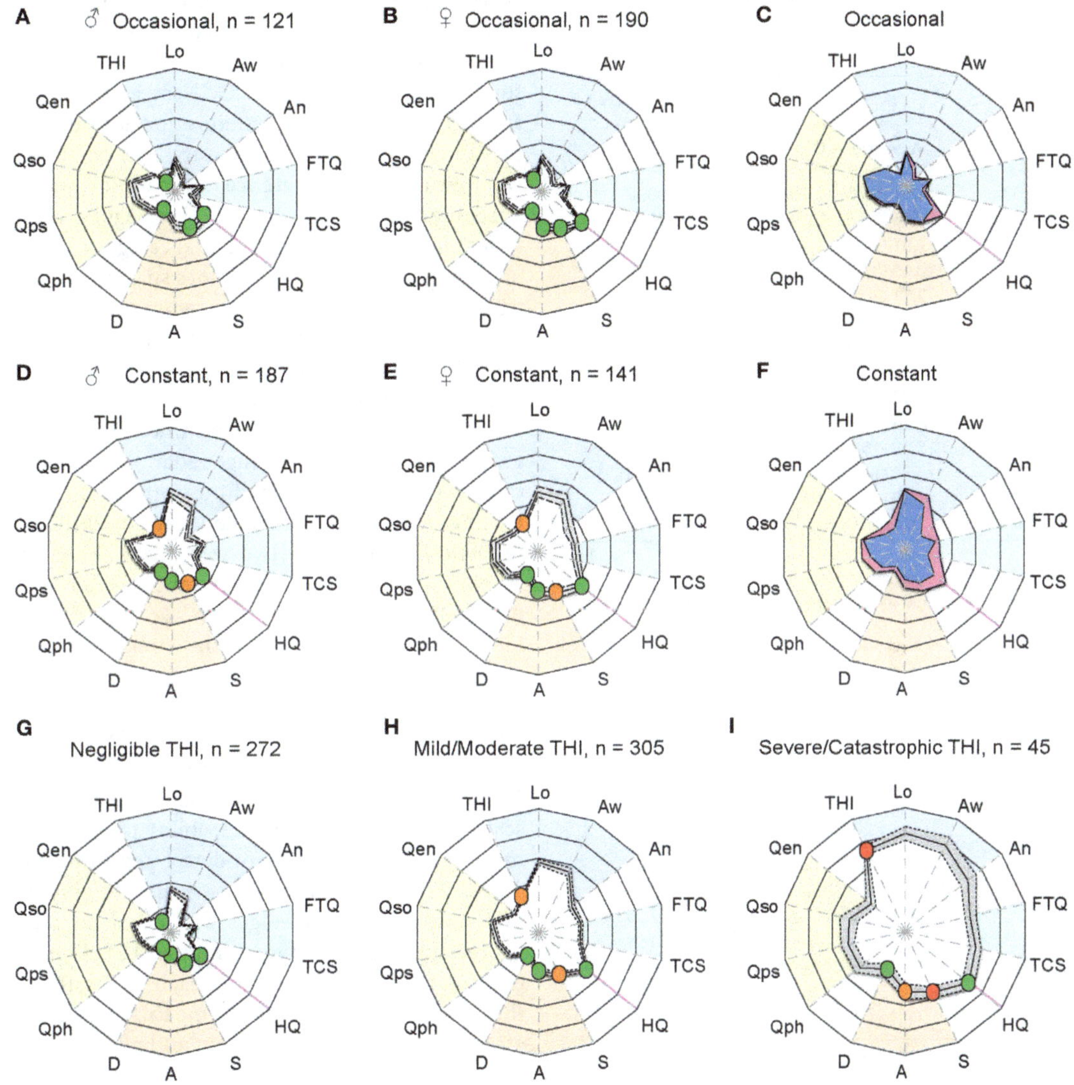

FIGURE 2 | Radar plot profiling that characterizes greater burden in women with tinnitus than in men. Radar plots illustrating the evaluation of global changes in tinnitus burden according to occasional tinnitus for men **(A)** and women **(B)** and constant tinnitus for men **(D)** and women **(E)**. In all four plots, a solid line shows the average, with the 95% confidence intervals represented by the dashed lines. Average tinnitus-associated burden, for men (blue) and women (pink) is shown for occasional **(C)** and constant **(F)** tinnitus. Measures from **(G)** negligible, **(H)** mild/moderate, and **(I)** severe/catastrophic THI groups from the STOP database. The blue background gathers the tinnitus domain assessed with the THI and several numerical rating scales, the light blue represents the tinnitus-associated fears, the hyperacusis domain is marked in purple, emotional affects are in orange, and the yellow background represents the quality of life domain evaluated with the WHOQoL-BREF. The continuous line shows the average scores, and the dashed lines illustrate the 95% confidence intervals. Instruments are labeled as follows: THI, tinnitus-related psychological distress; Lo, tinnitus loudness; Aw, tinnitus awareness; An, tinnitus annoyance; TCS, tinnitus catastrophizing; FTQ, tinnitus fears; HQ, hyperacusis questionnaire; S, stress; A, anxiety; D, depression scores; quality of life for physical (Qph), psychological (Qps), social (Qso), and environment (Qen). Color dots illustrate the severity score of those instruments with published severity category boundaries: negligible (green), moderate (orange), and severe (red).

(THI, WHOQoL-BREF, and tinnitus-related numeric rating scales). The mean age of the group was 53.3 years (SD 12.2) with an average tinnitus duration of 8.4 years (SD 8.87). Women made up 36.7% of the group. These patients were classified into different groups based on the CGI rating (**Table 3**). Only three patients rated their posttreatment state as "very much worse" and as a consequence this category was excluded from analysis ($N = 571$). We note that the size of the "very much better" and "much worse" groups were also rather small ($n = 18$ and $n = 24$, respectively).

We hypothesized that the surface area of the radar plots could be used to evaluate and quantify treatment efficacy. However, for a more sensitive measure of treatment outcome, one has to consider the order of the measures around the circumference since the surface area could be influenced depending on which instruments are situated next to each other. It is thus conceivable that a specific arrangement of the axis makes the radar plot tool more sensitive for displaying clinical changes than other possible arrangements. With the restriction that instruments forming part of the same domain should be displayed in vicinity

TABLE 1 | Raw scores from STOP participants with occasional or constant tinnitus according to gender.

Occasional tinnitus			
	♂ (*N* = 121)	♀ (*N* = 190)	Two-way ANOVA (*p* value)
	Average ± CI	Average ± CI	
THI	10.35 (8.07–12.63)	11.51 (9.76–13.26)	<0.9999
Lo	25.87 (22.43–29.3)	28.56 (25.62–31.49)	0.228
Aw	13.66 (10.76–16.56)	17.97 (14.8–21.13)	0.6937
An	6.97 (5–8.94)	10.65 (8.09–13.21)	0.8108
FTQ	3.76 (3.37–4.16)	3.61 (3.31–3.92)	>0.9999
TCS	7.02 (5.7–8.33)	8.61 (7.34–9.87)	>0.9999
HQ	12.32 (10.88–13.75)	16.6 (15.38–17.82)	***<0.0001
S	0.33 (0.3–0.36)	0.33 (0.31–0.36)	>0.9999
A	5.7 (5.01–6.39)	5.92 (5.33–6.51)	>0.9999
D	3.32 (2.77–3.86)	3.24 (2.75–3.73)	>0.9999
Qph	16.25 (15.83–16.67)	15.93 (15.53–16.32)	0.4321
Qps	14.98 (14.47–15.5)	14.84 (14.45–15.23)	0.9863
Qso	14.31 (13.77–14.85)	14.6 (14.18–15.02)	>0.9999
Qen	16.45 (16.06–16.84)	16.4 (16.09–16.7)	>0.9999
Constant tinnitus			
	♂ (*N* = 187)	♀ (*N* = 141)	Two-way ANOVA (*p* value)
	Average ± CI	Average ± CI	
THI	18.73 (16.47–20.99)	26.29 (23.19–29.38)	***0.0001
Lo	47.24 (43.78–50.69)	49.16 (45.05–53.26)	0.0031
Aw	40.23 (35.52–44.94)	47.84 (42.67–53.01)	***<0.0001
An	17.69 (14.48–20.9)	31.32 (26.73–35.9)	***<0.0001
FTQ	4.56 (4.19–4.93)	5.1 (4.66–5.54)	0.7674
TCS	10.55 (9.27–11.83)	16.24 (14.54–17.94)	***<0.0001
HQ	13.75 (12.55–14.96)	18.89 (17.35–20.44)	***<0.0001
S	0.3 (0.28–0.33)	0.37 (0.33–0.4)	**0.0046
A	5.15 (4.61–5.69)	6.54 (5.78–7.29)	***0.0002
D	3.24 (2.8–3.67)	3.94 (3.28–4.61)	0.6755
Qph	16.22 (15.88–16.57)	15.2 (14.71–15.69)	*0.0184
Qps	15.57 (15.23–15.91)	14.44 (13.95–14.92)	**0.0066
Qso	14.49 (14.08–14.89)	14.32 (13.76–14.89)	>0.9999
Qen	16.83 (16.55–17.12)	15.94 (15.54–16.35)	0.1123

See ***Figure 1*** *for a description of the abbreviations for each measure. Average values and 95% confidence intervals are shown. Pairwise comparisons using Bonferroni tests are reported.*
**p < 0.05.*
***p < 0.001.*
****p < 0.001.*

to each other (e.g., WHOQoL-BREF), we simulated the full set of possible permutations, which allowed a number of 34,560 different variants of the radar plot. For each of these variants, the following steps were repeated:

- Plots for all tinnitus patients were created and the surface area calculated.
- Patients were grouped to the CGI categories (see **Table 3**), the average surface area was calculated for each category to compute the mean distance between groups.
- Patients were grouped to the CGI categories (see **Table 3**) and the variance of the surface area within each category calculated.

The results of these calculations are displayed in **Figure 3A** with the mean surface difference between CGI categories plotted against the mean surface variance within categories. The goal of this step was to select a figure outline that minimized the surface variance within CGI categories and maximized the mean surface difference between CGI categories (marked with a red square). This radar plot configuration appeared as optimal to the set of instruments used within the TRI database. In **Figure 3B**, we show the mean difference in radar plot surface area pre- and post-intervention for each CGI category using the selected radar plot configuration. The CGI category "no change" showed on average no change in the plot's surface, while CGI categories with an improvement show a reduction, while CGI categories with a worsening of the patients' symptoms are characterized by an increase of the plot's surface.

Having determined the optimal configuration of the radar plot to visualize and score treatment-related changes in CGI groups, we plotted the average radar plots of each of the six CGI categories pretreatment and posttreatment (**Figures 4A,B**). All CGI groups in the improvement categories displayed significant reduction in surface [two-way ANOVA; very much better: $F_{(1,\ 374)} = 77.47$, $p < 0.0001$; much better: $F_{(1,\ 1,430)} = 155.3$, $p < 0.0001$, minimally better: $F_{(1,\ 2,860)} = 162.3$, $p < 0.0001$]. With increasing power in the "much better" and "minimally better" groups, significant improvement was detected for all instruments, with the exception of the quality of life domain (Table S2 in Supplementary Material). Conversely, in the "minimally worse" group, significant changes were observed [two-way ANOVA; $F_{(1,\ 506)} = 28.88$, $p < 0.0001$] in particular for the numeric rating scales of loudness, annoyance, ability to ignore, and unpleasantness, while the THI did not detect any worsening ($p > 0.9999$, Table S2 in Supplementary Material). Merging the pretreatment and posttreatment averages on the same radar plot helped appreciating these changes (**Figure 4C**). **Figure 4D** illustrates examples of individuals within each CGI category. As shown in these examples, changes over time can be displayed and appreciated by comparing pretreatment and posttreatment plots.

DISCUSSION

This article describes an innovative visualization method for displaying patient profiles, both to aid clinical assessment and evaluate the effects of treatment-related change, here applied in the context of tinnitus. The method can be adapted to individual patients (e.g., **Figures 1** and **4D**) as well as on a group level (e.g., **Figures 2** and **4A–C**). The present method uses data from a multi-dimensional set of relevant measurement instruments and integrates them into a radar plot. Both total scores on domain-specific questionnaires (e.g., the HQ, HADS, and WHOQoL-BREF) and single-item numeric rating scales as well as a psychoacoustic tests can be incorporated to provide an overview in a single plot. The data representation facilitates the visualization of both individual and group data and gives an understandable representation of burden status in a manner that is accessible to a range of observers. Moreover, the representation is sensitive to changes over time and enables the detection of clinically significant improvements in treatment outcome. Different coloring methods can be used such as in **Figures 1**, **2** and **4** to highlight specific aspects of the data. Usability studies

TABLE 2 | Raw scores from STOP participants according to different THI subgroups.

		THI severity subgroups		
Instruments	**Controls ($N = 1,223$)**	**Negligible ($N = 272$)**	**Mild/moderate ($N = 305$)**	**Severe/catastrophic ($N = 45$)**
THI		8.6 (8–9.2)	31.1 (29.9–32.2)[a]	72.4 (68.9–75.9)[a,b]
VAS Lo		34.9 (32.7–37.2)	56.8 (54.3–59.3)[a]	79.1 (73.9–84.3)[a,b]
VAS Aw		28.8 (25.5–32)	54.6 (51–58.2)[a]	77.3 (70.1–84.5)[a,b]
VAS An		9.8 (8–11.5)	33 (30.1–35.9)[a]	66.2 (58.5–73.9)[a,b]
FTQ		3.6 (3.4–3.8)	5.8 (5.5–6.1)	9.3 (8.6–10.1)[c]
TCS		6.8 (6.2–7.4)	17.4 (16.5–18.3)[a]	30.9 (28.5–33.2)[a,b]
HQ	11.4 (11–11.8)	12 (11.1–12.9)	20.1 (19.2–21)[a]	27.9 (25.5–30.3)[a,b]
S	0.3 (0.3–0.3)	0.3 (0.2–0.3)	0.4 (0.4–0.4)	0.5 (0.5–0.6)
A	4.8 (4.6–5)	4.1 (3.7–4.5)	6.5 (6.1–7)[d]	10.2 (8.9–11.5)[c]
D	2.6 (2.4–2.7)	2.5 (2.2–2.9)	4 (3.6–4.4)	7.1 (5.9–8.4)
Qph	16.9 (16.8–17)	16.7 (16.5–17)	15.3 (15–15.6)	12.5 (11.7–13.4)
Qps	15.7 (15.6–15.9)	16 (15.7–16.2)	14.6 (14.3–14.9)	12.4 (11.6–13.3)
Qso	14.9 (14.8–15.1)	15.1 (14.8–15.4)	13.9 (13.5–14.2)	12.6 (11.4–13.7)
Qen	17 (16.9–17.1)	17 (16.8–17.3)	16.1 (15.8–16.4)	14.3 (13.5–15.1)

See **Figure 1** *for a description of the abbreviations for each measure. Average values and 95% confidence intervals are shown. Multiple comparisons from Holm–Sidak's tests are reported in superscripts, where different letters represent a statistically significant difference.* [a]$p < 0.001$ *compared with negligible THI,* [b]$p < 0.001$ *compared with mild/moderate THI,* [c]$p < 0.01$ *compared with negligible THI,* [d]$p < 0.05$ *compared with negligible THI. Controls did not differ from negligible THI scores.*

TABLE 3 | Categorization of the 571 participants from the Tinnitus Research Initiative database according to their posttreatment CGI rating.

CGI rating	***N***
Very much better	18
Much better	66
Minimally better	131
No change	255
Minimally worse	77
Much worse	24

involving practitioners will be needed to decide which coloring method should be used to optimally display the clinical data.

Saary first proposed radar plots for their use of health-care data (24). Funabiki et al. applied this methodology in the context of the assessment of pervasive developmental disorder and attention-deficit/hyperactivity disorder (41). Similarly, Pierzycki et al. used radar plots to visualize factor structure and test–retest reliability of multiple baseline test scores in the context of tinnitus (19). However, all these studies did not apply this methodology in the context of the evaluation of treatment outcome. To the best of our knowledge, this is the first attempt in the medical area to design a comprehensive visualization tool of integrated measures over time. Here, we show the sensitivity of this tool for the assessment of tinnitus patients at their initial consultation at the clinic and for monitoring their progress under a specific treatment. The methodology presented here suggests that it could be applied for monitoring patients throughout their therapeutic intervention. In our examples, a decrease in the radar plot surface could be interpreted as a clinical improvement, while an increase of the surface could be interpreted as a worsening of clinical symptoms (see **Figure 4D** for individual examples). An important aspect of this use case is the graphical implementation of the minimal clinically important difference (MCID). Meaningful clinical differences need to be highlighted in order to dissociate them from differences that are not of clinical relevance. Further research will be needed to define and implement the MCID in the radar plots.

We also propose that this approach could be applied to other complex disorders where multiple measures are incorporated. We are not stating that the total surface of the area, which can be interpreted as a *global burden* score, can replace the use of a single primary outcome instrument. Rather such visualization tool can be used to appreciate global changes associated with the status of a patient and his responsiveness to a treatment. Although useful for group comparisons, this tool appears to have particular utility in individual patient management strategies. Additionally, specific color-coding methods can be implemented in order to highlight specific aspects of the plot and mark meaningful clinical differences on instruments that have known thresholds of severity. Further work will be needed to develop and standardize a radar plot that is designed to optimally display the clinical status of the tinnitus patients.

An important leverage is the order of the axis used to create the radar plot. As we showed, the selection of the axis order has a strong impact on the surface and surface difference between two time points. Whether instruments need to be grouped according to broad fields such as those used here (e.g., tinnitus, quality of life, emotional burden, and auditory profiles) or instead according to instrument subscales (sleep, cognitive, intrusiveness, relaxation, sense of control, and auditory performance) remains to be established. Furthermore, it is likely that varying the number of data points on the radar plots may also affect the precision and the sensitivity of the tool. The STOP data contain a greater number of instruments than in the TRI data; however, it does not contain treatment outcome data. The TRI data utilized in the present work are limited to (i) the THI, for which validity and reliability has been questioned, (ii) visual analog scales, for which precision is also subject to debate, and (iii) the WHOQoL, which usefulness in the evaluation of treatment outcome is unclear. As a consequence, to evaluate the influence of the number of data points on the precision of the radar plots, studies will have to be performed using a larger set of instruments. This will allow a greater flexibility in evaluating the effects of inclusion

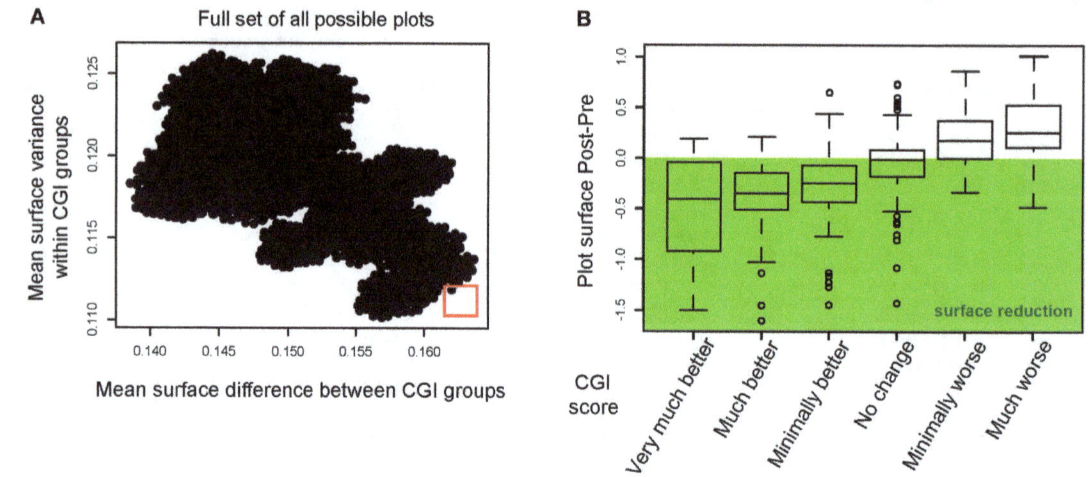

FIGURE 3 | Instrument permutations and alignment of the radar plot with improvements in Clinical Global Impression. **(A)** The full set of all possible radar plots with different surface outlines (i.e., different organization of axes) was simulated. The mean surface difference between CGI groups was calculated for all radar plots (abscissa). The mean surface variance within CGI groups was calculated and plotted on the ordinate. The red square highlights the radar plot outline optimized for maximum difference *between* CGI categories and minimum variance *within* CGI categories. **(B)** Radar plot surface differences (post-intervention minus pre-intervention) are displayed for the optimal outline. The mean surface difference is shown for each CGI category.

or exclusion of specific instruments on the sensitivity of the radar plots in measuring a successful treatment outcome.

The work presented here outlines a framework for this development, which can be used for tinnitus and for other chronic diseases. One important consideration for the optimal use of this visualization method is the selection of measurement instruments. For example, single-item visual analog or numeric rating scales tend to be viewed as inferior because (i) they are more vulnerable to random measurement errors, which are more likely to be eliminated with multiple items, (ii) the reliability statistic "internal consistency" cannot be computed, and (iii) they are more vulnerable to unknown biases in meaning and interpretation. Here, our selection was in part pragmatic since it was constrained by the data that were available in the STOP study and in the TRI database. The present methodology is generic in a sense that it can be adapted to include any measurement scales. Another important leverage will be the selection of instruments that measure unique and independent components of a complex health-care condition since this should maximize discriminability between patient profiles. The selection of the instruments is thus an important influencer of the radar plots' sensitivity to change. The choice of instruments is normally guided by the personal preference of the physician or investigator. However, future synthesis of data originating from multiple centers will require agreement from those heads and other key opinion leaders to use a common set of instruments; something that is challenging given the broad diversity of instruments in current use (22). In this regard, the COMiT initiative is currently in the process of establishing an international consensus-based recommendation of a minimum set of outcome domains and instruments considered critically important for performing clinical trials (23). Such international programs will help defining the core set of measurement instruments. A challenge emerging from such endeavors is to obtain instruments of equivalent reliability and efficiency in different languages and sensitive to culture context (42).

Whether such aggregated visualization of data using radar plots will prove useful to clinicians for the management of complex health-care conditions (e.g., tinnitus) will have to be tested. A preliminary evaluation of the radar plots shows mitigated opinions. Some physicians view it as extremely appealing and practical tool to picture the global status of a patient (tinnitus distress, fear of tinnitus, sensitivity to noise, emotional burden, and quality of life), while others do not foresee in what way the radar plots will enable an optimization of the treatment selection. We predict such opinions will also vary between countries where culture and average socioeconomic status differ, and also where different health-care systems apply (purely social-based health-care system versus insurance-based, clinical versus private practice). Furthermore, some physicians express concerns of exposing tinnitus patients to the long list of questionnaires such as those used in the STOP cohort, which could reinforce the negative thoughts and feelings about tinnitus. The participants in STOP originate from the general population and not from a clinical population, and thus whether such series of questionnaires can used on a clinical group will have to be tested. Future research will also have to evaluate the physician perspective in introducing multiple measures in the assessment of tinnitus burden and provide solid conclusions on the usefulness of such integrated measures in the management and treatment of tinnitus.

We personally view that with the increasing pressure over social health-care systems and the dissatisfaction of patients with regards to the quality of the care, novel methodologies are needed to assess patients at baseline and monitor individual response to a treatment. With the increasing development of value-based health care (43), and the distant monitoring of health conditions, smartphone applications could become routinely used in clinics to monitor patients at distance. In the context of tinnitus, the development of such distant monitoring has been recently initiated by Schlee et al. (44–46). This mobile platform could represent an ideal setting to collect patient data at different follow-up times, whereas the physician frontend would display an automated radar plot of the patient's status. Our hope is that such a tool would allow an immediate monitoring of treatment progress over time and enable the physician to rapidly readjust a treatment prescription depending on the responsiveness of a patient. Furthermore, the inclusion

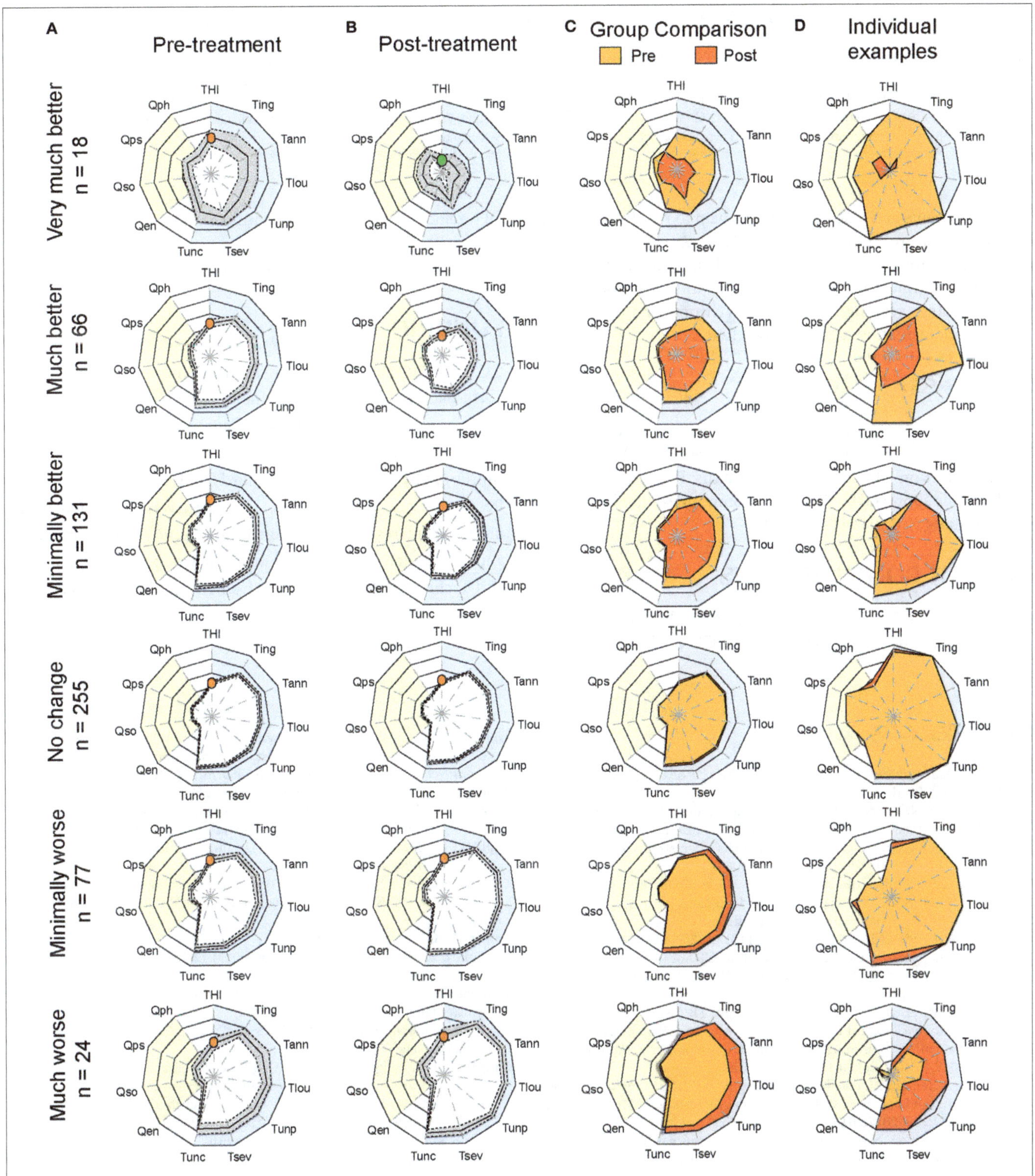

FIGURE 4 | Continued

FIGURE 4 | Continued
Plots of average pretreatment and posttreatment scores based on CGI ratings. Radar plots illustrating the evaluation of global changes in tinnitus burden according to measures from **(A)** baseline (pretreatment) and **(B)** follow-up (posttreatment) during the evaluation of various treatments within the TRI database. Patients were grouped according to Clinical Global Impression scores and their number is shown on the left. The yellow background represents the quality of life domain evaluated with the WHOQoL-BREF and the blue background gathers the tinnitus domain assessed with the THI and several numerical rating scales. The continuous line in the pretreatment and posttreatment shows the average scores, and the dashed lines illustrate the 95% confidence intervals. **(C)** Pretreatment (yellow) and posttreatment (orange) average values are presented on the same plot. The orange dot in the THI scale marks the moderate scores of the group for this instrument, whereas the green shows the progression of the group to negligible THI. Note the reduction of tinnitus-associated burden in the "very much better" group. **(D)** Example of individuals within each CGI category to illustrate changes before and after treatment for the same patient. Instruments are labeled as follows: THI, Tinnitus Handicap Inventory; Tign, Tinnitus Numeric Rating Scale (Ignore); Tann, Tinnitus Numeric Rating Scale (Annoyance); Tlou, Tinnitus Numeric Rating Scale (Loudness); Tunp, Tinnitus Numeric Rating Scale (Unpleasant); Tsev, Tinnitus Numeric Rating Scale (Severity); Tunc, Tinnitus Numeric Rating Scale (Uncomfortable); Qen, WHO Quality of Life (environment); Qso, WHO Quality of Life (social relationships); Qps, WHO Quality of Life (psychological); Qph, WHO Quality of Life (physical health). Statistical analyses comparing **(A,B)** are available in Table S2 in Supplementary Material.

of adverse events and side effects would help to rapidly terminate an intervention and address appropriate care. A better recognition of a patient status and its comorbidities will likely improve the priorities and treatment prescription. Overall, this work contributes to novel strategies for high quality care of chronic tinnitus patients and its implementation in the general clinic.

ETHICS STATEMENT

The STOP project was approved by the local ethics committee "Regionala etikprövningsnämnden" in Stockholm (#2014/1998-31/4). Collection of data for the Tinnitus Research Initiative database was approved by the Ethics Committee of the University of Regensburg, Germany (#08/046).

AUTHOR CONTRIBUTIONS

WS, CC, BL, and BC designed the study. NE collected, extracted, and processed the STOP data. WS and CC analyzed the data. DH helped to develop the scientific arguments and contributed to data interpretation. All authors played a role in writing the manuscript and approved the final version.

FUNDING

CC and BC have received funding from Vetenskapsrådet, Tysta Skolan, and Karolinska Institutet. CC has received funding from Lars Hiertas Minne, Magnus Bergvalls Stiftelserna, Hörselforskningsfonden, and Loo och Hans Ostermans. DH is supported by National Institute for Health Research Biomedical Research Centre programme. The work was supported by an independent research program funded under the Biomedicine and Molecular Biosciences European Cooperation in Science and Technology (COST) Action framework (TINNET BM1306).

REFERENCES

Hunter DJ. Gene-environment interactions in human diseases. *Nat Rev Genet* (2005) 6:287–98. doi:10.1038/nrg1578
Massa MS, Wang N, Bickerton WL, Demeyere N, Riddoch MJ, Humphreys GW. On the importance of cognitive profiling: a graphical modelling analysis of domain-specific and domain-general deficits after stroke. *Cortex* (2015) 71:190–204. doi:10.1016/j.cortex.2015.06.006
Tyler RS, Baker LJ. Difficulties experienced by tinnitus sufferers. *J Speech Hear Disord* (1983) 48:150–4. doi:10.1044/jshd.4802.150
Stouffer JL, Tyler RS. Characterization of tinnitus by tinnitus patients. *J Speech Hear Disord* (1990) 55:439–53. doi:10.1044/jshd.5503.439
Elgoyhen AB, Langguth B, De Ridder D, Vanneste S. Tinnitus: perspectives from human neuroimaging. *Nat Rev Neurosci* (2015) 16:632–42. doi:10.1038/nrn4003
Schecklmann M, Pregler M, Kreuzer PM, Poeppl TB, Lehner A, Cronlein T, et al. Psychophysiological associations between chronic tinnitus and sleep: a cross validation of tinnitus and insomnia questionnaires. *Biomed Res Int* (2015) 2015:461090. doi:10.1155/2015/461090
Tegg-Quinn S, Bennett RJ, Eikelboom RH, Baguley DM. The impact of tinnitus upon cognition in adults: a systematic review. *Int J Audiol* (2016) 55:533–40. d oi:10.1080/14992027.2016.1185168
Trevis KJ, McLachlan NM, Wilson SJ. Cognitive mechanisms in chronic tinnitus: psychological markers of a failure to switch attention. *Front Psychol* (2016) 7:1262. doi:10.3389/fpsyg.2016.01262
Gilles A, Schlee W, Rabau S, Wouters K, Fransen E, Van de Heyning P. Decreased speech-in-noise understanding in young adults with tinnitus. *Front Neurosci* (2016) 10:288. doi:10.3389/fnins.2016.00288
Hoare DJ, Kowalkowski VL, Kang S, Hall DA. Systematic review and meta-analyses of randomized controlled trials examining tinnitus manage- ment. *Laryngoscope* (2011) 121:1555–64. doi:10.1002/lary.21825
Baguley D, McFerran D, Hall D. Tinnitus. *Lancet* (2013) 382:1600–7. doi:10.1016/S0140-6736(13)60142-7
Cederroth CR, Canlon B, Langguth B. Hearing loss and tinnitus – are funders and industry listening? *Nat Biotechnol* (2013) 31:972–4. doi:10.1038/nbt.2736
Langguth B, Kreuzer PM, Kleinjung T, De Ridder D. Tinnitus: causes and clinical management. *Lancet Neurol* (2013) 12:920–30. doi:10.1016/ S1474-4422(13)70160-1
Dauman R, Tyler RS. *Some Considerations on the Classification of Tinnitus.* Amsterdam: Kugler Publications (1992).
Tyler RS. *Neurophysiological Models, Psychological Models, and Treatments for Tinnitus.* New York: Thieme (2006).
Langguth B, Goodey R, Azevedo A, Bjorne A, Cacace A, Crocetti A, et al. Consensus for tinnitus patient assessment and treatment outcome measurement: tinnitus research initiative meeting, Regensburg, July 2006. *Prog Brain Res* (2007) 166:525–36. doi:10.1016/S0079-6123(07)66050-6
Zeman F, Koller M, Schecklmann M, Langguth B, Landgrebe M; TRI Database Study Group. Tinnitus assessment by means of standardized self-report questionnaires: psychometric properties of the tinnitus questionnaire (TQ), the Tinnitus Handicap Inventory (THI), and their short versions in an

international and multi-lingual sample. *Health Qual Life Outcomes* (2012) 10:128. doi:10.1186/1477-7525-10-128

Milerova J, Anders M, Dvorak T, Sand PG, Koniger S, Langguth B. The influence of psychological factors on tinnitus severity. *Gen Hosp Psychiatry* (2013) 35:412–6. doi:10.1016/j.genhosppsych.2013.02.008

Pierzycki RH, McNamara AJ, Hoare DJ, Hall DA. Whole scalp resting state EEG of oscillatory brain activity shows no parametric relationship with psychoacoustic and psychosocial assessment of tinnitus: a repeated measures study. *Hear Res* (2016) 331:101–8. doi:10.1016/j.heares.2015.11.003

Tyler RS, Noble W, Coelho C. Considerations for the design of clinical trials for tinnitus. *Acta Otolaryngol Suppl* (2006) 126:44–9. doi:10.1080/03655230600895424

Tyler RS, Oleson J, Noble W, Coelho C, Ji H. Clinical trials for tinnitus: study populations, designs, measurement variables, and data analysis. *Prog Brain Res* (2007) 166:499–509. doi:10.1016/S0079-6123(07)66048-8

Hall DA, Haider H, Szczepek AJ, Lau P, Rabau S, Jones-Diette J, et al. Systematic review of outcome domains and instruments used in clinical trials of tinnitus treatments in adults. *Trials* (2016) 17:270. doi:10.1186/s13063-016- 1399-9

Hall DA, Haider H, Kikidis D, Mielczarek M, Mazurek B, Szczepek AJ, et al. Toward a global consensus on outcome measures for clinical trials in tinnitus: report from the first International Meeting of the COMiT initiative, November 14, 2014, Amsterdam, The Netherlands. *Trends Hear* (2015) 19: 1–7. doi:10.1177/2331216515580272

Saary MJ. Radar plots: a useful way for presenting multivariate health care data. *J Clin Epidemiol* (2008) 61:311–7. doi:10.1016/j.jclinepi.2007. 04.021

Müller K, Edvall NK, Idrizbegovic E, Huhn R, Cima RFF, Persson V, et al. Validation of online Swedish tinnitus questionnaires. *Front Aging Neurosci* (2016) 8:272. doi:10.3389/fnagi.2016.00272

Landgrebe M, Zeman F, Koller M, Eberl Y, Mohr M, Reiter J, et al. The tinnitus research initiative (TRI) database: a new approach for delineation of tinnitus subtypes and generation of predictors for treatment outcome. *BMC Med Inform Decis Mak* (2010) 10:42. doi:10.1186/1472-6947-10-42

Newman CW, Jacobson GP, Spitzer JB. Development of the Tinnitus Handicap Inventory. *Arch Otolaryngol Head Neck Surg* (1996) 122:143–8. doi:10.1001/archotol.1996.01890140029007

Newman CW, Sandridge SA, Jacobson GP. Psychometric adequacy of the Tinnitus Handicap Inventory (THI) for evaluating treatment outcome. *J Am Acad Audiol* (1998) 9:153–60.

Hesser H, Andersson G. Dimensional or categorical approach to tinnitus severity: an item response mixture modeling analysis of tinnitus handicap. *Int J Behav Med* (2014) 21:982–8. doi:10.1007/s12529-013-9375-1

McCombe A, Baguley D, Coles R, McKenna L, McKinney C, Windle-Taylor P, et al. Guidelines for the grading of tinnitus severity: the results of a working group commissioned by the British Association of Otolaryngologists, Head and Neck Surgeons, 1999. *Clin Otolaryngol Allied Sci* (2001) 26:388–93. doi:10.1046/j.1365-2273.2001.00490.x

Cima RF, Crombez G, Vlaeyen JW. Catastrophizing and fear of tinnitus predict quality of life in patients with chronic tinnitus. *Ear Hear* (2011) 32:634–41. doi:10.1097/AUD.0b013e31821106dd

Sullivan MJL, Bishop SC, Pivik J. The Pain Catastrophizing Scale: development and validation. *Psychol Assess* (1995) 7:524–32.

Zigmond AS, Snaith RP. The Hospital Anxiety and Depression Scale. *Acta Psychiatr Scand* (1983) 67:361–70. doi:10.1111/j.1600-0447.1983. tb09716.x

Levenstein S, Prantera C, Varvo V, Scribano ML, Berto E, Luzi C, et al. Development of the perceived stress questionnaire: a new tool for psychosomatic research. *J Psychosom Res* (1993) 37:19–32. doi:10.1016/0022-3999(93)90120-5

Fliege H, Rose M, Arck P, Walter OB, Kocalevent RD, Weber C, et al. The perceived stress questionnaire (PSQ) reconsidered: validation and reference values from different clinical and healthy adult samples. *Psychosom Med* (2005) 67:78–88. doi:10.1097/01.psy.0000151491.80178.78

Khalfa S, Dubal S, Veuillet E, Perez-Diaz F, Jouvent R, Collet L. Psychometric normalization of a hyperacusis questionnaire. *ORL J Otorhinolaryngol Relat Spec* (2002) 64:436–42. doi:10.1159/000067570

Fackrell K, Fearnley C, Hoare DJ, Sereda M. Hyperacusis questionnaire as a tool for measuring hypersensitivity to sound in a tinnitus research population. *Biomed Res Int* (2015) 2015:290425. doi:10.1155/2015/290425

The WHOQOL Group. Development of the World Health Organization WHOQOL-BREF quality of life assessment. *Psychol Med* (1998) 28:551–8. doi:10.1017/S0033291798006667

Busner J, Targum SD. The clinical global impressions scale: applying a research tool in clinical practice. *Psychiatry (Edgmont)* (2007) 4:28–37.

Clark JG. Uses and abuses of hearing loss classification. *ASHA* (1981) 23:493–500.

Funabiki Y, Kawagishi H, Uwatoko T, Yoshimura S, Murai T. Development of a multi-dimensional scale for PDD and ADHD. *Res Dev Disabil* (2011) 32:995–1003. doi:10.1016/j.ridd.2011.01.052

Wild D, Eremenco S, Mear I, Martin M, Houchin C, Gawlicki M, et al. Multinational trials-recommendations on the translations required, approaches to using the same language in different countries, and the approaches to support pooling the data: the ISPOR patient-reported outcomes translation and linguistic validation good research practices task force report. *Value Health* (2009) 12:430–40. doi:10.1111/j.1524-4733.2008.00471.x

Porter ME. What is value in health care? *N Engl J Med* (2010) 363:2477–81. doi:10.1056/NEJMp1011024

Probst T, Pryss R, Langguth B, Schlee W. Emotion dynamics and tinnitus: daily life data from the "TrackYourTinnitus" application. *Sci Rep* (2016) 6:31166. doi:10.1038/srep31166

Probst T, Pryss R, Langguth B, Schlee W. Emotional states as mediators between tinnitus loudness and tinnitus distress in daily life: results from the "TrackYourTinnitus" application. *Sci Rep* (2016) 6:20382. doi:10.1038/srep20382

Schlee W, Pryss RC, Probst T, Schobel J, Bachmeier A, Reichert M, et al. Measuring the moment-to-moment variability of tinnitus: the TrackYourTinnitus smart phone app. *Front Aging Neurosci* (2016) 8:294. doi:10.3389/fnagi.2016.00294

9

Cluster Analysis to Identify Possible Subgroups in Tinnitus Patients

Minke J. C. van den Berge[1,2], Rolien H. Free[1,2], Rosemarie Arnold[1], Emile de Kleine[1], Rutger Hofman[1], J. Marc C. van Dijk[2,3] and Pim van Dijk[1,2]*

[1] Department of Otorhinolaryngology/Head and Neck Surgery, University of Groningen, University Medical Center Groningen, Groningen, Netherlands, [2] Graduate School of Medical Sciences (Research School of Behavioural and Cognitive Neurosciences), University of Groningen, Groningen, Netherlands, [3] Department of Neurosurgery, University of Groningen, University Medical Center Groningen, Groningen, Netherlands

***Correspondence:**
Minke J. C. van den Berge
m.j.c.van.den.berge@umcg.nl

Introduction: In tinnitus treatment, there is a tendency to shift from a "one size fits all" to a more individual, patient-tailored approach. Insight in the heterogeneity of the tinnitus spectrum might improve the management of tinnitus patients in terms of choice of treatment and identification of patients with severe mental distress. The goal of this study was to identify subgroups in a large group of tinnitus patients.

Methods: Data were collected from patients with severe tinnitus complaints visiting our tertiary referral tinnitus care group at the University Medical Center Groningen. Patient-reported and physician-reported variables were collected during their visit to our clinic. Cluster analyses were used to characterize subgroups. For the selection of the right variables to enter in the cluster analysis, two approaches were used: (1) variable reduction with principle component analysis and (2) variable selection based on expert opinion.

Results: Various variables of 1,783 tinnitus patients were included in the analyses. Cluster analysis (1) included 976 patients and resulted in a four-cluster solution. The effect of external influences was the most discriminative between the groups, or clusters, of patients. The "silhouette measure" of the cluster outcome was low (0.2), indicating a "no substantial" cluster structure. Cluster analysis (2) included 761 patients and resulted in a three-cluster solution, comparable to the first analysis. Again, a "no substantial" cluster structure was found (0.2).

Conclusion: Two cluster analyses on a large database of tinnitus patients revealed that clusters of patients are mostly formed by a different response of external influences on their disease. However, both cluster outcomes based on this dataset showed a poor stability, suggesting that our tinnitus population comprises a continuum rather than a number of clearly defined subgroups.

Keywords: tinnitus, cluster analysis, subgroup identification, heterogeneity of tinnitus, principle component analysis

INTRODUCTION

Tinnitus is a prevalent condition, estimated to affect 5–18% of the adult population (1), which may lead to severe impairment in quality of life. Although many trials on tinnitus therapies have been conducted, hardly ever a treatment effect is demonstrated. A potential explanation for the lack of effectivity of these treatments might be the underlying heterogeneity of the disease. Therefore, consensus on the optimal treatment of tinnitus gradually shifts from a "one size fits all" approach to a more patient-tailored approach. Possibly, a particular group of patients would be more likely to respond to treatment, if a selection is made on etiology, tinnitus characteristics, or patient characteristics. It might be that in a specific subgroup of tinnitus patients a particular treatment is successful, while this treatment is not successful in another subgroup of tinnitus patients. Thus, insight in the heterogeneity of the tinnitus spectrum might improve the management of these patients.

Identification of tinnitus subgroups is also important with regard to concomitant mental distress. Hoekstra et al. demonstrated that patients who express certain characteristics (i.e., high percentage of experience of tinnitus during the day, self-reported depression or anxiety, and subjective experience of tinnitus loudness) are more at risk for a high tinnitus burden (2). This subgroup of patients with high tinnitus distress needs more extensive counseling and follow-up in order to prevent mental breakdown.

In an attempt to identify subgroups of tinnitus patients, cluster analysis was used in this study. Cluster analysis is a statistical technique that divides data into groups, or clusters, which are meaningful and/or useful. It is an explorative analysis that assigns patients to clusters based on certain characteristics, so that patients look very much alike within a cluster (high within-group homogeneity) and, at the same time, are very different from the other clusters (low between-group homogeneity) (3). In research, this cluster analysis method is not only used in medicine studies to identify groups of patients but also in marketing for finding customer segments for example.

In 2008, Tyler et al. performed a preliminary cluster analysis on 153 patients with tinnitus (4). The cluster analysis of Tyler et al. identified distinct cluster characteristics, which were described as: (1) "constant distressing tinnitus," (2) "varying tinnitus that is worse in noise," (3) "tinnitus patients who are copers and whose tinnitus is not influenced by somatic modulation," and (4) "tinnitus patients who are copers but whose tinnitus is worse in quiet environments." Tyler et al. did not report a statistic value to identify the degree to which patients are clustered in these groups.

In this paper, we report on an exploratory cluster analysis of patients from the tinnitus database of the University Medical Center Groningen ($n = 1,783$ patients). We initially attempted to replicate the cluster analysis reported by Tyler et al (4); however, this was not possible as many of the variables used in their analysis were not identical or not available in our database. Instead, we report on two further cluster analyses. In the first analysis, the choice of variables that were entered in the cluster analyses was fully guided by the statistical techniques. In the second analysis, the selection of variables was based on the expert opinions in our tinnitus clinic. The aim of this study was to identify subgroups of tinnitus using cluster analysis, based on a very large dataset of tinnitus patients.

MATERIALS AND METHODS

Tinnitus Population

This study was performed at the Otorhinolaryngology Department of the University Medical Center Groningen (The Netherlands), which has a specialized multidisciplinary care group for tinnitus patients since 2007. Patients with severe complaints of tinnitus can be referred to this care group for medical consultation and psychological support. Almost all patients who visit this care group have consulted an audiologist and/or otorhinolaryngologist earlier. However, these patients were referred to our specialized tertiary care group by these specialists, because of the severity and impact of the complaints. Consultation at our clinic consists of thorough evaluation by an otorhinolaryngologist, an audiologist, radiologist, a medical social worker, and/or a psychologist.

Variables

The variables that were available for this cluster analysis were demographic characteristics (e.g., sex and age), tinnitus characteristics (e.g., duration of tinnitus, onset, lateralization, pitch, variable loudness), factors of influence on patients tinnitus (e.g., influence of loud sounds, noisy environment, movement of head and neck), tinnitus and quality of life-related questionnaires [e.g., tinnitus handicap index (THI), visual analog scale (VAS), and hospital anxiety and depression scale (HADS)], and audiological characteristics [e.g., frequency matching, pure tone audiometry (PTAs), loudness matching of tinnitus]. Hearing loss was divided into categories based on the pure tone audiogram: (1) no or slight hearing loss (both ears thresholds <30 dB on PTA thresholds at 0.25–0.5–1–2–4–8 kHz), (2) asymmetrical hearing loss (≥30 dB difference between both ears on the mean PTA thresholds at 2–4–8 kHz), (3) bilateral high tone hearing loss (both ears thresholds ≥30 dB on PTA thresholds at 2–4–8 kHz), (4) bilateral severe hearing loss (PTA thresholds >30 dB on 0.25–0.5–1–2–4–8 kHz), and (5) others. The available variables are all listed in Table S1 in Supplementary Material. All patient-reported variables were completed by the patients in booklets during the visit at the tinnitus outpatient clinic. Physician reported data, such as audiological characteristics, were also reported in booklets by the physician. All these routinely collected data were anonymized and entered in a database. For the current analysis, these data were retrospectively analyzed. The collection of data was approved by the Institutional Reviewer Board of the UMCG. No full review was needed due to the retrospective nature of this study.

Selection of Variables for Cluster Analysis

All variables that were collected were entered in the database. However, not all of these variables could be entered in the cluster analysis. In cluster analysis, it is important to keep the sample size in mind when deciding how many variables to enter in the analysis. Formann recommends the number of variables (m) of 2^m = sample size (5). In our study, the sample size is $n = 1783$, implying that the number of variables should be 10 or 11. There are two ways to select appropriate variables for cluster analysis: (1) a statistical approach with the use of principal component analysis (PCA) and (2) selection of variables based on "expert opinion," i.e., variables that are presumed to be clinically relevant and thought to be discriminative in the total group. Both selection procedures were performed in this study, resulting in two different cluster analyses.

Variable Reduction by PCA

A PCA is a dimension reduction technique that condenses variables that are highly correlated into a set of factors, thereby removing overlap and redundancy. PCA with Varimax rotation was performed on all variables with missing values ≤20%. The PCA revealed several factors, and for each factor, the variable with the highest loading was selected for inclusion in the cluster analysis.

Variable Reduction by "Expert Panel"

After excluding variables with missing values >20%, variables were selected by a group of tinnitus care professionals and investigators [Minke J. C. van den Berge (otolaryngology resident, Ph.D. candidate in tinnitus research), Pim van Dijk (medical physicist, audiologist, involved in the tinnitus care group), and Emile de Kleine (medical physicist, audiologist, involved in the tinnitus care group)]. Based on clinical experience and knowledge, those variables were selected that were deemed important in discriminating subgroups of tinnitus.

Cluster Analysis

The "two-step" cluster analysis method was used as the analyses that contained both categorical and continuous variables (6). Continuous variables were standardized by default. For distance measures, the log-likelihood method was used, as both continuous and categorical variables were entered in the analysis. The number of clusters to be formed was not specified in advance. The "silhouette measure of cohesion and separation" is a measure for the overall goodness-of-fit of the cluster structure that was found. It ranges from −1 to 1 (<0.25: no substantial structure; 0.26–0.50: weak structure and could be artificial; 0.51–0.70: reasonable structure; 0.71–1.0: strong structure) (7).

Differences in characteristics between clusters were compared according to the cluster membership variable, using one-way ANOVA for continuous variables and Pearson Chi-square tests for categorical variables. SPSS version 23.0 (Chicago, IL, USA) was used for all tests. The significance level was set at $\alpha = 0.05$, and all tests were two tailed.

RESULTS

Subject Characteristics

For this study, data from 1,783 consecutive patients who visited the UMCG tinnitus clinic between July 2007 and June 2016 were collected. The baseline characteristics of this study population are shown in **Table 1**. Variables that had >20% missing values are not shown in this table. In this population, 39.3% were females and the mean age was 53.6 ± 13.5 years. Tinnitus was unilateral in 50.7% of the cases and bilateral or central in 48.2%. The mean THI in the total patient group was 42.5 ± 23.2.

Outcome of Cluster Analysis with Variables Selected by PCA

The PCA was performed to obtain eigen values for each factor. The Kaiser–Meyer–Olkin measure of sampling adequacy was

TABLE 1 | Demographic and tinnitus-related characteristic of included tinnitus patients (n = 1,783).

	Total *N*	
Demographic characteristics		
Mean age ± SD	1,783	53.6 ± 13.5
Female gender—no. (%)	1,783	701 (39.3)
Tinnitus characteristics		
Mean duration of tinnitus ± SD—in years	1,635	6.8 ± 8.7
Onset tinnitus—no. (%)	1,685	
Acute		813 (48.2)
Gradual		872 (51.8)
Lateralization of tinnitus—no. (%)	1,496	
Bilateral/central		738 (49.3)
Unilateral		758 (50.7)
Description of tinnitus—no. (%)	1,607	
Tonal		715 (44.5)
Noise		708 (44.1)
Other		184 (11.4)
Experience of tinnitus—no. (%)	1,645	
Continuous		1,512 (91.9)
Intervals		133 (8.1)
Pitch of tinnitus—no. (%)	1,620	
Low		79 (4.9)
Moderate		403 (24.9)
High		997 (61.5)
Other		141 (8.7)
Variable loudness of tinnitus—no. (%)	1,762	
Yes		1,271 (72.1)
No		491 (27.9)
Mean percentage of burden during awake time ± SD	1,671	74.7 ± 28.0
Preference for silence or noise—no. (%)	1,559	
Silence		697 (44.7)
Noisy environment		862 (55.3)
Highest burden at time of the day—no. (%)	1,522	
Waking up		131 (8.6)
Morning		38 (2.5)
Afternoon		34 (2.2)
Evening		282 (18.5)
Night		149 (9.8)
Other		888 (58.3)
Sound unpleasant—no. (%)	1,446	
Never		137 (9.5)
Seldom		192 (13.3)
Some times		590 (40.8)
Most of the time		357 (24.7)
Always		170 (11.8)
Factors of influence on tinnitus		
Influence of noisy background—no. (%)	1,551	
Tinnitus louder		212 (13.7)
No effect		753 (48.5)
Tinnitus less loud		586 (37.8)
Influence of loud sounds—no. (%)	1,539	
Tinnitus louder		693 (45.0)
No effect		523 (34.0)
Tinnitus less loud		323 (21.0)
Influence of movement of head and neck—no. (%)	1,559	
Tinnitus louder		479 (30.7)
No effect		995 (63.8)
Tinnitus less loud		85 (5.5)
Influence of nap in the afternoon—no. (%)	1,419	
Tinnitus louder		233 (16.4)
No effect		1,003 (70.7)
Tinnitus less loud		183 (12.9)

(Continued)

TABLE 1 | Continued

	Total *N*	
Influence of stress—no. (%)	1,508	
Tinnitus louder		937 (62.1)
No effect		552 (36.6)
Tinnitus less loud		19 (1.3)
Influence of sleep deprivation—no. (%)	1,491	
Tinnitus louder		847 (56.8)
No effect		629 (42.2)
Tinnitus less loud		15 (1.0)
Audiological characteristics		
Mean PTA over 1–2–4 kHz (mean ± SD)	1,764	29.7 ± 18.0
Difference in mean PTA over 1–2–4 kHz between both ears (mean ± SD)	1,764	11.5 ± 18.1
Frequency matching of tinnitus—no. (%)	1,469	
0–2,000 Hz		378 (24.0)
2,000–4,000 Hz		239 (15.5)
4,000–6,000 Hz		287 (18.6)
6,000–8,000 Hz		275 (17.9)
>8,000 Hz		290 (23.4)
Type of hearing loss—no. (%)	1,782	
No/slight hearing loss		989 (55.5)
Asymmetrical hearing loss		265 (14.9)
Bilateral high tone hearing loss		243 (13.6)
Bilateral severe hearing loss		246 (13.8)
Other		39 (2.2)
Tinnitus questionnaires		
VAS tinnitus loudness[a] (mean ± SD)	1,615	66.7 ± 20.9
VAS tinnitus annoyance[a] (mean ± SD)	1,641	69.1 ± 22.6
THI-score (mean ± SD)	1,505	42.5 ± 23.2
HADS-depression score ± SD	1,676	5.4 ± 4.3
Indication HADS-depression[b]—no. (%)	1,676	
No indication depression		1,321 (78.8)
Indication depression		355 (19.9)
HADS-anxiety score ± SD	1,690	6.9 ± 4.3
Indication HADS-anxiety[b]—no. (%)	1,690	
No indication anxiety		1,103 (65.3)
Indication anxiety		587 (34.7)

[a]*On visual analog scale (VAS) range from 0 to 100%.*
[b]*Range 0–21, indication for depression/anxiety with score >8.*
Range is 0–100 unless indicated otherwise.
dB, decibel; PTA, pure tone audiometry; THI, tinnitus handicap inventory; HADS, hospital anxiety and depression scale.

0.681 and the Bartlett's test of sphericity was significant [χ^2 (6,127) = 325, $p < 0.001$], both indicating an appropriate factor model. A total of eight factors were extracted (based on the eigenvalue >1 rule), which together explained 55% of the total variance. Variables with the highest loading on each factor were selected. Subsequently, these variables ($n = 8$) were entered in the cluster analysis. The clustering revealed a four-cluster solution. As the analysis excludes every case when there is any variable with a missing value (listwise exclusion), the analysis was based on $n = 976$ patients. The cluster outcome showed a "silhouette measure of cohesion and separation" of 0.20, indicating that it is a "no substantial" cluster solution (7). Characteristics of these four identified clusters are shown in **Table 2**. The variables in the table are ranked from most discriminative between groups (top of the table) to less discriminative (bottom of the table). All variables differed statistically significant between the four clusters, except for the variables "VAS tinnitus annoyance" and "frequency of the tinnitus" ($p = 0.925$ and $p = 0.478$, respectively).

Cluster 1 ($n = 293$) is characterized by the fact that tinnitus is not easily influenced: loud sounds, sleep deprivation, and nap in the afternoon have no effect on their tinnitus. These patients have a relatively high difference between hearing loss in the right and left ear. These patients have relatively low HADS-depression scores.

Cluster 2 ($n = 259$) is distinguished by a gradual onset of the tinnitus. Also in this group, tinnitus is easily negatively influenced, especially by loud sounds and sleep deprivation. Both make their tinnitus louder.

Cluster 3 ($n = 197$) is a group of patients who report that their tinnitus is less loud when they hear loud sounds. Sleep deprivation and a nap in the afternoon mostly have no effect on their tinnitus.

Cluster 4 ($n = 227$) is typically a group with tinnitus of acute onset. They report that their tinnitus is easily negatively influenced by loud sounds or sleep deprivation. They show relatively high HADS-depression scores.

Outcome of Cluster Analysis with Variables Selected by Expert Panel

For the alternative method of choosing variables for clustering, 11 variables were selected by a panel of experts in the field. The selected variables (see **Table 3**) were entered in the cluster analysis. The outcome was a three-cluster solution, with a "silhouette measure of cohesion and separation" of 0.20, again indicating a poor solution. Because of listwise exclusion as described earlier, this analysis was based on $n = 761$ patients. About 527 of these patients were also included in the first cluster analysis. Also in this table, variables are ranked according to their degree of discriminative value. All variables differed significantly between the clusters (all p-Values <0.001).

Cluster 1 ($n = 287$) is a group of patients whose tinnitus is not easily influenced: loud sounds, stress, or movement of head and neck have no effect on their tinnitus loudness. Patients prefer a noisy environment. Sounds are never to seldom experienced as uncomfortably loud. The tinnitus is mostly unilateral. Although most patients in this group have no or slight hearing loss, other types of hearing loss are present in this group as well. They are not very much bothered or depressed by their tinnitus, as the THI and HADS-depression scores are low.

Cluster 2 ($n = 247$) is a predominantly male group, whose tinnitus gets worse by stress, loud sounds, and movement of head and neck. These patients prefer to be in a noisy environment. Sometimes, sounds are experienced as uncomfortably loud. Most of the patients have no or slight hearing loss. Tinnitus is bilateral, and the loudness of the tinnitus is variable.

Cluster 3 ($n = 227$) is characterized by the fact that their tinnitus is easily negatively influenced: loud sounds and stress clearly make their tinnitus louder. These patients prefer a silent environment. Often, patients find sounds uncomfortably loud. Tinnitus is often bilateral with most patients having no or slight hearing loss or asymmetrical hearing loss. The loudness of the tinnitus is variable.

TABLE 2 | Characteristics of the four clusters identified by clustering with variable selection based on principal component analysis.

	Cluster 1 (n = 293)	Cluster 2 (n = 259)	Cluster 3 (n = 197)	Cluster 4 (n = 227)	p-Value
Influence of loud sound (%)					**<0.001**[a]
Tinnitus louder	37.5	54.4	0	68.7	
No effect	62.5	39.4	0	30.0	
Tinnitus less loud	0	6.2	100	1.3	
Influence of sleep deprivation (%)					**<0.001**[a]
Tinnitus louder	0	89.2	47.2	86.8	
No effect	100	10.8	49.7	11.5	
Tinnitus less loud	0	0.8	3.0	1.8	
Onset (%)					**<0.001**[a]
Acute	48.1	0	49.2	100	
Gradual	51.9	100	50.8	0	
Influence of nap afternoon (%)					**<0.001**[a]
Tinnitus louder	0	27.0	11.2	22.9	
No effect	100	56.8	84.3	52.4	
Tinnitus less loud	0	16.2	4.6	24.7	
Hospital anxiety and depression scale (mean)	4.6	5.6	5.5	6.0	**0.001**[b]
Difference in mean PTA ADS	13.1	10.8	7.9	11.9	**0.015**[b]
Frequency of tinnitus (%)					0.478[a]
0–2,000 Hz	23.2	23.2	21.8	25.1	
2,000–4,000 Hz	14.7	13.9	21.3	15.0	
4,000–6,000 Hz	18.8	20.5	20.3	15.0	
6,000–8,000 Hz	19.5	17.0	12.7	19.4	
>8,000 Hz	23.9	25.5	23.9	25.6	
Visual analog scale tinnitus annoyance (mean)	69.2	69.4	68.2	69.6	0.925[b]

[a]*Pearson Chi-square test.*
[b]*One-way ANOVA.*
ADS, both ears; PTA, pure tone audiometry.
Bold fonts represent a significant p-values (p < 0.05).

DISCUSSION

Key Results

In this study, we performed cluster analysis with the aim to identify subgroups in a population of tinnitus patients. Variable selection for cluster analysis was performed in two ways: by a strict methodological approach based on PCA, and by expert opinion. These analyses identified four- and three-patient clusters, where the clusters showed clearly different characteristics. However, the clustering solution in both analyses was not substantial, as indicated by a poor cluster solution quality.

Although both cluster analyses gave different outcomes, there were also interesting similarities. In both cluster solutions, the effects of "stress" and "loud sounds" on tinnitus have a relatively high discriminative value between groups. In each analysis, a group was revealed in which patients report that their tinnitus gets louder from loud sounds, and there was a group that reported that their tinnitus got less loud. In an earlier cluster analysis by Tyler et al., it is described that their found clusters differed by the effect of external factors on patients' tinnitus: some patients are easily and negatively influenced by external factors and, in others, this has no effect (4). On the contrary, Tyler et al. describe a group that is characterized by high scores on tinnitus questionnaires and the HADS depression and anxiety scale. However, this was not reflected in our cluster solutions.

In the cluster analysis based on variables selected by experts, there was a clear distinction between a group that preferred a silent environment for their tinnitus and another group that had a preference for a noisy environment. The fact that some patients with tinnitus prefer noise and others prefer silence has been described earlier (8). This is interesting, as one might speculate that the latter group may have a higher change of responding well to sound therapy than the other group.

When interpreting these results, it must be kept in mind that the "silhouette measure" of both analyses was only 0.2. This is lower than the critical boundary of 0.25, which implies that there was no substantial clustering in this patient cohort. A lack of clustering indicates that the transition from one cluster to another is relatively smooth, without clear-cut boundaries. As a comparison, consider a group of cities, where the coordinates of the cities would go into a cluster analysis. If one group of cities is clearly separated from another group by a stretch of open land, the silhouette value will be large (when viewed from a distance, the cities will have a distinct silhouette of their skyline). However, if there is no such open land between the clusters, the silhouette value is low, consistent with the absence of substantial clustering. In our patient cohort, there were clearly no distinct "open stretches of land" between the clusters, suggesting that patient form a continuum rather than a clear clustering. As discussed above, the cluster analysis of Tyler et al. identified clusters with characteristics that show some resemblance to the clusters reported here. Unfortunately, Tyler et al. do not report a silhouette value or other measure of clustering. Hence, at present, it is not possible to discuss the clustering strength in their cohort.

Cluster analysis has been upcoming in medical research. Recently, an interesting cluster analysis on bilateral Meniere disease was published to define clinical subgroups with potential

TABLE 3 | Characteristics of the four clusters identified by clustering with variables selected by expert opinion.

	Cluster 1 ($n = 287$)	Cluster 2 ($n = 247$)	Cluster 3 ($n = 227$)	*p*-Value
Influence of loud sound (%)				**<0.001**[a]
Tinnitus louder	16.0	27.9	96.9	
No effect	56.1	38.5	3.1	
Tinnitus less loud	27.9	33.6	0	
Influence of stress (%)				**<0.001**[a]
Tinnitus louder	24.4	87.4	78.4	
No effect	74.9	9.7	21.6	
Tinnitus less loud	0.7	2.8	0	
Preference for silence or noise (%)				**<0.001**[a]
Silence	28.2	25.5	89.9	
Noisy environment	71.8	74.5	10.1	
Are sounds uncomfortably loud? (%)				**<0.001**[a]
Never	18.8	6.9	0.4	
Seldom	28.9	13.4	3.1	
Sometimes	31.4	61.5	31.7	
Most of the time	14.6	13.4	43.2	
Always	6.3	4.9	21.6	
Lateralization of tinnitus (%)				**<0.001**[a]
Bilateral/central	31.0	84.2	38.3	
Unilateral	69.0	15.8	61.7	
Hearing loss category (%)				**<0.001**[a]
No hearing loss	51.9	72.5	44.9	
Asymmetrical hearing loss	15.7	2.4	35.2	
Bilateral high tone hearing loss	17.4	8.9	9.7	
Bilateral flat hearing loss	12.9	16.2	6.2	
Other	2.1	0	4.0	
Variable loudness (%)				**<0.001**[a]
No	49.8	15.0	18.1	
Yes	50.2	85.0	81.9	
Tinnitus handicap index-score (mean)	32.6	48.0	46.9	**<0.001**[b]
Influence of movement of head and neck (%)				**<0.001**[a]
Tinnitus louder	8.4	40.1	39.2	
No effect	84.3	55.5	55.9	
Tinnitus less loud	7.3	4.5	4.8	
Hospital anxiety and depression scale (mean)	4.2	5.9	5.4	**<0.001**[b]
Gender (%)				**<0.001**[a]
Male	59.9	74.1	55.9	
Female	40.1	25.9	44.1	

[a]*Pearson Chi-square test.*
[b]*One-way ANOVA.*
Bold fonts represent a significant p-values ($p < 0.05$).

similar etiologies. In this study, five clinical variants of bilateral Meniere disease were found based on six clinical variables and with a high silhouette measure of 0.8 (9). This study is not only beneficial to improve the selection of patients but also can explain the negative treatment effects of several treatment trials, as results can be biased by a heterogeneous patient group based on etiology (9). The difficulty in cluster analysis is that it is a type of analysis that is very sensitive to change of variables. The selection of variables is critical for the outcome of the cluster analysis (6). Generally, highly correlated variables should be avoided and it is important to select variables that can make a clear-cut differentiation between clusters (6). The systematic statistical approach of selecting variables using the highest factor loading on extracted factors by PCA is often used and has the advantage of choosing variables in a reproducible, transparent way. A downside of this technique is that the factor solution only explains a certain amount of variance and, therefore, much information is discarded. Eliminating factors with low loadings on the extracted factors has the same effect (10). This may lead to a reduced success of a subsequent cluster analysis. On the other hand, a disadvantage of selecting variables based on clinical knowledge or "gut feeling" is that it is less transparent. Also, unrecognized highly discriminating variables may remain undiscovered.

Strengths of the Study

For this study, a very large database of tinnitus patients was used with almost 1,800 patients. Even after exclusion of patients with missing values, $n = 976$ and $n = 761$ could be included in the cluster analyses. We expect that, if clear clustering would have existed with these variables, we would have been able to find it in these groups. There was an overlap of 527 patients who were included in both the first cluster outcome and the second cluster outcome. This is a substantial overlap, pointing out that it does not seem likely that the differences between both cluster analyses are caused by the differences in included patients.

Limitations

This study explored the patient cohort of a tertiary tinnitus referral center. Thus, the population described here consists of a group of tinnitus patients who were persistent in their search for treatments for their tinnitus. Our patient cohort may, therefore, be biased with a certain type of tinnitus patients. Potentially, a study including also less-persistent help seeking and non-help-seeking subjects would have identified a clearer clustering.

Although we had access to a large database of tinnitus patients (n = 1,783), over the years, there were changes in the variables that were collected because of changes made to the diagnostic protocol. Since the cluster analyses required a complete set of data for each patient, not all 1,783 patients could be included in the analysis, but 976 and 761.

Furthermore, it is debated internationally whether tinnitus is a disease or a symptom. One can look at it in both ways: when tinnitus is a result of an acoustic neuroma, then tinnitus can be a symptom. However, if we look at tinnitus as the result of defect on a cellular level of the auditory cortex, then tinnitus can be regarded as a disease. In most patients visiting our clinic, the etiology of the tinnitus is unclear. The fact is that these patients included in our dataset experience bothersome tinnitus. Within this group, we aimed to find subgroups such as patients with continuous central, loud tinnitus tend to have a high score on THI and VAS and find that their tinnitus gets worse in noisy environments. If we are able to find such patterns, may be we can adjust our treatment strategy to that (in this example, hearing aids might not be successful). Although the raised issue about tinnitus being a symptom or disease is important, we believe that this analysis looking for clusters of patients based on tinnitus characteristics transcends this issue.

Finally, the low silhouette value indicates that this patient cohort represents a heterogeneous group without clear clustering. Obviously, any cluster analysis outcome highly depends on the variables that we entered into the clustering algorithm. Our patient data consisted of mainly audiometry and questionnaire metrics. In these cluster analyses, tinnitus patients appear to represent a continuum rather than clearly defined subgroups, based on a low silhouette measure. However, it is possibly that other metrics (e.g., fMRI/EEG, genetic evaluation) are able to identify tinnitus subgroups. In other words, the lack of clustering in our analyses does not imply that clusters do not exist. However, if clusters exist, they cannot be identified with the variables that were considered here.

CONCLUSION

Two cluster analyses of a large patient cohort identified three and four groups of tinnitus patients, respectively. The clustering was not substantial, as a low silhouette measure of the cluster solutions was found. This indicates that in this particular cohort, tinnitus patients appear to represent rather a continuum than clearly defined subgroups. This finding may have consequences for future treatments: if clear subgroups would have been present, clearly distinct treatment might be developed in the future. However, for a continuum of patients, it may be necessary to use a number of treatments to find the optimum for each individual patient. Obviously, our conclusion is based on the set of variables that were at our disposal. Possibly, new future ways to characterize tinnitus patients may be able to find distinct subgroup in tinnitus patients.

AUTHOR CONTRIBUTIONS

Conception of study and design; writing of manuscript: MB and PD. Intellectual contribution to analyses: MB, PD, and EK. Critical revision of the manuscript: RF, RA, PD, and JD. Data acquisition: MB, PD, RA, RH, and EK.

FUNDING

There were no funding sources for this study.

REFERENCES

Savage J, Waddell A. Tinnitus. *BMJ Clin Evid* (2014) 2014:0506.

Hoekstra CE, Wesdorp FM, van Zanten GA. Socio-demographic, health, and tinnitus related variables affecting tinnitus severity. *Ear Hear* (2014) 35(5):544–54. doi:10.1097/AUD.0000000000000045

Clatworthy J, Buick D, Hankins M, Weinman J, Horne R. The use and reporting of cluster analysis in health psychology: a review. *Br J Health Psychol* (2005) 10(Pt 3):329–58. doi:10.1348/135910705X25697

Tyler R, Coelho C, Tao P, Ji H, Noble W, Gehringer A, et al. Identifying tinnitus subgroups with cluster analysis. *Am J Audiol* (2008) 17(2):S176–84. doi:10.1044/1059-0889(2008/07-0044)

Formann AK. *Die Latent-Class-Analyse: Einführungin Theorieund Anwendung.* Weinheim, Germany: Beltz (1984). Available from: http://catalog.hathitrust.org/api/volumes/oclc/16851238.html

Mooi E, Sarstedt M. Cluster analysis. *A Concise Guide to Market Research.* Berlin, Heidelberg: Springer-Verlag (2011). p. 237–84.

Kaufman L, Rousseeuw PJ, editors. *Finding Groups in Data: An Introduction to Cluster Analysis.* Hoboken, NJ: John Wiley & Sons, Inc. (1990).

Stouffer JL, Tyler RS. Characterization of tinnitus by tinnitus patients. *J Speech Hear Disord* (1990) 55(3):439–53. doi:10.1044/jshd.5503.439

Frejo L, Soto-Varela A, Santos-Perez S, Aran I, Batuecas-Caletrio A, Perez-Guillen V, et al. Clinical subgroups in bilateral Meniere disease. *Front Neurol* (2016) 7:182. doi:10.3389/fneur.2016.00182

Dolnicar S, Grunn B. Challenging "factor-cluster-segmentation". *J Travel Res* (2008) 47:63–71. doi:10.1177/0047287508318910

10

Does Chronic Tinnitus Alter the Emotional Response Function of the Amygdala?: A Sound-Evoked fMRI Study

Jeff E. Davies[1,2,3], Phillip E. Gander[2,3] and Deborah A. Hall[2,3]*

[1] Division of Audiology, Faculty of Health and Life Sciences, School of Allied Health Sciences, De Montfort University, Leicester, UK, [2] National Institute for Health Research, Nottingham Hearing Biomedical Research Unit, Nottingham, UK, [3] Otology and Hearing Group, Division of Clinical Neuroscience, School of Medicine, University of Nottingham, Nottingham, UK

***Correspondence:**
Jeff E. Davies
jeff.davies@dmu.ac.uk

Tinnitus is often associated with strong negative thoughts and emotions which can contribute to a distressing and chronic long-term condition. The amygdala, the "feeling and reacting" part of the brain, may play a key role in this process. Although implicated in several theoretical models of tinnitus, quantification of activity in the human amygdala has only been made possible more recently through neuroimaging methods such as functional magnetic resonance imaging (fMRI) but benefits from modified scanning parameters using a double-echo acquisition for improved BOLD sensitivity. This study thus examined the role of the amygdala in emotional sound processing in people with tinnitus using a novel double-echo imaging sequence for optimal detectability of subcortical activity. Our hypotheses were: (1) emotionally evocative sound clips rated as pleasant or unpleasant would elicit stronger amygdalar activation than sound clips rated as neutral, (2) people with tinnitus have greater amygdalar activation in response to emotionally evocative sounds (relative to neutral sounds) compared to controls.

Methods: Twelve participants all with chronic, constant tinnitus took part. We also recruited 11 age and hearing-matched controls. Participants listened to a range of emotionally evocative sound clips; rated as pleasant, unpleasant or neutral. A region-of-interest analysis was chosen to test our a priori hypotheses.

Results: Both groups displayed a robust and similar overall response to sounds vs. silence in the following ascending auditory pathways; inferior colliculus, medial geniculate body and the primary auditory cortex. In support of our first hypothesis, the amygdala's response to pleasant and unpleasant sound clips was significantly greater than neutral sounds. Opposing our second hypothesis, we found that the amygdala's overall response to pleasant and unpleasant sounds (compared to neutral sounds) was actually lower in the tinnitus group as compared to the controls.

Conclusions: The "muted" amygdala activation observed in the tinnitus group could reflect an internal modification of emotional response perhaps as a result of successful habituation to emotionally negative sound. This interpretation would predict a heightened amygdala emotional response in individuals with a more clinically bothersome tinnitus.

Keywords: amygdala, double echo, functional magnetic resonance imaging (fMRI), tinnitus, valence, emotion, distress, fMRI

INTRODUCTION

Tinnitus describes the phantom perception of sound, in the absence of an external sound source. Most individuals who experience tinnitus will habituate such that it does not impact on quality of life or emotional state (Davis and El Rafaie, 2000). However, for some the experience of tinnitus can be distressing, affecting sleep, concentration, and mood (Folmer et al., 1999; Cronlein et al., 2016; Tegg-Quinn et al., 2016). Interestingly, the amount of distress attributed to tinnitus is not predicted by its psychoacoustic composition e.g., perceived loudness (Jakes et al., 1985; Leaver et al., 2012). Instead, the emotional evaluation of stimuli appears strongly linked to the limbic system.

The limbic system is a convenient way of describing a number of functionally and anatomically connected brain structures that regulate autonomic and endocrine function, particularly in response to emotional stimuli (Le Doux, 2000). There is no universal agreement on the total list of structures which comprise the limbic system but it includes the cingulate gyrus, parahippocampal gyrus, hippocampal formation, amygdala, septal area, and hypothalamus (Rajmohan and Mohandas, 2007). The limbic system forms the "feeling and reacting brain" but many of the brain areas within the limbic system are also implicated in memory, particularly emotional memory (Rajmohan and Mohandas, 2007).

The amygdala may be particularly significant in its role of mediating emotional responses to sensory stimuli. To decipher specifically how information is relayed between the auditory cortex and amygdala, Kumar et al. (2012) used a range of aversive sound clips in a group of 16 young adults (aged 22–35) with normal hearing. Their analysis focused on the interactions between auditory cortex and amygdala (effective connectivity) using a technique known as dynamic causal modeling. According to the models tested, they concluded the following: unpleasant sound stimuli are first processed and decoded in the auditory cortex before any emotional response can be assigned by the amygdala. Forward connections from the auditory cortex to the amygdala are modulated by acoustic features. The amygdala then modulates the auditory cortex in accordance with the (un)pleasantness of sounds.

Irwin et al. (2011) compared responses to sound clips of real world soundscapes rated as pleasant, neutral or unpleasant to examine the role of auditory and limbic brain networks in normal hearing adults (aged 21–55 years). Irwin et al. (2011) found that highly pleasant or highly unpleasant soundscapes relative to neutral soundscapes evoked greater activation of a number of auditory brain regions including the auditory cortex and the posterior insula, and non-auditory brain regions such as the amygdala. A large response was found to emotionally evocative sounds, irrespective of whether they were pleasant or unpleasant. Irwin described this as a "U-shaped function." A direct between-hemisphere comparison of amygdala response activation revealed no differences.

The amygdala has been proposed in models of tinnitus to account for the emotional distress that can occur for some individuals in response to "phantom" sounds. Jastreboff's neurophysiological model of tinnitus (1990) includes the amygdala as a key component. Central to this model is the concept that sounds which evoke strong emotional reactions activate limbic and autonomic systems. Sounds can be real physical sounds or phantom sounds such as tinnitus. Typically, repeated exposure to the same sound results in habituation, where the person becomes less aware of that sound. However, when there is an emotional reaction to the sound, any subsequent exposure to the same sound stimulus maintains a conscious awareness of the sound, without habituation. For De Ridder et al. (2011, 2014), a key factor in chronic tinnitus concerns the role of emotional memories. Such memory mechanisms play a role in persistent tinnitus because they result in an extended state of hypervigilance which promotes a sustained state of awareness about the tinnitus. The amygdala is highlighted as a structure of major functional importance because it is not only part of the "distress network" but it also overlaps with brain areas involved in central control of the autonomic system, consistent with Jastreboff's neurophysiological model.

Despite its projected role in tinnitus, the involvement of the amygdala has not been directly measured until more recently (e.g., Shulman et al., 1995; Roy et al., 2009; Crippa et al., 2010; Irwin et al., 2011; Kumar et al., 2012). And even so has been considered as a single functional structure, rather than its known anatomical substructures. Generally these study findings are consistent with the view that the amygdala works with auditory brain regions in the perception of emotionally evocative sounds (both real sounds and phantom sounds). Emotional information (auditory and visual) can be described by two main factors (Bradley and Lang, 2000; Hall et al., 2013). The first factor relates to ratings of pleasantness (valence) and the second factor relates to ratings of vibrancy (arousal). While brain imaging research tends to focus on the coding of pleasantness, for example by measuring the differential response to stimuli that have previously been rated as unpleasant, neutral, or pleasant, Irwin et al. (2011) reported that vibrancy had little effect on the overall brain response.

A majority of the studies examining the response to the emotional dimension of stimulus processing have enrolled young healthy participants (Bradley and Lang, 2000; Costa et al., 2010; Irwin et al., 2011; Kumar et al., 2012). But there are a small number of relevant fMRI studies that have recruited people with tinnitus. Golm et al. (2013) used a non-auditory sentence reading task to stimulate cognitive emotional processing in individuals with varying degrees of tinnitus distress. The task comprised three sentence types, neutral (e.g., regularly I look at my watch), negative (e.g., I often feel sorry for myself), and tinnitus-related (e.g., I will never get rid of the noise). Compared to healthy age- and hearing-matched controls, tinnitus patients showed stronger activations when reading tinnitus-related sentences relative to neutral sentences in many parts of the limbic system: anterior cingulate cortex, mid-cingulate cortex, posterior cingulate cortex, retrosplenial cortex, and insula as well as frontal areas. The tinnitus group were also divided according to levels of perceived tinnitus distress. Individuals with a global score of 31 or higher on the Tinnitus Questionnaire (Hallam, 1996) were assigned into the high distress group. Direct group comparisons (high distress vs. low distress) revealed stronger activity in the left middle frontal gyrus in the high tinnitus distress group, a brain region which Jastreboff (1990) had previously implicated in the integration of sensory and emotional characteristics of tinnitus. Although this study showed some limbic activity, specific amygdala involvement was not found.

Carpenter-Thompson et al. (2014) used emotionally evocative sounds chosen from the International Affective Digital Sounds database (Bradley and Lang, 2007) to directly assess the effects of tinnitus on emotional processing. The authors were motivated by the hypothesis that alterations of the limbic system due to the presence of chronic aversive internal sounds (i.e., tinnitus) are also manifested when processing external affective sounds. They expected to observe an elevated response in the amygdala, parahippocampus, and insula regions of the tinnitus group in response to emotionally evocative sounds, relative to the control groups. They also hypothesized that the tinnitus group would show a heightened response in auditory regions relative to the other two groups. To examine these questions their stimulus set comprised 30 pleasant, 30 unpleasant, and 30 neutral sound clips. In an effort to control for hearing loss, three participant groups were included: "hearing loss with tinnitus" ($n = 13$), "hearing loss without tinnitus," ($n = 12$) and "normal hearing without tinnitus" ($n = 12$). All groups were gender matched and age matched (mean and SD). Contrary to the author's hypothesis, the tinnitus group did not show an elevated amygdala response in either the pleasant > neutral or unpleasant > neutral contrasts. Direct between-group comparisons failed to show any statistically significant differences in the amygdala response, but the authors highlighted a trend across groups such that "normal hearing without tinnitus" > "hearing loss without tinnitus" > "hearing loss with tinnitus" for the two statistical contrasts described above. And these reached statistical significance only at an uncorrected threshold level of $p < 0.001$ in the normal hearing group for emotionally evocative sounds. The authors suggested two reasons for this: (1) individuals with tinnitus might re-route their emotional signaling pathway to avoid the amygdala and its connections to the auditory cortex, (2) because their participants had mildly bothersome tinnitus, and so may have habituated to the tinnitus. However, we propose a third explanation; it is well known that detecting signal from the amygdala is challenging with fMRI due to its location leading to MR signal loss (Chen et al., 2003; Irwin et al., 2012). It is therefore conceivable that the sensitivity to detecting responses relevant for emotional coding may have been restricted by their choice of fMRI parameters, which were not optimally suited for detection Blood Oxygen Level Dependent (BOLD) contrast in the peri-amygdalar area of the brain.

The present study advances our understanding of how chronic tinnitus impacts upon emotional processing by seeking to conduct an independent confirmation of the previous findings reviewed here. For completeness of reporting, we describe the pattern of sound-related activity in the ascending auditory system, but the focus of this article is on two specific directional hypotheses:

1) Sound clips rated as pleasant and/or unpleasant elicit greater amygdalar activity than neutral sound clips.
2) Compared to age and hearing-matched controls, people with tinnitus have greater amygdalar activity in response to pleasant and unpleasant sounds, relative to neutral sounds.

Our study design sought to overcome several limitations of some of the previous studies. First, we took great care to match groups for age and hearing loss accounting for these known confounding effects (Adjamian et al., 2009). Second, we applied a novel double-echo Echo Planar Imaging (EPI) sequence to improve BOLD sensitivity. This sequence acquires two EPI images per pulse and a sum of these two datasets was created for image analysis (Marciani et al., 2006).

An exploratory research question explored whether differential responses could be detected within the three subdivisions of the amygdala. This was of interest because while previous studies (Golm et al., 2013; Carpenter-Thompson et al., 2014) consider the amygdala as a single homogenous body, this structure can be anatomically delineated into three major subdivisions (Amunts et al., 2005); the laterobasal nuclei (LB), the superficial subnuclei (SF), and the centromedial subnuclei (CM).

MATERIALS AND METHODS

Participants

Twelve participants (mean age 65.8 years) with chronic subjective tinnitus and 11 age- and hearing-matched controls (mean age 68.5 years) were recruited through Nottingham Audiology Services or the Ear, Nose and Throat (ENT) department, Queen's Medical Centre, Nottingham. All participants were aged 49–75 years without a history of neurological disorder. See **Table 1**. for participant demographics and tinnitus characteristics. This study was approved by the National Research Ethics Committee (REC: 09/H0407/8). All participants gave written informed consent prior to taking part. Participants reported in this current study are also described in a previous article (Davies et al., 2014).

Clinical Profile

All participants underwent extended frequency audiometry (125–14 kHz) prior to scanning. No participants presented with unilateral or asymmetrical hearing loss (as indicated by a between-ear air conduction threshold difference of 15 dB at two or more consecutive frequencies). The average hearing status of both groups could be described as a bilateral, mild to moderately severe sloping sensorineural hearing loss, typical of presbyacusis (see **Figure 1**). All participants were not considered to have hyperacusis, as indicated by a score of <29 on the hyperacusis questionnaire (Khalfa et al., 2002).

Questionnaire scores are given in **Table 1**. All participants completed the Hyperacusis Questionnaire (HQ: Khalfa et al., 2002), the Beck Anxiety Inventory (BAI: Beck et al., 1988) and the Beck Depression Inventory—Fast Screen (BDI-FS: Beck et al., 2000). Groups were comparable in terms of clinical profile of co-morbidities. No participant had a HQ score greater than the 28 point cut-off for hyperacusis (Khalfa et al., 2002). All participants had low anxiety, as evidenced by scores <21 on the BAI scale. And all but one participant in each group

TABLE 1 | Group demographics, questionnaire scores and tinnitus characteristics.

	No tinnitus group					Tinnitus group					Tinnitus characteristics			
	Sex	**Age**	**HQ**	**BAI**	**BDI-FS**	**Sex**	**Age**	**HQ**	**BAI**	**BDI-FS**	**Laterality**	**Duration (yrs)**	**THQ**	**TCHQ % annoy**
	F	68	6	2	0	M	72	24	10	4	L	15	25.1	28
	F	71	9	8	3	M	64	14	2	2	L&R	2	35.5	10
	M	58	13	2	0	M	72	14	2	2	L&R	2	60.4	70
	M	68	19	0	3	F	67	8	6	0	L&R	4	61.3	50
	M	75	8	3	0	F	73	11	4	2	IN HEAD	70	21.1	5
	M	68	9	0	0	F	57	18	11	0	IN HEAD	2	63.3	50
	M	60	2	0	0	M	71	22	3	0	IN HEAD	6	68.4	30
	F	75	18	13	4	M	71	11	5	0	L&R	10	32.2	20
	M	66	8	0	0	M	64	11	0	0	L&R	20	30	20
	M	74	2	0	1	F	72	17	3	0	R	13	50.6	35
	M	70	11	14	0	M	49	10	4	2	L&R	2	57.5	50
	~	~	~	~	~	F	58	15	1	1	L&R	40	18.7	25
MEAN	8M/3F	68.5	9.6	3.8	1	7M/5F	65.8	14.6	4.3	1.1	~	15.5	43.7	32.8
SD	~	~	5.54	5.34	1.55	~	~	4.9	3.36	1.31	~	20.4	18.32	

M, male; F, female; L, left; R, right; HEAD, central tinnitus; HQ, hyperacusis questionnaire; BAI, beck anxiety inventory; BDI-FS, beck depression inventory—fast screen; THQ, tinnitus handicap questionnaire; TCHQ, tinnitus case history questionnaire.

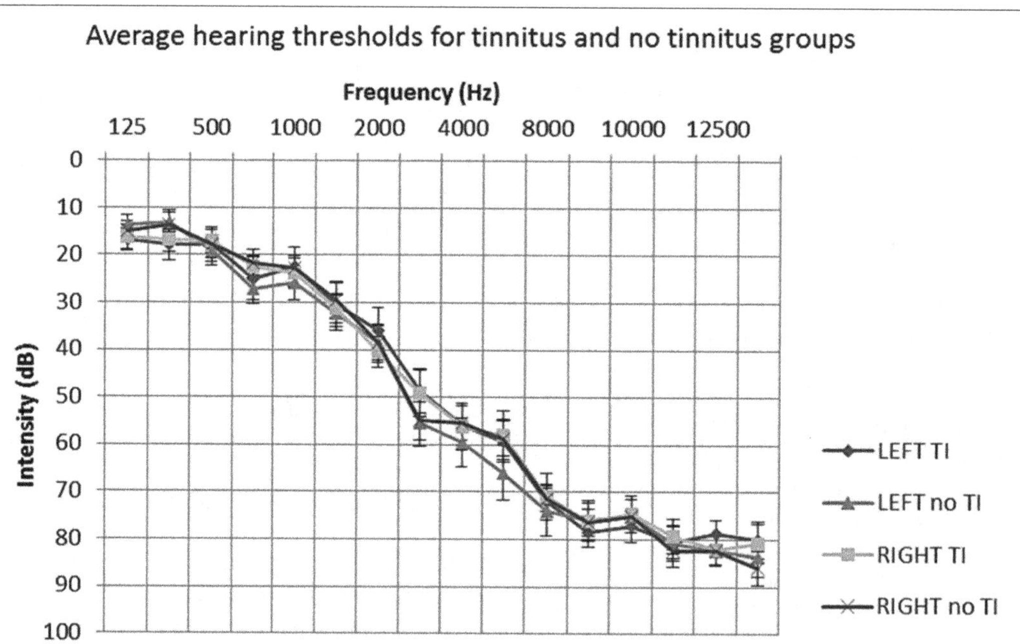

FIGURE 1 | Mean average audiometric thresholds for tinnitus and no tinnitus groups. *Post hoc t*-tests of average hearing thresholds found no significant differences between or within participant groups ($P > 0.05$). Error bars represent one standard error of the mean. TI, tinnitus.

had a minimal depression, as evidenced by scores ≤3 on the BDI-FS scale.

Tinnitus participants also completed the Tinnitus Handicap Questionnaire (THQ: Kuk et al., 1990) and the Tinnitus Case History Questionnaire (TCHQ: Langguth et al., 2007). The tinnitus group had an average global THQ score of 43.7 out of 100 and subjectively rated their tinnitus annoyance at 32.8 out of 100.

Sound Stimuli and Task

The present study used 84 sound clips derived from a previously published fMRI study (Irwin et al., 2011). This subset of sound clips were chosen to vary among natural and mechanical real-world sound sources and were previously rated as being pleasant e.g., bird song, unpleasant e.g., car crash or neutral e.g., footsteps. The strategy used to rate the sound clips (see Hall et al., 2013) was as follows; five raters (aged between 21 and 40) rated a total of 219 sound clips using a 9-point visual analog scale with anchor points at either end e.g., 1 = unpleasant/unhappy, 5 = neutral and 9 = pleasant/happy. Scores for each sound clip were comparable across the five raters. In the present study, these sound clips were further reduced down to 84 sound clips (28 pleasant, 28 neutral, and 28 unpleasant) by omitting sounds that were rated either between the anchor end-points (pleasant and unpleasant) or not in the center (neutral) of the 9-point scale. Although our study participants did not rate the sound clips, many of their subjective comments regarding their pleasantness aligned with the formal ratings. Furthermore, we did not expect people with tinnitus to rate sounds differently to that of individuals without tinnitus, for example see Carpenter-Thompson et al. (2014). The intensity of all sound clips was matched at 71 dB A by taking a root-mean-square level average over the 7.8 s clip duration. In an effort to preserve the ecological validity of the listener experience, frequency content was not altered to compensate for participant hearing levels.

Figure 2 shows an illustrative example of the sound clip sequence design which participants had to listen to whilst in the MRI scanner. Each sound clip had a 50 ms onset and offset ramp. Sound clips were presented to participants in a pseudo-randomized order, such that the three categories of sound (neutral, pleasant, and unpleasant) and silence period occurred within a single block that was repeated 16 times. Within each block two segments of sound clips of the same category (or silence) were played in succession (brief inter-stimulus gap of 450 ms) and no repeated sounds were allowed in the two segments. Each participant therefore listened to each sound category (and silent periods) a total of 32 times. The sequence of sounds was constrained to avoid two sequential blocks of the same sound category. Three different unique orderings of sounds were created (i.e., not similar within or across blocks) and randomized across subjects.

fMRI Acquisition

Data were obtained using a Philips Achieva 3.0 Tesla MR scanner (Philips Medical Systems, The Netherlands) and an 8-channel SENSE receiver head coil. For improved BOLD sensitivity in the peri-amygdala area, whole-brain EPI data were acquired by collecting two MR time-series at echo times of 20 and 45 ms after each radio-frequency (RF) pulse (see Marciani et al., 2006). Other EPI parameters were: $TR = 8250$ ms, acquisition time = 2,420 ms, 36 slices, 0 mm slice gap, $FOV = 240 \times 240$ mm along the AC-PC line, voxel size = $3 \times 3 \times 3$ mm, acquisition matrix = 80×77, 120 volumes, SENSE factor = 2.3, descending slice order). Slice acquisition angle was tilted in line with the axis of the supratemporal plane to capture as much of the brain as possible, with the same negative sloping pitch in the sagittal plane for each subject.

A sparse sampling sequence was adopted, which gave long periods of no scanner noise (5830 ms) in between acquisitions (Hall et al., 1999). Sound clips were presented as shown in **Figure 3**. Our previous methodological work supports our belief that the small overlap of the sound and the scan acquisition does not affect the BOLD response to the extent that it would affect the statistical contrasts of interest. A 5 min MPRAGE anatomical image was also acquired for each participant (160 slices, $FOV = 256$, voxel size $1 \times 1 \times 1$ mm).

The participants were instructed to keep still with their eyes closed and listen to the sounds. Scanning duration was approximately 16 min. Sound stimuli were delivered through customized circum-aural ear defenders which could provide up to 40 dB attenuation. The ear defenders also employed active noise cancelation, helping to reduce scanner noise by up to an additional 35 dB (Hall et al., 2009). The noise reduction procedures were considered critical for the perception of the sounds, but also to make the scanner environment more suitable for people with tinnitus, whose tinnitus sound could otherwise be masked by the scanner noise or even exacerbated.

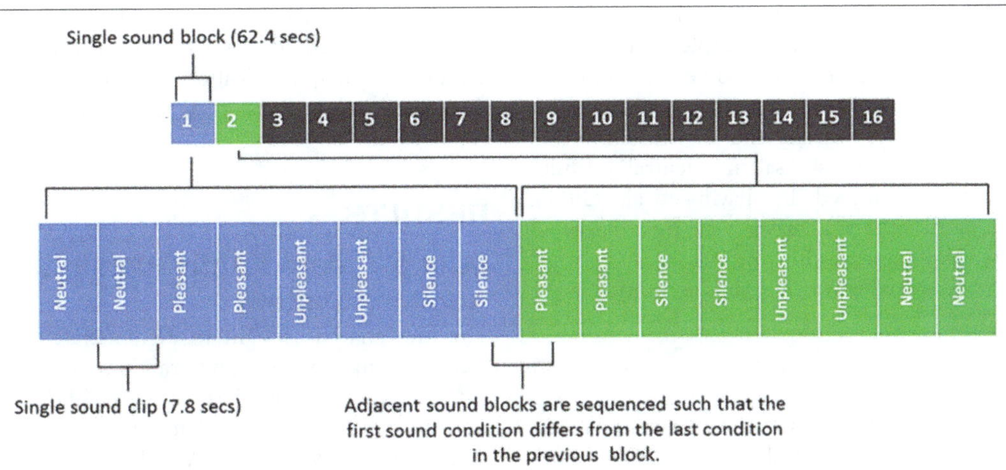

FIGURE 2 | Sound clip sequence, with blocks 1 and 2 being broken down into their component parts for illustrative purposes. Each sound block contains 4 different sound conditions/8 sound clips (each sound clip is repeated in quick succession; with a brief inter-stimulus gap of 450 ms). Total duration of all 16 sounds blocks was 16 min 38 s.

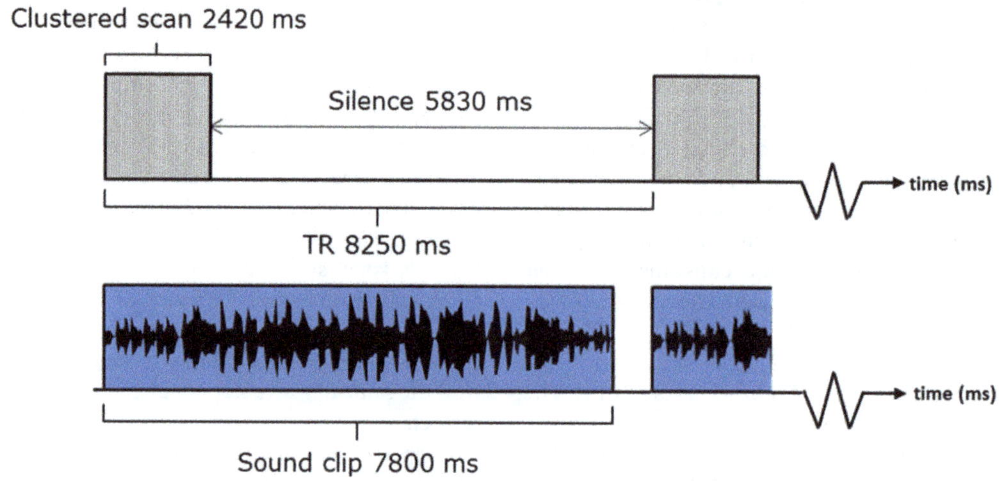

FIGURE 3 | fMRI listening task paradigm.

Preprocessing and Analysis

First, the two time-series (i.e., at 20 and 45 ms echo times) were combined using a weighted sum; with equal 50/50 weighting using a custom MATLAB script. The single functional time-series was then processed using statistical parametric mapping software SPM8 (http://www.fil.ion.ucl.ac.uk/spm/software/spm8/). Images were realigned, co-registered with the participant's high resolution anatomical scan, normalized to the Montreal Neurological Institute (MNI152) template and spatially smoothed (4 mm full-width at half maximum). A 4 mm smoothing kernel was chosen because of the desire to limit signal spread in small brain regions (Morawetz et al., 2008). The precision of the normalization process was checked visually using the inferior colliculus as a marker since this is easily visible as a discrete structure on both anatomical and functional images.

We adopted a random effects general linear model approach. A first-level fixed-effects analysis was performed on each individual's data, specifying the following t contrasts (sound>silence, pleasant>neutral, unpleasant>neutral, neutral>silence and salient>neutral). Here, "sound" is defined as the sum of all sound conditions. "Salient" is defined as the sum of both pleasant and unpleasant sound conditions such that the contrast "salient>neutral" defines the U-shaped function identified by Irwin et al. (2011). A second-level random effects analysis was then specified to interrogate the hypotheses, with the variance between individuals within a group and between groups accounted in the model.

Regions of Interest

The ascending auditory system comprises the inferior colliculus, medical geniculate nucleus, and auditory cortex in both hemispheres. Localization of activity in the inferior colliculus and medial geniculate body was guided by known co-ordinates (±SEM) for the center of each region. A single inferior colliculus has a volume of about 135 mm^3 (Kang et al., 2008) which, at our given acquisition resolution, corresponds to 5 voxels, with an MNI co-ordinate center of +/−4, −4, −10 mm. A single medical geniculate nucleus has a volume of about 129 mm^3 (Kitajima et al., 2015) which corresponds to 5 voxels with a center at ±15, −27, −7 mm.

To test our *a priori* hypotheses relating to sound-evoked activation, analysis targeted pre-defined regions relevant to the hypotheses concerning amygdala in both hemispheres. The average size of the "classic" amygdala is estimated to be 1.24 cm^3 ($SD = 0.14$), while the average size of the amygdala with wider borders was 1.63 cm^3 ($SD = 0.2$) (Brabec et al., 2010). At our given acquisition resolution, this corresponded to 23–53 voxels. To localize the amygdala, we used a probabilistic map of the amygdala and its subdivisions based on anatomical data and transformed into MNI space and implemented in the SPM anatomy toolbox v1.8 (Amunts et al., 2005; Eickhoff et al., 2005). This map defined a wide amygdala border as it was thresholded to include those voxels with a <10% probability. While this method reduces the impact of normalization errors on the quantification of overall amygdala activity, it does reduce the precision of segmenting the three amygdalar subdivisions.

RESULTS

Sound-Related Activation in the Ascending Auditory System

The first analysis sought to demonstrate sound-related brain activity using a second-level random effects one-sample *t*-test for the contrast "sound>silence" in SPM8 ($n = 23$). Results were whole-brain corrected for family wise error (FWE) and thresholded at $p < 0.05$. We observed robust sound-evoked activation within the inferior colliculus, medial geniculate body and primary auditory cortex, across both hemispheres (see **Figure 4**). There were no significant differences between groups ($p > 0.05$ FWE corrected).

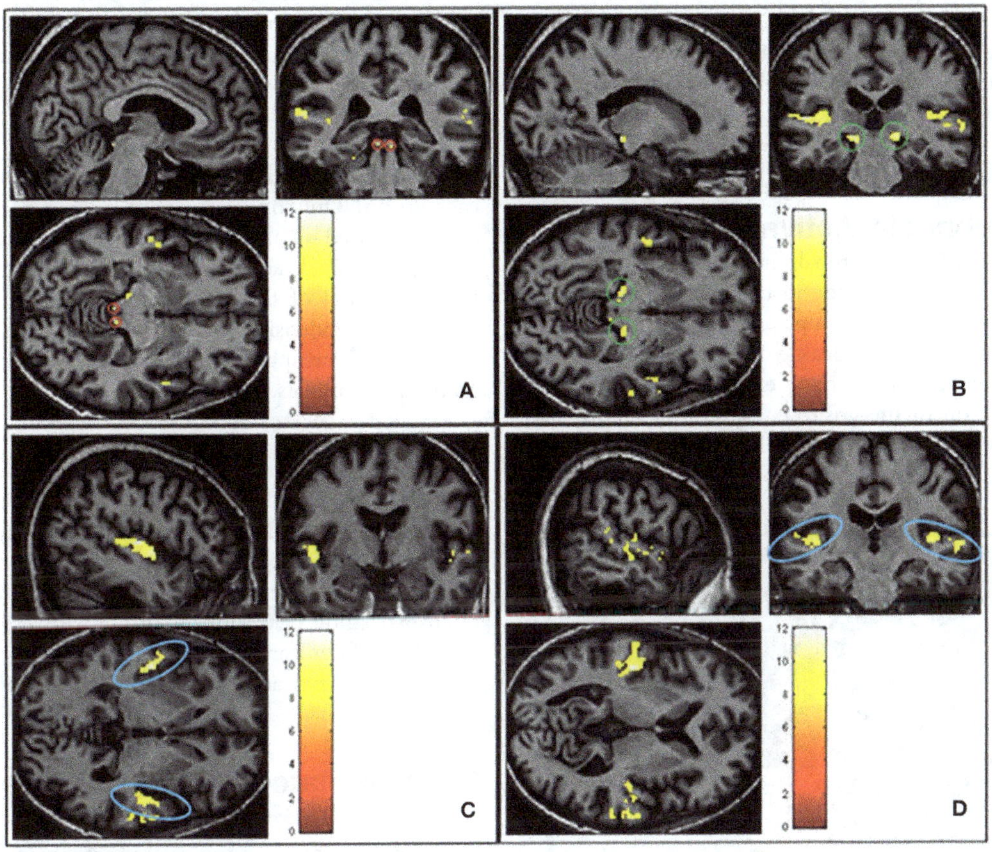

FIGURE 4 | Shows group averaged (n = 23) activation of ascending auditory structures in response to all sound conditions (pleasant, neutral and unpleasant) > silence (p < 0.05 FWE corrected). (A) Inferior colliculus circled in red. **(B)** Medial geniculate body circled in green. **(C)** Primary auditory cortex circled in blue. **(D)** Primary auditory cortex circled in blue.

Differential Sound-Evoked Activity in Amygdala

The next analysis addressed the first hypothesis by examining the data using a second-level random effects one-sample t-test for the contrast "salient>neutral" in SPM8 ($n = 23$). Because we were testing a specific hypothesis in a pre-defined region of the brain we report uncorrected p-values. Within the thresholded borders of the probabilistic map, bilateral amygdala activity was observed to be greater in response to pleasant sounds and unpleasant sounds compared with neutral sounds ($p < 0.05$, uncorrected), potentially consistent with a U-shaped function. The uncorrected result is shown in **Figure 5**. However, this did not survive statistical thresholding after implementing FWE small volume correction.

Effects of Tinnitus on the Response to Pleasant and Unpleasant Sounds

The second hypothesis predicted that people with tinnitus have greater amygdala activity in response to emotionally evocative sounds (relative to neutral sounds) compared to age and hearing-matched controls. Overall amygdala activity was quantified by selecting the peak maxima for the contrast "salient>neutral," separately in the left and right hemisphere for each individual. Peak maxima fell within the borders of the probabilistic map, as above. For each peak maxima, we extracted the general linear model beta values for each sound condition. These beta values were then submitted to a mixed model ANalysis Of VAriance (ANOVA) in SPSS, with two within-group factors; valence (pleasant, neutral, and unpleasant) and hemisphere (left and right) and one between-group factor (no tinnitus and tinnitus). Results are displayed in **Figure 6**. Again results in these selected voxels confirmed there was a strong effect of valence [$F_{(2, 42)} = 102.99$, $p < 0.0001$], with the amygdala showing the greatest response to pleasant sounds and unpleasant sounds compared with neutral sounds. However, the response was statistically equivalent in both people with tinnitus and no tinnitus controls [$F_{(1, 21)} = 3.58$, $p = 0.072$] and across hemispheres [$F_{(1, 42)} = 0.27, p = 0.608$]. There was no interaction between hemisphere and group [$F_{(1, 42)} = 2.06, p = 0.166$].

A significant interaction was observed between valence and group [$F_{(2, 42)} = 3.63, p = 0.035$]. *Post-hoc* testing showed that the no tinnitus group had a significantly greater amygdala response to pleasant>neutral sounds ($p = 0.024$) and unpleasant>neutral sounds ($p = 0.043$) compared to the tinnitus group. Direct comparison of the amygdala's response to the neutral>silence condition were not significantly different between groups ($p = 0.77$) suggesting that both groups had a similar "baseline response" to neutral sounds. These main effects and U-shaped pattern were confirmed even when a more conservative ANOVA was re-run to include only those participants with peaks confirmed within the amygdala according to the probabilistic atlas.

Amygdala Subnuclei Activation

The voxel-wise statistics and probability value associated with each peak maxima for the contrast "salient>neutral" are presented in **Table 2** (tinnitus group) and **Table 3** (no tinnitus controls). The assignment of peak voxel to subdivisions of the amygdala provides preliminary exploratory information about the distribution of the greatest response to emotionally evocative sounds (relative to neutral sounds) within this brain region. Whilst all peak voxel amygdala co-ordinates fell within the borders of the probabilistic map, we note that some contiguous voxel clusters extend beyond those borders.

Bilateral peak activity occurred in 9 out of 12 (75%) tinnitus participants and 9 out of 11 (81.8%) of the no tinnitus controls. Unilateral peak activity occurred in six participants (3 from each group). Only one participant (subject 85 in the no tinnitus group) showed no amygdala activation in either the left or right hemisphere. Peak activity was most likely to be found in the LB subdivision of the amygdala, and least likely to be found in the CM subdivision of the amygdala. This pattern was true across both hemispheres and both for people with tinnitus and no tinnitus controls.

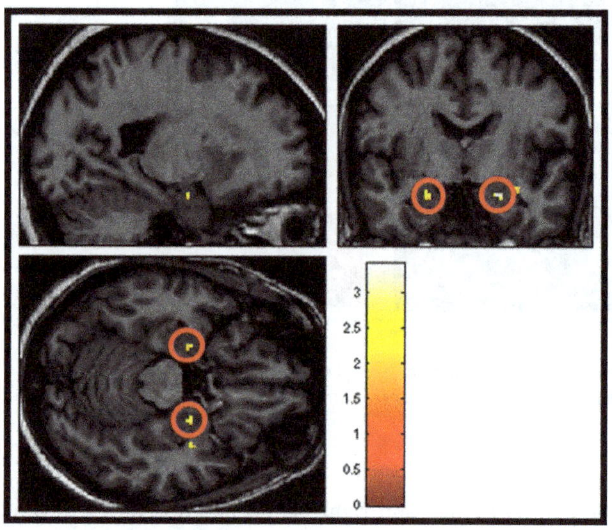

FIGURE 5 | Shows group averaged ($n = 23$) activation of amygdala structures (circled in red) in response to salience > neutral sound condition, masked with amygdala template ($p < 0.05$ uncorrected).

DISCUSSION

This study examined how the amygdala responds to emotionally evocative sounds in people with and without chronic tinnitus. Using an experimental protocol adapted from a previously published study (Irwin et al., 2011) we were able to measure activation of auditory brain areas and the amygdala in response to emotionally evocative sounds. The main findings of all analyses are now discussed.

Sound-Related Activation of Ascending Auditory Pathways

We found significant sound-related activity in several portions of the ascending auditory pathways including the inferior colliculus, medial geniculate body and the primary auditory cortex, across both brain hemispheres. As expected, this replicates the findings of several earlier sound-evoked studies (Hunter et al., 2010; Husain et al., 2011; Irwin et al., 2011; Carpenter-Thompson et al., 2014). Upon direct statistical comparison between groups, we found no differences in activation amongst auditory brain regions. This finding mimics that of Carpenter-Thompson et al. (2014) study which implemented a similar experimental design and also controlled for hearing loss.

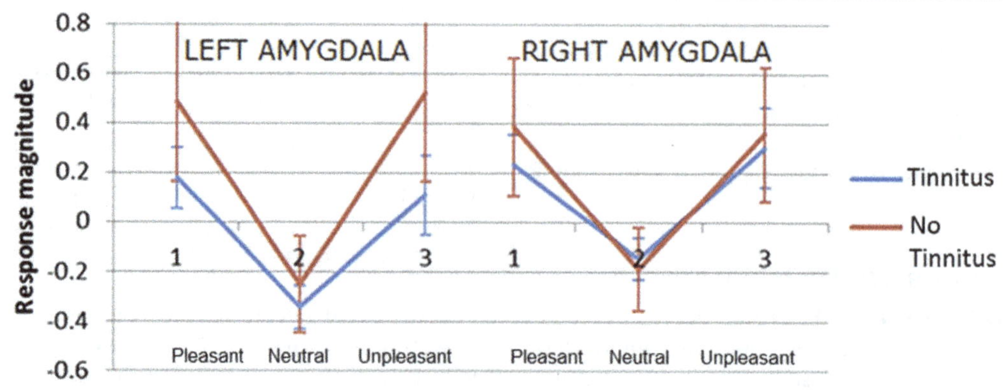

FIGURE 6 | Plots of mean response magnitude (beta values $p < 0.05$, uncorrected) for the left and right amygdala across three categories of pleasantness (1) pleasant (2) neutral (3) unpleasant. Error bars represent 95% confidence intervals.

TABLE 2 | Tinnitus group: Amygdala response to the "salient>neutral" contrast ($p < 0.05$ uncorrected).

Subject No.	Peak voxel co-ordinates and associated statistics							Localization probability		
	x	*y*	*z*	*T*-stat	*Z*-score	T2* intensity	Cluster size	LB	SF	CM
LEFT AMYGDALA										
1	−24	−14	−8	2.19	2.17	35.07	24	20	30	40
6	−26	−6	−30	2.75	2.7	26.95	7	50	0	0
17	−22	−10	−24	3.01	2.94	59.42	36	100	10	0
19	−20	−8	−12	2.41	2.38	29.54	10	80	100	20
24	−22	−6	−16	3.29	3.2	50.14	133	60	50	10
25	−26	2	−28	2.68	2.63	34.64	71	0	0	0
29	−26	−6	−24	1.93	1.91	20.62	2	100	0	0
30	−30	−2	−18	1.63 n.s	1.63 n.s	57.08	4	20	0	0
34	−34	−2	−22	2.4	2.36	40.93	4	0	0	0
45	−16	0	−18	2.94	2.87	55.26	9	10	0	0
54	−32	−6	−32	2.44	2.39	41.64	16	0	0	0
74	−28	−6	−20	3.88	3.72	57.78	134	100	0	0
Average						42.42				
SD						13.35				
RIGHT AMYGDALA										
1	26	−2	−18	2.4	2.37	55.21	17	10	10	0
6	32	−10	−10	2.55	2.51	55.45	3	60	20	0
17	18	−6	−20	2.44	2.4	65.28	17	0	10	0
19	28	−14	−8	2.83	2.77	43.75	10	40	20	20
24	32	−2	−36	3.41	3.31	37.96	42	10	0	0
25	30	2	−24	2.95	3.88	57.84	43	0	0	0
29	30	4	−32	1.49 n.s	1.49 n.s	0	2	10	0	0
30	28	−2	−18	1.84	1.83	69.45	3	30	10	0
34	30	−4	−22	3.05	2.97	49.25	79	70	0	0
45	24	−4	−12	2.47	2.43	60.07	10	20	60	0
54	20	−10	−12	2.23	2.19	59.98	10	10	80	0
74	20	−8	−12	2.27	2.23	45	15	0	80	0
Average						49.93				
SD						18.19				
(*T*-stat of 1.66/$p = 0.049$)										

Statistical outputs are reported for each individual's peak voxel amygdala co-ordinates (across hemispheres). Amygdala subnuclei: SF, superficial; CM, centromedial; LB, laterobasal. n.s, not significant ($p > 0.05$).

The Effects of Pleasantness on Amygdala Activity

In support of our first hypothesis we found that the amygdala's response to sound was significantly modulated by emotional valence. That is, compared with neutral sound clips, the amygdala's response to pleasant and unpleasant sound clips was significantly enhanced. This overall "U-shaped" response to pleasantness reflects the same amygdala response pattern found by Irwin et al. (2011) in young adults with normal hearing. Also in agreement with Irwin et al.'s (2011) data, we found no main effect of hemisphere, suggesting a lack of amygdala dominance. However, the distinctive amygdala U-shaped response pattern that has been independently replicated across both studies seems to suggest a genuine neurophysiological difference in amygdala function between sound conditions.

Contrary to our second hypothesis, we found no significant main effect of group, indicating that the amygdala's overall response to emotionally evocative sounds was similar between groups. Surprisingly however, a consistent trend for higher activation in response to salient sounds compared with neutral sounds was observed in the "no tinnitus group." Planned contrasts revealed the specific nature of this relationship. Compared to the "tinnitus group," the "no tinnitus" group had significantly greater amygdala response magnitude to both pleasant and unpleasant sounds (compared to neutral sounds). By comparing the neutral>silence conditions we determined that there was no difference in baseline activation to non-valent sound between our tinnitus and control groups, discounting the possibility of a ceiling effect caused by a raised baseline response from either group. Our findings are able to build

TABLE 3 | No tinnitus group: Amygdala response to the "salient>neutral" contrast ($p < 0.05$ uncorrected).

Subject No.	Peak voxel co-ordinates and associated statistics							Localization probability		
	x	*y*	*z*	*T*-stat	*Z*-score	T2* intensity	Cluster size	LB	SF	CM
LEFT AMYGDALA										
79	−22	−6	−16	2.6	2.54	41.7	23	60	50	10
80	−22	0	−22	3.18	3.09	137.02	60	20	10	0
81	−20	0	−22	4.07	3.88	31.85	53	10	10	0
82	−22	−8	−20	3.2	3.1	39.82	55	90	30	0
83	−24	−2	−22	3.08	2.99	53.07	50	30	10	0
84	−22	−6	−28	2.5	2.45	38.23	12	50	0	0
85	−26	2	−26	1.8	1.78	48.41	3	0	0	0
86	−20	−4	−10	1.57 n.s	1.57 n.s	30.39	1	0	70	10
88	−22	−6	−14	3	2.92	46.41	24	20	50	20
89	−20	−6	−6	2.89	2.82	22.56	5	10	80	20
90	−26	−6	−28	2.55	2.5	40.54	23	60	0	0
Average						48.14				
SD						30.70				
RIGHT AMYGDALA										
79	20	−6	−12	2.23	2.2	77.17	9	0	80	0
80	32	−2	−22	2.5	2.45	62.82	17	60	0	0
81	32	0	−20	2.41	2.36	54.44	8	0	0	0
82	36	−4	−32	2.7	2.64	39.77	15	10	0	0
83	28	−16	−8	2.63	2.57	45.23	6	30	20	20
84	24	−4	−30	3.21	3.11	35.56	27	0	0	0
85	28	2	−26	1.8	1.78	37.39	1	0	0	0
86	30	−8	−14	1.88	1.87	35.71	3	80	30	0
88	34	−6	−20	2.62	2.57	52.74	14	80	10	0
89	34	2	−26	2.38	2.34	28.96	14	0	0	0
90	30	−2	−20	2.43	2.39	62.67	10	50	0	0
Average						48.40				
SD						14.84				
(*T* stat of 1.66/$p = 0.049$)										

Statistical outputs are reported for each individual's peak voxel amygdala co-ordinates (across hemispheres). Amygdala subnuclei: SF, superficial; CM, centromedial; LB, laterobasal. n.s, not significant ($p > 0.05$).

on this uncertainty discussed by Carpenter-Thompson et al. (2014) who did not use a silence condition. In opposition to our original hypothesis, these findings seems to indicate a "muting" of the amygdala response amongst individuals with tinnitus. This finding agrees with Carpenter-Thompson et al. (2014) who observed a decreasing trend in amygdala response activation for NH>HL>TIN groups (note this trend was not statistically significant). Two potential interpretations of this finding include: (1) given the chronic nature of tinnitus, amygdala resources could be automatically be recruited to process the valent tinnitus sound, or (2) people with tinnitus may be actively controlling their emotional response to tinnitus. It may therefore be plausible that in an effort to reduce one's emotional reaction to tinnitus, affected individuals suppress amygdala activation through self-modulation in an effort to divert attention away from the experience of chronic tinnitus. In doing so, this leaves less available "resources" for assignment to other emotional stimuli. Supporting this notion, Domes et al. (2010) found that a group of healthy adults were able to modulate activation of their amygdala up or down by increasing or decreasing their emotional response to affective visual stimuli. Notably, our participants had mild to moderate tinnitus distress and may be better / more successful tinnitus habituators.

Amygdala Subnuclei Activation

Amygdala activation was found in the vast majority of participants ($n = 22/23$). This number is considerably higher than Irwin et al. (2011) study from which this experimental protocol was adapted, where only 3/16 participants demonstrated suprathreshold amygdala activity. This large difference in amygdala detectability between studies may reflect our application of a double echo imaging sequence, which is known to provide improved signal contrast across the brain and improved BOLD sensitivity across a range of tissues (Posse et al., 1999; Marciani et al., 2006).

In our exploratory research question which explored whether differential responses could be detected within the three subdivisions of the amygdala, we found that peak activity was most likely to be found in the LB subdivision of the amygdala, and least likely to be found in the CM subdivision of the amygdala. This pattern was consistent across both hemispheres and for both study groups. Within the animal literature, it is well known that the LB nuclei acts as the "gateway" for sensory information to the amygdala, receiving input from both the auditory thalamus and from association areas of the auditory cortex (Bordi and LeDoux, 1992). Support for similar involvement of the LB nuclei when processing emotionally evocative auditory stimuli has been presented in more recent human neuroimaging studies (Ball et al., 2007; Kumar et al., 2012). Kumar et al. (2012) found both the LB and the SF nucleus to encode acoustic features necessary for attributing valence. An earlier study by Ball et al. (2007) also found activation of the LB nuclei but in response to both pleasant and unpleasant sounds. Here, the authors thought this finding may reflect a predominance of auditory inputs to LB subnuclei. In line with this literature, our observed decreasing trend of LB>SF>CM subnuclei activation seems to suggest that the LB nuclei played the most active role in processing the emotional auditory stimuli. However, Ball et al. (2007) discuss an important caveat regarding the choice of voxel resolution. Given that the centers of the different amygdala nuclei are at most 1 cm apart (Mai et al., 1997), subdivision-level investigation of the human amygdala is not optimized at 3 mm^3 resolution. This finding should therefore be interpreted cautiously.

CONCLUSION

To summarize, this study used a double-echo imaging sequence to optimally detect amygdala response patterns to emotionally evocative sounds in people with mild to moderately distressing tinnitus. Our main results show a strong modulatory effect of emotional valence on the amygdala's response. This pattern of activation was reduced in individuals with tinnitus, contrary to our expectations.

By using micro-anatomically defined probabilistic maps, we were able to estimate the origins of amygdala peak level activity. In line with previous research, this found the LB nucleus to be most active when processing emotional auditory stimuli. Based on these findings, the amygdala does appear to provide some useful information which could help in the identification and objectification of tinnitus. However, such activation patterns are, up to now, unlikely to be able to differentiate between the true presence or absence of tinnitus on a single subject level. Future studies targeting amygdala function should carefully consider fMRI parameters to ensure sufficient signal quality from the amygdala regions.

AUTHOR CONTRIBUTIONS

JD, PG, and DH conceived the study. JD and PG collected the data. JD analyzed the data and wrote the article. PG and DH supervised and provided guidance.

ACKNOWLEDGMENTS

This research was supported by a Deafness Research UK PhD studentship awarded to the first author JD.

REFERENCES

Adjamian, P., Magdalena, S., and Hall, D. (2009). The mechanisms for tinnitus: perspectives from human functional neuroimaging. *Hear. Res.* 253, 15–31. doi: 10.1016/j.heares.2009.04.001

Amunts, K., Kedo, O., Kindler, M., Pieperhoff, P., Mohlberg, H., Shah, N., et al. (2005). Cytoarchitectonic mapping of the human amygdala, hippocampal region and entorhinal cortex: intersubject variability and probability maps. *Anatomy Embryol.* 210, 343–352. doi: 10.1007/s00429-005-0025-5

Ball, T., Rahm, B., Eickhoff, S. B., Schulze-Bonhage, A., Speck, O., and Mutschler, I. (2007). Response properties of human amygdala subregions: evidence based on functional MRI combined with probabilistic anatomical maps. *PLoS ONE* 2:e307. doi: 10.1371/journal.pone.0000307

Beck, A. T., Epstein, N., Brown, G., and Steer, R. A., (1988). An inventory for measuring clinical anxiety: psychometric properties. *J. Consult. Clin. Psychol.* 56, 893–897. doi: 10.1037/0022-006X.56.6.893

Beck, A. T., Steer, R. A., and Brown, G. K. (2000). *BDI-Fast Screen for Medical Patients: Manual.* San Antonio, TX: Psychological Corporation.

Bordi, F., and LeDoux, J. (1992). Sensory tuning beyond the sensory system: an initial analysis of auditory response properties of neurons in the lateral amygdaloid nucleus and overlying areas of the striatum. *J. Neurosci.* 12, 2493–2503.

Brabec, J., Rulseh, A., Hoyt, B., Vizek, M., Horinek, D., Hort, J., et al. (2010). Volumetry of the human amygdala - an anatomical study. *Psychiatry Res.* 182, 67–72. doi: 10.1016/j.pscychresns.2009.11.005

Bradley, M. M., and Lang, P. J. (2000). Affective reactions to acoustic stimuli. *Psychophysiology* 37, 204–215. doi: 10.1111/1469-8986.3720204

Bradley, M. M., and Lang, P. J. (2007). *The International Affective Digitized Sounds (IADS-2): Affective Ratings of Sounds and Instruction Manual.* Gainesville, FL: University of Florida.

Carpenter-Thompson, J. R., Akrofi, K., Schmidt, S. A., Dolcos, F., and Husain, F. T. (2014). Alterations of the emotional processing system may underlie preserved rapid reaction time in tinnitus. *Brain Res.* 1567, 28–41. doi: 10.1016/j.brainres.2014.04.024

Chen, N. K., Dickey, C. C., Yoo, S.-S., Guttman, C. R. G., and Panych, L. P. (2003). Selection of voxel size and slice orientation for fMRI in the presence of susceptibility field gradients: application to imaging of the amygdala. *NeuroImage* 19, 817–825. doi: 10.1016/S1053-8119(03)00091-0

Costa, V. D., Lang, P. J., Sabatinelli, D., Versace, F., and Bradley, M. M. (2010). Emotional imagery: assessing pleasure and arousal in the brain's reward circuitry. *Hum. Brain Mapp.* 31, 1446–1457. doi: 10.1002/hbm.20948

Crippa, A., Lanting, C. P., van Dijk, P., and Roerdink, J. B. (2010). A diffusion tensor imaging study on the auditory system and tinnitus. *Open Neuroimage J.* 4, 16–25. doi: 10.2174/1874440001004010016

Cronlein, T., Langguth, B., Pregler, M., Kreuzer, P. M., Wetter, T. C., and Schecklmann, M. (2016). Insomnia in patients with chronic tinnitus: Cognitive and emotional distress as moderator variables. *J. Psychosom. Res.* 83, 65–68. doi: 10.1016/j.jpsychores.2016.03.001

Davies, J., Gander, P. E., Andrews, M., and Hall, D. A. (2014). Auditory network connectivity in tinnitus patients: a resting-state fMRI study. *Int. J. Audiol.* 53, 192–198. doi: 10.3109/14992027.2013.846482

Davis, A., and El Rafaie, A. (2000). "Epidemiology of tinnitus," in *Tinnitus Handbook*, ed R. S. Tyler (San Diego, CA: Singular Thomson Learning), 1–23.

De Ridder, D., Elgoyhen, A. B., Romo, R., and Langguth, B. (2011). Phantom percepts: tinnitus and pain as persisting aversive memory networks. *Proc. Natl. Acad. Sci. U.S.A.* 108, 8075–8080. doi: 10.1073/pnas.1018466108

De Ridder, D., Vanneste, S., Weisz, N., Londero, A., Schlee, W., Elgoyhen, A., et al. (2014). An integrative model of auditory phantom perception: tinnitus as a unified percept of interacting separable subnetworks. *Neurosci. Biobehav. Rev.* 44, 16–32. doi: 10.1016/j.neubiorev.2013.03.021

Domes, G., Schulze, L., Bottger, M., Grossmann, A., Hauenstein, K., Wirtz, P. H., et al. (2010). The neural correlates of sex differences in emotional reactivity and emotion regulation. *Hum. Brain Mapp.* 31, 758–769. doi: 10.1002/hbm.20903

Eickhoff, S., Stephan, K. E., Mohlberg, H., Grefkes, C., Fink, G. R., Amunts, K., et al. (2005). A new SPM toolbox for combining probabilistic cytoarchitectonic maps and functional imaging data. *NeuroImage* 25, 1325–1335. doi: 10.1016/j.neuroimage.2004.12.034

Folmer, R., Griest, S., Meikle, M., and Martin, W. (1999). Tinnitus severity, loudness, and depression. *Otolaryngol. Head Neck Surg.* 121, 48–51.

Golm, D., Schmidt-Samoa, C., Dechent, P., and Kroner-Herwig, B. (2013). Neural correlates of tinnitus related distress: an fMRI-study. *Hear. Res.* 295, 87–99. doi: 10.1016/j.heares.2012.03.003

Hall, D. A., Chambers, J., Akeroyd, M. A., Foster, J. R., Coxon, R., and Palmer, A. R. (2009). Acoustic, psychophysical, and neuroimaging measurements of the effectiveness of active cancellation during auditory functional magnetic resonance imaging. *J. Acoust. Soc. Am.* 125, 347–359. doi: 10.1121/1.3021437

Hall, D. A., Haggard, M. P., Akeroyd, M. A., Palmer, A. R., Summerfield, A. Q., Elliott, M. R., et al. (1999). Sparse temporal sampling in auditory fMRI. *Hum. Brain Mapp.* 7, 213–223. doi: 10.1002/(SICI)1097-0193(1999)7:3<213::AID-HBM5>3.0.CO;2-N

Hall, D. A., Irwin, A., Edmondson-Jones, M., Phillips, S., and Poxon, J. E. W. (2013). An exploratory evaluation of perceptual, psychoacoustic and acoustical properties of urban soundscapes. Special Issue. *Appl. Acoust.* 74, 248–254. doi: 10.1016/j.apacoust.2011.03.006

Hallam, R. S. (1996). *Manual of the Tinnitus Questionnaire*. London: The Psychological Corporation.

Hunter, M. D., Eickhoff, S. B., Pheasant, R. J., Douglas, M. J., Watts, G. R., Farrow, T. F., et al. (2010).The state of tranquility: subjective perception is shaped by contextual modulation of auditory connectivity. *Neuroimage* 53, 611–618. doi: 10.1016/j.neuroimage.2010.06.053

Husain, F. T., Pajor, N. M., Smith, J. F., Kim, J. H., Rudy, S., Zalewski, C., et al. (2011). Discrimination task reveals differences in neural bases of tinnitus and hearing impairment. *PLoS ONE* 6:e26639. doi: 10.1371/journal.pone.0026639

Irwin, A., Gander, P. E., and Hall, D. A. (2012). "Listening to emotion: auditory processing and the amygdala," in *Insights into the Amygdala: Structure Function and Implications for Disorders,* ed D. Yilmazer-Hanke (New York, NY: Nova Science Publishers Inc.), 255–275.

Irwin, A., Hall, D. A., Peters, A., and Plack, C. J. (2011). Listening to urban soundscapes: physiological validity of perceptual dimensions. *Psychophysiology* 48, 258–268. doi: 10.1111/j.1469-8986.2010.01051.x

Jakes, S. C., Hallam, R. S., Chambers, C., and Hinchcliffe, R. (1985). A factor analytical study of tinnitus complaint behaviour. *Int. J. Audiol.* 24, 195–206. doi: 10.3109/00206098509070103

Jastreboff, P. J. (1990). Phantom auditory perception (tinnitus): mechanisms of generation and perception. *Neurosci. Res.* 8, 221–254. doi: 10.1016/0168-0102(90)90031-9

Kang, D., Kwon, K., Gu, B., Choi, J., Jang, J., and Kwon, J. (2008). Structural abnormalities of the right inferior colliculus in schizophrenia. *Psychiatry Res.* 164, 160–165. doi: 10.1016/j.pscychresns.2007.12.023

Khalfa, S., Dubal, S., Veuillet, E., Perez-Diaz, F., Jouvent, R., and Collet, L. (2002). Psychometric normalization of a hyperacusis questionnaire. *ORL J. Otorhinolaryngol. Relat. Spec.* 64, 436–442. doi: 10.1159/000067570

Kitajima, M., Hirai, T., Yoneda, T., Iryo, Y., Azuma, M., Tateishi, M., et al. (2015). Visualization of the medial and lateral Geniculate nucleus on phase difference enhanced imaging. *Am. J. Neuroradiol.* 36, 1669–1674. doi: 10.3174/ajnr.A4356

Kuk, F. K., Tyler, R. S., Russell, D., and Jordan, H. (1990). The psychometric properties of a tinnitus handicap questionnaire. *Ear Hear.* 11, 434–445. doi: 10.1097/00003446-199012000-00005

Kumar, S., von Kriegstein, K., Friston, K., and Griffiths, T. D. (2012). Features versus feelings: dissociable representations of the acoustic features and valence of aversive sounds. *J. Neurosci.* 32, 14184–14192. doi: 10.1523/JNEUROSCI.1759-12.2012

Langguth, B., Goodey, R., Azevedo, A., Bjorne, A., Cacace, A., Crocetti, A., et al. (2007). Consensus for tinnitus patient assessment and treatment outcome measurement: tinnitus research initiative meeting, Regensburg, July 2006. *Prog. Brain Res.* 166, 525–536. doi: 10.1016/S0079-6123(07)66050-6

Leaver, A. M., Seydell-Greenwald, A., Turesky, T. K., Morgan, S., Kim, H. J., and Rauschecker, J. P. (2012). Cortico-limbic morphology separates tinnitus from tinnitus distress. *Front. Syst. Neurosci.* 6:21. doi: 10.3389/fnsys.2012.00021

Le Doux, J. E. (2000). Emotion circuits in the brain. *Annu. Rev. Neurosci.* 23, 155–184. doi: 10.1146/annurev.neuro.23.1.155

Mai, J. K., Assheuer, J., and Paxinos, G. (1997). *Atlas of the Human Brain*. San Diego, CA: Academic Press.

Marciani, L., Pfeiffer, J. C., Hort, J., Head, K., Bush, D., Taylor, A. J., et al. (2006). Improved methods for fMRI studies of combined taste and aroma stimuli. *J. Neurosci. Methods* 158, 186–194. doi: 10.1016/j.jneumeth.2006.05.035

Morawetz, C., Holz, P., Lange, C., Baudewig, J., Weniger, G., Irle, E., et al. (2008). Improved functional mapping of the human amygdala using a standard functional magnetic resonance imaging sequence with simple modifications. *Magn. Reson. Imaging* 26, 45–53. doi: 10.1016/j.mri.2007.04.014

Posse, S., Wiese, S., Gembris, D., Mathiak, K., Kessler, C., Grosse-Ruyken, M., et al. (1999). Enhancement of BOLD-contrast sensitivity by single-shot multi-echo functional MR imaging. *Magn. Reson. Med.* 42, 87–97. doi: 10.1002/(SICI)1522-2594(199907)42:1<87::AID-MRM13>3.0.CO;2-O

Rajmohan, V., and Mohandas, E. (2007). The limbic system. *Indian J. Psychiatry* 49, 132–139. doi: 10.4103/0019-5545.33264

Roy, A. K., Shehzad, Z., Margulies, D. S., Kelly, A. M., Uddin, L. Q., Gotimer, K., et al. (2009). Functional connectivity of the human amygdala using resting state fMR. *NeuroImage* 45, 614–626. doi: 10.1016/j.neuroimage.2008.11.030

Shulman, A., Strashun, A. M., Afriyie, M., Aronson, F., Abel, W., and Goldstein, B. (1995). SPECT imaging of brain and tinnitus–neurotologic/neurologic implications. *Int. Tinnitus J.* 1, 13–29.

Tegg-Quinn, S., Bennett, R., Eikelboom, R., and Baguley, D. (2016). The impact of tinnitus upon cognition in adults: A systematic review. *Int. J. Audiol.* 55, 533–540. doi: 10.1080/14992027.2016.1185168

11

Validation of the Italian Tinnitus Questionnaire Short Form (TQ 12-I) as a Brief Test for the Assessment of Tinnitus-Related Distress: Results of a Cross-Sectional Multicenter-Study

Roland Moschen[1], Alessandra Fioretti[2], Alberto Eibenstein[2,3], Eleonora Natalini[2], Domenico Cuda[4], Giuseppe Chiarella[5], Gerhard Rumpold[1] and David Riedl[1]**

[1] University Clinic of Medical Psychology, Medical University of Innsbruck, Innsbruck, Austria, [2] Tinnitus Center, European Hospital, Rome, Italy, [3] Department of Applied Clinical and Biotechnological Sciences, University of Aquila, L'Aquila, Italy, [4] Department of Otorhinolaryngology, Guglielmo da Saliceto Hospital, Piacenza, Italy, [5] Department of Experimental and Clinical Medicine, Unit of Audiology and Phoniatrics, Magna Græcia University, Catanzaro, Italy

***Correspondence:**
David Riedl
david.riedl@tirol-kliniken.at
Roland Moschen
roland.moschen@tirol-kliniken.at

Objectives: The use of reliable and valid psychometric tools to assess subjectively experienced distress due to tinnitus is broadly recommended. The purpose of the study was the validation of the Italian version of Tinnitus Questionnaire 12 item short form (TQ 12-I) as a brief test for the assessment of patient reported tinnitus-related distress.

Design: Cross-sectional multicenter questionnaire study.

Setting: Tinnitus Center, European Hospital (Rome), the Department of Otorhinolaryngology, "Guglielmo da Saliceto" Hospital (Piacenza), and the Department of Audiology and Phoniatry, "Mater Domini" University Hospital (Catanzaro).

Participants: One hundred and forty-three outpatients with tinnitus treated at one of the participating medical centers.

Main Outcome Measures: Tinnitus Questionnaire Short Form (TQ 12-I), compared to the Tinnitus Handicap Inventory (THI), Brief Symptom Inventory (BSI), and Short Form (SF-36) Health Survey.

Results: Our factor analysis revealed a two-factor solution (health anxiety, cognitive distress), accounting for 53.5% of the variance. Good internal consistency for the total score (α = 0.86) and both factors (α = 0.79–0.87) was found. Moderate correlations with the THI ($r = 0.65$, $p < 0.001$) indicated good convergent validity. Tinnitus distress was further correlated to increased psychological distress ($r = 0.31$, $p < 0.001$) and reduced emotional well-being ($r = -0.34$, $p < 0.001$).

Conclusion: The study clearly showed that the TQ 12-I is a reliable and valid instrument to assess tinnitus-related distress which can be used in clinical practice as well as for research.

Keywords: Tinnitus Questionnaire, TQ 12, validation, tinnitus, tinnitus distress

INTRODUCTION

Tinnitus is defined as a subjective acoustic perception in the absence of any external source (Hallam et al., 1984). Epidemiological studies reported a prevalence of 10–16% for chronic tinnitus in the adult population that increases with age (Davis and El Refaie, 2000; Shargorodsky et al., 2010; McCormack et al., 2014). The majority of people with tinnitus do not suffer from it strongly. Yet, about 0.5–3% of the general population develop severe distress and experience impairment in everyday life, sleep, mood, concentration and daily work (Davis and El Refaie, 2000; Gopinath et al., 2010). Because the subjectively experienced distress due to tinnitus cannot sufficiently be explained by psychoacoustic parameters (e.g., tinnitus loudness) (Henry and Meikle, 2000), psychological factors like depression, anxiety or catastrophizing have been assumed to be adjuvant to explain tinnitus distress (Milerová et al., 2013; Weise et al., 2013; McKenna et al., 2014).

National and international guidelines recommend using psychometrically and clinically validated questionnaires for the assessment of tinnitus severity (Langguth et al., 2007; AWMF, 2015). In order to be applicable during routine clinical practice a questionnaire for the assessment of tinnitus severity should not only be psychometrically and clinically validated but also quickly administered to minimize the patients' burden. Several reliable and internationally validated tools for the assessment of tinnitus severity have been developed. One of the most commonly used tools is the Tinnitus Questionnaire (TQ) (Goebel and Hiller, 1998), which assesses different aspects of tinnitus related distress (emotional and cognitive distress, intrusiveness, auditory perceptual difficulties, sleep disturbance and somatic complaints). The TQ has been translated and validated in several different languages, including German, Dutch, French, and Chinese. To enable a faster but equally reliable assessment of tinnitus related distress the TQ 12 was initially developed by Hiller and Goebel (2004). The TQ 12 was validated in German (Hiller and Goebel, 2004), Portuguese (Cerejeira et al., 2009), Greek (Panagiotopoulos et al., 2015), Chinese (Kam, 2012), Dutch (Vanneste et al., 2011), and Arabic (El Beaino and Eter, 2017). Good psychometric properties were reported for all of the translated versions of the TQ 12: the psychometric analyses across various validations showed good reliability (internal consistency: α = 0.86–0.90; retest-reliability: k = 0.89–0.91) and high correlation with the TQ total score (r = 0.90–0.93) (Hiller and Goebel, 2004; Kam, 2012; Zeman et al., 2012; Panagiotopoulos et al., 2015). The TQ 12 total score allows the classification of the patients as compensated (0–7), moderately distressed (8–12), severely distressed (13–18), and most severely distressed (19–24) (Hiller and Goebel, 2004). Yet, conflicting evidence was found for the factorial structure: most of the validations presumed a single global factor, whereas Panagiotopoulos et al. (2015) reported a three factor solution (Distress, Health pre-occupation, and Depression). So far, neither the TQ nor the TQ 12 have been validated in Italian. The aim of the present study was to evaluate the reliability, validity and factorial structure of the Italian TQ 12-I.

MATERIALS AND METHODS

Sample and Setting

The sample of this cross-sectional multi-center study consisted of 143 outpatients, which were include from the following healthcare institutions: Tinnitus Center, European Hospital (Rome), the Department of Otorhinolaryngology, "Guglielmo da Saliceto" Hospital (Piacenza), and the Department of Experimental and Clinical Medicine, Unit of Audiology and Phoniatrics, University "Magna Graecia" (Catanzaro). Patients were included in the study if they (a) had tinnitus for at least 3 months, (b) were older than 18 years, (c) spoke Italian fluently and (d) had no apparent cognitive impairment. The patients completed the questionnaires as part of the routine clinical practice. Written informed consent was obtained by all patients.

Measures

Tinnitus Sample Case History (TSCH)

Sociodemographic and clinical data were assessed with the Italian version of the TSCH. It was developed by the Tinnitus Research Initiative as in attempt to standardize the assessment of sociodemographic and clinical data in tinnitus research (Langguth et al., 2007). The questionnaire consists of 35 items on background (i.e., age, gender), tinnitus history (i.e., loudness, pitch, percentage of awake time aware of tinnitus, hyperacusis) and related conditions (i.e., hearing impairment, noise annoyance, vertigo/dizziness).

Tinnitus Questionnaire (TQ 12)

The TQ 12 consists of 12 items, which can be scored on a three point ordinal Likert Scale ranging from 0 to 2. The total score has a range of 0–24 points with higher values indicating higher tinnitus distress. The items of the TQ 12 correlated highly with the TQ total score, were reliable and showed good responsiveness (Hiller and Goebel, 2004). The Italian translation of the English TQ 12 was provided by an Italian native speaker, fluent in the source language and expert in the medical field of tinnitus. This forward translation was checked by a second independent person with the same level of expertise.

Tinnitus Handicap Inventory (THI)

The Tinnitus Handicap Inventory (Newman et al., 1996) is a one of the most commonly used questionnaires to assess tinnitus distress. The THI consists of 25 items that can be divided in a functional, emotional and catastrophic scale. Patients can score the frequency/intensity of these symptoms on a three point ordinal Likert Scale ranging from 0 to 4. The total score ranges from 0 to 100 points with higher values indicating higher tinnitus distress The total score the THI can be graduated in five grades of tinnitus severity: slight (0–16), mild (18–36), moderate (38–56), severe handicap (58–76), and catastrophic (78–100) (Zeman et al., 2014). Good reliability (α = 0.94) and validity were reported for the total score of the Italian THI version (Passi et al., 2008; Salviati et al., 2013).

Brief Symptom Inventory (BSI)

Mental health symptoms and psychological distress were assessed with the Brief Symptom Inventory (BSI; Derogatis, 1993). The BSI consists of 53 items, which can be divided into nine subscales and three scales to capture global psychological distress. Good reliability and validity for the subscales and total score were reported (De Leo et al., 1993).

Short Form (36) Health Survey

The health status was measured with the Short Form (36) Health Survey (SF-36) (Ware and Sherbourne, 1992), a broadly used, well established instrument to assess the Health-Related Quality of Life (HRQOL). The SF-36 consists of 36 items which can be divided into eight subscales and a physical and psychological total score. The subscale's internal consistencies were tested in nine samples, showing a Cronbach's α between 0.77 and 0.93. Good validity has been reported in several studies (Apolone and Mosconi, 1998).

Statistical Analysis

Psychometric values (means, standard deviations, item-total correlations) of the items are presented. The floor and ceiling effect, defined as the highest and lowest 15% of the scale were also calculated. A factor analyses (maximum likelihood, direct oblimin) with a fixed number of factors was conducted to investigate the three-factor solution proposed by Panagiotopoulos et al. (2015). Based on the results of this initial analysis an additional exploratory factor analysis was calculated. Scree plots and Eigenvalues were used to determine the ideal number of factors. Reliability was evaluated by calculating Cronbach's α (internal consistency) and item-total correlations. The convergent validity was evaluated by two-sided Pearson correlations with the THI and the discriminant validity was examined by correlations with BSI and SF-36 scores. To test if the proposed TQ 12-I severity grades differentiated well enough between different levels of tinnitus distress, analyses of variances (ANOVAs) with Bonferroni-corrected *post hoc* analyses were calculated. Statistical analyses were conducted using IBM SPSS (v.22).

RESULTS

A total sample of 146 patients were included in the study, of which 46.5% were recruited in Piacenza, 36.1% in Rome, and 17.4% in Catanzaro. The sample had a mean age of 53.6 years and 54% were men. The mean tinnitus duration was 7.5 years and a large proportion of the sample reported tinnitus in both ears (41.0%). More than half of the sample (57.5%) had subjective hearing problems and about a third (36.3%) reported physical discomfort because of surrounding sounds (hyperacusis). About 21% of the sample had undergone several or many treatments due to their tinnitus. Based on the THI total score patients' tinnitus distress was graded as follows: 19.9% very mild, 26.2% mild, 31.9% moderate, 15.6% severe, and 6.4% catastrophic. About 5% of the sample reported to be currently under treatment for psychiatric disorders. For details see **Table 1**.

Psychometric Values

The mean, standard deviation and item-total correlation of each item are presented in **Table 2**. The mean TQ 12-I total score was 10.8 (*SD*: 5.8). No floor or ceiling effect was found.

We initially tested the proposed factor solution of Panagiotopoulos et al. (2015) by factor analysis (main component analysis and maximum likelihood). Bartlett's test of sphericity [χ^2 (66) = 827.9, $p < 0.001$] was significant and the Kaiser–Meyer–Olkin measure verified the sampling adequacy for the analysis (KMO = 0.85). Initial Eigenvalues indicated that the first three factors explained 41.7%, 19.1%, and 7.9% of the variance, respectively. The three-factor-solution explained 58.4% of the variance, the diagonals of the anti-image correlation matrix were between 0.69 and 0.93.

TABLE 1 | Clinical properties of the sample.

TN loudness: 0–100 (*SD*)	53.2 (28.9)
Missing	10 (6.8%)
Duration: years (*SD*)	7.5 (10.3)
Family history of tinnitus complaints	37 (25.3%)
Missing	1 (0.7%)
Subjective hearing problem	84 (57.5%)
Missing	1 (0.7%)
Hearing aid	19 (13.7%)
Missing	1 (0.7%)
Hyperacusis	53 (36.3%)
Missing	1 (0.7%)
Tinnitus loudness varies during the day:	
Yes	96 (65.8%)
No	48 (32.9%)
Missing	2 (1.4%)
Pulsatile tinnitus	41 (27.5%)
If yes: with heartbeat	15 (38.5%)
If yes: different from heartbeat	24 (61.5%)
Location	
Right ear	30 (20.5%)
Left ear	36 (24.7%)
Both ears	60 (41.0%)
Inside the head	11 (7.5%)
Missing	9 (6.2%)
Pitch	
Very high frequency	20 (13.7%)
High frequency	58 (39.7%)
Medium frequency	49 (33.6%)
Low frequency	12 (8.2%)
Missing	7 (4.8%)
Number of treatments for tinnitus	
None	78 (53.4%)
One	37 (25.3%)
Several	23 (15.8%)
Many	6 (4.1%)
Missing	2 (1.4%)

TABLE 2 | Mean, standard deviations, and variance of the TQ 12-I.

	Mean	*SD*	Item-total correlation
1. I am aware of the noises from the moment I get up to the moment I sleep	1.34	0.75	0.14
2. Because of the noises I worry that there is something seriously wrong with my body	0.61	0.80	0.50
3. If the noises continue my life will not be worth living	0.48	0.80	0.44
4. I am more irritable with my family and friends because of the noises	0.82	0.72	0.66
5. I worry that the noises might damage my physical health	0.74	0.76	0.61
6. I find it harder to relax because of the noises	0.99	0.74	0.65
7. My noises are often so bad that I cannot ignore them	1.14	0.75	0.57
8. It takes me longer to get to sleep because of the noises	0.99	0.82	0.53
9. I am more liable to feel low because of the noises	0.90	0.78	0.71
10. I often think about whether the noises will ever go away	1.19	0.80	0.32
11. I am a victim of my noises	0.73	0.82	0.62
12. The noises have affected my concentration	0.92	0.76	0.70

Item-total correlations were corrected for the individual contribution of each item.

The factorial structure was examined with oblique rotation (oblimin), but we were not able to replicate the proposed three-factor-solution. Furthermore, the scree plot and the Eigenvalues supported a two-factor-solution (**Figure 1**). Therefore we also calculated an exploratory factor analysis (maximum likelihood) without a predefined number of factors. The results clearly supported the two-factor solution, explaining 53.5% of the variance. **Table 3** shows the factor loadings after rotation. Based on these results the remaining calculations were conducted for the two-factor solution. The content analysis for naming the extracted factors was independently conducted by two researchers, differences were resolved by consensus (reconciliation process). The items clustered on the same component suggest that factor 1 represents 'health anxiety,' while factor 2 represents 'cognitive distress' related to tinnitus.

Good internal consistency was found for the total score ($\alpha = 0.86$) as well as for factor 1 'health anxiety' ($\alpha = 0.87$) and factor 2 'cognitive distress' ($\alpha = 0.79$). The item-total correlations were acceptable for all items, except item 1. Also, the Cronbach's α would be slightly higher for the total scale if item 1 was excluded ($\alpha = 0.87$), but not for factor 2.

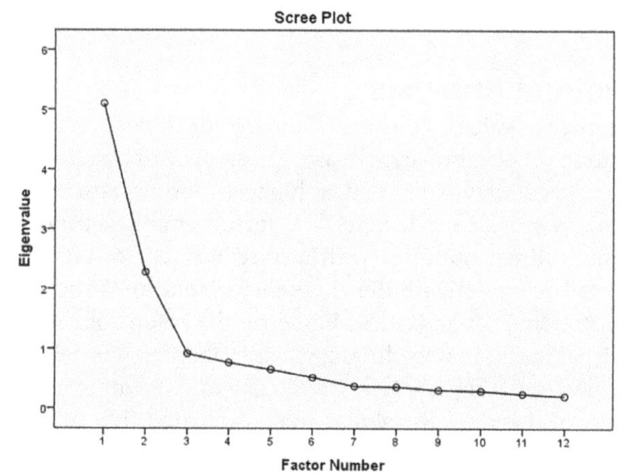

FIGURE 1 | Scree plot for the TQ 12-I.

Validity Analysis

The TQ 12-I correlated moderately with the THI-total score and its subscales, which indicated good convergent validity. Furthermore elevated tinnitus distress measured by the TQ 12-I total score was correlated positively with higher global psychological distress (BSI total score) and negatively with emotional well-being (SF-36 emotional score). Details are presented in **Table 4**. The correlations with the BSI and SF-36 were significantly lower than with the THI, which indicates good discriminant validity. No significant correlation was found between tinnitus distress and physical well-being.

We found no correlation between the TQ 12-I total score and age ($p = 0.57$), gender ($p = 0.23$) or symptom duration ($p = 0.72$). Yet, patients who had higher scores on the TQ 12-I also reported a subjectively louder ear noise ($r = 0.27$, $p = 0.002$). The presence of subjective hearing problems were more present in patients with higher age ($p = 0.04$). In our sample patients with subjective hearing problems did not differ in their perceived tinnitus loudness from patients without subjective hearing problems ($p = 0.41$).

According to the proposed cut-off values by Hiller and Goebel (2004) for the German TQ 12 31.9% of the present sample reported no clinically relevant tinnitus distress (1–7 points), 27.0% were moderately distressed (8–12 points), 32.6% were severely distressed (13–18 points) and 8.5% were most severely distressed (>19 points). The ANOVA showed significant differences between the TQ 12-I severity groups regarding the THI-total score ($F = 31.86$, $p < 0.001$). *Post hoc* analyses revealed significant differences between all severity groups, except severely and most severely distressed patients (**Figure 2**).

DISCUSSION

For use in busy clinical practice, a questionnaire for the assessment of tinnitus severity should not only be

TABLE 3 | Results of the factor analysis (Pattern Matrix).

	Factor	
	Health anxiety	**Cognitive distress**
1. I am aware of the noises from the moment I get up to the moment I sleep	−0.188	**0.534**
2. Because of the noises I worry that there is something seriously wrong with my body	**0.765**	0.054
3. If the noises continue my life will not be worth living	**0.827**	−0.025
4. I am more irritable with my family and friends because of the noises	**0.654**	0.490
5. I worry that the noises might damage my physical health	**0.751**	0.232
6. I find it harder to relax because of the noises	0.409	**0.776**
7. My noises are often so bad that I cannot ignore them	0.217	**0.812**
8. It takes me longer to get to sleep because of the noises	0.414	**0.508**
9. I am more liable to feel low because of the noises	**0.639**	0.508
10. I often think about whether the noises will ever go away	0.080	**0.460**
11. I am a victim of my noises	**0.700**	0.311
12. The noises have affected my concentration	0.531	**0.715**

Extraction Method: Maximum Likelihood; Rotation Method: Oblimin with Kaiser Normalization; bold values indicate which factor the item was assigned.

TABLE 4 | Correlations between TQ 12-I, THI, BSI, and SF-36.

	TQ 12-I total score	TQ 12-I health anxiety	TQ 12-I cognitive distress
THI total score	0.65***	0.44***	0.66***
THI functional subscale	0.60***	0.39***	0.64***
THI emotional subscale	0.58***	0.42***	0.56***
THI catastrophic subscale	0.59***	0.41***	0.61***
BSI total score	0.31***	0.21**	0.32***
SF-36 – physical subscale	−0.14	−0.07	−0.17
SF-36 – emotional subscale	−0.34***	−0.22**	−0.36***

$^{*}p < 0.05$, $^{**}p < 0.01$, $^{***}p < 0.001$, two-tailed

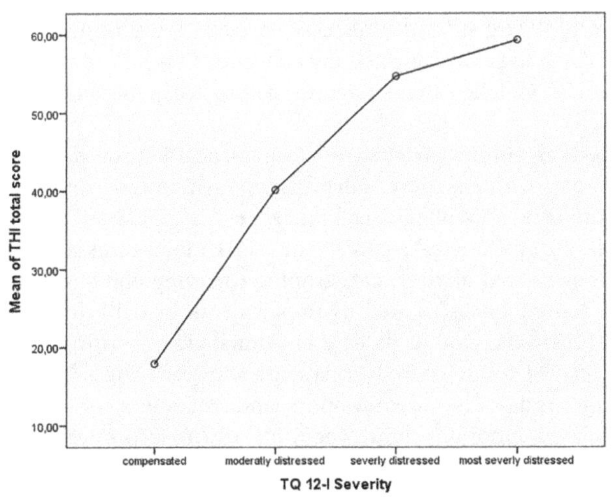

FIGURE 2 | Comparison of TQ 12-I severity groups with THI total score.

psychometrically and clinically validated, but also quickly to use to minimize the patients' burden. For the TQ 12 good psychometric and clinical values have been reported in several languages (Hiller and Goebel, 2004; Cerejeira et al., 2009; Vanneste et al., 2011; Kam, 2012; Zeman et al., 2012; Panagiotopoulos et al., 2015). Thus far the psychometric properties of the Italian translation of the TQ 12 have not been investigated. The aim of the present study therefore, was to evaluate the Italian short version of the Tinnitus Questionnaire, the TQ 12-I, in a multicenter study in which 143 patients with tinnitus complaints from three study centers participated. The results of our study showed that the TQ 12-I is a reliable and valid measure for assessing tinnitus-related distress and its severity.

The psychometric evaluation of the individual items showed no floor- or ceiling effects, which indicates that all items are well suited to discriminate between low and high levels of tinnitus distress. We found item-total correlations from acceptable to good (values higher than 0.3) for all items, except for item 1 ('I am aware of the noises from the moment I get up to the moment I sleep'), which had a value of 0.14. This was somehow surprising since item 1 had good item-total correlations (values of 0.3–0.6) in all other versions of the TQ 12 (Hiller and Goebel, 2004; Cerejeira et al., 2009; Vanneste et al., 2011; Kam, 2012; Panagiotopoulos et al., 2015). The translation of the items was independently checked by native-speakers in the course of translation and confirmed by further native speaking researches in the course of the data interpretation. Because of the good psychometric properties in previous studies and the high content validity of the item, we recommend to retain the item in the questionnaire.

It has been pointed out that the factorial structure of the TQ is a weak spot of the otherwise well suited questionnaire. Thus far, only one study has investigated the factorial structure of the TQ 12 (Panagiotopoulos et al., 2015). In that study, with three hundred and one adult Greek patients, the authors reported a three-factor solution, which could not be replicated in our sample. An additional exploratory factor analysis showed that a two-factor solution was better suited for the patients in our sample. Apart from intercultural differences, a possible explanation for the conflicting findings might be the comparatively low mean TQ 12 score in the Greek validation study compared to our study and other validation studies (Hiller and Goebel, 2004; Cerejeira et al., 2009; Kam, 2012).

The two factors were named 'health anxiety' and 'cognitive distress,' based on a thorough content analysis. The factor **'health anxiety'** included questions that depicted tinnitus-related anxiety, for example catastrophic assumptions regarding one's own future life if the tinnitus persisted (item 3 'If the noises continue my life will not be worth living'), fears about an underlying severe physical illness (item 2: 'Because of my noises I worry that there is something seriously wrong with my body') or about threatening consequences of tinnitus (item 5: 'I worry that the noises might damage my physical health'). Additionally, the questions also cover the influence of the tinnitus on the patients' mood (item 9: 'I am more liable to feel low because of the noises') and feelings of helplessness or resignation toward tinnitus (item 11: 'I am a victim of my noises').

The factor **'cognitive distress'** includes questions that address experienced impairments in daily life, such as difficulties to distract oneself from the tinnitus (item 7: 'My noises are often so bad that I cannot ignore them'), to relax or to concentrate (item 6: 'I find it harder to relax because of the tinnitus'; item 12: 'The noises have affected my concentration'), or to fall asleep (item 8: 'It takes me longer to get to sleep because of the noises').

Several studies showed a close association of distressing tinnitus with anxiety, depressive symptoms and sleep disturbances (Wallhausser-Franke et al., 2012; Cronlein et al., 2016; Ziai et al., 2017). The TQ 12-I captures aspects of tinnitus-related anxiety, catastrophic worrying about its causes and consequences as well as impairments in daily life, mood and functions. Due to its easy and intelligible wording the TQ 12-I can be administered to patients with differing educational backgrounds. The identification and reduction of tinnitus-associated emotional and cognitive distress through patient education, reassurance and demystification of tinnitus promote the habituation process of tinnitus (Moschen et al., 2015). The TQ 12-I provides indications for a subsequent differentiated assessment of comorbid disorders by validated psychopathology questionnaires (Wallhausser-Franke et al., 2012) and may serve for the assessment of therapeutic outcomes.

In our study, the total score of the TQ 12-I had a good internal consistency of $\alpha = 0.86$, which was comparable with previous studies (Hiller and Goebel, 2004; Cerejeira et al., 2009; Vanneste et al., 2011; Kam, 2012; Zeman et al., 2012; Panagiotopoulos et al., 2015). The internal consistency of the two subscales was also good (health anxiety: $\alpha = 0.87$; cognitive distress: $\alpha = 0.80$). The previously problematic item 1 did not lower the factor's Cronbach α.

We furthermore investigated the validity of the TQ 12-I and its subscales through correlations with tinnitus distress (THI), general psychological distress (BSI), and quality of life (SF-36). As expected, the correlation between the two tinnitus related questionnaires was strong and highly significant, which indicated good convergent validity. Higher tinnitus distress as measured by the TQ 12-I was correlated with higher psychological distress and with lower emotional quality of life. These findings are in accordance with a large body of previous research (Shargorodsky et al., 2010; Milerová et al., 2013; Riedl et al., 2015). The two factors also showed significant correlations with the THI and its subscales as well as psychological distress and emotional quality of life.

In their initial development of the TQ 12 Hiller and Goebel (2004) proposed four grades of tinnitus severity, based on the total score of the TQ 12. To increase the usability of the TQ 12-I in a clinical context we have evaluated the severity grades for the TQ 12-I. Our analysis confirmed the proposed cut-offs, although the differences between the 'severely distress' and 'most severely distressed' groups were not statistically significant. This might be caused by the comparatively small size of the group with the most severely distressed patients (n = 12). The results indicate, that the proposed cut-off values may be used for the Italian TQ 12-I.

Limitations

In our sample the group of highly distressed patients was comparatively small, although the mean score was comparable to, or even higher than in previous validation studies (Hiller and Goebel, 2004; Vanneste et al., 2011; Panagiotopoulos et al., 2015). The small sample size may have influenced the results of the factor analysis. The proposed factorial structure should be further validated with confirmatory factor analysis in an international sample. In addition, we did not evaluate divergent validity of tinnitus severity with other comorbidity like hearing loss. The cross-sectional design of the present study did not allow us to evaluate the sensitivity to change (responsiveness) or the retest-reliability of the TQ 12-I. Previous studies have shown promising results regarding retest-reliability (Kam, 2012; Panagiotopoulos et al., 2015) and responsiveness (Hiller and Goebel, 2004; Zeman et al., 2012) of the TQ 12.

CONCLUSION

The present study showed that the TQ 12-I is a reliable and valid tool to assess the severity of tinnitus distress. The items of the TQ 12-I can be used in everyday clinical practice and research and permit a compact, quick and economical assessment of the most important aspects of subjective tinnitus distress. The provided cutoffs facilitate the interpretation of individual scores and provide indications for a multidisciplinary therapeutic approach.

ETHICS STATEMENT

All procedures performed in studies involving human participants were in accordance with the ethical standards of the institutional and/or national research committee and with the 1964 Helsinki declaration and its later amendments or comparable ethical standards. The study was performed in three ENT centers in Italy, namely Rome, Catanzaro, and Piacenza. Heads of these centers (AE, GC, and DC) agreed on the procedures and provided access to tinnitus patients. Participation was voluntary and every patient gave written consent before filling out the questionnaires.

AUTHOR CONTRIBUTIONS

RM and AF designed the study; GC collected the data at the ENT center in Catanzaro; AF, EN, and AE collected the data at the Tinnitus Center in Rome; DC collected the data at the ENT center in Piacenza; AF and EN consulted on the redaction of the manuscript at all stages and contributed to the revision of the manuscript; RM, GR, and DR analyzed the data, wrote the paper and commented on the manuscript at all stages; DR provided the statistical expertise and revised the manuscript at several stages.

ACKNOWLEDGMENTS

The authors thank *COST Action* BM1306 "*TINNET - Better Understanding the Heterogeneity of Tinnitus to Improve and Develop New Treatments*" for supporting this study with a Short Term Scientific Mission to the Tinnitus Center in Rome, Italy.

REFERENCES

Apolone, G., and Mosconi, P. (1998). The Italian SF-36 Health Survey: translation, validation and norming. *J. Clin. Epidemiol.* 51, 1025–1036. doi: 10.1016/S0895-4356(98)00094-8

AWMF (2015). *Treatment of Chronic Tinnitus. S3 – Guideline of the German Society of Otolaryngoly.* Available at: http://www.awmf.org/uploads/tx_szleitlinien/017-064l_S3_Chronischer_Tinnitus_2015-02.pdf

Cerejeira, R., Cerejeira, J., Paiva, S., Goncalves, P., Firmino, H., Quartilho, M., et al. (2009). The Portuguese version of Mini-Tinnitus Questionnaire: brief screening test for assessment of tinnitus-induced stress. *Otol. Neurotol.* 30, 112–115. doi: 10.1097/MAO.0b013e31818de749

Cronlein, T., Langguth, B., Pregler, M., Kreuzer, P. M., Wetter, T. C., and Schecklmann, M. (2016). Insomnia in patients with chronic tinnitus: cognitive and emotional distress as moderator variables. *J. Psychosom. Res.* 83, 65–68. doi: 10.1016/j.jpsychores.2016.03.001

Davis, A., and El Refaie, A. (2000). "Epidemiology of tinnitus," in *Tinnitus Handbook*, ed. R. S. Tyler (San Diego, CA: Singular), 1–21.

De Leo, D., Frisoni, G. B., Rozzini, R., and Trabucchi, M. (1993). Italian community norms for the brief symptom inventory in the elderly. *Br. J. Clin. Psychol.* 32(Pt 2), 209–213. doi: 10.1111/j.2044-8260.1993.tb01045.x

Derogatis, L. R. (1993). *Brief Symptom Inventory (BSI): Administration, Scoring and Procedures Manual.* Minneapolis, MN: Pearson.

El Beaino, M., and Eter, E. (2017). Arabic validation of the tinnitus handicap inventory and the mini-tinnitus questionnaire on 100 adult patients. *Clin. Otolaryngol.* doi: 10.1111/coa.12980 [Epub ahead of print].

Goebel, G., and Hiller, W. (1998). *Tinnitus-Fragebogen (TF). Ein Instrument zur Erfassung von Belastung und Schweregrad bei Tinnitus.* Göttingen: Hogrefe.

Gopinath, B., Mcmahon, C. M., Rochtchina, E., Krapa, M. J., and Mitchell, P. (2010). Incidence, persistence and progression of tinnitus symptoms in older adults: the blue mountains hearing study. *Ear Hear.* 31, 407–412. doi: 10.1097/AUD.0b013e3181cdb2a2

Hallam, R. S., Rachman, S., and Hinchcliffe, R. (1984). "Psychological aspects of tinnitus," in *Contributions to Medical Psychology*, ed. S. Rachman (Oxford: Pergamon), 31–53.

Henry, J. A., and Meikle, M. B. (2000). Psychoacoustic measures of tinnitus. *J. Am. Acad. Audiol.* 11, 138–155.

Hiller, W., and Goebel, G. (2004). Rapid assessment of tinnitus-related psychological distress using the Mini-TQ. *Int. J. Audiol.* 43, 600–604. doi: 10.1080/14992020400050077

Kam, A. C. (2012). A screening tool for tinnitus-related distress - the Chinese version of mini tinnitus questionnaire: our experience in one hundred and fourteen adult patients. *Clin. Otolaryngol.* 37, 234–237. doi: 10.1111/j.1749-4486.2012.02479.x

Langguth, B., Goodey, R., Azevedo, A., Bjorne, A., Cacace, A., Crocetti, A., et al. (2007). Consensus for tinnitus patient assessment and treatment outcome measurement: tinnitus research initiative meeting, Regensburg, July 2006. *Prog. Brain Res.* 166, 525–536. doi: 10.1016/S0079-6123(07)66050-6

McCormack, A., Edmondson-Jones, M., Fortnum, H., Dawes, P., Middleton, H., Munro, K. J., et al. (2014). The prevalence of tinnitus and the relationship with neuroticism in a middle-aged UK population. *J. Psychosom. Res.* 76, 56–60. doi: 10.1016/j.jpsychores.2013.08.018

McKenna, L., Handscomb, L., Hoare, D. J., and Hall, D. A. (2014). A scientific cognitive-behavioral model of tinnitus: novel conceptualizations of tinnitus distress. *Front. Neurol.* 5:196. doi: 10.3389/fneur.2014.00196

Milerová, J., Anders, M., Dvořák, T., Sand, P. G., Königer, S., and Langguth, B. (2013). The influence of psychological factors on tinnitus severity. *Gen. Hosp. Psychiatry* 35, 412–416. doi: 10.1016/j.genhosppsych.2013.02.008

Moschen, R., Riedl, D., Schmidt, A., Kumnig, M., Bliem, H. R., and Rumpold, G. (2015). The development of Acceptance of chronic tinnitus in the course of a cognitive-behavioral group therapy. *Z. Psychosom. Med. Psychother.* 61, 237–245. doi: 10.13109/zptm.2015.61.3.238

Newman, C. W., Jacobson, G. P., and Spitzer, J. B. (1996). Development of the Tinnitus Handicap Inventory. *Arch. Otolaryngol. Head Neck Surg.* 122, 143–148. doi: 10.1001/archotol.1996.01890140029007

Panagiotopoulos, G., Galanakis, M., Varvogli, L., Chrousos, G., and Darviri, C. (2015). Validation of the Greek version of mini tinnitus questionnaire as a brief screening test for assessment of tinnitus-related distress: our experience in 301 adult patients. *Clin. Otolaryngol.* 40, 363–369. doi: 10.1111/coa.12383

Passi, S., Ralli, G., Capparelli, E., Mammone, A., Scacciatelli, D., and Cianfrone, G. (2008). The THI questionnaire: psychometric data for reliability and validity of the Italian version. *Int. Tinnitus J.* 14, 26–33.

Riedl, D., Rumpold, G., Schmidt, A., Zorowka, P. G., Bliem, H. R., and Moschen, R. (2015). The influence of tinnitus acceptance on the quality of life and psychological distress in patients with chronic tinnitus. *Noise Health* 17, 374–381. doi: 10.4103/1463-1741.165068

Salviati, M., Macrì, F., Terlizzi, S., Melcore, C., Provenzano, A., Capparelli, E., et al. (2013). The tinnitus handicap inventory as a screening test for psychiatric comorbidity in patients with tinnitus. *Psychosomatics* 54, 248–256. doi: 10.1016/j.psym.2012.05.007

Shargorodsky, J., Curhan, G. C., and Farwell, W. R. (2010). Prevalence and characteristics of tinnitus among US adults. *Am. J. Med.* 123, 711–718. doi: 10.1016/j.amjmed.2010.02.015

Vanneste, S., Plazier, M., Van Der Loo, E., Ost, J., Meeus, O., Van De Heyning, P., et al. (2011). Validation of the Mini-TQ in a Dutch-speaking population: a rapid assessment for tinnitus-related distress. *B-ENT* 7, 31–36.

Wallhausser-Franke, E., Brade, J., Balkenhol, T., D'amelio, R., Seegmuller, A., and Delb, W. (2012). Tinnitus: distinguishing between subjectively perceived loudness and tinnitus-related distress. *PLOS ONE* 7:e34583. doi: 10.1371/journal.pone.0034583

Ware, J. E. Jr., and Sherbourne, C. D. (1992). The MOS 36-item short-form health survey (SF-36). I. Conceptual framework and item selection. *Med. Care* 30, 473–483. doi: 10.1097/00005650-199206000-00002

Weise, C., Hesser, H., Andersson, G., Nyenhuis, N., and Zastrutzki, S. (2013). The role of catastrophizing in recent onset tinnitus: its nature and association with tinnitus distress and medical utilization. *Int. J. Audiol.* 52, 177–188. doi: 10.3109/14992027.2012.752111

Zeman, F., Koller, M., Langguth, B., and Landgrebe, M. (2014). Which tinnitus-related aspects are relevant for quality of life and depression: results from a large international multicentre sample. *Health Qual. Life Outcomes* 12:7. doi: 10.1186/1477-7525-12-7

Zeman, F., Koller, M., Schecklmann, M., Langguth, B., and Landgrebe, M. (2012). Tinnitus assessment by means of standardized self-report questionnaires: psychometric properties of the Tinnitus Questionnaire (TQ), the Tinnitus Handicap Inventory (THI), and their short versions in an international and multi-lingual sample. *Health Qual. Life Outcomes* 10:128. doi: 10.1186/1477-7525-10-128

Ziai, K., Moshtaghi, O., Mahboubi, H., and Djalilian, H. R. (2017). Tinnitus patients suffering from anxiety and depression: a review. *Int. Tinnitus J.* 21, 68–73. doi: 10.5935/0946-5448.20170013

12

Call for an Evidence-Based Consensus on Outcome Reporting in Tinnitus Intervention Studies

Alain Londero[1] and Deborah A. Hall[2,3]*

[1] Service ORL et CCF, Hôpital Européen G. Pompidou, Paris, France, [2] NIHR Nottingham Biomedical Research Centre, Nottingham, UK, [3] Otology and Hearing Group, Division of Clinical Neuroscience, School of Medicine, University of Nottingham, Nottingham, UK

Keywords: tinnitus, Delphi survey, trial reporting, core outcome set, patient-reported complaints

***Correspondence:**
Alain Londero
alain.londero@egp.aphp.fr

Tinnitus is a very common symptom affecting 5.1–42.7% of the population (1) and is frequently seen in family medicine and primary care settings. Despite its considerable socioeconomic relevance (2), real progress in developing an effective cure for tinnitus has been fruitless (3). In most of the cases, the proposed therapies remain palliative; aiming at alleviating the negative consequences of tinnitus. Although the need for effective management options for tinnitus is clear, methodological and reporting quality of clinical trials have been low (4, 5) making useful recommendations and practical guidelines for family medicine and primary health-care practitioners almost impossible to draw. Indeed, Baguley and colleagues (6) concluded that, with the exception of cognitive behavior therapy for tinnitus, evidence for the effectiveness of different treatment strategies is insufficient (pp. 1605).

The CONSORT statement[1] is perhaps the most well-known guideline for solving problems arising from inadequate reporting of randomized controlled trials, but other tinnitus-specific statements have been around since the 1990s. Unfortunately, these recommendations have not yet transformed standards in the tinnitus field so far. Indeed, recent systematic reviews of published clinical trials aiming at evaluating tinnitus therapeutic interventions have shown that reporting is still flawed by poor methodology and poor reporting (4, 5).

In this opinion, we discuss the selection and reporting of outcomes; perhaps, the most important aspect of determining whether a treatment works for patients and whether this treatment should be implemented in the medical practice either in primary or secondary settings. Selecting an appropriate outcome for determining clinical efficacy is one of those key trial design decisions. As Noble eloquently put it: "critical to any form of treatment for tinnitus is the reliance placed on measures to assess the effectiveness of the intervention" (pp. 20) (7). Just over 10 years later, Landgrebe et al. (8) made the same point stressing that "assessment of outcome is probably the single most important factor in conducting a clinical trial in tinnitus" (pp. 9). This is so because in clinical trials, therapeutic benefit is evaluated according to its effect on primary (and secondary) outcome measures that should be purposefully chosen according to the complaints (domains) of tinnitus considered to be most important from the perspective of determining therapeutic benefit (9). More specifically, the primary outcome measure is that which confirms whether or not the primary hypothesis is supported by the data. It is typically a variable relating to clinical efficacy but could also be one relating to safety, tolerability, or quality of life, if that is the primary research question. Generally speaking, the primary outcome should also be the endpoint that is clinically relevant from the patients' perspective and to health-care providers' in their everyday practice, not just significant from a statistical point of view. In support of this, the ICH E9 states that "The primary variable should be that variable capable of providing the most clinically relevant and convincing evidence directly related to the primary objective of the trial" (pp. 5) (10).

[1] www.consort-statement.org/.

Bearing in mind that tinnitus is a subjective condition for which patients experience a diversity of complaints, there is no straightforward outcome instrument. Outcome reporting typically relies on self-report, often in the form of a multi-item tinnitus questionnaire that asks questions about a range of complaints (not all of which are the same across existing questionnaires). A number of important issues have been raised and debated over the years, but many of those concerns remain unresolved. **Table 1** summarizes conclusions/recommendations about clinical trial outcomes in tinnitus. Although this may not be exhaustive, it nevertheless serves to illustrate the status of the field spanning across three decades.

Our observations are as follows:

(i) Are instruments really validated for use in assessing tinnitus treatment-related change?

While early conclusions implied that questionnaires are the "best" primary outcomes and that adequate "validated" questionnaires exist for this purpose, by 2007 some researchers were

TABLE 1 | Concluding remarks or recommendations about clinical trial outcomes in tinnitus made in various review articles.

Reference	Conclusions and recommendations concerning outcomes
Tyler (29)	Benefit should be measured with established questionnaires and with measures of the magnitude of tinnitus. A persuasive tinnitus treatment will be one that shows a large treatment effect, can be generalized across patients and clinicians, is specific and credible, and changes the way we think about tinnitus
Tyler et al. (9)	Several scaling procedures are available, but we believe a 100-point interval scale is superior. Several validated and reliable questionnaires are available and can serve as adequate primary measures. Secondary measures that quantify the magnitude of the tinnitus should also be obtained
Langguth et al. (15)	It was generally agreed that a questionnaire is required that is specifically designed for the assessment of treatment outcomes, and which is validated in many languages and in many cultural and socioeconomic groups. The consensus agreement is that at the present time one validated questionnaire, which can be Tinnitus Handicap Inventory (THI), Tinnitus Handicap Questionnaire (THQ), TRQ, or Tinnitus Questionnaire (TQ), is an essential part of patient assessment. Therapeutic trials should use one of these questionnaires also as outcome measurement. Assessment of tinnitus severity with at least one additional questionnaire is highly recommended
Meikle et al. (11)	While the tinnitus questionnaires that are currently available provide valuable information on which to base diagnostic and screening decisions, they were not originally developed in such a way as to maximize their sensitivity to treatment-related changes in tinnitus. As a result, their construct validity for measuring treatment benefit has not received appropriate attention
Tyler et al. (9)	When the treatment is intended to reduce the tinnitus, we recommend measuring the magnitude of the tinnitus. We provide arguments and data to support the use of the THQ as a measure of the reaction to the tinnitus. We suggest that the current quality of life measures are not valid for measuring lifestyle effects of alleviating tinnitus. A clinically meaningful effect should represent a valid and reliable statistical change for an individual
Meikle et al. (13)	It is to be hoped that investigators will address the need for information about the responsiveness of all the various types of tinnitus measures. The fact that measures of sensory impairment versus functional disability and handicap each provide unique insights into treatment-related changes in tinnitus reinforces the notion that both approaches are needed for insightful assessment of tinnitus treatment outcomes
Hesser (30)	If we restrict the assessment to one particular aspect of tinnitus-related disability, definitive claims about overall treatment benefits will be difficult to make. Moreover, the measures we use need to be validated and psychometrically robust. Although several psychometrically examined measures are available to assess tinnitus impact and severity (e.g., THI, Tinnitus Reaction Questionnaire), there is no standard outcome measure that is obligatory to include in a trial. I do believe that treatment evaluations within the field would not only benefit from calculating and reporting average effects but also must rely on data on the individual level, e.g., as clinical significant change, in determining the effects of treatment
Kamalski et al. (12)	The Health-Related-Quality of Life (HR-QoL) instruments used in tinnitus trials (THI, TQ, TRQ, TSI, THQ, and TSQ) appear not to be validated to measure effectiveness of interventions. Using tests or instruments that are valid and reliable is a crucial component of research quality, and both should therefore be studied before final conclusions can be drawn from the questionnaires in upcoming clinical trials. The validity, reliability, and responsiveness of each tinnitus-specific HR-QoL should be studied before final conclusions can be drawn regarding the utility of these questionnaires in future clinical studies
Landgrebe et al. (8)	Basic requirements for clinical trials in tinnitus include: - Definition of one or more main outcome measure(s) (i.e., a validated tinnitus questionnaire). - THI should be included in every trial at least as secondary outcome to improve inter-study comparability
Newman et al. (31)	Although psychometrically robust measures of tinnitus HR-QoL do exist, there is no unanimity in, for example, what tests should be included in the tinnitus assessment, and how studies of HR-QoL should be conducted. The current authors suggest that future studies employ more rigorous designs and contain (minimally) the following characteristics: (1) utilization of randomized control groups and blinding; (2) appropriate statistical testing including "dropouts" that should be used in an "intention to treat" analysis rather than elimination from the final data set; (3) long-term follow-up assessment to evaluate responsiveness; (4) appropriate inclusion criteria to avoid "ceiling" and "floor" effects; and (5) suitable sample sizes based on the application of power analyses
Fackrell et al. (14)	- We recommend that the "gold standard" would be to carry out a systematic review of the literature before selecting any given tinnitus questionnaire for a service audit or clinical trial. - In addition to the measurement properties, selection might also give consideration to the suitability of the tinnitus questionnaire for the study population, the potential burden of completing the questionnaire (e.g., length, question difficulty, emotional impact of certain questions), and the practical aspects (e.g., copyright costs, complexity of scoring method)

(Continued)

TABLE 1 | **Continued**

Reference	Conclusions and recommendations concerning outcomes
Hall et al. (27)	The overall ambition of the working group is to establish an international standard for outcome measurements in clinical trials of tinnitus. The standard will be achieved by a two-step effort to produce core outcome sets of domains and instruments that harmonize viewpoints across both professional and patient stakeholder groups. A roadmap has been proposed, which sets out a provisional plan for delivery. This roadmap reflects the two-step process with Stage 1 identifying and agreeing on outcome domains and Stage 2 identifying and agreeing on outcome instruments
Plein et al. (4)	(There is) a need in the literature for high-quality tinnitus research that is adequately randomized, ensures adequate follow-up, and does not exclude a large range of common otologic conditions that can result in tinnitus, which would result in improved external validity. Analysis of external validity is essential to the development of further guidelines and should be taken into account if we hope to develop recommendations that are of most benefit to clinicians and patients
Hall et al. (5)	- Generic names and terms such as "handicap" and "severity" perpetuate the difficulty that many trialists experience in understanding what construct(s) a particular questionnaire instrument measures. - Safety, tolerability, side effects, and withdrawals might be domains that all inform the measurement of adverse events. To improve trial reporting, we draw attention to the specialized CONSORT guidelines for reporting harms-related issues in a randomized controlled trial. - We advise caution if pooling findings from the THI in a meta-analysis since it is unclear whether all translations achieve equivalence with the British original

beginning to challenge the validity of existing tinnitus questionnaires for use in assessing treatment-related change (11). In 2010, a particularly critical evaluation of the psychometric properties of six of the commonly used multi-item questionnaires assessing tinnitus burden, including the Tinnitus Handicap Inventory, TQ, and Tinnitus Handicap Questionnaire, was published by Kamalski et al. (12). For each identified tinnitus-specific Health-Related-Quality of Life questionnaire, they systematically searched for published details regarding the questionnaire's test characteristics including number of domains, construct validity, internal consistency, reproducibility, and responsiveness. Like Meikle et al. (13), they were critical that none of the six questionnaires assessed had been validated for evaluative purposes, which is necessary to be useful in clinical trials. In particular, responsiveness, which measures the ability to detect a clinically important change over time, had not been reported for any of the six instruments.

Fackrell et al. (14) raised a new issue about the dynamic nature of psychometric properties. What questionnaire properties hold for one patient population might not for another. Indeed, for this reason we prefer the term psychometric "exploration" not "validation," and we hope that questionnaire developers might be sympathetic to adaptations in order to maintain equivalence across cultures [see also Ref. (15)].

(ii) Can we reduce the diversity of outcome instruments?

Two recent systematic reviews of outcome instruments in tinnitus trials have confirmed unacceptable heterogeneity in measurement tools (4, 5) For example, we found 78 different primary outcome instruments across 228 trials (5). This makes comparisons between studies elusive.

(iii) What is a clinically meaningful effect?

Tyler et al. (9) highlighted the importance of benefit from the individual patient experience, although this psychometric property of tinnitus questionnaires has generally not been investigated or quantified [see Meikle et al. (16), for a good example].

In the race to develop and utilize tinnitus questionnaires in our research, we are losing sight of understanding "what" it is that needs to be measured at the expense of "how" it is measured. Do we really know which tinnitus-related complaints are the most relevant both from the first and second line health-care providers' and patients' perspectives? We would argue not. Primary care physicians and patients in particular have been left out of the questionnaire development process.

Involving primary care physicians and patients in developing outcome reporting standards would go a long way to resolving heterogeneity in outcome assessment and ensuring its relevance. It could then help the tinnitus community to focus efforts on conducting an appropriate psychometric exploration of whatever are the preferred instruments. As an important first step, we are therefore leading a consensus exercise to develop an agreed minimum reporting set of outcomes for trials of interventions in tinnitus. What is urgently needed are targeted discussions around "what" needs to be measured for each therapeutic approach (sound therapies, pharmacological therapies, psychological interventions, and neuromodulation) since not all interventions seek to alleviate the same tinnitus-related complaints.

Such consensus for a minimal (core) set of outcome measurements that should be used in every clinical trial clearly calls for a predefined, multidisciplinary (including patients and primary care professionals), international, and methodologically driven clinimetric approach (17). The rationale underpinning this scientific approach of outcome assessment has already been theorized. For example, the Core Outcome Measures in Effectiveness Trials (COMET) initiative brings together from all over the world researchers interested in the development and application of agreed standardized "Core Outcome Sets" (COS) (18). A COS represents the minimum that should be measured and reported in all clinical trials for a specific condition (19). COS could also be suitable for a use in clinical audit or research other than randomized trials. One should note that COS are not limitative. If necessary, other outcomes might be added to those in the relevant COS in a particular trial. But, it is recommended that all the COS items should be collected and reported, making it easier for the

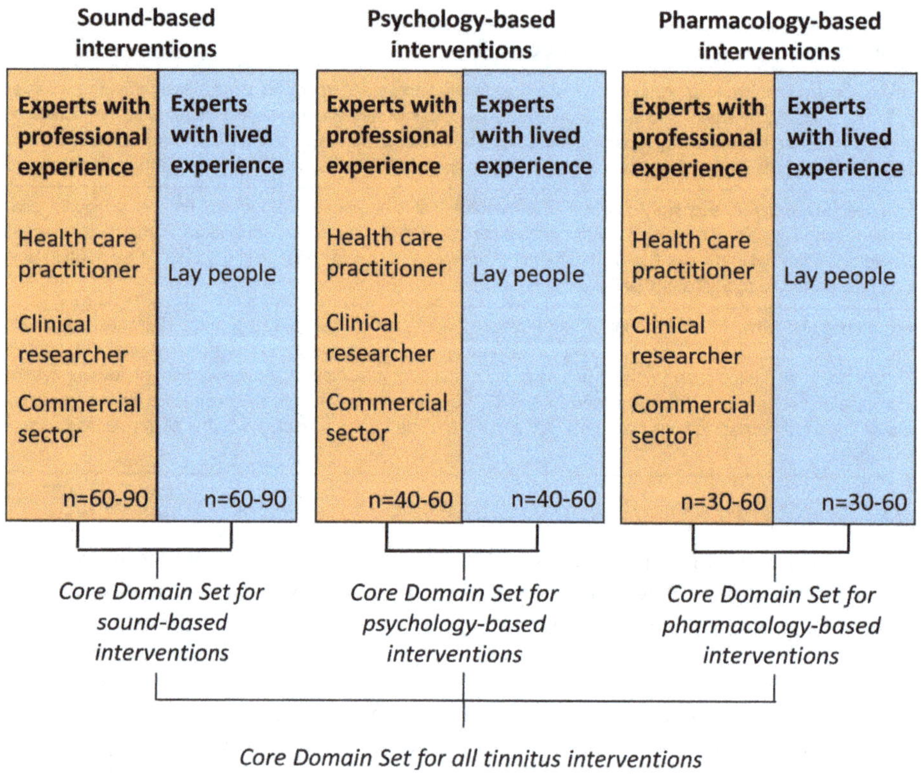

FIGURE 1 | Proposed Delphi survey strategy to identify different core outcome sets that are appropriately tailored according to different tinnitus interventions.

results to be compared, contrasted, and merged as appropriate. Indeed, similar international initiatives aiming at harmonizing outcome assessment are already existing such as for eczema (HOME for Harmonizing Outcome Measures for Eczema) (20) or, in the auditory field, for hearing loss (ICF for International Classification of Functioning, disability, and health core sets for hearing loss) (21). Then, we urge the tinnitus community to adopt and adapt these international standards of outcome definition and evaluation to the tinnitus field.

Deciding which outcome domains should be in this minimal core set requires a great deal of interactions and collaboration between stakeholders, professionals, and patients. This objective lends itself well to an international and multidisciplinary effort. We propose to follow a Delphi methodology to reach this goal. Delphi might be defined as "a method for structuring a group communication process so that the process is effective in allowing a group of individuals, as a whole, to deal with a complex problem" (22). Delphi methodology has been already proposed with success to reach a consensus in a variety of complex medical issues [e.g., see Ref. (23–25)]. Delphi methodology has also been used in the tinnitus field (26). Adapting a Delphi protocol to define a consensus core set of domains and a core set of instruments for tinnitus assessment in clinical trials is the aim of the recently launched Core Outcome Measures in Tinnitus (COMiT) initiative on behalf of the EU COST BM1306 action.[2] The activities of our COMiT initiative are registered on the website of the COMET initiative[3] according to roadmap that plans out a program of work. The first step is aimed at identifying and agreeing on core domains (27). It has started with two systematic reviews in order to establish existing knowledge and practice: the first review reflects the view of professional stakeholders by systematically looking at the current reported outcome domains in tinnitus intervention studies. The results of this review have already been published according to the PRISMA checklist of items to include when reporting a systematic review (5) establishing which outcome domains and outcome instruments have been measured in recent registered and published clinical trials. The second one represents the opinion of tinnitus people who experience the condition and/or their significant others by systematically searching in the literature and the internet the dimensions or domains that relate to tinnitus perceived intrusiveness. This second study will summarize the findings of narrative syntheses of qualitative data to establish which domains are important to patient and their significant others (28).

The data synthesis arising from both of these reviews will inform our online Delphi process, which will seek a consensus about what outcome domains are important both from healthcare professionals' and patients' perspectives. The methods for reaching consensus will use an iterative series of questionnaires, with an international multidisciplinary panel of patients, clinicians, and other professional stakeholder groups (such as

[2]http://www.cost.eu/COST_Actions/bmbs/BM1306.

[3]www.comet-initiative.org.

industry) all contributing with their views. We plan to conduct three independent Delphi processes devoted to different types of interventions (sound-, psychology-, and pharmacology-based interventions) that may require different COS. This Delphi process is illustrated in **Figure 1**. It is expected that the whole Delphi process will cover the 4-year period of the COST Action BM1306 grant. Our strong belief is that this innovative effort will improve not only trial reporting in the tinnitus domain but also the practical guidelines recommended in primary or secondary care settings for this common condition mistakenly considered to be always untreatable.

AUTHOR CONTRIBUTIONS

AL and DAH participated in conceiving, drafting, and revising the article and gave final approval of the version to be submitted.

FUNDING

This is an independent research program funded under the Biomedicine and Molecular Biosciences European Cooperation in Science and Technology (COST) Action framework (TINNET BM1306).

REFERENCES

McCormack A, Edmondson-Jones M, Somerset S, Hall D. A systematic review of the reporting of tinnitus prevalence and severity. *Hear Res* (2016) 337:70–9. doi:10.1016/j.heares.2016.05.009

Vio MM, Holme RH. Hearing loss and tinnitus: 250 million people and a US$10 billion potential market. *Drug Discov Today* (2005) 10(19):1263–5. doi:10.1016/S1359-6446(05)03594-4

Langguth B. Treatment of tinnitus. *Curr Opin Otolaryngol Head Neck Surg* (2015) 23(5):361–8. doi:10.1097/MOO.0000000000000185

Plein CT, Harounian J, Floyd E, Irizarry R, Ferzli G, Kidwai S, et al. A systematic review of eligibility and outcomes in tinnitus trials: reassessment of tinnitus guideline. *Otolaryngol Head Neck Surg* (2016) 154(1):24–32. doi:10.1177/0194599815608160

Hall DA, Haider H, Szczepek AJ, Lau P, Rabau S, Jones-Diette J, et al. Systematic review of outcome domains and instruments used in clinical trials of tinnitus treatments in adults. *Trials* (2016) 17(1):270. doi:10.1186/s13063-016-1399-9

Baguley D, McFerran D, Hall D. Tinnitus. *Lancet* (2013) 382(9904):1600–7. doi:10.1016/S0140-6736(13)60142-7

Noble W. Tinnitus self-assessment scales: domains of coverage and psychometric properties. *Hear J* (2001) 54(11):20–6. doi:10.1097/01.HJ.0000293150.63349.c7

Landgrebe M, Azevedo A, Baguley D, Bauer C, Cacace A, Coelho C, et al. Methodological aspects of clinical trials in tinnitus: a proposal for an international standard. *J Psychosom Res* (2012) 73(2):112–21. doi:10.1016/j.jpsychores.2012.05.002

Tyler RS, Oleson J, Noble W, Coelho C, Ji H. Clinical trials for tinnitus: study populations, designs, measurement variables, and data analysis. *Prog Brain Res* (2007) 166:499–509. doi:10.1016/S0079-6123(07)66048-8

Guideline for Good Clinical Practice – E9_Guideline. (1998). Available from: http://www.ich.org/fileadmin/Public_Web_Site/ICH_Products/Guidelines/Efficacy/E9/Step4/E9_Guideline.pdf

Meikle MB, Stewart BJ, Griest SE, Martin WH, Henry JA, Abrams HB, et al. Assessment of tinnitus: measurement of treatment outcomes. *Prog Brain Res* (2007) 166:511–21. doi:10.1016/S0079-6123(07)66049-X

Kamalski DM, Hoekstra CE, van Zanten BG, Grolman W, Rovers MM. Measuring disease-specific health-related quality of life to evaluate treatment outcomes in tinnitus patients: a systematic review. *Otolaryngol Head Neck Surg* (2010) 143(2):181–5. doi:10.1016/j.otohns.2010.03.026

Meikle MB, Stewart BJ, Griest SE, Henry JA. Tinnitus outcomes assessment. *Trends Amplif* (2008) 12(3):223–35. doi:10.1177/1084713808319943

Fackrell K, Hall DA, Barry JG, Hoare DJ. Psychometric properties of the Tinnitus functional index (TFI): assessment in a UK research volunteer population. *Hear Res* (2016) 335:220–35. doi:10.1016/j.heares.2015.09.009

Langguth B, Goodey R, Azevedo A, Bjorne A, Cacace A, Crocetti A, et al. Consensus for tinnitus patient assessment and treatment outcome measurement: Tinnitus research initiative meeting, Regensburg, July 2006. *Prog Brain Res* (2007) 166:525–36. doi:10.1016/S0079-6123(07)66050-6

Meikle MB, Henry JA, Griest SE, Stewart BJ, Abrams HB, McArdle R, et al. The tinnitus functional index: development of a new clinical measure for chronic, intrusive tinnitus. *Ear Hear* (2012) 33(2):153–76. doi:10.1097/AUD.0b013e31822f67c0

de Vet HCW, Terwee CB, Mokkink LB, Knol DL. *Measurement in Medicine: a Practical Guide*. Cambridge, New York, NY: Cambridge University Press (2011). 338 p.

Prinsen CAC, Vohra S, Rose MR, King-Jones S, Ishaque S, Bhaloo Z, et al. Core outcome measures in effectiveness trials (COMET) initiative: protocol for an international Delphi study to achieve consensus on how to select outcome measurement instruments for outcomes included in a "core outcome set". *Trials* (2014) 15:247. doi:10.1186/1745-6215-15-247

Williamson P, Altman D, Blazeby J, Clarke M, Gargon E. Driving up the quality and relevance of research through the use of agreed core outcomes. *J Health Serv Res Policy* (2012) 17(1):1–2. doi:10.1258/jhsrp.2011.011131

Chalmers JR, Simpson E, Apfelbacher CJ, Thomas KS, von Kobyletzki L, Schmitt J, et al. Report from the fourth international consensus meeting to harmonize core outcome measures for atopic eczema/dermatitis clinical trials (HOME initiative). *Br J Dermatol* (2016) 175(1):69–79. doi:10.1111/bjd.14773

Granberg S, Swanepoel DW, Englund U, Möller C, Danermark B. The ICF core sets for hearing loss project: international expert survey on functioning and disability of adults with hearing loss using the international classification of functioning, disability, and health (ICF). *Int J Audiol* (2014) 53(8):497–506. doi:10.3109/14992027.2014.900196

Linstone HA, Turoff M, editors. *The Delphi Method: Techniques and Applications*. Reading, MA: Addison-Wesley Pub. Co., Advanced Book Program (1975). 620 p.

Potter S, Brookes ST, Holcombe C, Ward JA, Blazeby JM. Exploring methods for the selection and integration of stakeholder views in the development of core outcome sets: a case study in reconstructive breast surgery. *Trials* (2016) 17(1):463. doi:10.1186/s13063-016-1591-y

Hughes A-M, Bouças SB, Burridge JH, Alt Murphy M, Buurke J, Feys P, et al. Evaluation of upper extremity neurorehabilitation using technology: a European Delphi consensus study within the EU cost action network on robotics for neurorehabilitation. *J Neuroeng Rehabil* (2016) 13(1):86. doi:10.1186/s12984-016-0192-z

Casini A, de Moerloose P; The Congenital Fibrinogen Disorders Group. Management of congenital quantitative fibrinogen disorders: a Delphi consensus. *Haemophilia* (2016) 22(6):898–905. doi:10.1111/hae.13061

Sereda M, Hoare DJ, Nicholson R, Smith S, Hall DA. Consensus on hearing aid candidature and fitting for mild hearing loss, with and without Tinnitus: Delphi review. *Ear Hear* (2015) 36(4):417–29. doi:10.1097/AUD.0000000000000140

Hall DA, Haider H, Kikidis D, Mielczarek M, Mazurek B, Szczepek AJ, et al. Toward a global consensus on outcome measures for clinical trials in Tinnitus: report from the first International Meeting of the COMiT initiative, November 14, 2014, Amsterdam, The Netherlands. *Trends Hear* (2015) 4:19. doi:10.1177/2331216515580272

Haider H, Fackrell K, Kennedy V, Hall DA. Dimensions of tinnitus-related complaints reported by patients and their significant others: protocol for a systematic review. *BMJ Open* (2016) 6(10):e009171. doi:10.1136/bmjopen-2015-009171

Tyler RS. The use of science to find successful tinnitus treatments. *Proceedings of the Sixth International Tinnitus Seminar*; Cambridge, UK; 1999 September 5–9. London: The Tinnitus and Hyperacusis Centre. (1999). 3 p.

Hesser H. Methodological considerations in treatment evaluations of tinnitus distress: a call for guidelines. *J Psychosom Res* (2010) 69(3):305–7.

13

A Quantitative Electroencephalography Study on Cochlear Implant-Induced Cortical Changes in Single-Sided Deafness with Tinnitus

Jae-Jin Song[1], Kyungsoo Kim[2], Woongsang Sunwoo[1], Griet Mertens[3], Paul Van de Heyning[3], Dirk De Ridder[4], Sven Vanneste[5], Sang-Youp Lee[1], Kyung-Joon Park[2]*, Hongsoo Choi[6]* and Ji-Woong Choi[2]**

[1] Department of Otorhinolaryngology-Head and Neck Surgery, Seoul National University Bundang Hospital, Seongnam, South Korea, [2] Department of Information and Communication Engineering, Daegu Gyeongbuk Institute of Science and Technology, Daegu, South Korea, [3] Department of Otorhinolaryngology and Head and Neck Surgery, University Hospital Antwerp, Edegem, Belgium, [4] Department of Surgical Sciences, Section of Neurosurgery, Dunedin School of Medicine, University of Otago, Dunedin, New Zealand, [5] Lab for Clinical and Integrative Neuroscience, School of Behavioral and Brain Sciences, The University of Texas at Dallas, Richardson, TX, USA, [6] Department of Robotics Engineering, Daegu Gyeongbuk Institute of Science and Technology, Daegu, South Korea

***Correspondence:**
Jae-Jin Song
jjsong96@snubh.org;
jjsong96@gmail.com
Kyung-Joon Park
kjp@dgist.ac.kr
Hongsoo Choi
mems@dgist.ac.kr
Ji-Woong Choi
jwchoi@dgist.ac.kr

The mechanism of tinnitus suppression after cochlear implantation (CI) in single-sided deafness (SSD) is not fully understood. In this regard, by comparing pre- and post-CI quantitative electroencephalography (qEEG), we explored cortical changes relevant to tinnitus improvement. In SSD patients who underwent CI, qEEG data were collected: (1) before CI, (2) 6 months post-operatively with CI-on, and (3) 30 min after CI-off and source-localized cortical activity/functional connectivity analyses were performed. Compared to the pre-operative baseline, the CI-on condition demonstrated significantly decreased activity in the right auditory- and orbitofrontal cortices (OFC) for the delta frequency band as well as decreased connectivity between the auditory cortex/posterior cingulate cortex for the delta/beta2 bands. Meanwhile, compared to the CI-off condition, the CI-on condition displayed decreased activity in the right auditory cortices/OFC for the delta band, and in bilateral auditory cortices, left inferior frontal cortex/OFC for the gamma band. However, qEEG analyses showed no significant differences between the CI-off and baseline conditions. CI induced overall decreased cortical activity and functional connectivity. However, judging from no differences between the CI-off and baseline conditions, CI-induced cortical activity and functional connectivity changes are not by cortical plastic changes, but by dynamic peripheral reafferentation.

Keywords: single side deafness, tinnitus, cochlear implantation, electroencephalography, dynamic peripheral reafferentation

INTRODUCTION

Tinnitus, the conscious perception of sound in the absence of a corresponding external acoustic stimulus (Baguley et al., 2013), afflicts 10–15% of the adult population and interferes severely with the quality of life of 5–26% of the affected population (Heller, 2003; Krog et al., 2010). The development of tinnitus is frequently deemed to be a neuroplastic response to sensory deprivation (Eggermont and Roberts, 2004; Song et al., 2012). This assumption is supported by a transient perception of tinnitus after experimentally induced partial (Schaette et al., 2012) and complete (Del Bo et al., 2008) temporary auditory deprivation in normal subjects, and was further reinforced by lack of tinnitus in congenitally deaf animal models (Eggermont and Kral, 2016). Furthermore, analogous to phantom limb pain, the tinnitus spectrum corresponds to auditory deprived frequencies (Norena et al., 2002).

In patients with severe peripheral auditory deafferentation, reafferentation of the ascending auditory nervous system with cochlear implants (CI) may abate tinnitus. Indeed, CI improved tinnitus significantly in 66–100%of CI users with bilateral profound hearing loss (Ruckenstein et al., 2001). Also, improvement of tinnitus by CI was reported in patients with single-sided deafness (SSD) and ipsilesional debilitating tinnitus (Punte et al., 2011). In a recent meta-analysis, CI showed a statistically significant improvement in the severity of tinnitus (Blasco and Redleaf, 2014). In this regard, CI is a promising treatment option for patients with SSD and combined severe tinnitus.

However, the mechanism of tinnitus suppression after CI in patients with SSD is not fully understood. In previous literature, several mechanisms of CI-mediated tinnitus suppression have been suggested. Some researchers have claimed that acoustic masking provided by CI is the primary mechanism of tinnitus suppression, by distracting attention from tinnitus (Andersson et al., 2009; Kleinjung et al., 2009), while others have suggested that plastic changes in the central auditory system by prolonged CI stimulation (Giraud et al., 2001) and electrical stimulation resulting in contralateral residual inhibition (Souliere et al., 1992) are possible mechanisms of tinnitus suppression. These assumptions are, however, based on inferential reasoning rather than data-driven analysis.

From this perspective, a study to explore post-CI changes in patients with SSD with regard to ongoing cortical activity may be of help in further understanding the mechanism of tinnitus alterations in SSD subjects after CI. By comparing pre- and post-CI source-localized quantitative electroencephalography (qEEG) findings, we attempted to find CI-driven cortical activity changes that may have abated subjective tinnitus in patients with SSD. Additionally, by analyzing changes in functional connectivity, we sought to reveal changes in functional connections of remote brain areas that may be responsible for the improvement of tinnitus after CI.

MATERIALS AND METHODS

Participants

Four patients (three men and one woman) with unilateral acquired SSD (pure tone threshold >90 dB at 0.5, 1, 2, and 4 kHz) and ipsilateral tinnitus underwent pre-operative EEG and subsequent CI with a Med-EL device (Med-EL, Innsbruck, Austria). All patients presented with left-sided SSD and the median duration of deafness was 4.5 years (range, 9 months to 5 years). All four patients' etiology of SSD was idiopathic sudden sensorineural hearing loss. The detailed demographic characteristics of the patients are summarized in **Table 1**.

The criteria for CI in patients with SSD and tinnitus were: (1) a duration of SSD < 10 years, (2) tinnitus development after SSD onset, and (3) tinnitus loudness on a numeric rating scale (NRS) ≥ 6 of 10 for at least 6 months that was intractable to conventional therapies including medication, tinnitus retraining therapy, and non-invasive neuromodulation such as transcranial magnetic stimulation or transcranial direct current stimulation. The exclusion criteria were: (1) severe depression with a Beck Depression Index (Beck and Steer, 1984) score > 16, and (2) a presumed etiology of tinnitus other than SSD. With regard to tinnitus loudness and tinnitus-related distress, all patients were evaluated using a NRS loudness score and a tinnitus questionnaire (TQ) (Goebel and Hiller, 1994) score.

This study and all related documents were approved by the ethics committee of Antwerp University Hospital. All patients gave written informed consent before enrollment. The study procedures were carried out in accordance with the relevant guidelines and regulations.

EEG Recording

Pre-operative and 6-month post-operative EEGs were performed in all four patients. Pre-operative EEGs were recorded during resting-state for 5 min, while post-operative EEGs were recorded for 5 min under the following two conditions: (1) CI switch-on with a music stimulus (classical music from a radio channel) to the CI ear presented directly to the external audio processor via an audio cable at the most comfortable loudness level for each patient (CI-on); and (2) CI switch-off with no sound stimulus (CI-off).

Electroencephalograms were measured using the WinEEG software version 2.84.44 (Mitsar, St. Petersburg, Russia) in a room shielded against sound and stray electric fields with patients sitting upright with their eyes closed to reduce resting-state skin conductance levels in overall frequency bands (Barry et al., 2007, 2009). The EEG was sampled with 19 electrodes in the standard 10–20 International placements referenced to linked ears. While recording, impedance was maintained below 5 kΩ at all electrodes. Data were recorded with a sampling rate of 1,024 Hz using a 0.15 Hz high-pass filter and a 200 Hz low-pass filter. After initial recording, the data were processed offline by resampling to 128 Hz and band-pass filtering at 2–44 Hz by employing a fast Fourier transform filter with application of a Hanning window, and then imported into the Eureka! Software (Sherlin and Congedo, 2005) for precise artifact rejection before source-localization. All artifacts in the recorded EEG stream were removed meticulously by manual inspection.

The vigilance of all participants was checked by monitoring EEG streams to prevent unwanted changes, caused by drowsiness, such as alpha rhythm slowing or the appearance of spindles (Moazami-Goudarzi et al., 2010); no enrolled participant exhibited drowsiness-related EEG changes.

TABLE 1 | Demographic characteristics of the included subjects.

Subject number	Age (years)/sex	Contralateral hearing threshold (average of 0.5, 1, 2, and 4 kHz) (dB HL)	Duration of single-sided deafness	Etiology	Psychoacoustic characteristics of tinnitus	Frequency matching (Hz)	Perceived tinnitus loudness (dB SL)	Side of the cochlear implant	Name of the implanted device
1	53/female	20	4 years	Sudden sensorineural hearing loss	Pure tone	6000	20	Left	MED-EL Sonata ti 100 FLEX Soft electrode
2	64/male	23	5 years	Sudden sensorineural hearing loss	Pure tone	3000	10	Left	MEDEL Sonata ti 100 FLEX Soft electrode
3	47/male	15	9 months	Sudden sensorineural hearing loss	Pure tone	8000	30	Left	MED-EL Sonata ti 100 FLEX 24 electrode
4	49/male	15	5 years	Sudden sensorineural hearing loss	Narrow band noise	6000	40	Left	MED-EL Pulsar ci 100 Standard electrode

dB HL, dB hearing level; dB SL, dB sensation level.

Artifact Removal by Band-Limited Independent Component Analysis

Localization of the cortical resting-state or auditory evoked potentials in CI users via qEEG is confounded by stimulus artifacts produced by the implanted device itself. In a previous article, we described a successful method of CI artifact removal from specific bands in the EEG streams of patients with CIs using band-limited independent component analysis [BL-ICA, for further information, please refer to Kim et al. (2015)]. BL-ICA successfully removes artifacts by applying a narrow band-pass filter, which limits the number of sources and enhances the signal to noise ratio, thus allowing CI artifacts to be clearly detected and separated from other brain sources. By applying BL-ICA, all post-operative EEG data measured while listening to music were cleaned.

Source Localization Analysis

Low-resolution brain electromagnetic tomography (LORETA)-KEY software[1], dedicated to functional localization of current densities based on certain electrophysiological and neuroanatomical constraints, (Pascual-Marqui, 2002) was utilized to localize the cortical sources that generated the scalp-recorded electrical activity in each of the following eight frequency bands: delta (2–3.5 Hz), theta (4–7.5 Hz), alpha 1 (8–10 Hz), alpha 2 (10–12 Hz), beta 1 (13–18 Hz), beta 2 (18.5–21 Hz), beta 3 (21.5–30 Hz), and gamma (30.5–44 Hz) (Song et al., 2013a,b, 2014, 2015a,b; Vanneste et al., 2013; Kim et al., 2015, 2016). This software implements the lead field of Fuchs et al. (2002) that was derived from standard electrode positions realigned to a standard Montreal Neurological Institute (MNI)-152 head in combination with a boundary element method derived from the same standard anatomy (Jurcak et al., 2007). The LORETA-KEY anatomical template divides the neocortical MNI-152 volume, including the hippocampus and anterior cingulate cortex, into 6,239 voxels with dimensions of 5 mm × 5 mm × 5 mm, based on the Daemon Atlas (Lancaster et al., 2000). Anatomical labeling of significant clusters was performed automatically by a toolbox implemented in LORETA-KEY. The locations of significant clusters were initially investigated using the Anatomy toolbox (Eickhoff et al., 2005), and were reconfirmed using the Talairach and Tournoux atlas (Talairach and Tornoux, 1988). Renders were generated using the BrainNet Viewer[2] (Xia et al., 2013).

Functional Connectivity

Using the pre- and post-operative qEEG data, the extent of phase synchronization and coherence between the time series corresponding to different regions of interest (ROIs) were calculated to analyze functional connectivity. To calculate functional connectivity, we employed the built-in connectivity toolbox of the LORETA-KEY. This toolbox defines measures of linear- and non-linear dependence (i.e., coherence and phase synchronization) between multivariate time series. In the

[1] http://www.uzh.ch/keyinst/NewLORETA/Software/Software.htm

[2] http://www.nitrc.org/projects/bnv/

current study, we have calculated lagged linear coherence that excludes non-lagged parts of coherence which comprises effects of volume conduction, and effects of non-recorded sources that simultaneously drive recorded sources (Milz et al., 2014). For lagged linear coherence connectivity analysis, a total of 28 ROIs defined by Brodmann areas (BA) were selected as possible nodes based on previous literature on tinnitus: bilateral primary and secondary auditory cortices (A1s and A2s) (Rolls, 2004; Kringelbach, 2005), bilateral parahippocampus (PHC) (Landgrebe et al., 2009), bilateral dorsal/pregenual/subgenual anterior cingulate cortices (dACC/pgACC/sgACC) (Vanneste et al., 2010; De Ridder et al., 2011), bilateral posterior cingulate cortices (PCC) (Vanneste et al., 2010; Schecklmann et al., 2011), bilateral insula, bilateral precuneus, and bilateral orbitofrontal cortices (OFC) (Vanneste et al., 2010; De Ridder et al., 2011).

Statistical Analysis

To identify cortical activity differences between pre-operative resting-state and post-operative sound stimuli-induced cortical activity, between pre-operative resting-state and post-operative device-off state activity, and between post-operative device-on with sound stimuli and device-off state activity ("CI-on - CI-off"), voxel-by-voxel analysis using LORETA-KEY was performed for the eight frequency band between-condition comparisons of the current density distribution. Also, regression analyses were performed to compare between "CI-on - CI-off" and percent improvement in tinnitus loudness and between "CI-on - CI-off" and percent improvement in TQ score. For source-localized group comparison analyses, statistical non-parametric mapping (SnPM) of LORETA-KEY images was performed for each contrast using LORETA-KEY's built-in voxelwise randomization tests (5000 permutations) and employing a log-F-ratio statistic for independent groups with a threshold of $P < 0.01$. A correction for multiple comparisons in SnPM using random permutations (5000 permutations in the current study) has been proven to give results similar to those obtained from a comparable Statistical Parametric Mapping approach using a general linear model with multiple comparison corrections derived from random field theory (Holmes et al., 1996; Nichols and Holmes, 2002). Additionally, power spectral density (PSD) was calculated by EEGLAB toolbox (Delorme and Makeig, 2004). Topography was described based on PSD in 19 channels. The red, green, and blue colors in the topography represent maximum, mean, and minimum power, respectively, in specific bands such as delta and gamma.

For lagged linear connectivity differences, we compared differences between the pre-operative baseline, post-operative CI-off, and post-operative CI-on with music stimuli conditions, employing the t-statistics for groups with a threshold of $P < 0.05$, and also corrected for multiple comparisons by performing LORETA-KEY-built-in voxelwise randomization tests (5000 permutations).

All other descriptive statistical analyses were performed using the SPSS software version 20.0 (SPSS Inc., Chicago, IL, USA). For all analyses, descriptive statistical significance was set at $P < 0.05$.

RESULTS

Comparison of Changes in Visual Analog Scale Tinnitus Loudness and Tinnitus Questionnaire Scores in all Patients

Table 2 summarizes the pre- and post-operative comparisons of NRS tinnitus loudness and TQ scores. All four patients showed improved NRS loudness and TQ scores under the post-operative CI-on state compared with the pre-operative baseline. Also, compared to pre-operative NRS loudness (median, 8.5; range, 7–9) and TQ scores (median, 61; range, 52–78), the post-operative CI-on state showed improved NRS loudness (median, 4; range, 3–6) and TQ scores (median, 42.5; range, 29–56) with a trend-level significance ($P = 0.068$; $Z = 1.826$ for both comparisons, Wilcoxon signed rank test). When we compared the post-operative CI-on and off states, the CI-on state showed tinnitus alleviation with regard to NRS loudness and TQ score compared with CI-off NRS loudness (median, 8.5; range, 6–9) and TQ score (median, 61; range, 52–76) with a trend-level significance ($P = 0.068$; $Z = 1.826$ for both comparisons, Wilcoxon signed rank test). However, the comparison between the pre-operative baseline and the post-operative CI-off state showed no differences with regard to NRS loudness and TQ score ($P = 0.317$; $Z = 1.00$ and $P = 0.564$; $Z = 0.577$, respectively, Wilcoxon signed rank test) (**Table 2**).

Meanwhile, regression analyses comparing between "CI-on - CI-off" and percent improvement in tinnitus loudness and between "CI-on - CI-off" and percent improvement in TQ score did not reveal any significant correlations between cortical activity changes and percent improvement in tinnitus loudness or TQ score.

Group Comparison with Regard to Source-Localized Activity and Functional Connectivity

Post-operative CI-On versus Pre-operative Baseline

Compared with the pre-operative baseline, the post-operative CI-on condition resulted in significantly decreased activity in the right A1 (BAs 41 and 42) and A2 (BAs 21 and 22) and in the right OFC (BAs 10 and 11) for the delta frequency band ($P < 0.01$) (**Figure 1**). For the other seven frequency bands, no significant differences with regard to source-localized activity were found between the two conditions.

On lagged linear connectivity comparison, the patients showed decreased functional connectivity between the PCC and A1 for the delta frequency band and between the PCC and A2 for the beta 2 band for the post-operative CI-on state compared with pre-operative baseline (**Figure 2**).

Post-Operative CI-On versus CI-Off

Compared to the cortical activity of the CI-off condition, the subjects demonstrated significantly decreased activity in the right A1 (BAs 41 and 42) and A2 (BAs 21 and 22) and right OFC (BAs 10 and 11) for the delta frequency band, and in the right A1 and A2, left A2, left temporopolar cortex (TPC, BA 38), left inferior

TABLE 2 | Pre- and post-operative comparison of numeric rating scale tinnitus loudness and tinnitus questionnaire scores in all patients (the order of the subjects are the same as Table 1).

Subject number	Pre-operative NRS loudness	Pre-operative TQ score	Post-operative NRS loudness (CI-on with music stimuli)	Post-operative TQ score (CI-on with music stimuli)	Post-operative NRS loudness (CI-off)	Post-operative TQ score (CI-off)
1	8	78	3	41	8	76
2	7	60	5	44	6	58
3	9	52	3	29	9	52
4	9	62	6	56	9	64

NRS, numeric rating scale; TQ, tinnitus questionnaire.

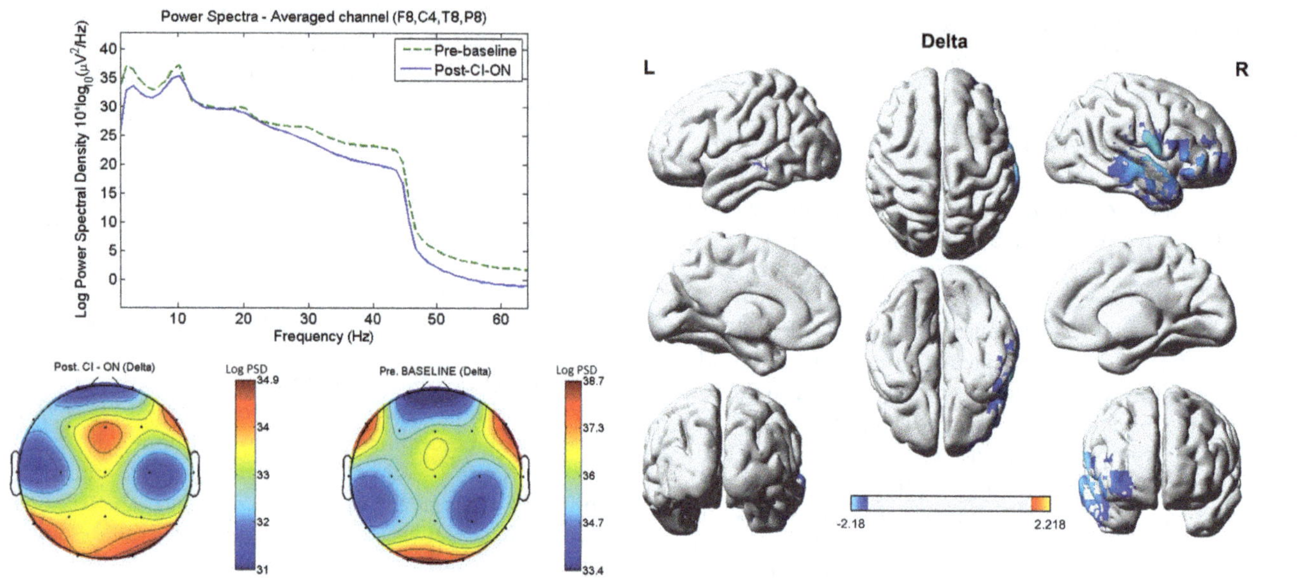

FIGURE 1 | Comparisons between the post-operative cochlear implant (CI)-on condition and the pre-operative baseline with regard to power spectra, sensor topography, and source-localized activity. As compared with the pre-operative baseline, the post-operative CI-on condition resulted in significantly decreased activity in the right primary (BAs 41 and 42) and secondary (BAs 21 and 22) auditory cortices, and in the right orbitofrontal cortex (BAs 10 and 11) for the delta frequency band ($P < 0.01$). L, left; R, right. Color bar (right bottom) presents t-value. PSD, power spectral density.

frontal cortex (IFC, BA 47), and left OFC for the gamma band of the CI-on condition ($P < 0.01$) (**Figure 3**).

On lagged linear connectivity comparison, no significant differences were found between the two conditions for all eight frequency bands.

Post-operative CI-Off versus Pre-operative Baseline

Neither source-localized cortical activity comparisons nor lagged linear functional connectivity analysis showed statistically significant differences between the CI-off and pre-operative baseline conditions for all eight frequency bands.

DISCUSSION

In the current study, we investigated post-CI changes in patients with SSD with regard to source-localized cortical activity and functional connectivity. In short, the CI-on condition resulted in decreased cortical activity as compared with both the CI-off and pre-operative baseline conditions, but the CI-off and pre-operative baseline conditions showed no significant differences.

Alleviation of Tinnitus and Tinnitus-Related Distress by Peripheral Reafferentation-Induced Cortical Deactivation

All four subjects in the current study showed improvements in NRS tinnitus loudness and TQ score. Although these improvements were only marginally significant both for NRS tinnitus loudness and TQ score ($P = 0.068$ for both parameters), considering the small number of included subjects, the improvements can be regarded to indicate a meaningful alleviation of tinnitus and tinnitus-related loudness.

On source-localized cortical activity analysis, as compared with the pre-operative baseline, the post-operative CI-on condition demonstrated significantly decreased activity in the right A1 and A2, and in the right OFC for the delta frequency

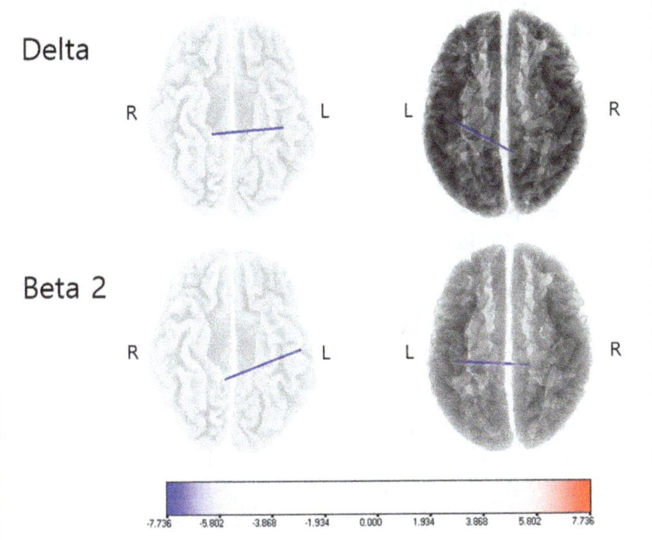

FIGURE 2 | Lagged linear connectivity comparisons between the post-operative cochlear implant (CI)-on condition and the pre-operative baseline. The patients showed decreased functional connectivity between the PCC and A1 for the delta frequency band and between the PCC and A2 for the beta 2 band for the post-operative CI-on state, as compared with the pre-operative baseline. Color bar presents *t*-value.

band. Previous studies both in animals (Engineer et al., 2011) and in human subjects (van der Loo et al., 2009) have demonstrated that the auditory cortex (AC) plays an important role in tinnitus perception. A recent meta-analysis on positron emission tomography (PET) studies in tinnitus patients has also reported increased regional cerebral blood flow in the A1 and A2 (Song et al., 2012). Moreover, perceived tinnitus loudness is correlated with increased contralateral source-localized activity in the AC (van der Loo et al., 2009). In this regard, the significantly decreased activity in the A1 and A2 in patients with SSD after CI, compared with the pre-operative baseline, may be associated with the improvement of tinnitus loudness in these subjects.

Moreover, significantly decreased functional connectivity between the A1 and PCC for the delta frequency band and between the A2 and PCC for the beta 2 band under the CI-on condition, as compared to those under the pre-operative baseline, may also be related to the improvement of tinnitus loudness in these SSD subjects. PCC has been posited to be an important component of the brain's default mode network (DMN) (Raichle et al., 2001; Raichle and Snyder, 2007), which is a set of cortical areas activated when a subject is occupied with internally focused tasks (Schlee et al., 2012). In persistent vegetative state patients, auditory stimulation-induced cortical activation is restricted to the A1, without functional connectivity to the areas comprising the DMN, including the PCC (Laureys et al., 2000; Boly et al., 2004). In other words, functional connectivity between the A1 and the PCC is crucial for conscious auditory perception. In a recent study that evaluated the correlation between pre-CI cortical activity and the extent of tinnitus improvement, increased activity of the PCC for the delta band and increased functional connectivity between the A1 and the PCC for the delta band were negatively correlated with the percent improvement of tinnitus loudness (Song et al., 2013b). This is in line with the current results showing the significantly decreased functional connectivity between the A1 and PCC for the delta frequency band under the CI-on condition as compared to those under the pre-operative baseline. That is, functional decoupling between the A1 and PCC for the delta band by CI may be associated with the improvement of tinnitus under the CI-on condition as compared with the pre-operative baseline condition. Also, the delta and beta 2 frequency bands has been found to be important in the integrity of the

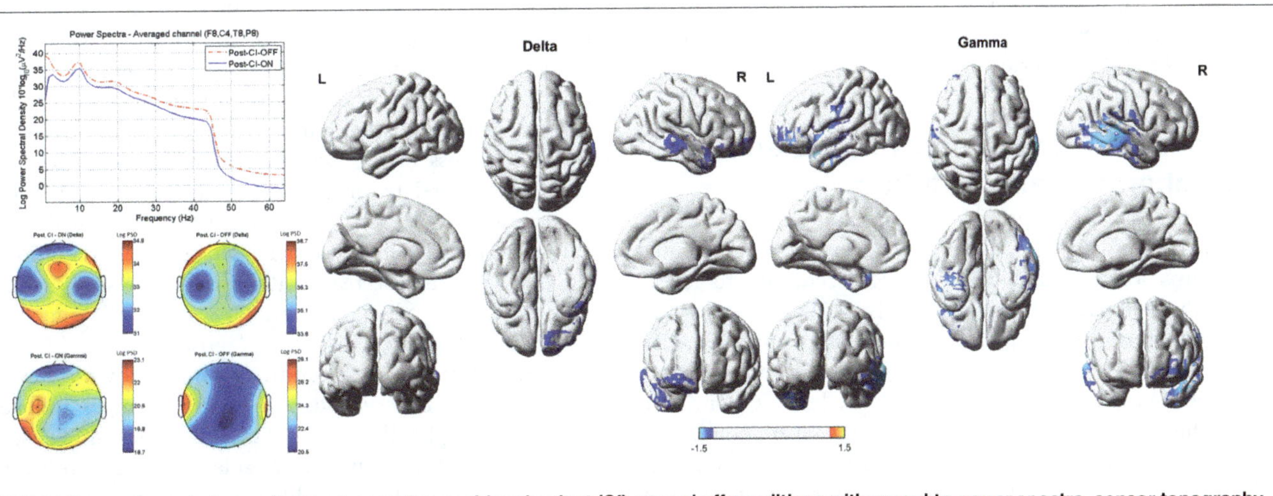

FIGURE 3 | Comparisons between the post-operative cochlear implant (CI)-on and off conditions with regard to power spectra, sensor topography, and source-localized activity. Compared to the cortical activity of the CI-off condition, the subjects demonstrated significantly decreased activity in the right primary (BAs 41 and 42) and secondary (BAs 21 and 22) auditory cortices (A1 and A2), and right orbitofrontal cortex (OFC, BAs 10 and 11) for the delta frequency band and in the right A1 and A2, left A2, left temporopolar cortex (BA 38), left inferior frontal cortex (BA 47), and left OFC for the gamma band for the CI-on with music stimulus condition. L, left; R, right. Color bar (right bottom) presents *t*-value. PSD, power spectral density.

DMN in previous EEG studies (Neuner et al., 2014; Thatcher et al., 2014). Considering this, functional decoupling of the A1/A2 from a component of DMN for the delta and beta 2 frequency bands may have hindered conscious perception of the abnormal activity in the auditory cortices and thus associated with the improvement of tinnitus loudness. Thus, decreased functional connectivity between the A1/A2 and the PCC may be associated with the improvement of tinnitus loudness in these subjects.

Meanwhile, significantly decreased activity in the right OFC for the delta frequency band after CI compared with the pre-operative baseline may be associated with the improvement of the TQ score (i.e., tinnitus-related distress). The OFC has been suggested to be important for emotional processing of sounds (Blood et al., 1999; Vanneste and De Ridder, 2012) and also plays an important role in the top-down modulation of peripheral physiological responses to emotional experiences (Critchley et al., 2004). Additionally, the aforementioned correlation study between pre-CI cortical activity and the amount of post-CI tinnitus improvement revealed that increased pre-CI connectivity between the AC and the OFC is a predictor of poor response to the improvement of tinnitus-related distress (Song et al., 2013b). In particular, a previous qEEG study has demonstrated that the OFC were more activated in highly distressed tinnitus patients than in less distressed patients for the delta band (Song et al., 2015b). In this regard, decreased activity in the OFC for the delta band after CI may be associated with the improvement of the TQ score in our case series.

One possible bias that might be crucial in the interpretation of the comparison between the CI-on condition and pre-operative baseline is the baseline activity of the subjects. In other words, the differences detected in the analysis above might also be partly affected by the changes in the baseline activity in the subjects that might have not be detected in the analysis comparing the CI-off condition and pre-operative baseline. To further clarify this issue, future studies comparing these conditions repeatedly in a larger number of subjects or comparing the CI-off condition and pre-operative baseline serially at different time points after turning the device off should be performed.

"Dynamic" Cortical Activity Modulation by Peripheral Reafferentation

Although CIs starkly improved tinnitus and distress in our current patients with SSD, when they were turned off, the NRS tinnitus loudness and the TQ score returned to levels close to those measured pre-operatively. Moreover, the CI-on condition resulted in significantly decreased activity in the right A1 and A2 and the right OFC for the delta band and in the right A1 and A2, left A2, left TPC, left IFC, and left OFC for the gamma band, compared with the CI-off condition. In addition to the role of A1/A2 in tinnitus perception and of the OFC in tinnitus-related distress described above, the left TPC and IFC were significantly deactivated when the CI was on. The TPC contributes to the processing of auditory concepts (Bonner and Price, 2013) and increased pre-operative activity of the TPC was found to be a negative predictor of tinnitus loudness improvement in SSD patients after CI (Song et al., 2013b). The aggravation of tinnitus loudness after turning off the CI device may be partly due to reactivation of the left TPC. Meanwhile, the left IFC is involved in non-spatial auditory cognition and congruity (Michelon et al., 2003) or cognitive reappraisal (Wager et al., 2008). In a previous meta-analysis of PET studies in tinnitus, the IFC, or the ventrolateral prefrontal cortex, has been found to be commonly activated in tinnitus patients (Song et al., 2012). Therefore, cognitive processing of tinnitus may have been disinhibited in the current subjects after turning off the CI device, and this disinhibition may have manifested as the aggravation of tinnitus loudness.

When the pre-operative baseline and post-operative CI-off conditions were compared, neither subjectively perceived tinnitus loudness/distress nor source-localized activity showed statistically significant differences. CI-induced peripheral reafferentation was effective in alleviating tinnitus only when the device was actively functioning, at least until 6 months post-operatively. In other words, CI-related improvements in tinnitus may be associated with peripheral auditory reafferentation-induced dynamic suppression of tinnitus-related maladaptive cortical activity.

Limitations of the Current Study and Proposed Future Studies

To our knowledge, this is the first study comparing pre- and post-operative cortical activity and functional connectivity in SSD patients who underwent CI. Although we found several significant findings, there are several limitations that should be further investigated in future studies. First, only four patients were included in this study. Although we found several cortical areas that showed significantly decreased activity and functional connectivity for the post-operative CI-on condition, as compared to the pre-operative baseline or post-operative CI-off conditions, we may have failed to discover other crucial areas that also contribute to the improvement of tinnitus, due to the limited statistical power. Additionally, the lack of differences between CI-off and baseline conditions or no significant correlations between cortical activity changes and percent improvement in tinnitus loudness or TQ score might have been due to small subject number-related insufficient statistical power inherent in the current study. Second, the current study revealed dynamic tinnitus suppression by peripheral sensory reafferentation, and these results should be reevaluated in a future study with both a larger number of subjects and a longer follow-up period. In the current study, the subjects' post-operative EEGs were measured 6 months post-operatively, which may not have been long enough to observe possible central changes induced by continuous peripheral stimulus. Further studies in SSD subjects with CI, with follow-up periods of at least 12–24 months, should be performed to explore possible plastic changes. Third, all four subjects in the current study were coincidentally left SSD subjects. This may have affected the results because previous researchers reported that cortical activity differences from normal hearing peers are reported to be larger when the hearing loss occurred in the left ear compared with the right ear (Ponton et al., 2001; Hanss et al., 2009), and left and right unilateral sensorineural hearing loss subjects show different cortical activation patterns to sound stimuli (Schmithorst et al., 2005). Further studies comparing left- and right-SSD subjects with tinnitus after CI should be performed to further explore possible differences. Fourth, the lack of control group, composed of SSD subjects without tinnitus who underwent CI, limits the value of comparison between the CI-on and CI-off conditions. Future studies enrolling SSD subjects without tinnitus who underwent CI as a control group should be performed to further compare CI-on and CI-off conditions. Fifth, BL-ICA-based cleaning of the CI-on condition might have resulted in power decrease in the cleaned bands, and thus the direct comparison between the CI-on and CI-off conditions has inherent limitations. Future studies using auditory stimulation of the non-deaf side may give information on what extent the BL-ICA itself has an adverse effect on the interpretation of the results, and thus give us more precise results. Also, future studies using a similar study paradigm to the current study while measuring cortical activity changes by PET may give us additional precise information, as PET is not affected by device-related artifacts.

CONCLUSION

Taken together, our data demonstrated that the CI-on condition resulted in decreased cortical activity compared with both the CI-off and pre-operative baseline conditions, particularly in areas such as the A1/A2 and the OFC. Also, decreased functional connectivity between the A1/A2 and the PCC were observed in the CI-on condition compared with pre-operative baseline. However, the CI-off and pre-operative baseline conditions showed no significant differences with regard to source-localized activity and functional connectivity. In this regard, CI may alleviate tinnitus in patients with SSD not by sound stimuli-induced cortical plastic changes, but by suppressing abnormally active tinnitus-related cortical regions by dynamic peripheral reafferentation.

AUTHOR CONTRIBUTIONS

J-JS led the analysis and interpretation of the results, and drafted the first manuscript. K-JP, HC, and J-WC conceived the investigation, revised the manuscript for important intellectual content. KK, WS, S-YL, GM, PVdH, DDR, and SV contributed to all aspects of the investigation, including methodological design, data collection and analysis, interpretation of the results, and revision of the manuscript for important intellectual content. All authors approved the final version of the manuscript and agree to be accountable for all aspects of the work.

FUNDING

This work was supported by the National Research Foundation of Korea (NRF) grant funded by the Korea government (MSIP) (No. 2016R1C1B2007911) and Institute for Information and communications Technology Promotion (IITP) grant funded by the Korea government (MSIP; 2014-0-00065, Resilient Cyber-Physical Systems Research) (http://www.nrf.re.kr/nrf_eng_cms/).

ACKNOWLEDGMENTS

The English in this document has been checked by at least two professional editors, both native speakers of English. For a certificate, please see: http://www.textcheck.com/certificate/T7mAyC.

REFERENCES

Andersson, G., Freijd, A., Baguley, D. M., and Idrizbegovic, E. (2009). Tinnitus distress, anxiety, depression, and hearing problems among cochlear implant patients with tinnitus. *J. Am. Acad. Audiol.* 20, 315–319. doi: 10.3766/jaaa.20.5.5

Baguley, D., McFerran, D., and Hall, D. (2013). Tinnitus. *Lancet* 382, 1600–1607. doi: 10.1016/s0140-6736(13)60142-7

Barry, R. J., Clarke, A. R., Johnstone, S. J., and Brown, C. R. (2009). EEG differences in children between eyes-closed and eyes-open resting conditions. *Clin. Neurophysiol.* 120, 1806–1811. doi: 10.1016/j.clinph.2009.08.006

Barry, R. J., Clarke, A. R., Johnstone, S. J., Magee, C. A., and Rushby, J. A. (2007). EEG differences between eyes-closed and eyes-open resting conditions. *Clin. Neurophysiol.* 118, 2765–2773. doi: 10.1016/j.clinph.2007.07.028

Beck, A. T., and Steer, R. A. (1984). Internal consistencies of the original and revised Beck Depression Inventory. *J. Clin. Psychol.* 40, 1365–1367. doi: 10.1002/1097-4679(198411)40:6<1365::AID-JCLP2270400615>3.0.CO;2-D

Blasco, M. A., and Redleaf, M. I. (2014). Cochlear implantation in unilateral sudden deafness improves tinnitus and speech comprehension: meta-analysis and systematic review. *Otol. Neurotol.* 35, 1426–1432. doi: 10.1097/MAO.0000000000000431

Blood, A. J., Zatorre, R. J., Bermudez, P., and Evans, A. C. (1999). Emotional responses to pleasant and unpleasant music correlate with activity in paralimbic brain regions. *Nat. Neurosci.* 2, 382–387. doi: 10.1038/7299

Boly, M., Faymonville, M. E., Peigneux, P., Lambermont, B., Damas, P., Del Fiore, G., et al. (2004). Auditory processing in severely brain injured patients: differences between the minimally conscious state and the persistent vegetative state. *Arch. Neurol.* 61, 233–238. doi: 10.1001/archneur.61.2.233

Bonner, M. F., and Price, A. R. (2013). Where is the anterior temporal lobe and what does it do? *J. Neurosci.* 33, 4213–4215. doi: 10.1523/JNEUROSCI.0041-13.2013

Critchley, H. D., Wiens, S., Rotshtein, P., Ohman, A., and Dolan, R. J. (2004). Neural systems supporting interoceptive awareness. *Nat. Neurosci.* 7, 189–195. doi: 10.1038/nn1176

De Ridder, D., Vanneste, S., and Congedo, M. (2011). The distressed brain: a group blind source separation analysis on tinnitus. *PLoS ONE* 6:e24273. doi: 10.1371/journal.pone.0024273

Del Bo, L., Forti, S., Ambrosetti, U., Costanzo, S., Mauro, D., Ugazio, G., et al. (2008). Tinnitus aurium in persons with normal hearing: 55 years later. *Otolaryngol. Head Neck Surg.* 139, 391–394. doi: 10.1016/j.otohns.2008.06.019

Delorme, A., and Makeig, S. (2004). EEGLAB: an open source toolbox for analysis of single-trial EEG dynamics including independent component analysis. *J. Neurosci. Methods* 134, 9–21. doi: 10.1016/j.jneumeth.2003.10.009

Eggermont, J. J., and Kral, A. (2016). Somatic memory and gain increase as preconditions for tinnitus: insights from congenital deafness. *Hear. Res.* 333, 37–48. doi: 10.1016/j.heares.2015.12.018

Eggermont, J. J., and Roberts, L. E. (2004). The neuroscience of tinnitus. *Trends Neurosci.* 27, 676–682. doi: 10.1016/j.tins.2004.08.010

Eickhoff, S. B., Stephan, K. E., Mohlberg, H., Grefkes, C., Fink, G. R., Amunts, K., et al. (2005). A new SPM toolbox for combining probabilistic cytoarchitectonic maps and functional imaging data. *Neuroimage* 25, 1325–1335. doi: 10.1016/j.neuroimage.2004.12.034

Engineer, N. D., Riley, J. R., Seale, J. D., Vrana, W. A., Shetake, J. A., Sudanagunta, S. P., et al. (2011). Reversing pathological neural activity using targeted plasticity. *Nature* 470, 101–104. doi: 10.1038/nature09656

Fuchs, M., Kastner, J., Wagner, M., Hawes, S., and Ebersole, J. S. (2002). A standardized boundary element method volume conductor model. *Clin. Neurophysiol.* 113, 702–712. doi: 10.1016/S1388-2457(02)00030-5

Giraud, A. L., Price, C. J., Graham, J. M., and Frackowiak, R. S. (2001). Functional plasticity of language-related brain areas after cochlear implantation. *Brain* 124(Pt 7), 1307–1316. doi: 10.1093/brain/124.7.1307

Goebel, G., and Hiller, W. (1994). [The tinnitus questionnaire. A standard instrument for grading the degree of tinnitus. Results of a multicenter study with the tinnitus questionnaire]. *HNO* 42, 166–172.

Hanss, J., Veuillet, E., Adjout, K., Besle, J., Collet, L., and Thai-Van, H. (2009). The effect of long-term unilateral deafness on the activation pattern in the auditory cortices of French-native speakers: influence of deafness side. *BMC Neurosci.* 10:23. doi: 10.1186/1471-2202-10-23

Heller, A. J. (2003). Classification and epidemiology of tinnitus. *Otolaryngol. Clin. North Am.* 36, 239–248. doi: 10.1016/S0030-6665(02)00160-3

Holmes, A. P., Blair, R. C., Watson, J. D., and Ford, I. (1996). Nonparametric analysis of statistic images from functional mapping experiments. *J. Cereb. Blood Flow Metab.* 16, 7–22. doi: 10.1097/00004647-199601000-00002

Jurcak, V., Tsuzuki, D., and Dan, I. (2007). 10/20, 10/10, and 10/5 systems revisited: their validity as relative head-surface-based positioning systems. *Neuroimage* 34, 1600–1611. doi: 10.1016/j.neuroimage.2006.09.024

Kim, K., Punte, A. K., Mertens, G., Van de Heyning, P., Park, K. J., Choi, H., et al. (2015). A novel method for device-related electroencephalography artifact suppression to explore cochlear implant-related cortical changes in single-sided deafness. *J. Neurosci. Methods* 255, 22–28. doi: 10.1016/j.jneumeth.2015.07.020

Kim, S. H., Jang, J. H., Lee, S. Y., Han, J. J., Koo, J. W., Vanneste, S., et al. (2016). Neural substrates predicting short-term improvement of tinnitus loudness and distress after modified tinnitus retraining therapy. *Sci. Rep.* 6:29140. doi: 10.1038/srep29140

Kleinjung, T., Steffens, T., Strutz, J., and Langguth, B. (2009). Curing tinnitus with a Cochlear Implant in a patient with unilateral sudden deafness: a case report. *Cases J.* 2:7462. doi: 10.1186/1757-1626-2-7462

Kringelbach, M. L. (2005). The human orbitofrontal cortex: linking reward to hedonic experience. *Nat. Rev. Neurosci.* 6, 691–702. doi: 10.1038/nrn1747

Krog, N. H., Engdahl, B., and Tambs, K. (2010). The association between tinnitus and mental health in a general population sample: results from the HUNT Study. *J. Psychosom. Res.* 69, 289–298. doi: 10.1016/j.jpsychores.2010.03.008

Lancaster, J. L., Woldorff, M. G., Parsons, L. M., Liotti, M., Freitas, C. S., Rainey, L., et al. (2000). Automated Talairach atlas labels for functional brain mapping. *Hum. Brain Mapp.* 10, 120–131. doi: 10.1002/1097-0193(200007)10:3<120::AID-HBM30>3.0.CO;2-8

Landgrebe, M., Langguth, B., Rosengarth, K., Braun, S., Koch, A., Kleinjung, T., et al. (2009). Structural brain changes in tinnitus: grey matter decrease in auditory and non-auditory brain areas. *Neuroimage* 46, 213–218. doi: 10.1016/j.neuroimage.2009.01.069

Laureys, S., Faymonville, M. E., Degueldre, C., Fiore, G. D., Damas, P., Lambermont, B., et al. (2000). Auditory processing in the vegetative state. *Brain* 123(Pt 8), 1589–1601. doi: 10.1093/brain/123.8.1589

Michelon, P., Snyder, A. Z., Buckner, R. L., McAvoy, M., and Zacks, J. M. (2003). Neural correlates of incongruous visual information. An event-related fMRI study. *Neuroimage* 19, 1612–1626. doi: 10.1016/S1053-8119(03)00111-3

Milz, P., Faber, P. L., Lehmann, D., Kochi, K., and Pascual-Marqui, R. D. (2014). sLORETA intracortical lagged coherence during breath counting in meditation-naive participants. *Front. Hum. Neurosci.* 8:303. doi: 10.3389/fnhum.2014.00303

Moazami-Goudarzi, M., Michels, L., Weisz, N., and Jeanmonod, D. (2010). Temporo-insular enhancement of EEG low and high frequencies in patients with chronic tinnitus. QEEG study of chronic tinnitus patients. *BMC Neurosci.* 11:40. doi: 10.1186/1471-2202-11-40

Neuner, I., Arrubla, J., Werner, C. J., Hitz, K., Boers, F., Kawohl, W., et al. (2014). The default mode network and EEG regional spectral power: a simultaneous fMRI-EEG study. *PLoS ONE* 9:e88214. doi: 10.1371/journal.pone.0088214

Nichols, T. E., and Holmes, A. P. (2002). Nonparametric permutation tests for functional neuroimaging: a primer with examples. *Hum. Brain Mapp.* 15, 1–25. doi: 10.1002/hbm.1058

Norena, A., Micheyl, C., Chery-Croze, S., and Collet, L. (2002). Psychoacoustic characterization of the tinnitus spectrum: implications for the underlying mechanisms of tinnitus. *Audiol. Neurootol.* 7, 358–369. doi: 10.1159/000066156

Pascual-Marqui, R. D. (2002). Standardized low-resolution brain electromagnetic tomography (sLORETA): technical details. *Methods Find. Exp. Clin. Pharmacol.* 24(Suppl. D), 5–12.

Ponton, C. W., Vasama, J. P., Tremblay, K., Khosla, D., Kwong, B., and Don, M. (2001). Plasticity in the adult human central auditory system: evidence from late-onset profound unilateral deafness. *Hear. Res.* 154, 32–44. doi: 10.1016/S0378-5955(01)00214-3

Punte, A. K., Vermeire, K., Hofkens, A., De Bodt, M., De Ridder, D., and Van de Heyning, P. (2011). Cochlear implantation as a durable tinnitus treatment in single-sided deafness. *Cochlear Implants Int.* 12(Suppl. 1), S26–S29. doi: 10.1179/146701011X13001035752336

Raichle, M. E., MacLeod, A. M., Snyder, A. Z., Powers, W. J., Gusnard, D. A., and Shulman, G. L. (2001). A default mode of brain function. *Proc. Natl. Acad. Sci. U.S.A.* 98, 676–682. doi: 10.1073/pnas.98.2.676

Raichle, M. E., and Snyder, A. Z. (2007). A default mode of brain function: a brief history of an evolving idea. *Neuroimage* 37, 1083–1090; discussion 1097–1089. doi: 10.1016/j.neuroimage.2007.02.041

Rolls, E. T. (2004). The functions of the orbitofrontal cortex. *Brain Cogn.* 55, 11–29. doi: 10.1016/S0278-2626(03)00277-X

Ruckenstein, M. J., Hedgepeth, C., Rafter, K. O., Montes, M. L., and Bigelow, D. C. (2001). Tinnitus suppression in patients with cochlear implants. *Otol. Neurotol.* 22, 200–204. doi: 10.1097/00129492-200103000-00014

Schaette, R., Turtle, C., and Munro, K. J. (2012). Reversible induction of phantom auditory sensations through simulated unilateral hearing loss. *PLoS ONE* 7:e35238. doi: 10.1371/journal.pone.0035238

Schecklmann, M., Landgrebe, M., Poeppl, T. B., Kreuzer, P., Manner, P., Marienhagen, J., et al. (2011). Neural correlates of tinnitus duration and Distress: a positron emission tomography study. *Hum. Brain Mapp.* 34, 233–240. doi: 10.1002/hbm.21426

Schlee, W., Leirer, V., Kolassa, I. T., Weisz, N., and Elbert, T. (2012). Age-related changes in neural functional connectivity and its behavioral relevance. *BMC Neurosci.* 13:16. doi: 10.1186/1471-2202-13-16

Schmithorst, V. J., Holland, S. K., Ret, J., Duggins, A., Arjmand, E., and Greinwald, J. (2005). Cortical reorganization in children with unilateral sensorineural hearing loss. *Neuroreport* 16, 463–467. doi: 10.1097/00001756-200504040-00009

Sherlin, L., and Congedo, M. (2005). Obsessive-compulsive dimension localized using low-resolution brain electromagnetic tomography (LORETA). *Neurosci. Lett.* 387, 72–74. doi: 10.1016/j.neulet.2005.06.069

Song, J. J., De Ridder, D., Schlee, W., Van de Heyning, P., and Vanneste, S. (2013a). "Distressed aging": the differences in brain activity between early- and late-onset tinnitus. *Neurobiol. Aging* 34, 1853–1863. doi: 10.1016/j.neurobiolaging.2013.01.014

Song, J. J., De Ridder, D., Van de Heyning, P., and Vanneste, S. (2012). Mapping tinnitus-related brain activation: an activation-likelihood estimation metaanalysis of PET studies. *J. Nucl. Med.* 53, 1550–1557. doi: 10.2967/jnumed.112.102939

Song, J. J., De Ridder, D., Weisz, N., Schlee, W., Van de Heyning, P., and Vanneste, S. (2014). Hyperacusis-associated pathological resting-state brain oscillations in the tinnitus brain: a hyperresponsiveness network with paradoxically inactive auditory cortex. *Brain Struct. Funct.* 219, 1113–1128. doi: 10.1007/s00429-013-0555-1

Song, J. J., Punte, A. K., De Ridder, D., Vanneste, S., and Van de Heyning, P. (2013b). Neural substrates predicting improvement of tinnitus after cochlear implantation in patients with single-sided deafness. *Hear. Res.* 299, 1–9. doi: 10.1016/j.heares.2013.02.001

Song, J. J., Vanneste, S., and De Ridder, D. (2015a). Dysfunctional noise cancelling of the rostral anterior cingulate cortex in tinnitus patients. *PLoS ONE* 10:e0123538. doi: 10.1371/journal.pone.0123538

Song, J. J., Vanneste, S., Schlee, W., Van de Heyning, P., and De Ridder, D. (2015b). Onset-related differences in neural substrates of tinnitus-related distress: the anterior cingulate cortex in late-onset tinnitus, and the frontal cortex in early-onset tinnitus. *Brain Struct. Funct.* 220, 571–584. doi: 10.1007/s00429-013-0648-x

Souliere, C. R. Jr., Kileny, P. R., Zwolan, T. A., and Kemink, J. L. (1992). Tinnitus suppression following cochlear implantation. A multifactorial investigation. *Arch. Otolaryngol. Head Neck Surg.* 118, 1291–1297. doi: 10.1001/archotol.1992.01880120017004

Talairach, J., and Tornoux, P. (1988). *Co-Planar Stereotaxic Atlas of the Human Brain: 3-Dimensional Proportional System: An Approach to Cerebral Imaging.* Stuttgart: Georg Thieme.

Thatcher, R. W., North, D. M., and Biver, C. J. (2014). LORETA EEG phase reset of the default mode network. *Front. Hum. Neurosci.* 8:529. doi: 10.3389/fnhum.2014.00529

van der Loo, E., Gais, S., Congedo, M., Vanneste, S., Plazier, M., Menovsky, T., et al. (2009). Tinnitus intensity dependent gamma oscillations of the contralateral auditory cortex. *PLoS ONE* 4:e7396. doi: 10.1371/journal.pone.0007396

Vanneste, S., and De Ridder, D. (2012). The auditory and non-auditory brain areas involved in tinnitus. An emergent property of multiple parallel overlapping subnetworks. *Front. Syst. Neurosci.* 6:31. doi: 10.3389/fnsys.2012.00031

Vanneste, S., Plazier, M., der Loo, E., de Heyning, P. V., Congedo, M., and De Ridder, D. (2010). The neural correlates of tinnitus-related distress. *Neuroimage* 52, 470–480. doi: 10.1016/j.neuroimage.2010.04.029

Vanneste, S., Song, J. J., and De Ridder, D. (2013). Tinnitus and musical hallucinosis: the same but more. *Neuroimage* 82, 373–383. doi: 10.1016/j.neuroimage.2013.05.107

Wager, T. D., Davidson, M. L., Hughes, B. L., Lindquist, M. A., and Ochsner, K. N. (2008). Prefrontal-subcortical pathways mediating successful emotion regulation. *Neuron* 59, 1037–1050. doi: 10.1016/j.neuron.2008.09.006

Xia, M., Wang, J., and He, Y. (2013). BrainNet viewer: a network visualization tool for human brain connectomics. *PLoS ONE* 8:e68910. doi: 10.1371/journal.pone.0068910

14

Polish Translation and Validation of the Tinnitus Handicap Inventory and the Tinnitus Functional Index

Małgorzata Wrzosek[1], Eugeniusz Szymiec[2], Wiesława Klemens[3], Piotr Kotyło[4], Winfried Schlee[5], Małgorzata Modrzyńska[2], Agnieszka Lang-Małecka[2], Anna Preis[6] and Jan Bulla[7]*

[1] Department of Logic and Cognitive Science, Adam Mickiewicz University, Poznań, Poland, [2] ENT Department, University of Medical Sciences, Poznań, Poland, [3] ENT Private Practice, Gdynia, Poland, [4] Audiology and Phoniatrics Clinic, Nofer Institute of Occupational Medicine in Łódź, Łódź, Poland, [5] Department of Psychiatry and Psychotherapy, University of Regensburg, Regensburg, Germany, [6] Institute of Acoustics, Adam Mickiewicz University, Poznań, Poland, [7] Department of Mathematics, University of Bergen, Bergen, Norway

***Correspondence:**
Jan Bulla
jan.bulla@uib.no

Objective: The need for validated measures enabling clinicians to classify tinnitus patients according to the severity of tinnitus and screen the progress of therapies in our country led us to translate into Polish and to validate two tinnitus questionnaires, namely the Tinnitus Handicap Inventory (THI) and the Tinnitus Functional Index (TFI).

Design: The original English versions of the questionnaires were translated into Polish and translated back to English by three independent translators. These versions were then finalized by the authors into a Polish THI (THI-Pl) and a Polish TFI (TFI-Pl). Participants from three laryngological centers in Poland anonymously answered the THI-Pl (N = 98) and the TFI-Pl (N = 108) in addition to the Polish versions of the Center for Epidemiologic Studies Depression Scale as a measure of self-perceived level of depression, and the Satisfaction With Life Scale to assess self-perceived quality of life. Both were used to determine discriminant validity. Two Visual Analog Scales were used to measure tinnitus annoyance and tinnitus loudness in order to determine convergent validity.

Results: Similar to the original version of the THI, the THI-Pl showed a high internal consistency (Cronbach's α = 0.93). The exploratory factor analysis revealed that the questionnaire has a three-factorial structure that does not correspond to the original division for functional, catastrophic, and emotional subscales. Convergent and discriminant validities were confirmed. The TFI-Pl showed high internal consistency (Cronbach's α = 0.96) with the reliability ranging from 0.82 to 0.95 for its different subscales. Factor analysis confirmed an eight-factorial structure with factors assigning all items to appropriate subscales reported in the original version of the questionnaire. Discriminant and convergent validities were also confirmed for the TFI-Pl.

Conclusion: We translated and validated the Polish versions of the THI and the TFI to make them suitable for clinical use in Poland.

Keywords: Tinnitus Handicap Inventory, THI, Tinnitus Functional Index, TFI, Polish, adaptation

INTRODUCTION

Tinnitus ("ringing in the ears") is described as the perception of sound without any external stimulation. Chronic tinnitus is a common condition, affecting around 10% of the general population, and for some people this condition is debilitating (Langguth et al., 2011). As for the Polish adult population, Skarżyński et al. (2000) estimated that 20% experienced tinnitus lasting more than 5 min, around 5% were affected by chronic tinnitus, and for 4% (almost 1.6 million adults) tinnitus caused severe annoyance. Moreover, Polish children are affected by this problem as well. The study by Raj-Koziak et al. (2011) reports that more than 5% of 55201 7-year-old children tested reported their perception of tinnitus to be often or very often.

Tinnitus can seriously affect quality of life and, in extreme cases, even lead to suicide (Jastreboff and Hazell, 2004). Among tinnitus related comorbidities we can distinguish anxiety (Udupi et al., 2013; Kehrle et al., 2016), depression (Langguth et al., 2011), or sleep disorders (Crönlein et al., 2016). Tinnitus may be closely linked to hearing loss (Martines et al., 2010; Schecklmann et al., 2012). Different therapeutic approaches offer the use of hearing aids, tinnitus maskers, or tinnitus instruments that combine both (Vernon and Meikle, 2003); counseling sessions (e.g., cognitive behavior therapy, see Cima et al., 2014); counseling combined with the use of sound generators [e.g., Tinnitus Retraining Therapy (TRT), see Jastreboff and Hazel, 1993]; relaxation techniques (e.g., Mindfulness Based Stress Reduction, see Roland et al., 2015); neuromodulation (e.g., the Acoustic Coordinated Reset Neuromodulation, see Tass et al., 2012); or brain stimulation (e.g., Repetitive Transcranial Magnetic Stimulation Treatment, see Folmer et al., 2015). There are many possible options for treatment; however, none of these provides immediate and constant relief for tinnitus (for further details see, e.g., Baguley et al., 2013; Maldonado Fernández et al., 2015).

At the moment, no valid and standardized questionnaire for the assessment of tinnitus is available in Poland. As of yet, clinicians in Poland rely on self-made, non-validated translations of the original version of the questionnaire, which limits the reliability of patient assessment, but also prevents the comparison of therapeutic outcomes with other clinics using validated instruments.

We decided to translate and validate the Tinnitus Handicap Inventory (THI) and the Tinnitus Functional Index (TFI) developed by Newman et al. (1996) and Meikle et al. (2012), respectively. Our choice of the THI was based on two observations: firstly, it is a well-known questionnaire that has been extensively used in clinical and scientific practice to measure tinnitus distress and to test potential reduction of the THI score as a consequence of applied therapy (see, e.g., Landgrebe et al., 2010; Shekhawat et al., 2013; Roland et al., 2015; Wilson et al., 2015; Wise et al., 2015; Zobay et al., 2015). It was determined that a clinically meaningful change is achieved with a reduction of 20 or more points of the total score of the THI (Newman et al., 1996, 1998; Fackrell et al., 2014). Secondly, the THI is integrated into the Tinnitus Research Initiative database, which contains standardized data collected from different tinnitus research centers and countries (Landgrebe et al., 2010). A validated Polish version of the tool would enable clinicians not only to classify tinnitus patients according to severity, but would also create a possibility for Polish scientists to contribute to international research projects.

Our second choice—the TFI—was based on its unique feature; precisely, the possibility to evaluate therapeutic outcomes (Meikle et al., 2012). In addition, this questionnaire may be used by clinicians and researchers to classify patients according to tinnitus severity. Nevertheless, our goal was to provide to Polish ENT centers a tool which enables the evaluation of the effectiveness of applied treatments (see, e.g., Krings et al., 2014; Folmer et al., 2015; Overdevest et al., 2015; Roland et al., 2015; Wilson et al., 2015; Fackrell et al., 2016).

MATERIALS AND METHODS

Participants

The study was performed in three clinics in Polish cities—namely Poznań, Gdańsk and Łódź —where paper versions of the questionnaires were filled out anonymously by 98 patients (for the THI-Pl) and 108 patients (for the TFI-PI) who reported tinnitus as either a primary complaint or secondary complaint after hearing loss (defined by hearing loss exceeding 25 dB HL for at least one of the frequencies tested in the audiological pre-interview). Ten of 108 patients tested with the TFI-Pl questionnaire did not fill out the THI-Pl. Participation was voluntary, all participants gave oral consent before filling out the questionnaire, and data was stored and analyzed completely anonymously. The sample was heterogeneous and included a large variety of patients visiting our clinics. This range included, for example, patients with different degrees of hearing loss and self-reported tinnitus severity visiting the ENT doctor for the first time, but also those who had already undergone particular treatments and patients currently in the therapeutic process (Poznań: mainly TRT or electrostimulation; Gdańsk: TRT; Łódź: TRT, counseling sessions). A study information sheet was provided and all volunteers were informed about the aim of the study as well as the estimated time for completing the questionnaires. The participants filled out the questionnaires while waiting for their consultation with an ENT specialist. Descriptive measures of patients who filled in the THI-Pl and TFI-Pl questionnaires are shown in Supplementary Tables S1 and S2, respectively.

Tinnitus Handicap Inventory

The THI (Newman et al., 1996) is a self-reported measure consisting of 25 items divided into three subscales: functional (11 items measuring the functional aspects of tinnitus such as mental, social/occupational, and physical functioning), catastrophic (five items reflecting catastrophic responses to tinnitus, including depression, and sleep disturbance), and emotional (nine items representing affective responses to tinnitus). There are three possible answers to each item (and 25 items in total): "yes" (four points), "sometimes" (two points), and "no" (zero points). Scores are calculated for the THI total scale (range 0–100 points) as well as for the three subscales: functional (THIf), catastrophic (THIc), and emotional (THIe)—ranges 0–44, 0–20, and 0–36 points, respectively). It is noteworthy that some researchers proposed a unifactorial structure of the questionnaire, with no division for subscales (Baguley and Andersson, 2003; Fackrell et al., 2014).

The THI has been widely validated and translated, for example, into Danish (Zachariae et al., 2000), Korean (Kim et al., 2002), Italian (Monzani et al., 2008), Chinese (Kam et al., 2009), German (Kleinstäuber et al., 2015), Persian (Jalali et al., 2015), and Russian (Oron et al., 2015).

Tinnitus Functional Index

The TFI (Meikle et al., 2012) is a self-report measure used for the evaluation of tinnitus severity, measuring clinically important changes. It consists of 25 items divided into 8 subscales addressing different domains of tinnitus severity: intrusive (three items, TFIint), sense of control (three items, TFIsoc), cognitive (three items, TFIcog), sleep (three items, TFIsleep), auditory (three items, TFIaud), relaxation (three items, TFIrelax), quality of life (four items, TFIqol) and emotional (three items, TFIem). The TFI-Pl uses a 10-point scale in the range 0–10 or 0–100%. The scores are calculated for the total scale and all subscales (range 0–100 each). Detailed scoring instructions are provided by the authors (Meikle et al., 2012).

The TFI is currently translated and validated by scientists from Holland (Rabau et al., 2014) and England (Fackrell et al., 2016).

Translation Procedure

The original versions of the questionnaires were translated into Polish by the authors fluent in English. These authors agreed to the translated version being further forwarded to three independent translators who performed translations back into English. Two of these translators were native English speakers and one was an English teacher who studied English philology. They were unfamiliar with the original version of the questionnaire. After comparing the original and the translated versions, the authors constructed the final versions of the THI-Pl and TFI-Pl (see "Supplementary Material 1" which displays the Polish versions of the THI and information on how to obtain the TFI), based on a simple frequency criterion. More precisely, when discrepancies between the three translations provided were observed, the authors chose the version preferred by two of the three translators. Other forms of discrepancies were not observed. The questionnaires were pre-tested by the authors themselves and with hospital staff who volunteered for this task.

Additional Measures

Participants were additionally asked to complete the Polish version of The Centre for Epidemiological Studies Depression Scale (CES-D; Radloff, 1977; Polish adaptation: Dojka et al., 2003; Kaniasty, 2003; Ziarko et al., 2013) and the Polish version of The Satisfaction With Life Scale (SWLS; Diener et al., 1985; Pavot and Diener, 1993; Polish adaptation: Juczyński, 2001). We also used two versions of the Visual Analog Scale as a measure of self-perceived tinnitus annoyance and tinnitus loudness.

The CES-D is a tool which is free of charge and widely used in clinical practice to estimate the number and intensity of depressive symptoms after the diagnosis of depression (Ziarko et al., 2013). It consists of 25 items divided into four subscales measuring: (1) depressive affect (depressive mood), (2) lack of positive affect (well-being), (3) somatic symptoms and inhibition of activity (somatic symptoms), and (4) attitude to other people (intrapersonal affect) (Radloff, 1977; Ziarko et al., 2013). The structure of the Polish version of the tool is internally compliant with the theoretical assumptions and its temporal stability was confirmed in the longitudinal studies (Ziarko et al., 2013).

The SWLS assesses self-perceived quality of life. The tool includes five statements with which patients have to express their degree of agreement (1–"I totally disagree," 7–"I totally agree"). The total score of the Polish and original version of this tool is a general indicator of a participant's satisfaction with their life (Juczyński, 2001).

The Visual Analog Scales (VAS; assessing self-perceived tinnitus anxiety and tinnitus loudness) were chosen, because they are considered to be valid and effective tools for measuring reductions in tinnitus severity in people with chronic tinnitus (Adamchic et al., 2012). The Visual Analog Scale was used in order to ascertain the severity of tinnitus (tinnitus annoyance and tinnitus loudness). The VAS scales consisted of two 10 cm lines with marked endpoints. There were two faces drawn: a smiling one indicating lack of annoyance or no perception of tinnitus (painted under the left endpoint of a line) and a sad one indicating extreme annoyance or extremely loud tinnitus (painted under the right endpoint of a line).

Statistical Analysis

Statistical analyses of data were performed with the Statistical Package for Social Sciences (v22; SPSS, Inc., Chicago, IL, USA). Since the majority of our samples were non-Gaussian (indicated by the Shapiro–Wilk test), we relied mainly on non-parametric techniques. More specifically, whenever the normality assumption was rejected, we used the Wilcoxon–Mann–Whitney for comparisons of two (unpaired) groups. Alternatively, the *t*-test was preferred for Gaussian samples. Similarly, the Kruskal–Wallis test served to compare larger numbers of groups when the normality hypothesis was rejected. For the Gaussian sample, we used a one-way ANOVA. Spearman's rank correlation coefficient (rho) was used for measuring associations. Internal consistency was evaluated by measuring Cronbach's alpha coefficient in order to assess questionnaire reliability and the item-total correlation. The Kaiser-Meyer-Olkin (KMO) Measure of Sampling Adequacy and Bartlett's Test of Sphericity were assessed to assure that our data was eligible for our exploratory factor analysis. Correlations between the factors were calculated, and factor analysis was carried out using the oblique Oblimin rotation. In addition, two orthogonal rotations (Varimax, Quartimax) were investigated. For increased robustness, we selected the Unweighted Least Squares method as an estimation technique. Confirmatory factor analysis (CFA) was performed using IBM SPSS AMOS 22. Statistical significance was set for p-values smaller than 0.05.

In order to determine the discriminant validity, we asked participants to complete the Polish version of The Centre for Epidemiological Studies Depression Scale (CES-D; Radloff, 1977; Polish adaptation: Dojka et al., 2003; Kaniasty, 2003; Ziarko et al., 2013) and the Polish version of The Satisfaction With Life

Scale (SWLS; Diener et al., 1985; Pavot and Diener, 1993; Polish adaptation: Juczyński, 2001). We assumed that discriminant validity would be confirmed when at most moderate ($\rho < 0.6$) correlations between the THI and TFI total score and CES-D and SWLS scores were observed (Newman et al., 1996; Fackrell et al., 2014).

To access the convergent validity, we used two versions of the Visual Analog Scale as a measure of the self-perceived tinnitus annoyance and tinnitus loudness. We assumed that convergent validity would be confirmed when at least strong correlations ($\rho > 0.6$) between the THI and TFI total score and VAS annoyance and VAS loudness scores were observed.

Five TFI-Pl questionnaires from two female and three male respondents with seven or more omitted responses were removed from the analysis, according to the recommendation by Meikle et al. (2012). We did not have to exclude any THI-Pl questionnaires. Thus, the final number of questionnaires retained was $N = 98$ and $N = 103$ for the THI and TFI analysis, respectively. Note that our THI-Pl sample contained a total of 35 missing observations, and the TFI-Pl sample contained a total of 22 missing observations (after the exclusion of five participants), resulting from questions skipped by responders. Since this constitutes only ~1% of the data, we applied a mean-replacement for reliability analysis as well as a factor analysis.

RESULTS

The Polish version of the THI

Descriptive Statistics, Intergroup Differences, and Correlations

The average age of patients who filled in the THI-Pl questionnaire was 51.72 years ($SD = 13.06$) and the mean duration of tinnitus was 6.56 years ($SD = 11.64$). Responses given to particular items of the THI-Pl are presented in Supplementary Table S3. **Table 1** shows average scores obtained by participants for the THI-Pl, VAS scales, CES-D, and SWLS. **Table 2** summarizes correlations between the different scales. The highest correlations were found for the THI total score and VAS annoyance. The relation between the THI total score (or its subscales) and gender was not significant, as shown by the Wilcoxon–Mann–Whitney test. In addition, the Kruskal–Wallis test did not reveal any significant differences for THI total score (or its subscales) resulting from variations in tinnitus pitch, localization, or character. The Wilcoxon–Mann–Whitney test showed significant influence of hearing loss on the total THI score ($p = 0.044$). Participants subject to hearing loss obtained higher scores than normal hearing patients (41.6 vs. 33.4). There were no significant correlations between the THI-Pl and age or duration of tinnitus.

Convergent validity was confirmed by strong positive Spearman's correlations for the total THI score and the VAS annoyance and loudness scales. Discriminant validity was assessed by weak negative correlations ($\rho < 0.4$) for the SWLS and moderate positive correlations ($\rho < 0.6$) for the CES-D total score.

Internal Consistency

The THI-Pl has the same high internal consistency reliability as the original version of the questionnaire ($\alpha = 0.93$; from Newman et al., 1996, which serves as a reference for all statistical

TABLE 1 | Average scores and their standard deviations for THI-Pl and additional measures obtained from the Polish participants.

	Scale							
	THI-Pl	**THIf**	**THIc**	**THIe**	**VASa**	**VASl**	**CES-D**	**SWLS**
Mean	38.6	17.7	8.8	12.1	48.9	50.0	15.6	21.5
SD	22.9	10.3	5.1	9.5	26.3	26.2	10.6	5.8

THI, Tinnitus Handicap Inventory; Pl, Polish; f, functional; c, catastrophic; e, emotional; VAS, Visual Analog Scale; a, annoyance; l, loudness; SWLS, The Satisfaction With Life Scale; CES-D, The Centre for Epidemiological Studies Depression Scale.

TABLE 2 | Correlations (Spearman's rho) between the THI-Pl and other measures used in the adaptation procedure.

Measure	VASa	VASl	CES-D	SWLS
THI-Pl	0.799***	0.610***	0.528***	−0.300**

****p < 0.001; **p < 0.01; THI, Tinnitus Handicap Inventory; Pl, Polish; VAS, Visual Analog Scale; a, annoyance; l, loudness; CES-D, The Centre for Epidemiological Studies Depression Scale; SWLS, The Satisfaction With Life Scale.*

TABLE 3 | Corrected item total correlation for all items of the THI-Pl.

Scale/Item	Corrected item-total correlation
F 1	0.706
F 2	0.303
E 3	0.514
F 4	0.514
C 5	0.673
E 6	0.668
F 7	0.405
C 8	0.481
F 9	0.720
E 10	0.682
C 11	0.486
F 12	0.720
F 13	0.627
E 14	0.711
F 15	0.536
E 16	0.694
E 17	0.628
F 18	0.495
C 19	0.246
F 20	0.674
E 21	0.713
E 22	0.743
C 23	0.632
F 24	0.266
E 25	0.748

F, functional; E, emotional; C, catastrophic.

measures in the following as well, if not stated otherwise). **Table 3** presents the corrected item total correlation. Further details concerning Cronbach's alpha coefficient if an item is deleted are included in Supplementary Table S4. Items 2, 19, and 24 had the lowest possible corrected item total correlation, with values lower than 0.4–0.30, 0.25, and 0.27, respectively. The analysis revealed that the removal of these items would only slightly elevate Cronbach's alpha coefficient from $\alpha = 0.933$ to $\alpha = 0.935$. We therefore decided to preserve the original number of items in the questionnaire. For the other 22 items, the corrected item total correlation was high ($r = 0.6$). When compared to the original version of questionnaire, internal consistency reliability was slightly lower for the functional subscale ($\alpha = 0.83$ vs. $\alpha = 0.86$) and slightly higher for the catastrophic ($\alpha = 0.70$ vs. $\alpha = 0.68$) and emotional ($\alpha = 0.90$ vs. $\alpha = 0.87$) subscales. Supplementary Table S5 lists the reliability coefficients of the THI-Pl and other adaptations. The last two columns report the average internal consistency reliability of all adaptations excluding the Polish and the original English version and the sample standard deviation. Cronbach's alpha determined for the Polish adaptation fell within the estimated 95% quantile of all questionnaires as presented in Supplementary Table S5.

Factor Analysis

We started with an exploratory factor analysis, assuming the original structure of the questionnaire (Newman et al., 1996) with three factors. All factors were moderately correlated with each other, as can be seen in the lower part of **Table 4**, supporting the choice of an oblique rotation. The first main factor with an eigenvalue of 10.2 explained 41.0% of the variance; the second with an eigenvalue of 1.9–7.5% and the third with an eigenvalue of 1.4–5.5% together explained 54.1% of the total variance. Supplementary Figure S1 shows a scree plot of factors with corresponding eigenvalues. On the one hand, the first factor is dominant, which at first glance supports a unifactorial questionnaire structure. **Table 4** represents the rotated factor loadings of the described solution and the factor correlations. Investigation of the factor loadings and their corresponding eigenvalues led us to three conclusions. Firstly, three factors contribute to the loadings of the 25 items, but these factors do not correspond to the subscales of the questionnaire. Except for three items, all of these loadings can be considered important as they have values greater than 0.4 (Floyd and Widaman, 1995; Baguley and Andersson, 2003). In addition, the remaining items carry loadings higher than 0.27 and two of these are greater than 0.3. Secondly, of the first factor loads on 15 items, six belong to the emotional subscale, four to the catastrophic subscale, and five to the functional one. In our opinion, these items may be considered to be referring to the impact of tinnitus on everyday functioning and the emotional state of the patient. Five questions are loaded by the second factor, four of which originally belonged to the functional and one to the emotional subscale. These items could be viewed as describing the aspect of "helplessness" resulting from the perception of tinnitus. The third factor also loads five items, two belonging to the functional, two to the emotional, and one to the catastrophic subscale. Four of these questions refer either to relationships with other people or to social activities. Item number 12 concerns satisfaction with life ("Does your tinnitus make it difficult for you to enjoy life?") and, in our belief, can be linked with satisfaction from social relations. Taking into consideration loadings greater than 0.3, only three items (5, 22, and 23) are double-loaded. Two of them—item 5 ("Because of your tinnitus, do you feel desperate?") and item 23 ("Do you feel that you can no longer cope with your tinnitus?")—are additionally loaded by the third factor, which seems to be appropriate in the context of "helplessness." The question "Does your tinnitus make you feel anxious?" (item 22) is loaded by the third factor, but also by the first one. Since this item refers to the emotional state of the patient, an observation of double-loading seems to be justified.

Thirdly, the first factor alone explains less than half of the total variance. Taking this and the factor loadings of the second and

TABLE 4 | Rotated factor loading matrices of the predefined-factor models.

Scale/Item	Factor		
	1	**2**	**3**
	10.25	**1.88**	**1.38**
E 16	**0.672**		
F 15	**0.641**		
F 20	**0.637**		
F 7	**0.627**		
C 8	**0.534**		
F 18	**0.516**		
C 23	**0.511**		0.359
E 25	**0.494**		
F 1	**0.494**		
E 10	**0.477**		
E 14	**0.465**		
E 6	**0.447**		
C 19	**0.435**		
C 5	**0.425**		0.355
E 3	**0.280**		
E 17		**−0.886**	
F 13		**−0.744**	
F 9		**−0.586**	
F 2		**−0.472**	
F 12		**−0.452**	
E 21			**0.699**
F 24			**0.556**
E 22	0.464		**0.473**
F 4			**0.319**
C 11			**0.310**
Correlations			
Factor 1	1.000	−0.433	0.317
Factor 2	−0.433	1.000	−0.442
Factor 3	0.317	−0.442	1.000

Eigenvalues are presented below the names of factors. Lower part of the table shows correlations between the factors. Loadings > 0.30 displayed (with exception of Item 3). Loadings assigned to particular factors in bold; F, functional; E, emotional; C, catastrophic.

third factors into account, it may be advisable to consider at least a two- or even three-factorial structure for attaining approximately 50% explained variation.

Moreover, we also investigated the effect of using orthogonal rotations for exploratory purposes (Supplementary Table S6 reports the results). Then the results changed substantially: on the one hand, the Varimax solution suggests a structure similar to that obtained by the Oblimin solution. On the other hand, the Quartimax rotation leads to one main factor carrying the highest load for 22 of the 25 items, suggesting a unifactorial structure.

Lastly, we carried out a CFA for investigating if we can confirm the original three-factorial structure suggested by Newman et al. (1996). Some of the values of our fit indices were not too far from those obtained by Kleinstäuber et al. (2015); for example, Kleinstäuber et al. (2015) obtained an RMSEA of 0.060, whereas our corresponding value equals 0.084. However, the overall results did not permit us to conclude an acceptable fit with the data, which is also in line with Kleinstäuber et al. (2015). Supplementary Table S14 presents details of the estimation results. Due to our comparably low sample size and the resulting lower reliability of all χ^2-based statistics, we refrained from investigating further modifications of our factor model.

The Polish version of the TFI

Descriptive Statistics, Intergroup Differences, and Correlations

Supplementary Table S7 presents responses to particular items of the TFI-Pl. **Table 5** shows the average scores obtained by participants for the TFI-Pl, VAS scales, CES-D, and SWLS. **Table 6** summarizes the correlations between the different scales (correlations between THI-Pl and TFI-Pl are included). Lastly, Supplementary Table S8 presents more details on correlations of all THI and TFI scales with other measures.

TABLE 5 | Average scores and their standard deviations for TFI-Pl, the original version of the TFI (values in brackets), and additional measures obtained from the Polish participants.

Scale	Mean	*SD*
TFI	46.7 (54.4)	22.5 (24.7)
TFIint	53.1 (67.8)	25.9 (24.3)
TFIsoc	64.0 (64.7)	27.0 (25.0)
TFIcog	40.2 (48.0)	25.0 (29.0)
TFIsleep	42.6 (51.5)	31.5 (35.3)
TFIaud	40.0 (53.1)	29.3 (30.2)
TFIrelax	50.5 (59.9)	28.9 (30.3)
TFIqol	36.4 (46.3)	29.4 (29.9)
TFIem	45.6 (47.2)	29.0 (31.8)
VASa	4.8	2.6
VASl	4.9	2.6
CES-D	15.2	10.3
SWLS	21.8	5.8

TFI, Tinnitus Functional Index; int, intrusive; soc, sence of control; cog, cognitive; aud, auditory; relax, relaxation; qol, quality of life; em, emotional; VAS, Visual Analog Scale; a, annoyance; l, loudness; CES-D, The Centre for Epidemiological Studies Depression Scale; SWLS, The Satisfaction With Life Scale.

We did not discover any impact of gender or hearing loss on the TFI-Pl score or its subscales (all p-values from t-test were non-significant). The Wilcoxon–Mann–Whitney test showed significant influence of hearing loss presence on the scores obtained in the auditory, quality of life, and emotional subscales ($p = 0.017$, $p = 0.020$, and $p = 0.024$, respectively). The group with participants subject to hearing loss obtained higher scores than normal hearing patients. In addition, the Kruskal–Wallis test revealed significant differences for the quality of life ($p = 0.03$) and emotional ($p = 0.049$) subscales and tinnitus pitch as well as for the sense of control subscale and tinnitus characteristics (tonal vs. non-tonal tinnitus). The highest scores in both the quality of life and emotional subscales were obtained by participants whose tinnitus pitch corresponded to a sound of 125 Hz; the lowest score corresponded to 500 Hz. The lowest sense of control was reported for patients experiencing a mixed type of tinnitus. A one-way ANOVA did not confirm any significant differences for the TFI-Pl total score (or its subscales) resulting from variations in tinnitus localization or character. Significant differences were observed for the relaxation subscale and tinnitus pitch ($p = 0.012$). A tinnitus pitch of 125 Hz interfered with relaxation particularly strongly, whereas 250 Hz corresponded to the lowest score obtained on the relaxation subscale. Weak but significant correlations were found between the auditory subscale and age or duration of tinnitus.

Convergent validity was confirmed with strong positive Spearman's correlations for the total TFI-Pl score and VAS loudness scale and very strong correlations with the VAS annoyance scale. Moreover, strong correlations were found between the THI-Pl and TFI-Pl. Discriminant validity was shown with no significant correlations for the SWLS and weak positive correlations for the CES-D. The lowest correlations were found for the TFI auditory subscale.

Internal Consistency

The TFI-Pl has almost the same high internal consistency reliability as the original version of the questionnaire ($\alpha = 0.96$ vs. 0.97). Consistency reliability of the TFI subscales ranged from 0.83 (sense of control subscale) to 0.95 (emotional subscale). **Table 7** shows the corrected-item total correlation; Supplementary Table S9 section contains additional information about Cronbach's alpha when a particular item is deleted. Supplementary Table S10 section presents Cronbach's alpha coefficients for the TFI total and all subscales for the TFI-Pl and other adapted versions.

TABLE 6 | Correlations (Spearman's rho) for TFI-Pl and other measures used in the adaptation procedure.

Measure	THI-Pl	VASa	VASl	CES-D	SWLS
TFI-Pl	782***	0.837***	0.761***	0.361***	−0.223*

****$p < 0.001$; *$p < 0.05$; TFI, Tinnitus Functional Index; THI, Tinnitus Handicap Inventory; Pl, Polish; VAS, Visual Analog Scale; a, annoyance; l, loudness; CES-D, The Centre for Epidemiological Studies Depression Scale; SWLS, The Satisfaction With Life Scale.*

Factor Analysis

Similar to the THI, we carried out an exploratory factor analysis based on the oblique Oblimin rotation, since several factors showed moderate correlation (see lower part of **Table 8**). The resulting eigenvalues greater than or equal 1 indicated that five factors are sufficient for explaining the total variance (the fifth factor had an eigenvalue of 0.999). The first factor explained 52.7% of variance, the second 10.8%, the third 5.7%, and the two remaining 5.2% and 4.0%, respectively. The following three factors had eigenvalues of lower than 1 (0.87, 0.67, and 0.51), explaining altogether 8.2% of variance. Meikle et al. (2012) obtained similar results in the factor analysis of their first prototype of the TFI with 43 items, where the eigenvalues of factors five to eight were also lower than 1. However, these authors considered eight factors meaningful and decided to retain all of them. They then performed further confirmatory analysis of a second prototype as well as the final version of the TFI with a specified number (8) of factors. In their analysis of the final version, 79.5% of the total variance was explained, whereas in our case eight factors are explained 86.7%. It may be noted that we performed our factor analysis using the Unweighted Least Squares method with oblique Oblimin rotation, since factors were correlated. The Kaiser-Meyer-Olkin (KMO) Measure of Sampling Adequacy was high (KMO = 0.903) and Bartlett's Test of Sphericity was statistically significant ($p < 0.001$).

Table 8 presents the pattern matrix of an eight-factor solution. All factors contribute to the loadings of the 25 items and correspond to the respective subscales of the questionnaire. Except for three items, all loadings have values greater than 0.5. The remaining items (TFI 20, TFI 19, and TFI 2) carry loadings higher than 0.3 and are loaded by two factors. The decision to assign item TFI 2 to the intrusive subscale seems arbitrary, since it is equally loaded (0.305) by the factor referring to the sense of control subscale. However, assignment of this item to any other factor would leave only two items remaining in the subscale, which is not recommended (Meikle et al., 2012).

In summary, our investigation of the factor loadings and their corresponding eigenvalues led to the conclusion that the original structure of the questionnaire should be replicated.

For exploratory purposes, we also investigated the results of a factor analysis with orthogonal rotations (Supplementary Tables S12 and S13 show the results). The loadings obtained from the Varimax solution suggest a seven-factorial structure; for the Quartimax solution, the corresponding number reduces to five.

Moreover, we carried out a CFA for investigating if we can confirm the original eight-factorial structure suggested by Meikle et al. (2012). The results, on the one hand, were not fully satisfactory in terms of fit indices and thus did not permit us to conclude an acceptable fit with the data (Supplementary Table S14 presents details on the estimation results). On the other hand, some of these values were not much lower than those obtained by Fackrell et al. (2016); e.g., TLI (0.915 vs. 0.939) or RMSEA (0.084 vs. 0.064). Obviously, the same limitations caused by our comparably low sample size apply.

TABLE 7 | Corrected item total correlation for all items of the TFI-Pl.

Item	Corrected item-total correlation
1	0.585
2	0.736
3	0.666
4	0.374
5	0.669
6	0.717
7	0.747
8	0.740
9	0.772
10	0.609
11	0.655
12	0.642
13	0.604
14	0.487
15	0.599
16	0.739
17	0.715
18	0.728
19	0.769
20	0.833
21	0.780
22	0.721
23	0.784
24	0.798
25	0.798

DISCUSSION

Objectives

The main goal of our study was to provide Polish clinicians and researchers with validated translations of the THI and the TFI questionnaires that could facilitate the classification of tinnitus patients according to severity and potential evaluation of therapeutic outcomes. The results of the presented work show that valid and reliable Polish versions of the THI and TFI questionnaires were constructed. The THI-Pl and TFI-Pl are satisfactory in terms of construct and criterion validity. They may be used by Polish clinicians working with people who have tinnitus and by Polish scientists working on international scientific research reports. Moreover, the TFI-Pl provides a decent psychometric tool and may be used by Polish clinicians working with patients suffering from tinnitus by enabling the detection of treatment-related changes. Polish scientists working in the tinnitus field may consider scores and subscores to identify factors potentially influencing results obtained during their research. For the THI-Pl one may focus stronger on the total score in clinical and scientific reports.

Limitations

We would also like to address two issues, which could be considered as limitations of our study. The size of our sample was not very large (98 patients for the THI-Pl, 108 patients for the TFI-Pl), and that created natural limits, for instance, for performing the CFA which could be of potential interest for some professional researchers working on adaptations or construction of questionnaires. On the other hand, only four among the 19 adaptations of THI cited in this paper were based on larger amounts of questionnaires (Brazilian/Portuguese–180, French–174, German–373, Japanese–182; Shinden et al., 2002; Ferreira et al., 2005; Schmidt et al., 2006; Ghulyan-Bédikian et al., 2010; Kleinstäuber et al., 2015, respectively), and only the German version of the THI included a presentation of the CFA results. In that study the CFA was justified by a sufficient number of patients. Six studies recruited a similar number of participants (Chinese–114, Persian–102, Italian–100, Korean–111, Turkish–110, and Arabic–100; Kim et al., 2002; Aksoy et al., 2007; Monzani et al., 2008; Kam et al., 2009; Jalali et al., 2015; Barake et al., 2016), and the remaining nine studies tested much fewer tinnitus patients. As far as the TFI is concerned, both the Dutch and English adaptations recruited more participants (263 and 294; Fackrell et al., 2014; Rabau et al., 2014, respectively). In the first case, the authors performed an EFA; in the second a CFA. Our aim was to adapt already existing tools in a manner that would enable the comparison of the THI-Pl and the TFI-Pl with other language versions. We believe that our choice of sample size and factor analysis has good justification in light of the mentioned literature. Future work will be needed to

TABLE 8 | Rotated factor loading matrix of the predefined-factor model.

	Factor							
	1	**2**	**3**	**4**	**5**	**6**	**7**	**8**
Item	**13.2**	**2.7**	**1.4**	**1.3**	**1.0**	**0.9**	**0.7**	**0.5**
21	**0.793**							
22	**0.713**							
20	**0.399**					0.305		
19	**0.315**					0.305		
14		**−0.993**						
13		**−0.828**						
15		**−0.763**						
7			**0.842**					
8			**0.807**					
9			**0.642**					
11				**−0.913**				
12				**−0.790**				
10				**−0.684**				
1					**0.995**			
3					**0.537**			
23						**0.789**		
25						**0.720**		
24						**0.685**		
5							**0.901**	
4							**0.670**	
6							**0.507**	
2					**0.305**		0.305	
17								**0.961**
18								**0.735**
16								**0.734**
				Correlations				
Factor 1	1.000	−0.609	0.511	−0.331	0.326	0.604	0.250	0.531
Factor 2	−0.609	1.000	−0.485	0.172	−0.286	−0.397	−0.149	−0.245
Factor 3	0.511	−0.485	1.000	−0.491	0.385	0.447	0.471	0.543
Factor 4	−0.331	0.172	−0.491	1.000	−0.437	−0.328	−0.470	−0.565
Factor 5	0.326	−0.286	0.385	−0.437	1.000	0.353	0.492	0.422
Factor 6	0.604	−0.397	0.447	−0.328	0.353	1.000	0.411	0.492
Factor 7	0.250	−0.149	0.471	−0.470	0.492	0.411	1.000	0.402
Factor 8	0.531	−0.245	0.543	−0.565	0.422	0.492	0.402	1.000

Eigenvalues are presented below the names of factors. Lower part of the table shows correlations between the factors. Loadings > 0.30 displayed. Loadings assigned to particular factors in bold.

assess the test-retest reliability, which, when confirmed would add important value to Polish versions of the THI and TFI questionnaires.

The Polish version of the THI

Conclusions from the THI-Pl factor analysis are ambiguous since the scree-plot shows a clear dominance of the first factor and limited contribution of the second and third factors in terms of explained variation, which supports a unifactorial structure. On the other hand, multiple factor loadings above the threshold of 0.4 attributed to the second and third factors suggest that a three-factorial structure should not be discarded. Therefore, our results are between those of Newman et al. (1996) and the more recent findings suggesting a unifactorial structure (Baguley and Andersson, 2003; Fackrell et al., 2014). Consequently, one could eventually consider the current subscale division or alternatively simply treat the THI-Pl as a homogenous tool.

Lastly, one aspect is particularly noteworthy in the context of the factor analysis results. Since all factors are moderately correlated with each other, an oblique rotation seems appropriate. However, ignoring the correlation and using the orthogonal Quartimax rotation may lead to substantially different results, with loadings clearly supporting a unifactorial structure. It may be possible that related phenomena may be, in part, responsible for varying results on the factorial structure obtained by different studies.

High correlations between the THI subscales observed in the original version of the questionnaire were also observed in the Polish THI adaptation. Similarly, as far as the total and subscale scores are concerned, the THI-Pl has high internal reliability. Convergent validity was confirmed by strong correlations with the VAS scale accessing tinnitus severity annoyance and the VAS loudness scale. Discriminant validity was assessed by moderate associations between the THI and the CES-D measuring the self-perceived level of depression, and weak associations for the SWLS scale measuring the self-perceived quality of life. Thus, our expectations concerning convergent and discriminant validity were confirmed.

The Polish version of the TFI

During the development of the first version of the TFI containing 43 items, Meikle et al. (2012) reported four factors with eigenvalues higher or equal to 1 when performing the factor analysis. Nevertheless, they decided to preserve eight subscales in the TFI and continued further analysis on a second prototype and the final version of the questionnaire with a specified number (8) of factors. For statistical purposes only—i.e., considering factors with eigenvalues greater or equal to one—we decided to perform an additional factor analysis with five factors. This approach was also motivated by the scree plot (Supplementary Figure S2), which does not support an eight-factorial structure, but rather suggests three to four factors, thus encouraging the exclusion of factors with eigenvalues smaller than 1. Moreover, the five factors contributed to 78.4% of the explained variation, which can be considered satisfactory. Note that for the sake of comparability with our eight-factor solution, we chose a similar setting (Unweighted Least Squares, oblique Oblimin rotation). In the five-factorial solution the first and main factor loaded 10 items, and the second, third, fourth, and fifth factors loaded five, four, three, and three items, respectively. The relaxation, quality of life, and emotional subscales were assigned to one factor, and the intrusive subscale was separated into sense of control (two items) and sleep (one item) subscales. This observation is in line with concerns described by Meikle et al. (2012). These authors state that the intrusive, quality of life, and emotional subscales may reflect only a general tinnitus severity factor or both general and specific factors. Our conclusions from five- and eight-factorial solutions seem to confirm this reflection. The rotated factor matrix of this solution is available in Supplementary Table S11. Furthermore, for the TFI-Pl both orthogonal transformations investigated suggest factorial structures with a lower number of factors. This suggests, in particular, that the popular Varimax rotation should be used with care for analyzing the TFI-Pl (and potentially the TFI in other languages).

The TFI-Pl presents excellent internal consistency reliability and is satisfactory in terms of convergent and discriminant validity. As for the factor analysis results, an eight-factorial solution assigns all items to appropriate subscales for both the TFI-Pl and the original version of the TFI.

Finally, we would like to emphasize the importance of the fact that Polish versions of tinnitus questionnaires will provide Polish researchers with the possibility to become active within international scientific networks. In light of the complex nature of tinnitus, the collaboration between different communities seems to be of very great importance. Using the THI-Pl and TFI-Pl, Polish scientists will not only be able to compare and report results of their studies dedicated to tinnitus, but also become valued contributors on international scientific platforms.

ETHICS STATEMENT

The study was performed in three ENT centers in Poland, namely Poznan, Gdansk, and Lodz. Heads of these centers (MD Eugeniusz Szymiec, MD Wiesława Klemens and MD Piotr Kotylo) agreed on the procedures and provided access to tinnitus patients. Participation was voluntary and completely anonymous, all procedures were non-intrusive. Every patient gave oral consent before filling out the questionnaire. Patients visiting one of the three ENT centers in Poland were informed about the aim of the study as well as the estimated time for completing the questionnaires. Once a patient agreed to volunteer, a study information sheet was provided.

AUTHOR CONTRIBUTIONS

MW translated the questionnaire, designed and performed experiments, analyzed data and wrote the paper; ES, AL-M, and MM performed experiments at the ENT center in Poznań; WK performed experiments at the ENT Private Practice in Gdynia; PK performed experiments at the ENT center in Łódź; WS consulted on the redaction of the manuscript at all stages, and contributed to the revision of the manuscript; AP commented on the manuscript at all stages; JB provided statistical expertise and revised the manuscript at several stages.

ACKNOWLEDGMENTS

We thank *COST Action* BM1306 "*TINNET – Better Understanding the Heterogeneity of Tinnitus to Improve and Develop New Treatments*" for supporting this study with a Short Term Scientific Mission to the University of Bergen, Norway. In addition, we thank Christopher R. Cederroth for providing insightful comments on this paper.

REFERENCES

Adamchic, I., Langguth, B., Hauptmann, C., and Tass, P. A. (2012). Psychometric evaluation of visual analog scale for the assessment of chronic tinnitus. *Am. J. Audiol.* 21, 215–225. doi: 10.1044/1059-0889(2012/12-0010)

Aksoy, S., Firat, Y., and Alpar, R. (2007). The Tinnitus Handicap Inventory: a study of validity and reliability. *Int. Tinnitus J.* 3, 94–98.

Baguley, D., McFerran, D., and Hall, D. (2013). Tinnitus. *Lancet* 382, 1600–1607. doi: 10.1016/S0140-6736(13)60142-7

Baguley, D. M., and Andersson, G. (2003). Factor analysis of the Tinnitus Handicap Inventory. *Am. J. Audiol.* 12, 31–34. doi: 10.1044/1059-0889(2003/007)

Barake, R., Rizk, S. A., Ziade, G., Zaytoun, G., and Bassim, M. (2016). Adaptation of the arabic version of the Tinnitus Handicap Inventory. *Otolaryngol. Head Neck Surg.* 154, 508–512. doi: 10.1177/0194599815621551

Cima, R. F., Andersson, G., Schmidt, C. J., and Henry, J. A. (2014). Cognitive-behavioral treatments for tinnitus: a review of the literature. *J. Am. Acad. Audiol.* 25, 29–61. doi: 10.3766/jaaa.25.1.4

Crönlein, T., Langguth, B., Pregler, M., Kreuzer, P. M., Wetter, T. C., and Schecklmann, M. (2016). Insomnia in patients with chronic tinnitus: cognitive and emotional distress as moderator variables. *J. Psychosom. Res.* 83, 65–68. doi: 10.1016/j.jpsychores.2016.03.001

Diener, E., Emmons, R. A., Larsen, R. J., and Griffin, S. (1985). The satisfaction with life scale. *J. Pers. Assess.* 49, 71–75. doi: 10.1207/s15327752jpa4901_13

Dojka, E., Gorkiewicz, M., and Pajak, A. (2003). Psychometric value of CES-D scale for the assessment of depression in polish population. *Psychiatr. Pol.* 37, 281–292.

Fackrell, K., Hall, D. A., Barry, J., and Hoare, D. J. (2014). "Tools for tinnitus measurement: development and validity of questionnaires to assess handicap and treatment effects," in *Tinnitus: Causes Treatment and Short & Long-Term Health Effects*, eds F. Signorelli and F. Turjman (New York, NY: Nova Science Publishers Inc), 13–60.

Fackrell, K., Hall, D. A., Barry, J. G., and Hoare, D. J. (2016). Psychometric properties of the Tinnitus Functional Index (TFI): assessment in a UK research volunteer population. *Hear. Res.* 335, 220–235. doi: 10.1016/j.heares.2015.09.009

Ferreira, F. E., Cunha, F., Onishi, E. T., Barreiro, F., and Gananca, F. (2005). Tinnitus Handicap Inventory: cross-cultural adaptation to Brazilian Portuguese. *Pro Fono* 17, 303–310. doi: 10.1590/S0104-56872005000300004

Floyd, F. J., and Widaman, K. F. (1995). Factor analysis in the development and refinement of clinical assessment instruments. *Psychol. Assess.* 7, 286–299. doi: 10.1037/1040-3590.7.3.286

Folmer, R. L., Theodoroff, S. M., Casiana, L., Shi, Y., Griest, S., and Vachhani, J. (2015). Repetitive transcranial magnetic stimulation treatment for chronic tinnitus: a randomized clinical trial. *JAMA Otolaryngol. Head Neck Surg.* 141, 716–722. doi: 10.1001/jamaoto.2015.1219

Ghulyan-Bédikian, V., Paolino, M., Giorgetti-D'Esclercs, F., and Paolino, F. (2010). Propriétés psychométriques d'une version francaise du Tinnitus Handicap Inventory [Psychometric properties of a French adaptation of the Tinnitus Handicap Inventory]. *L'Encéphale.* 36, 390–396.

Jalali, M. M., Soleimani, R., Fallahi, M., Aghajanpour, M., and Elahi, M. (2015). Psychometric properties of the persian version of the Tinnitus Handicap Inventory (THI-P). *Iran J. Otorhinolaryngol.* 27, 83–94.

Jastreboff, P. J., and Hazel, J. W. P. (1993). A neurophysiological approach to tinnitus. Clinical implications. *Br. J. Audiol.* 27, 7–17. doi: 10.3109/03005369309077884

Jastreboff, P. J., and Hazell, J. W. P. (2004). *Tinnitus Retraining Therapy: Implementing the Neurophysiological Model.* Cambridge: Cambridge University Press.

Juczyński, Z. (2001). *Narzędzia Pomiaru w Promocji i Psychologii Zdrowia [Measurement Tools in Health Promotion and Health Psychology].* Warszawa: Pracownia Testów Psychologicznych Polskiego Towarzystwa Psychologicznego.

Kam, A. C. S., Cheung, A. P. P., Chan, P. Y. B., Leung, E. K. S., Wong, T. K. C., Van Hasselt, C. A., et al. (2009). Psychometric properties of the Chinese (Cantonese) Tinnitus Handicap Inventory. *Clin. Otolaryngol.* 34, 309–315. doi: 10.1111/j.1749-4486.2009.01946.x

Kaniasty, K. (2003). *Klęska Żywiołowa czy Katastrofa Społeczna? Psychospołeczne Konsekwencje Polskiej Powodzi 1997 Roku [Natural or Social Catastrophy? Psychosocial Consequences of 1997 Flood in Poland].* Gdańsk: Gdańskie Wydawnictwo Psychologiczne.

Kehrle, H. M., Sampaio, A. L., Granjeiro, R. C., Oliveira, T. S., and Oliveira, C. A. (2016). Tinnitus annoyance in normal-hearing individuals correlation with depression and anxiety. *Ann. Otol. Rhinol. Laryngol.* 125, 185–194. doi: 10.1177/0003489415606445

Kim, J. H., Lee, S. Y., Kim, C. H., Lim, S. L., Shin, J., Chung, W. H., et al. (2002). Reliability and validity of a Korean adaptation of the Tinnitus Handicap Inventory. *Korean J. Otolaryngol.* 45, 328–334.

Kleinstäuber, M., Frank, I., and Weise, C. (2015). A confirmatory factor analytic validation of the Tinnitus Handicap Inventory. *J. Psychosom. Res.* 78, 277–284. doi: 10.1016/j.jpsychores.2014.12.001

Krings, J. G., Wineland, A., Kallogjeri, D., Rodebaugh, T. L., Nicklaus, J., Lenze, E. J., et al. (2014). A novel treatment for tinnitus and tinnitus-related cognitive difficulties using computer-based cognitive training and D-Cycloserine. *JAMA Otolaryngol. Head Neck Surg.* 141, 18–26. doi: 10.1001/jamaoto.2014.2669

Landgrebe, M., Zeman, F., Koller, M., and Eberl, Y. (2010). The Tinnitus Research Initiative (TRI) database: a new approach for delineation of tinnitus subtypes and generation of predictors for treatment outcome. *BMC Med. Inform. Decis. Mak.* 10:42. doi: 10.1186/1472-6947-10-42

Langguth, B., Landgrebe, M., Kleinjung, T., Sand, G. P., and Hajak, G. (2011). Tinnitus and depression. *World J. Biol. Psychiatry* 12, 489–500. doi: 10.3109/15622975.2011.575178

Maldonado Fernández, M., Shin, J., Scherer, R. W., and Murdin, L. (2015). Interventions for tinnitus in adults: an overview of systematic reviews. *Cochrane Database Syst. Rev.* 2015:CD011795. doi: 10.1002/14651858.CD011795

Martines, F., Bentivegna, D., Martines, E., Sciacca, V., and Martinciglio, G. (2010). Characteristics of tinnitus with or without hearing loss: clinical observations in Sicilian tinnitus patients. *Auris Nasus Larynx* 37, 685–693. doi: 10.1016/j.anl.2010.03.008

Meikle, M. B., Henry, J. A., Griest, S. E., Stewart, B. J., Abrams, H. B., McArdle, R., et al. (2012). The Tinnitus Functional Index: development of a new clinical measure for chronic intrusive tinnitus. *Ear Hear.* 33, 153–176. doi: 10.1097/AUD.0b013e31822f67c0

Monzani, D., Genovese, E., Marrara, A., Gherpelli, C., Pingani, L., Forghieri, M., et al. (2008). Validity of the Italian adaptation of the Tinnitus Handicap Inventory; focus on quality of life and psychological distress in tinnitus-sufferers. *Acta Otorhinolaryngol. Ital.* 28, 126–134.

Newman, C. W., Jacobson, G. P., and Spitzer, J. B. (1996). Development of the Tinnitus Handicap Inventory. *Arch Otolayrngol. Head Neck Surg.* 122, 143–148. doi: 10.1001/archotol.1996.01890140029007

Newman, C. W., Sandridge, S. A., and Jacobson, G. P. (1998). Psychometric adequacy of the Tinnitus Handicap Inventory (THI) for evaluating treatment outcome. *J. Am. Acad. Audiol.* 9, 153–160.

Oron, Y., Sergeeva, N., Kazlak, M., Barbalat, I., Spevak, S., Lopatin, A. S., et al. (2015). Russian adaptation of the Tinnitus Handicap Inventory. *Int. J. Audiol.* 54, 485–489. doi: 10.3109/14992027.2014.996823

Overdevest, J. B., Pross, S. E., and Cheung, S. W. (2015). Tinnitus following treatment for sporadic acoustic neuroma. *Laryngoscope* 126, 1639–1643. doi: 10.1002/lary.25672

Pavot, W., and Diener, E. (1993). Review of the satisfaction with life scale. *Psychol. Assess.* 5, 164–172. doi: 10.1037/1040-3590.5.2.164

Rabau, S., Wouters, K., and Van de Heyning, P. (2014). Validation and translation of the dutch tinnitus functional index. *B-ENT.* 10, 251–258.

Radloff, L. S. (1977). The CES-D Scale: a selfreport depression scale for research in the general population. *Appl. Psychol. Meas.* 1, 385–401. doi: 10.1177/014662167700100306

Raj-Koziak, D., Kochanek, K., Piłka, A., Bartnik, G., Fabijańska, A., and Skarżyński, H. (2011). Ocena częstości występowania szumów usznych u dzieci z prawidłowym wynikiem badania przesiewowego słuchu [Tinnitus in children with normal results of hearing screening test]. *Otolaryngologia* 10, 171–175.

Roland, L. T., Lenze, E. J., Hardin, F. M., Kallogjeri, D., Nicklaus, J., Wineland, A. M., et al. (2015). Effects of mindfulness based stress reduction therapy on subjective bother and neural connectivity in chronic tinnitus. *Otolaryngol. Head Neck Surg.* 152, 919–926. doi: 10.1177/0194599815571556

Schecklmann, M., Vielsmeier, V., Steffens, T., Landgrebe, M., Langguth, B., and Kleinjung, T. (2012). Relationship between audiometric slope and tinnitus pitch in tinnitus patients: insights into the mechanisms of tinnitus generation. *PLoS ONE* 7:e34878. doi: 10.1371/journal.pone.0034878

Schmidt, L. P., Teixeria, V. N., Dall'Igna, C., Dallagnol, D., and Smith, M. M. (2006). Brazilian Portuguese language version of the "Tinnitus Handicap Inventory"; validity and reproducibility. *Rev. Bras. Otorrinolaringol.* 72, 808–810.

Shekhawat, G. S., Searchfield, G. D., Kobayashi, K., and Stinear, C. M. (2013). Prescription of hearing-aid output for tinnitus relief. *Int. J. Audiol.* 52, 617–625. doi: 10.3109/14992027.2013.799787

Shinden, S., Ogawa, K., Inoue, Y., Tazoe, M., and Asano, K. (2002). Tinnitus annoyance and difficulty in activities of daily life evaluated by the Tinnitus Handicap Inventory (THI). *Audiol. Japan.* 45, 685–691. doi: 10.4295/audiology.45.685

Skarżyński, H., Rogowski, M., Bartnik, G., and Fabijańska, A. (2000). Organization of Tinnitus Management in Poland. *Acta Otolaryngol.* 120, 225–226. doi: 10.1080/000164800750000973

Tass, A. P., Adamchic, I., Freund, H. J., von Stackelberg, T., and Hauptmann, C. (2012). Counteracting tinnitus by acoustic coordinated reset neuromodulation. *Restor. Neurol. Neurosci.* 30, 137–159. doi: 10.3233/RNN-2012-110218

Udupi, V. A., Uppunda, A. K., Mohan, K. M., Alex, J., and Mahendra, M. H. (2013). The relationship of perceived severity of tinnitus with depression, anxiety, hearing status, age and gender in individuals with tinnitus. *Int. Tinnitus J.* 18, 29–34. doi: 10.5935/0946-5448.20130005

Vernon, J. A., and Meikle, M. B. (2003). Tinnitus: clinical measurement. *Otolaryngol. Clin. North Am.* 36, 293–305. doi: 10.1016/S0030-6665(02)00162-7

Wilson, M. B., Kallogjeri, D., Joplin, C. N., Gorman, M. D., Krings, J. G., Lenze, E. J., et al. (2015). Ecological momentary assessment of tinnitus using smartphone technology. A pilot study. *Otolaryngol. Head Neck Surg.* 152, 897–903. doi: 10.1177/0194599815569692

Wise, K., Kobayashi, K., and Searchfield, G. D. (2015). Feasibility study of a game integrating assessment and therapy of tinnitus. *J. Neurosci. Methods* 15, 1–7. doi: 10.1016/j.jneumeth.2015.04.002

Zachariae, R., Mirz, F., Johansen, L. V., Andersen, S. E., Bjerring, P., and Pedersen, C. B. (2000). Reliability and validity of a Danish adaptation of the Tinnitus Handicap Inventory. *Scand. Audiol.* 29, 37–43. doi: 10.1080/010503900424589

Ziarko, M., Kaczmarek, ŁD., and Haładziński, P. (2013). Polish version of Center for Epidemiological Studies Depression Scale (CES-D): results of a preliminary study on the psychometric properties of the scale. *Curr. Issues Personal. Psychol.* 1, 51–61. doi: 10.5114/cipp.2013.40637

Zobay, O., Palmer, A. R., Hall, D. A., Sereda, M., and Adjamian, P. (2015). Source space estimation of oscillatory power and brain connectivity in tinnitus. *PLoS ONE* 10:e0120123. doi: 10.1371/journal.pone.0120123

15

Tinnitus Patients with Comorbid Headaches: The Influence of Headache Type and Laterality on Tinnitus Characteristics

Berthold Langguth[1]*, Verena Hund[1], Michael Landgrebe[1,2] and Martin Schecklmann[1]

[1] Department of Psychiatry and Psychotherapy, University of Regensburg, Regensburg, Germany,

[2] Department of Psychiatry, Psychosomatics and Psychotherapy, kbo-Lech-Mangfall-Klinik Agatharied, Hausham, Germany

Correspondence:
Berthold Langguth
berthold.langguth@medbo.de

Background: Both clinical experience and clinical studies suggest a relationship between tinnitus and headache. Here, we aimed to investigate the influence of comorbid headache type and headache laterality on tinnitus characteristics.

Method: The Tinnitus Research Initiative database was screened for patients of the Tinnitus Center of the University Regensburg who reported comorbid headaches. These patients were contacted to complete additional validated questionnaires. Based on these data, patients were categorized according to headache type and headache laterality, and their clinical characteristics were compared with tinnitus patients, who did not report comorbid headaches.

Results: Data from 193 patients with tinnitus and comorbid headaches were compared with those from 765 tinnitus patients without comorbid headaches. Tinnitus patients with comorbid headache have higher scores in tinnitus questionnaires, a lower quality of life and more frequently comorbidities such as painful sensation to loud sounds, vertigo, pain (neck, temporomandibular, and general), and depressive symptoms when compared with tinnitus patients without headaches. Both headache laterality and headache type interact with the degree of comorbidity with higher impairment in patients with left-sided and bilateral headaches as well as in patients with migraine or cluster headache.

Conclusion: The observed increased impairment in tinnitus patients with comorbid headache can be explained as an additive effect of both disorders on health-related quality of life. The more frequent occurrence of further comorbidities suggests a generally increased amplification of sensory signals in a subset of tinnitus patients with comorbid headaches.

Keywords: migraine, cluster headache, trigeminus, phantom sound, laterality, comorbidity

INTRODUCTION

Tinnitus, the perception of sound in the absence of a corresponding sound source, is a frequent disorder. In some forms of tinnitus, there is an internal sound source like sounds from abnormal blood flow because of vascular anomalies or palatal myoclonus. These forms are defined as objective tinnitus. In contrast, in subjective tinnitus, there exist neither external nor internal sound sources.

Subjective tinnitus can vary in its perceptual characteristics (loudness, pitch, number of tones, tonal or noise-like, pulsatile vs. non-pulsatile), its laterality (unilateral, bilateral, in the head), its maskability, its etiology, and its comorbidities. Accordingly, it has been assumed that there exist many different forms of tinnitus that also may differ in their pathophysiology. The identification of relevant criteria for subtyping different forms represents a major challenge in tinnitus research (1, 2). Specific comorbidities such as hyperacusis (3) or temporomandibular joint (TMJ) disorders (4) have turned out to represent potentially relevant criteria for subtyping. As an example patients with tinnitus and comorbid TMJ disorders were younger, more frequently female and suffered from less hearing loss (4), indicating that this group represents a clinically relevant tinnitus subtype.

Moreover, comorbidities such as hyperacousis (3), hearing loss (5), insomnia (6, 7), depression (8, 9), and pain syndromes (10) play a major role for tinnitus-related impairment in quality of life. Tinnitus-related health burden can be measured by specific validated tinnitus questionnaires (TQs) like the TQ (11) or the tinnitus handicap inventory (12), but also by numeric rating scales (13).

In the previous studies, an association between tinnitus and headaches has been demonstrated (14–16). These studies indicate that between 26 and 47% of patients with tinnitus also suffer from headache. Particularly frequent among tinnitus patients are unilateral headache syndromes (16). Since unilateral headaches and unilateral tinnitus symptoms occur in the majority of cases on the same side and headache and tinnitus are interacting over time, alterations in the trigeminal nerve activity have been proposed as a potentially relevant overlapping pathophysiological factor (16). Based on this reasoning, one may assume that headache as a comorbidity may represent a relevant factor for subtyping of tinnitus.

In order to investigate comorbid headache as potential criterion for tinnitus subtyping, we retrospectively analyzed clinical data from patients who presented at the multidisciplinary Tinnitus Center at the University of Regensburg. Patients who reported the existence of headaches in the Tinnitus Sample Case History Questionnaire (TSCHQ) (17) and who completed an additional headache questionnaire (18) were compared in their clinical and demographic characteristics with those patients who had tinnitus without headaches. In detail, we investigated whether tinnitus patients with specific forms or laterality of headache differ in demographic or other clinical characteristics from those tinnitus patients without headaches.

MATERIALS AND METHODS

Sample

The analysis was based on datasets of all patients, who presented at the multidisciplinary Tinnitus Center of the University of Regensburg between 2003 and 2011 and whose data were included in the Tinnitus Research Initiative database (19) ($n = 1,817$). All patients who reported the existence of headaches in the TSCHQ [answer "yes" to the question "Do you suffer from headaches?" (17)] ($n = 489$) were contacted by mail and asked to complete additional questionnaires (16). In these additional questions, patients were asked about the laterality of tinnitus and headache (Is your headache on one or predominantly one-sided? Is your tinnitus on one or predominantly one-sided?) and about the relationship between tinnitus and headache (time of onset of tinnitus and headache, respectively, and interaction between tinnitus and headache intensity). Completed headache and TQs were obtained from 193 patients, and this sample was compared with patients from the database who answered "no" to the question "Do you suffer from headaches?" in the TSCHQ ($n = 765$). Please note that three patients did not indicate the site of the headaches and were not included for the statistical analyses of headache laterality. Informed consent was obtained from all patients participating in the study. The study was approved by the Ethic committee of the University of Regensburg (11-101-0286), and all data were pseudonymized for analysis.

To exclude sample bias, we compared the patients with completed questionnaires with the group of patients with headache who did not respond to the mail ($n = 235$). Both groups did not differ significantly with respect to age at tinnitus onset ($t = 0.805$; df = 395; $p = 0.421$), gender ($\chi^2 = 0.566$; df = 1; $p = 0.452$), tinnitus duration ($t = 0.693$; df = 395; $p = 0.489$), tinnitus distress as indicated by TQ ($t = 0.114$; df = 405; $p = 0.909$) and tinnitus handicap inventory ($t = 0.072$; df = 413; $p = 0.943$), and mean hearing threshold ($t = 0.513$; df = 304; $p = 0.608$).

Assessment of Headaches and Tinnitus Severity

For the classification of headaches, the headache questionnaire by Fritsche et al. (18) was used, which was developed and validated according to the 2nd version of the classification criteria of the International Headache Society. The questionnaire enables to differentiate migraine, tension headache, cluster headache, combination of migraine and tension headache, and combination of tension- and cluster headache and non-classifiable headache.

Clinical and demographic information was obtained from available data of the investigated patients in the TRI database (19). Available data included the TSCHQ (17), the TQ (11), the Tinnitus Handicap Inventory (20, 21), various numeric tinnitus rating scales (13), the Beck depression inventory (BDI) (22), and the WHO Quality of Life Questionnaire (23).

Statistical Analysis

The relationship between the different demographic and clinical characteristics of tinnitus and the existence of comorbid headache, its laterality and its type was analyzed by using chi-square tests for categorical clinical variables and with analyses of variance (ANOVAs) for metric clinical variables. *Post hoc* tests were done for significant effects using least significant difference tests for ANOVAs and adjusted residuals ($z > 1.96$ was indicated as significant) for the chi-square tests and are indicated in **Tables 1** and **2**.

All analyses were performed with SPSS (Statistical Package for Social Studies, Version 19; SPSS Inc., USA). All tests were performed as two-sided tests, and the level of significance was set at 0.001 to correct for the fact that 56 comparisons were performed.

TABLE 1 | Influence of headache laterality on sample characteristics.

	Headache left	Headache right	Headache bilateral	No headache	Statistics
N	49	43	98	765	n.a.
Age at tinnitus onset (years)	44.8 ± 15.3 (*n* = 47)	42.4 ± 11.9 (*n* = 41)	41.6 ± 13.3 (*n* = 89)	44.0 ± 14.3 (*n* = 715)	$F = 0.937$; df = 3,888; $p = 0.422$
Duration of tinnitus (months)	89.9 ± 85.3 (*n* = 47)	100.7 ± 119.2 (*n* = 41)	97.5 ± 118.6 (*n* = 89)	100.7 ± 106.4 (*n* = 714)	$F = 0.165$; df = 3,887; $p = 0.920$
Gender (female/male)	**22/27**[a]	**22/21**[a]	**31/67**	**208/557**[a]	**$\chi^2 = 17.413$; df = 3; $p < 0.001$**
Tinnitus questionnaire	**47.4 ± 19.7 (*n* = 46); >no**	**40.6 ± 18.3 (*n* = 40)**	**46.9 ± 16.8 (*n* = 96) >no**	**38.8 ± 17.2 (*n* = 736)**	**$F = 10.964$; df = 3,914; $p < 0.001$**
Tinnitus handicap inventory	**54.3 ± 23.8 (*n* = 46); >no**	**48.8 ± 24.2 (*n* = 42)**	**56.2 ± 21.9 (*n* = 97); >no**	**44.0 ± 22.3 (*n* = 737)**	**$F = 10.983$; df = 3,918; $p < 0.001$**
Beck depression inventory	**14.2 ± 9.8 (*n* = 44); >no**	**12.0 ± 9.1 (*n* = 42); >no**	**14.5 ± 8.8 (*n* = 96); >no**	**9.1 ± 7.4 (*n* = 731)**	**$F = 19.545$; df = 3,909; $p < 0.001$**
Numeric rating scale loudness	6.7 ± 2.5 (*n* = 44)	6.5 ± 1.8 (*n* = 40)	6.8 ± 2.1 (*n* = 98)	6.2 ± 2.2 (*n* = 726)	$F = 3.262$; df = 3,904; $p = 0.021$
Numeric rating scale discomfort	**7.6 ± 2.0 (*n* = 43); >no**	**7.0 ± 2.2 (*n* = 41)**	**7.6 ± 2.1 (*n* = 97); >no**	**6.6 ± 2.3 (*n* = 725)**	**$F = 7.241$; df = 3,902; $p < 0.001$**
Numeric rating scale annoyance	7.1 ± 2.4 (*n* = 43)	6.7 ± 2.7 (*n* = 40)	7.1 ± 2.2 (*n* = 98)	6.4 ± 2.4 (*n* = 728)	$F = 3.402$; df = 3,905; $p = 0.017$
Numeric rating scale unpleasentness	6.9 ± 2.3 (*n* = 44)	6.7 ± 2.6 (*n* = 40)	7.1 ± 2.2 (*n* = 98)	6.4 ± 2.4 (*n* = 728)	$F = 2.858$; df = 3,906; $p = 0.036$
Numeric rating scale ignorability	7.0 ± 2.6 (*n* = 44)	7.0 ± 2.8 (*n* = 41)	7.0 ± 2.4 (*n* = 98)	6.6 ± 2.7 (*n* = 728)	$F = 0.872$; df = 3,907; $p = 0.455$
WHO quality of live—physical health	**13.6 ± 2.9 (*n* = 33); <no**	**14.3 ± 3.0 (*n* = 27); <no**	**13.4 ± 3.0 (*n* = 66); <no**	**15.5 ± 2.6 (*n* = 515)**	**$F = 16.543$; df = 3,537; $p < 0.001$**
WHO quality of live—psychological factors	**13.0 ± 3.6 (*n* = 33); <no**	**14.0 ± 2.8 (*n* = 28)**	**13.3 ± 2.7 (*n* = 66); <no**	**14.7 ± 2.6 (*n* = 417)**	**$F = 8.243$; df = 3,540; $p < 0.001$**
WHO quality of live—social relationships	14.2 ± 3.7 (*n* = 33)	13.6 ± 3.7 (*n* = 27)	14.0 ± 2.6 (*n* = 66)	15.0 ± 3.1 (*n* = 417)	$F = 3.614$; df = 3,539; $p = 0.013$
WHO quality of live—environment	15.7 ± 2.4 (*n* = 33)	15.9 ± 2.0 (*n* = 28)	15.7 ± 2.0 (*n* = 65)	16.5 ± 2.1 (*n* = 418)	$F = 3.916$; df = 3,540; $p = 0.009$
Sensitivity to loud sounds	3.4 ± 1.2 (*n* = 47)	3.3 ± 1.2 (*n* = 40)	3.3 ± 1.2 (*n* = 96)	3.2 ± 1.2 (*n* = 744)	$F = 1.329$; df = 3.923; $p = 0.264$
Painful sensations by loud sounds (yes/no)	**28/14**	**26/13**	**68/23**[a]	**354/314**	**$\chi^2 = 19.053$; df = 3; $p < 0.001$**
Pulsatile tinnitus (no/yes with.../yes different from heartbeat)	33/7/7	28/7/5	80/10/6	605/72/64	$\chi^2 = 7.863$; df = 6; $p = 0.248$
Tinnitusquality (tonal/noise/cricket/other)	25/6/11/4	27/3/7/5	61/14/17/5	449/76/144/72	$\chi^2 = 5.686$; df = 9; $p = 0.771$
Influence by noise (yes/no)	31/12	32/5	63/21	493/158	$\chi^2 = 2.658$; df = 3; $p = 0.447$
Somatic modulation (yes/no)	24/24	17/25	42/55	258/486	$\chi^2 = 7.045$; df = 3; $p = 0.070$
Mean hearing threshold	26 ± 13 (*n* = 44)	19 ± 11 (*n* = 42)	18 ± 12 (*n* = 96)	23 ± 15 (*n* = 731)	$F = 3.890$; df = 3,682; $p = 0.009$
Side of worse hearing (left/left = right/right)	20/2/10	13/2/7	35/5/33	284/35/228	$\chi^2 = 2.914$; df = 6; $p = 0.820$
Vertigo (yes/no)	**28/19**[a]	**23/20**[a]	**52/43**[a]	**158/585**[a]	**$\chi^2 = 87.258$; df = 3; $p < 0.001$**
Temporomandibular joint complaints (yes/no)	**17/31**[a]	**11/31**	**29/68**[a]	**124/620**[a]	**$\chi^2 = 19.471$; df = 3; $p < 0.001$**
Neck pain (yes/no)	**42/7**[a]	**32/10**[a]	**69/29**[a]	**341/402**[a]	**$\chi^2 = 56.552$; df = 3; $p < 0.001$**
General pain (yes/no)	**25/22**[a]	**25/18**[a]	**58/39**[a]	**249/480**[a]	**$\chi^2 = 35.427$; df = 3; $p < 0.001$**
Current psychiatric treatment (yes/no)	**12/36**[a]	**8/32**	**26/70**[a]	**89/659**[a]	**$\chi^2 = 21.608$; df = 3; $p < 0.001$**

Bold printed lines indicate significant effects.

[a]The number of cases in this cell is significant different from the number of expected cases under the assumption of independence of variables.

< or > indicate significant post hoc contrasts.

Please note that high values in quality of life mean high quality of life and that high values in the other measures mean high burden.

TABLE 2 | Influence of headache type on sample characteristics.

	Non-classifiable headache	Migraine	Tension-type headache	Tension-type headache and migraine	Cluster headache	No headache	Statistics
N	63	86	25	11	8	765	n.a.
Age at tinnitus onset (years)	44.0 ± 14.2 (*n* = 59)	41.4 ± 12.8 (*n* = 81)	41.3 ± 12.5 (*n* = 24)	40.0 ± 17.7 (*n* = 8)	52.1 ± 12.1 (*n* = 7)	44.0 ± 14.2 (*n* = 715)	*F* = 1.260; df = 5,888; *p* = 0.279
Duration of tinnitus (months)	84.7 ± 107.3 (*n* = 59)	104.1 ± 114.1 (*n* = 81)	111.9 ± 119.5 (*n* = 24)	61.0 ± 82.3 (*n* = 8)	94.0 ± 95.9 (*n* = 7)	100.7 ± 106.4 (*n* = 714)	*F* = 0.544; d = 5,887; *p* = 0.743
Gender (female/male)	19/44	33/53	13/12[a]	6/5	5/3[a]	208/557[a] (*n* = 715)	χ^2=18.761; df = 5; *p* = 0.002
Tinnitus questionnaire	**44.7 ± 18.2 (*n* = 60); >no**	**45.8 ± 18.4 (*n* = 81); >no**	**45.8 ± 17.7 (*n* = 24); >no**	**38.5 ± 14.7 (*n* = 11); <cluster**	**56.6 ± 15.4 (*n* = 8); >migraine + tension; >no**	**38.0 ± 17.2 (*n* = 736)**	***F* = 6.561; df = 5,914; *p* < 0.001**
Tinnitus handicap inventory	**52.0 ± 23.4 (*n* = 61); >no**	**54.9 ± 23.2 (*n* = 84); >no**	**55.5 ± 23.2 (*n* = 25); >no**	**43.9 ± 21.3 (*n* = 10)**	**61.9 ± 21.7 (*n* = 8); >no**	**44.0 ± 22.3 (*n* = 737)**	***F* = 6.379; df = 5,919; *p* < 0.001**
Beck depression inventory	**12.5 ± 8.4 (*n* = 59); >no**	**14.8 ± 9.2 (*n* = 83); >no**	**12.9 ± 10.3 (*n* = 25); >no**	**11.8 ± 8.5 (*n* = 10)**	**17.0 ± 10.4 (*n* = 8); >no**	**9.1 ± 7.4 (*n* = 731)**	***F* = 11.813; df = 5,910; *p* < 0.001**
Numeric rating scale loudness	6.5 ± 2.3 (*n* = 59)	6.8 ± 2.1 (*n* = 84)	7.0 ± 2.1 (*n* = 25)	7.0 ± 2.1 (*n* = 10)	6.6 ± 2.2 (*n* = 7)	6.2 ± 2.1 (*n* = 726)	*F* = 1.973; df = 5,905; *p* = 0.080
Numeric rating scale discomfort	**7.1 ± 2.2 (*n* = 60)**	**7.6 ± 2.1 (*n* = 83); >no**	**8.0 ± 1.8 (*n* = 24); >no**	**7.3 ± 2.3 (*n* = 10)**	**7.0 ± 1.6 (*n* = 7)**	**6.6 ± 2.3 (*n* = 725)**	***F* = 4.593; df = 5,903; *p* < 0.001**
Numeric rating scale annoyance	6.9 ± 2.4 (*n* = 59)	7.0 ± 2.3 (*n* = 83)	7.7 ± 2.2 (*n* = 25)	6.7 ± 2.5 (*n* = 10)	6.2 ± 2.2 (*n* = 7)	6.4 ± 2.4 (*n* = 728)	*F* = 2.406; df = 5,906; *p* = 0.035
Numeric rating scale unpleasentness	6.9 ± 2.2 (*n* = 59)	7.0 ± 2.4 (*n* = 84)	7.3 ± 2.5 (*n* = 25)	6.6 ± 2.4 (*n* = 10)	6.3 ± 2.2 (*n* = 7)	6.4 ± 2.4 (*n* = 728)	*F* = 1.728; df = 5,907; *p* = 0.126
Numeric rating scale ignorability	6.8 ± 2.3 (*n* = 60)	7.3 ± 2.7 (*n* = 84)	6.9 ± 2.7 (*n* = 25)	6.4 ± 2.6 (*n* = 10)	6.1 ± 2.2 (*n* = 7)	6.6 ± 2.7 (*n* = 728)	*F* = 0.961; df = 5,908; *p* = 0.441
WHO quality of live—physical health	**13.4 ± 3.3 (= 44); <no**	**13.5 ± 3.0 (*n* = 56); <no**	**14.8 ± 2.1 (*n* = 19)**	**15.7 ± 1.8 (*n* = 4)**	**12.8 ± 1.8 (*n* = 6); <no**	**15.5 ± 2.6 (*n* = 415)**	***F* = 10.764; df = 5,538; *p* < 0.001**
WHO quality of live—psychological factors	**13.5 ± 3.4 (*n* = 45); <no**	**13.2 ± 2.8 (*n* = 56); <no**	**13.8 ± 2.6 (*n* = 19)**	**15.8 ± 0.7 (*n* = 4); >no**	**12.3 ± 2.4 (*n* = 6); <tension + migraine; < no**	**14.7 ± 2.6 (*n* = 417)**	***F* = 5.556; df = 5,541; *p* < 0.001**
WHO quality of live—social relationships	14.3 ± 3.7 (*n* = 44)	13.8 ± 2.8 (*n* = 56)	14.4 ± 3.1 (*n* = 19)	14.7 ± 2.9 (*n* = 4)	11.6 ± 3.5 (*n* = 6)	15.0 ± 3.1 (*n* = 417)	*F* = 2.940; df = 5,540; *p* = 0.012
WHO quality of live—environment	15.9 ± 2.4 (*n* = 45)	15.5 ± 1.9 (*n* = 55)	16.6 ± 1.6 (*n* = 19)	15.1 ± 1.1 (*n* = 4)	14.4 ± 2.3 (*n* = 6)	16.5 ± 2.1 (*n* = 418)	*F* = 3.635; df = 5,541; *p* = 0.003
Sensitivity to loud sounds	3.1 ± 1.3 (*n* = 61)	3.5 ± 1.2 (*n* = 83)	3.2 ± 1.1 (*n* = 24)	3.1 ± 1.6 (*n* = 10)	4.0 ± 0.9 (*n* = 8)	3.2 ± 1.2 (*n* = 744)	*F* = 1.929; df = 5,924; *p* = 0.087
Painful sensations by loud sounds (yes/no)	**38/21**	**57/20[a]**	**15/6**	**9/1[a]**	**5/3**	**354/314[a]**	**χ^2=21.061; df = 5; *p* < 0.001**
Pulsatile tinnitus (no/yes with…/yes different from heartbeat)	50/4/7	60/15/7	20/3/2	9/1/0	4/2/2	605/72/64	χ^2=13.263; df = 10; *p* = 0.209
Tinnitusquality (tonal/noise/cricket/other)	40/11/8/4	52/9/16/6	14/4/5/1	6/0/3/1	2/0/3/3	449/76/144/72	χ^2=19.358; df = 15; *p* = 0.198
Influence by noise (yes/no)	43/14	58/16	17/7	7/1	3/1	493/158	χ^2=1.193; df = 5; *p* = 0.946
Somatic modulation (yes/no)	26/37	42/42	8/17	3/7	6/2	258/486	χ^2=13.751; df = 5; *p* = 0.017
Mean hearing threshold	18.5 ± 12.3 (*n* = 47)	21.3 ± 13.4 (*n* = 55)	18.9 ± 10.5 (*n* = 16)	16.4 ± 6.7 (*n* = 8)	30.5 ± 9.1 (*n* = 7)	22.8 ± 14.5 (*n* = 555)	*F* = 1.807; df = 5,682; *p* = 0.109
Side of worse hearing (left/left = right/right)	25/2/107	28/6/20	8/0/8	3/1/4	5/0/1	284/35/228	χ^2 = 7.197; df = 10; *p* = 0.639
Vertigo (yes/no)	**29/31[a]**	**52/33[a]**	**12/12[a]**	**5/6**	**6/2[a]**	**158/585[a]**	**χ^2=91.328; df = 5; *p* < 0.001**

(Continued)

TABLE 2 | Continued

	Non-classifiable headache	Migraine	Tension-type headache	Tension-type headache and migraine	Cluster headache	No headache	Statistics
Temporomandibular joint complaints (yes/no)	**21/41[a]**	**25/59[a]**	**5/20**	**3/8**	**4/4[a]**	**124/620[a]**	**χ^2=22.777; df = 5; p < 0.001**
Neck pain (yes/no)	**48/14[a]**	**62/24[a]**	**19/6[a]**	**9/2[a]**	**8/0[a]**	**341/402[a]**	**χ^2=58.133; df = 5; p < 0.001**
General pain (yes/no)	**31/30[a]**	**52/34[a]**	**15/10[a]**	**7/3[a]**	**4/4**	**249/480[a]**	**χ^2=36.522; df = 5; p < 0.001**
Current psychiatric treatment (yes/no)	**11/50**	**28/55[a]**	**4/21**	**1/9**	**2/6**	**89/659[a]**	**χ^2=30.493; df = 5; p < 0.001**

Bold printed lines indicate significant effects.

[a]The number of cases in this cell is significant different from the number of expected cases under the assumption of independence of variables.

< or > indicate significant post hoc contrasts.

Please note that high values in quality of life mean high quality of life and that high values in the other measures mean high burden.

RESULTS

For evaluation of clinical and demographic characteristics of patients with tinnitus and headaches, patients with left-sided, right-sided, and bilateral headaches were compared with patients with tinnitus, but without headaches from the TRI database (see **Table 1**).

About 27% of the tinnitus patients in our database answered "yes" to the question "do you suffer from headaches." Even if comparisons with population-based studies are difficult, as results depend strongly on the method of assessment, a proportion of 27% is not indicative of a substantially altered prevalence of headaches among tinnitus patients.

There was no significant interaction between headache laterality and age at tinnitus onset or tinnitus duration, but a significant interaction between headache laterality and gender, with women suffering more frequently from unilateral headache.

Analyses of tinnitus distress, depressive symptoms, numeric ratings scales, and quality of life showed similar results for all of these measures with increased burden for the group of patients with bilateral and left-sided headaches in contrast to patients with no headaches. The group of patients with right-sided headache showed no difference to the group of patients without headaches or ranged in between the left-sided/bilateral groups and the group with no headaches. This pattern could be seen descriptively in all variables but falling below the significance threshold for TQ, tinnitus handicap inventory, BDI, the numeric rating scale discomfort, and the quality of life domains physical and psychological health. As an exploratory analysis, the TQ score (TQ of the database entry: $r = 0.321$; $n = 175$; $p < 0.001$; TQ by response to mail: $r = 0.356$; $n = 184$; $p < 0.001$) also correlated with the headache frequency (number of days with headache/month).

Painful sensations through loud sounds were more frequently reported by patients with bilateral headache in contrast to patients with unilateral or no headaches. There were no significant effects concerning sensitivity to loud sounds, pulsatile character, tonal versus noise-like character, the ability to mask tinnitus through other sounds, duration of tinnitus, and the ability to modulate tinnitus through neck or jaw movements. There was no significant relationship between headache laterality and hearing function (measured as mean hearing threshold across all frequencies and both sides) nor with the side of worse hearing.

Patients with all headache forms (bilateral, right-sided, and left-sided) reported more frequently comorbid vertigo, TMJ complaints (except right-sided headaches), neck pain as well as pain in general. Patients with headaches were also more frequently treated by psychiatrists (except right-sided headaches). In separate analyses, differences in tinnitus characteristics between patients with specific types of comorbid headaches and no headaches were analyzed. Detailed results are provided in **Table 2**.

The headache type had no significant influence on age at tinnitus onset nor on tinnitus duration. However, there was a non-significant trend toward an interaction between gender and headache type with women suffering more frequently from comorbid tension-type and cluster headache.

Tinnitus patients with comorbid migraine, tension-type headache, cluster headache, and non-classifiable headache had all higher scores in the TQ, the THI, and the BDI when compared with tinnitus patients without comorbid headaches. Descriptively, highest scores were found for patients with comorbid cluster headache. Patients with combined tension-type headache and migraine did not differ from the other groups except for the TQ showing lower values in contrast to cluster headache.

In the different numeric rating scales, there were statistically significant differences for tinnitus discomfort (higher scores for patients with migraine and tension-type headaches in contrast to patients without headaches), whereas there were no differences for tinnitus severity, unpleasantness, and ability to ignore the tinnitus. The headache type had a significant influence on two domains of the WHOQoL (somatic, psychological) with impairment in quality of life in patients with comorbid unclassifiable headache, migraine, and cluster headaches in contrast to patients without headaches.

Headache type had no influence on the sensitivity to loud sounds, but on the induction of painful sensations by sounds, which was significantly more frequent in patients with migraine and in patients with combined migraine and tension-type headache.

There was no significant influence of headache type on the proportion of patients with hearing function, pulsatile tinnitus, tone or noise-like tinnitus, maskability of tinnitus by environmental sounds, or the ability to modulate tinnitus by somatic maneuvers.

Comorbid headaches had a significant influence on comorbid vertigo, neck pain, TMJ complaints, and pain in general. A higher prevalence of neck pain was found in all headache types and a higher prevalence of vertigo in all headache types apart from combined migraine and tension-type headache. TMJ complaints were more frequent in non-classifiable headache, migraine, and cluster headache, and general pain complaints were more frequent in all patients apart from cluster headache. Patients with comorbid migraine were also more frequently psychiatrically treated.

DISCUSSION

The main findings of this study are that tinnitus patients with comorbid headache have higher scores in TQs, a lower quality of life and more frequently comorbidities such as painful sensation to loud sounds, vertigo, neck pain, TMJ complaints, general pain, and depressive symptoms when compared with tinnitus patients without headaches. The higher impairment in quality of life in patients who suffer from both tinnitus and headache can be easily explained by a pure additive effect of both disorders on disease burden.

Both headache laterality and headache type interact with the degree of morbidity.

In detail, higher impairment is reported by patients with left-sided and bilateral headaches as well as by patients with migraine or cluster headache. We are aware that there is a certain interaction between headache type and headache laterality, which has to be considered in the interpretation of the results (see **Table 3**).

Our findings are in line with earlier studies, which demonstrated that tinnitus severity is higher in patients with comorbid headache (24) and correlates with headache frequency (25). A potential interaction between tinnitus and migraine (26–30) or other trigeminoautonomal headache syndromes (31, 32) has been described in many studies.

An important question is, whether the co-occurrence of tinnitus and headaches is pure co-incidence or whether there is a pathophysiological interaction. Several potential mechanisms for such a pathophysiological interaction have been proposed. First, increased excitability of the trigeminal system could link tinnitus and headache syndromes (16). Second, central sensitization in the context of migraine could provide an explanation for the development of tinnitus (28). Third, tinnitus could represent a symptom of vestibular migraine (33–35) or vestibular migraine could be related to a specific subtype of Meniere's disease (36). Fourth, migraine might cause pulsatile tinnitus by vascular alterations during Migraine attacks (30). Fifth, TMJ or neck pain could represent a common cause of comorbid headache and tinnitus. However, due to the cross-sectional design of our study, we can only describe symptom associations and cannot draw any firm conclusions about potential causal interactions between headaches and tinnitus.

In this study, patients with comorbid cluster headache demonstrated highest scores in TQs and most pronounced impairment in quality of life. Induction of painful sensations by loud sounds, general pain syndromes, and psychiatric treatment was most frequent in migraine patients. These findings do not necessarily indicate a specific pathophysiological interaction between headache syndromes and tinnitus, as an increased sensitivity to loud sounds is similar like vertigo a typical feature of migraine. The increased prevalence of psychiatric treatment can be easily explained by the well-known association of headache disorders with anxiety and depression (37). Patients who suffer from tinnitus and headache are more impaired in their quality of life and the higher scores in the TQs may purely reflect a higher health-related handicap, as many questions in the TQ and THI are not tinnitus specific. This fits with the finding that scores were most pronounced in patients with cluster headaches, which are known to be extremely debilitating. The higher comorbidities for pain syndromes, vertigo, sound-induced painful sensations,

TABLE 3 | Interaction between headache type and laterality.

	Non-classifiable headache	Migraine	Tension-type headache	Tension-type headache and migraine	Cluster headache
Headache left	14	24	2[a]	3	6[a]
Headache right	11	19	8	3	2
Headache bilateral	36	42	15	5	0[a]

Chi-square of independence indicates a significant association of headache type and laterality with decreased number of left-sided tension-type and bilateral cluster headache and increased frequency of left-sided cluster headache (χ^2=17.926; df = 8; p = 0.022).

[a]The number of cases in this cell is significant different from the number of expected cases under the assumption of independence of variables.

< or > indicate significant post hoc contrasts.

depressive syndromes, and the higher proportion of psychiatric treatment in this patient group could be explained by a generally increased amplification of sensory signals, which is, for example, encountered in patients with somatoform disorder.

Hints for specific interactions (e.g., a particular high proportion of vertigo in patients with migraine, which could point to vestibular migraine) could not be observed. However, our study cannot exclude that such specific interactions occur, as they can be missed by the statistical analysis, if they occur only in a small group of patients. However, our data also show hints against single additive effects. General pain is not increased in patients with cluster headaches and combination of migraine and tension-type headache did not result in higher burden as indicated by measures of tinnitus distress and discomfort, depressive syndrome, and quality of life.

In addition to headache type also headache laterality had an impact on patients' characteristics. Comorbid left-sided and bilateral headache had a particular impact on tinnitus severity, on quality of life, and on comorbid disorders such as vertigo, pain, depressive symptoms, and on the frequency of psychiatric treatment. Likewise for headache type, this pattern mainly reflects that patients with comorbid bilateral or left-sided headache are more severely impaired and more frequently suffer also from other somatic, somatoform, and psychiatric symptoms. An earlier analysis of the same sample revealed that left-sided headaches are also frequently associated with left-sided tinnitus and bilateral headaches more frequently with bilateral tinnitus (16). The finding of higher impairment of patients with left-sided symptoms is in line with the literature that shows a slight left-sided preponderance (55–60%) in somatoform disorders (38) and in somatoform pain (39). With respect to headaches, a relatively small study suggests that left-sided migraine is more frequently associated with psychiatric symptoms than right-sided migraine (40). Thus, among tinnitus patients with left-sided headaches, there might be a higher proportion of patients with a somatoform disorder, which can explain the higher impairment in this group. The same explanation may hold true for patients with bilateral headaches, as this group includes also all patients with a rather unspecific description of their headaches, and among patients with rather unspecific description of their headache syndrome a higher proportion of comorbid somatoform disorders is expected as well.

An alternative, but rather speculative explanation for our findings of higher impairment in patients with left-sided symptoms, is provided by a pilot study that investigated the relevance of laterality in able-bodied individuals desiring amputation of a limb (41). In most cases, these individuals desired amputation of a left-sided limb, the disorder was associated with elementary and complex somatosensory disturbances of the affected limb and the most frequent neurological comorbidity was migraine headache. Left-sidedness, limb specificity, and somatosensory disturbances of the affected limb were interpreted as hints for disturbed integration of multi-sensory information of the affected body parts into a coherent cerebral representation of the own body and suggestive of abnormal brain mechanisms in right frontoparietal cortex.

Tinnitus occurs also more frequently on the left side, is tonotopically specific, related to sensory disturbances (42, 43) and an incongruence between visual and auditory input (44), and might therefore be conceptualized as a symptom that compensates an otherwise incoherent cerebral representation of the acoustic environment in relation to the own body.

We are aware of methodological limitations of this study as all data come from one university center and may therefore not be representative. Moreover, data were solely collected by questionnaires and not verified by clinical examination. Thus, further research involving clinical evaluations will be needed to further explore the relationship between different forms of headaches and tinnitus. Nevertheless, our study revealed a greater impairment for tinnitus patients suffering from comorbid headaches and a hint for the occurrence of further comorbidities such as vertigo, pain syndromes, depression, and psychiatric disorders.

ETHICS STATEMENT

This study was carried out in accordance with the recommendations of the ethics committee of the University Hospital Regensburg with written informed consent from all subjects. All subjects gave written informed consent in accordance with the Declaration of Helsinki. The protocol was approved by the ethics committee of the University Hospital Regensburg.

AUTHOR CONTRIBUTIONS

VH gathered the data and entered the data in a database. MS performed the statistical analysis. BL and MS drafted the manuscript. All the authors designed the study, interpreted the data, and approved the final version of the manuscript.

ACKNOWLEDGMENTS

We thank Susanne Staudinger and Sandra Pfluegl for their assistance with data management.

FUNDING

The study has been performed by using the Tinnitus Research Initiative Database, which has been funded by the Tinnitus Research Initiative Foundation and the University of Regensburg.

REFERENCES

Elgoyhen AB, Langguth B, De Ridder D, Vanneste S. Tinnitus: perspectives from human neuroimaging. *Nat Rev Neurosci* (2015) 16(10):632–42. doi:10.1038/ nrn4003

Langguth B, Kreuzer PM, Kleinjung T, De Ridder D. Tinnitus: causes and clinical management. *Lancet Neurol* (2013) 12(9):920–30. doi:10.1016/ S1474- 4422(13)70160-1

Schecklmann M, Landgrebe M, Langguth B. Phenotypic characteristics of hyperacusis in tinnitus. *PLoS One* (2014) 9(1):e86944. doi:10.1371/journal. pone.0086944

Vielsmeier V, Strutz J, Kleinjung T, Schecklmann M, Kreuzer PM, Landgrebe M, et al. Temporomandibular joint disorder complaints in tinnitus: further hints for a putative tinnitus subtype. *PLoS One* (2012) 7(6):e38887. doi:10.1371/ journal.pone.0038887

Mazurek B, Olze H, Haupt H, Szczepek AJ. The more the worse: the grade of noise-induced hearing loss associates with the severity of tin- nitus. *Int J Environ Res Public Health* (2010) 7(8):3071–9. doi:10.3390/ ijerph7083071

Cronlein T, Langguth B, Geisler P, Hajak G. Tinnitus and insomnia. *Prog Brain Res* (2007) 166:227–33. doi:10.1016/S0079-6123(07)66021-X

Cronlein T, Langguth B, Pregler M, Kreuzer PM, Wetter TC, Schecklmann M. Insomnia in patients with chronic tinnitus: cognitive and emotional distress as moderator variables. *J Psychosom Res* (2016) 83:65–8. doi:10.1016/j.jpsychores.2016.03.001

Langguth B, Landgrebe M, Kleinjung T, Sand GP, Hajak G. Tinnitus and depression. *World J Biol Psychiatry* (2011) 12(7):489–500. doi:10.3109/15622975.2011.575178

Milerova J, Anders M, Dvorak T, Sand PG, Koniger S, Langguth B. The influence of psychological factors on tinnitus severity. *Gen Hosp Psychiatry* (2013) 35(4):412–6. doi:10.1016/j.genhosppsych.2013.02.008

Kreuzer PM, Landgrebe M, Vielsmeier V, Kleinjung T, De Ridder D, Langguth B. Trauma-associated tinnitus. *J Head Trauma Rehabil* (2014) 29(5):432–42. doi:10.1097/HTR.0b013e31829d3129

Hallam RS, Jakes SC, Hinchcliffe R. Cognitive variables in tinnitus annoy- ance. *Br J Clin Psychol* (1988) 27(Pt 3):213–22. doi:10.1111/j.2044-8260.1988.tb00778.x

Newman CW, Jacobson GP, Spitzer JB. Development of the tinnitus handicap inventory. *Arch Otolaryngol Head Neck Surg* (1996) 122(2):143–8. doi:10.1001/ archotol.1996.01890140029007

Zeman F, Koller M, Langguth B, Landgrebe M. Which tinnitus-related aspects are relevant for quality of life and depression: results from a large international multicentre sample. *Health Qual Life Outcomes* (2014) 12:7. doi:10.1186/1477-7525-12-7

Rubinstein B, Axelsson A, Carlsson GE. Prevalence of signs and symptoms of craniomandibular disorders in tinnitus patients. *J Craniomandib Disord* (1990) 4(3):186–92.

Lainez MJ, Ponz A. Tinnitus with headaches. In: Moller ALB, De Riddeer D, Kleinjung T, editors. *Textbook of Tinnitus*. New York: Springer (2011). p. 487–90.

Langguth B, Hund V, Busch V, Jurgens TP, Lainez JM, Landgrebe M, et al. Tinnitus and headache. *Biomed Res Int* (2015) 2015:797416. doi:10.1155/2015/797416

Langguth B, Goodey R, Azevedo A, Bjorne A, Cacace A, Crocetti A, et al. Consensus for tinnitus patient assessment and treatment outcome measurement: Tinnitus Research Initiative meeting, Regensburg, July 2006. *Prog Brain Res* (2007) 166:525–36. doi:10.1016/S0079-6123(07)66050-6

Fritsche G, Hueppe M, Kukava M, Dzagnidze A, Schuerks M, Yoon MS, et al. Validation of a German language questionnaire for screening for migraine, tension-type headache, and trigeminal autonomic cephalgias. *Headache* (2007) 47(4):546–51. doi:10.1111/j.1526-4610.2007.00758.x

Landgrebe M, Zeman F, Koller M, Eberl Y, Mohr M, Reiter J, et al. The Tinnitus Research Initiative (TRI) database: a new approach for delineation of tinnitus subtypes and generation of predictors for treatment outcome. *BMC Med Inform Decis Mak* (2010) 10:42. doi:10.1186/1472-6947-10-42

Newman CW, Sandridge SA, Jacobson GP. Psychometric adequacy of the Tinnitus Handicap Inventory (THI) for evaluating treatment outcome. *J Am Acad Audiol* (1998) 9(2):153–60.

Kleinjung T, Fischer B, Langguth B, Sand PG, Hajak G, Dvorakova J, et al. [Validation of the German-Version Tinnitus Handicap Inventory (THI)]. *Psychiatr Prax* (2007) 34(S1):140–2. doi:10.1055/s-2006-940218

Beck AT, Steer RA. Internal consistencies of the original and revised Beck depression inventory. *J Clin Psychol* (1984) 40(6):1365–7. doi:10.1002/1097-4679(198411)40:6<1365::AID-JCLP2270400615>3.0.CO;2-D

The WHOQOL Group. Development of the World Health Organization WHOQOL-BREF quality of life assessment. *Psychol Med* (1998) 28(3):551–8. doi:10.1017/S0033291798006667

Lindberg P, Lyttkens L, Melin L, Scott B. Tinnitus – incidence and handicap. *Scand Audiol* (1984) 13(4):287–91. doi:10.3109/01050398409042138

Erlandsson SI, Hallberg LR, Axelsson A. Psychological and audiological correlates of perceived tinnitus severity. *Audiology* (1992) 31(3):168–79. doi:10.3109/00206099209072912

Sindhusake D, Golding M, Newall P, Rubin G, Jakobsen K, Mitchell P. Risk factors for tinnitus in a population of older adults: the blue mountains hearingstudy. *Ear Hear* (2003) 24(6):501–7. doi:10.1097/01.AUD.0000100204. 08771.3D

Evans RW, Ishiyama G. Migraine with transient unilateral hearing loss and tinnitus. *Headache* (2009) 49(5):756–8. doi:10.1111/j.1526-4610.2008.01075.x

Volcy M, Sheftell FD, Tepper SJ, Rapoport AM, Bigal ME. Tinnitus in migraine: an allodynic symptom secondary to abnormal cortical functioning? *Headache* (2005) 45(8):1083–7. doi:10.1111/j.1526-4610.2005.05193_2.x

Guichard E, Montagni I, Tzourio C, Kurth T. Association between headaches and tinnitus in young adults: cross-sectional study. *Headache* (2016) 56(6):987–94. doi:10.1111/head.12845

Weinreich HM, Carey JP. Prevalence of pulsatile tinnitus among patients with migraine. *Otol Neurotol* (2016) 37(3):244–7. doi:10.1097/MAO.0000000000000968

Chan CC, Ghosh S. Red ear syndrome precipitated by a dietary trigger: a case report. *J Med Case Reports* (2014) 8:338. doi:10.1186/1752-1947-8-338

Kreuzer PM, Vielsmeier V, Poeppl TB, Langguth B. A case report on red ear syndrome with tinnitus successfully treated with transcranial random noise stimulation. *Pain Physician* (2017) 20(1):E199–205.

Chen J, Gong D, Cai S, Wu Z, Lin X, Ma X, et al. [Clinical characteristics of 100 vestibular migraine cases]. *Lin Chung Er Bi Yan Hou Tou Jing Wai Ke Za Zhi* (2016) 30(5):399–401.

Lopez-Escamez JA, Dlugaiczyk J, Jacobs J, Lempert T, Teggi R, von Brevern M, et al. Accompanying symptoms overlap during attacks in Menière's disease and vestibular migraine. *Front Neurol* (2014) 5:265. doi:10.3389/fneur.2014.00265

Eggers SD, Neff BA, Shepard NT, Staab JP. Comorbidities in vestibular migraine. *J Vestib Res* (2014) 24(5–6):387–95. doi:10.3233/VES-140525

Frejo L, Soto-Varela A, Santos-Perez S, Aran I, Batuecas-Caletrio A, Perez-Guillen V, et al. Clinical subgroups in bilateral meniere disease. *Front Neurol* (2016) 7:182. doi:10.3389/fneur.2016.00182

Peres MFP, Mercante JPP, Tobo PR, Kamei H, Bigal ME. Anxiety and depression symptoms and migraine: a symptom-based approach research. *J Headache Pain* (2017) 1(18):37. doi:10.1186/s10194-017-0742-1

Stone J, Sharpe M, Carson A, Lewis SC, Thomas B, Goldbeck R, et al. Are functional motor and sensory symptoms really more frequent on the left? A systematic review. *J Neurol Neurosurg Psychiatry* (2002) 73(5):578–81. doi:10.1136/jnnp.73.5.578

Min SK, Lee BO. Laterality in somatization. *Psychosom Med* (1997) 59(3): 236–40. doi:10.1097/00006842-199705000-00005

Cologno D, Buzzi MG, Carlesimo GA, Cicinelli P, Costa A, Fadda L, et al. Psychiatric disorders and pain location in unilateral migraineurs. *J Headache Pain* (2005) 6(4):227–30. doi:10.1007/s10194-005-0192-z

Blanke O, Morgenthaler FD, Brugger P, Overney LS. Preliminary evidence for a fronto-parietal dysfunction in able-bodied participants with a desire for limb amputation. *J Neuropsychol* (2009) 3(Pt 2):181–200. doi:10.1348/174866408X318653

Norena A, Micheyl C, Chery-Croze S, Collet L. Psychoacoustic characterization of the tinnitus spectrum: implications for the underlying mechanisms of tinnitus. *Audiol Neurootol* (2002) 7(6):358–69. doi:10.1159/000066156

Schecklmann M, Vielsmeier V, Steffens T, Landgrebe M, Langguth B, Kleinjung T. Relationship between audiometric slope and tinnitus pitch in tinnitus patients: insights into the mechanisms of tinnitus generation. *PLoS One* (2012) 7(4):e34878. doi:10.1371/journal.pone.0034878

De Ridder D, Elgoyhen AB, Romo R, Langguth B. Phantom percepts: tinnitus and pain as persisting aversive memory networks. *Proc Natl Acad Sci U S A* (2011) 108(20):8075–80. doi:10.1073/pnas.1018466108

16

Resting-State Brain Abnormalities in Chronic Subjective Tinnitus

Yu-Chen Chen[1†], Fang Wang[1†], Jie Wang[2], Fan Bo[1], Wenqing Xia[3], Jian-Ping Gu[4] and Xindao Yin[1*]*

[1]Department of Radiology, Nanjing First Hospital, Nanjing Medical University, Nanjing, China, [2]Department of Otolaryngology, Nanjing First Hospital, Nanjing Medical University, Nanjing, China, [3]Department of Endocrinology, Nanjing First Hospital, Nanjing Medical University, Nanjing, China, [4]Department of Vascular and Interventional Radiology, Nanjing First Hospital, Nanjing Medical University, Nanjing, China

***Correspondence:**
Yu-Chen Chen
chenyuchen1989@126.com
Xindao Yin
y.163yy@163.com

Purpose: The neural mechanisms that give rise to the phantom sound of tinnitus have not been fully elucidated. Neuroimaging studies have revealed abnormalities in resting-state activity that could represent the neural signature of tinnitus, but there is considerable heterogeneity in the data. To address this issue, we conducted a meta-analysis of published neuroimaging studies aimed at identifying a common core of resting-state brain abnormalities in tinnitus patients.

Methods: A systematic search was conducted for whole-brain resting-state neuroimaging studies with SPECT, PET and functional MRI that compared chronic tinnitus patients with healthy controls. The authors searched PubMed, Science Direct, Web of Knowledge and Embase databases for neuroimaging studies on tinnitus published up to September 2016. From each study, coordinates were extracted from clusters with significant differences between tinnitus subjects and controls. Meta-analysis was performed using the activation likelihood estimation (ALE) method.

Results: Data were included from nine resting-state neuroimaging studies that reported a total of 51 distinct foci. The meta-analysis identified consistent regions of increased resting-state brain activity in tinnitus patients relative to controls that included, bilaterally, the insula, middle temporal gyrus (MTG), inferior frontal gyrus (IFG), parahippocampal gyrus, cerebellum posterior lobe and right superior frontal gyrus. Moreover, decreased brain activity was only observed in the left cuneus and right thalamus.

Conclusions: The current meta-analysis is, to our knowledge, the first to demonstrate a characteristic pattern of resting-state brain abnormalities that may serve as neuroimaging markers and contribute to the understanding of neuropathophysiological mechanisms for chronic tinnitus.

Keywords: tinnitus, neuroimaging, meta-analysis, resting-state fMRI, brain networks

INTRODUCTION

Tinnitus is the conscious perception of sound in the absence of an internal or external acoustic signal (Jastreboff, 1990). In the United States, an estimated 50 million adults have experienced tinnitus occasionally, and 16 million adults are estimated to experience frequent tinnitus (Shargorodsky et al., 2010). The central nervous system is believed to play a major role in its development and maintenance of tinnitus (Rauschecker et al., 2010; Leaver et al., 2011; De Ridder et al., 2014b; Chen et al., 2015a). Previous electrophysiological and neuroimaging studies (Lockwood et al., 1998; Kaltenbach et al., 2005) suggest that tinnitus may arise from aberrant firing patterns or high levels of spontaneous neural activity in the central auditory pathway rather than the cochlea. However, evidences suggest that other brain regions outside the classical auditory pathway may involve attentional mechanisms that contribute to the persistent awareness of the phantom sound as well as the development of anxiety and distress leading to disabling features of chronic tinnitus (Mirz et al., 2000; Schmidt et al., 2013; Henry et al., 2014). Despite extensive research, the brain abnormalities and neuropathophysiological mechanisms underlying chronic tinnitus remain poorly understood. One of the major questions is what regions of the human brain are involved in tinnitus, a question that has been explored in numerous imaging studies (Jastreboff et al., 1994; Lockwood et al., 1998; Mirz et al., 2000; Rauschecker et al., 2010; De Ridder et al., 2014b).

A number of existing neurophysiological mechanisms and models have been proposed to account for the pathophysiology of tinnitus patients, such as central gain (Schaette and McAlpine, 2011), neural synchrony (Seki and Eggermont, 2003), frontostriatal gating (Rauschecker et al., 2015), thalamocortical dysrhythmia (Llinás et al., 1999), noise-canceling deficit (Rauschecker et al., 2010; Leaver et al., 2011), global workspace (De Ridder et al., 2014b), and precision/predictive coding models (Sedley et al., 2016). However, there is a lack of consensus as to which neural mechanism(s) and what regions of the central nervous system are common to the diverse population of tinnitus patients participating in the imaging studies. Human neuroimaging studies have revealed augmented activity in tinnitus patients in several brain regions within and/or beyond classical auditory pathways. According to the model of De Ridder et al. (2014b) tinnitus is underpinned by the integration of multiple nonspecific subnetworks of the brain involving general components of cognition, emotion and memory. Communication between these different subnetworks occurs at specific hubs, brain areas that are involved in multiple subnetworks simultaneously. These different subnetworks, which interact at different oscillatory frequencies, communicate with one another at partially overlapping hubs. Nonetheless, the role of the potential hubs involved in multiple subnetworks of tinnitus still remains unclear.

Since about 85% of chronic tinnitus patients perceived the phantom sound constantly (Schecklmann et al., 2014), the resting-state fMRI measurements seem well suited to identify the neural structures, subnetworks and hubs involved in tinnitus. A growing number of studies have used resting-state fMRI to investigate tinnitus (Husain and Schmidt, 2014) and multiple brain networks implicated in tinnitus have been identified, such as the auditory network (Burton et al., 2012; Kim et al., 2012; Maudoux et al., 2012a,b; Schmidt et al., 2013; Hinkley et al., 2015; Minami et al., 2015; Leaver et al., 2016b), default mode network (DMN; Schmidt et al., 2013; Chen et al., 2014, 2015d; Leaver et al., 2016b), dorsal attention network (DAN; Burton et al., 2012; Schmidt et al., 2013), ventral attention network (VAN; Burton et al., 2012), and visual network (Burton et al., 2012; Chen et al., 2014, 2015d). As such, tinnitus can be seen as the interaction of multiple brain subnetworks, each contributing to different aspects of tinnitus such as its acoustic features, emotional affect and awareness or attention. However, these studies reported relatively inconsistent results. For instance, most researches demonstrated the increased resting-state brain activity between tinnitus patients and healthy controls (Maudoux et al., 2012a; Chen et al., 2014, 2016; Laureano et al., 2014; Yang et al., 2014; Ueyama et al., 2015), while others failed to identify any regions of increased brain activity (Geven et al., 2014; Leaver et al., 2016b). Moreover, several studies have failed to detect any differences in network processing between tinnitus patients and controls (Wineland et al., 2012; Davies et al., 2014). These reported discrepancies can potentially be attributed to the limited sample size, variable clinical demographics and use of different methods. Furthermore, in many studies tinnitus groups were not compared to an appropriate control group (Leaver et al., 2011; Schecklmann et al., 2013; Lanting et al., 2014).

Tinnitus is a very heterogeneous condition with respect to the characteristics of the perceived sound, degree of associated awareness and distress, duration and comorbidities (Landgrebe et al., 2012). Given the high heterogeneity, it is not surprising that inconsistencies across studies are encountered. Nevertheless, there may be some commonalities across these diverse studies. One approach to identifying a common core is to perform a meta-analysis of the existing resting-state studies of patients with chronic tinnitus with the goal of identifying brain network hubs in tinnitus patients common to neuroimaging studies of tinnitus. Activation likelihood estimation (ALE) is the most common coordinate-based meta-analytic method used to analyze the neuroimaging literature; this approach seeks to identify brain locations with a consistent pattern of response across experiments. This approach is based on the collection of peak coordinates from each study included in the meta-analysis rather than the input of raw images (Turkeltaub et al., 2002; Wager et al., 2004; Laird et al., 2005a; Eickhoff et al., 2009). ALE technique has been successfully applied to neuroimaging studies of various neurological or psychiatric disorders, such as epilepsy (Li et al., 2012), Parkinson's disease (Shao et al., 2015), schizophrenia (Ellison-Wright and Bullmore, 2010), and narcolepsy (Weng et al., 2015). Song et al. (2012) performed a meta-analysis exclusively of PET studies of tinnitus using the ALE method to retrieve the most consistent activation areas across different task dimensions. However, this meta-analysis did not include the large body of fMRI studies that might prove useful in detecting resting-state brain abnormalities in tinnitus patients. Therefore the goal of the current study was to conduct a quantitative meta-analysis of several different types of resting state neuroimaging data in the tinnitus literature that met our inclusion criterion. To accomplish this, we used the ALE algorithm to determine the resting-state brain abnormalities in tinnitus patients compared to healthy controls. Our working hypothesis was that the ALE analysis would identify a common core of brain regions linked to tinnitus generation despite the heterogeneity of the patients and experimental methods.

MATERIALS AND METHODS

Search Strategies and Study Selection

Our analysis was performed according to the Meta-Analysis of Observational Studies in Epidemiology (MOOSE) criteria (Stroup et al., 2000). A comprehensive literature search up to September, 2016 was conducted in PubMed, Science Direct, Web of Knowledge, and Embase using the following search terms: (1) "neuroimaging" <OR> "PET" <OR> "fMRI"; (2) "resting state"; and (3) "tinnitus". Our search was restricted to humans. In addition, we manually reviewed the references cited in articles that were retrieved.

Studies were selected according to the following inclusion criteria: (1) published as an article (and not a letter or an abstract); (2) comparisons of tinnitus patients with healthy control groups on a whole-brain level; and (3) clearly reported Montreal Neurological Institute (MNI) or Talairach coordinates of the activation areas (*x*, *y*, *z*). Studies reporting only findings for specific ROIs were not included in the present meta-analysis. In accordance with many previous ALE meta-analyses (Laird et al., 2005b; Petacchi et al., 2005; Li et al., 2010; Kühn and Gallinat, 2013), we included coordinates resulting from fMRI as well as from PET data. We included data from PET and fMRI studies and other data analysis techniques despite the fact that they have different physiological bases and theoretical assumptions since both methods have been used to identify differences between the intrinsic brain function in patients compared with controls. The rationale was to provide an all-encompassing overview of attempts to identify resting-state abnormalities in tinnitus patients. Our search criteria yielded a total of 67 peer-reviewed published articles. Of the 67 studies, 26 studies were excluded as these studies were not about comparisons between tinnitus patients and healthy controls; nine articles were excluded since these were electroencephalography (EEG) or magnetoencephalography (MEG) studies; another four pulsatile tinnitus studies and four animal studies were excluded. Fifteen studies were further excluded since these did not report detailed peak coordinates over the whole brain. Finally, nine resting-state neuroimaging studies, six fMRI, two SPECT and one PET, were included in the ALE meta-analysis (**Figure 1** and **Table 1**).

Two independent reviewers (CYC and FW) evaluated the methodology and the risk of bias of the eligible studies. First, they assessed the titles of the search results and retrieved the relevant articles. Second, the articles that remained eligible were assessed based on their abstract to determine whether any of the inclusion criteria were not met. The full text of all remaining articles was then assessed with a data extraction template, which was constructed for the purpose of organizing and extracting information from the included articles and excluding articles without peak values. The reviewers analyzed all articles in terms of patient selection and their comparable controls, blinding, diagnostic criteria and regression methods. Any disagreements were assessed by the third reviewer (FB). The demographic data were extracted from each article, including the first author's name, year of publication, total patient number, sex distribution, mean patient age and range, statistic thresholds, hearing and psychological status.

Data Extraction

The *x*, *y*, and *z* peak activation coordinates of all eligible contrasts constituted the meta-analysis input. The data originally reported in Talairach spaces were converted to MNI coordinates (Lancaster et al., 2007). The data from MNI coordinates were texted and implemented in GingerALE 2.3.3[1], Research Imaging Institute of the University of Texas Health Science Center, San Antonio, TX, USA). Coordinates in each study were independently extracted by two authors (CYC and FW).

ALE Meta-Analysis

Ginger ALE software was used to analyze the resting-state brain activity between tinnitus patients and healthy controls. The reported loci of maximal anatomical differences were modeled as the peaks of three-dimensional Gaussian probability density functions defined by the full-width at half-maximum (FWHM), which was set according to a quantitative uncertainty model (Laird et al., 2005a; Eickhoff et al., 2009). ALE values were calculated on a voxel-by-voxel basis by measuring the union model activation maps modeled above. This revised analysis tested for convergence by studies (random effects) instead of foci (fixed effects). Following the method described by Turkeltaub et al. (2002, 2012), 1000 permutations were used to determine which tests were statistically significant and threshold determined for the resultant ALE map. A whole-brain histogram was computed in which the null hypothesis of uniformly distributed foci was rejected for voxels with an ALE value greater than the critical threshold, defined as the $100(1-\alpha)$th percentile of the permutation distribution, where α refers to the desired level of significance. The analyses were performed at a cluster forming threshold (reported with each p value and ALE thresholds in the results, ALE values greater than this threshold are statistically significant) computed using a $p < 0.05$, corrected for multiple comparisons using false-discovery rate (FDR; Genovese et al., 2002; Laird et al., 2005a). The volume of the minimum cluster threshold was set at 200 mm^3. The coordinates of the weighted center were generated for each cluster. The resulting significant anatomical areas were labeled based on probabilistic cytoarchitectonic maps of the human brain using the SPM Anatomy Toolbox v2.1 (Eickhoff et al., 2005). Results were visualized with Mango software[2], using the Colin brain template in the MNI space[3].

RESULTS

Using our inclusion/exclusion criteria, we identified nine eligible neuroimaging studies utilizing different methods, including

[1]http://brainmap.org/ale/
[2]http://ric.uthscsa.edu/mango/mango.html
[3]http://www.brainmap.org/ale

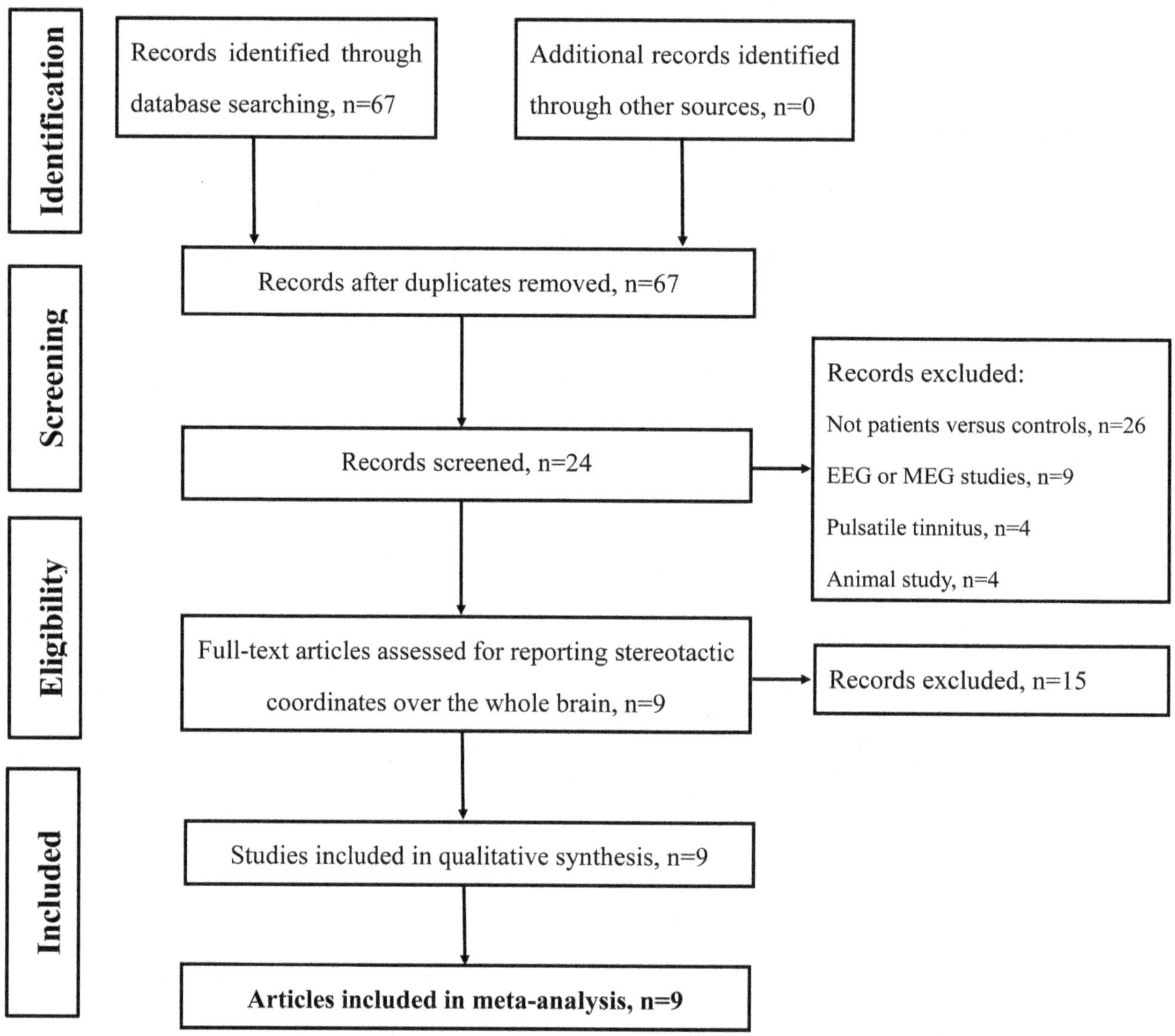

FIGURE 1 | Flow diagram of the literature search. Flow diagram shows the results of the systematic search for the selected studies in this meta-analysis.

SPECT (Laureano et al., 2014; Ueyama et al., 2015), PET (Geven et al., 2014), and fMRI (Maudoux et al., 2012a; Chen et al., 2014, 2015d, 2016; Leaver et al., 2016b). **Figure 1** is a flow diagram showing the steps in the identification, exclusion and inclusion of the studies. The clinical and demographic data of the participants from all recruited studies are presented in **Table 1**. The subjects of patients and controls from each study are generally comparable by age, sex, and education. The hearing and psychological status are also shown in **Table 2**.

As illustrated in **Figure 2**, a total of 13 peak foci were reported in this meta-analysis. Compared with healthy controls, tinnitus patients showed increased resting-state neural activity bilaterally in the middle temporal gyrus (MTG), inferior frontal gyrus (IFG), parahippocampal gyrus, insula, cerebellar posterior lobe and right superior frontal gyrus (SFG). Moreover, decreased brain activity was also observed in the left cuneus and right thalamus. **Table 3** displays the coordinates of cluster maxima.

DISCUSSION

The current study is the first whole-brain meta-analysis exploring the resting-state brain abnormalities in chronic tinnitus patients compared to healthy controls. By analyzing nine neuroimaging studies, the meta-analysis identified consistent regions of aberrant neural activity mainly in the non-auditory brain regions, including the MTG, frontal cortex, parahippocampus, insula, cerebellum, cuneus, and thalamus, in different aspects of tinnitus. Surprisingly, the auditory cortex was not detected in this study. This may be due to the fact that most patients in these studies had little or mild hearing loss.

TABLE 1 | List of all studies included in the meta-analysis: subjects' demographic and clinical characteristics.

Study	Journal	Modality/ Method of analysis	Male: Female		Mean age ± SD		Reported contrasts	Foci NO.	Scanner	Processing software	Smoothing kernel (mm)	Statistical threshold	MNI or Tal
			Patients	Control	Patients	Control							
Maudoux et al. (2012a)	Plos One	fMRI/ICA	7:6	9:6	52 ± 11	51 ± 13	TIN > HC HC > TIN	11 6	Siemens 3.0T	Brain Voyager	8	$P < 0.05$, FDR corrected	Tal
Geven et al. (2014)	Neuroscience	PET	10:10	9:10	51.0 ± 10.0	50.8 ± 9.5	HC > TIN	2	Siemens	SPM5	8	$p < 0.001$, uncorrected	MNI
Laureano et al. (2014)	Plos One	SPECT	6:14	6:11	42.95 ± 9.03	41.41 ± 9.98	TIN > HC	1	GE	SPM8	8	$P < 0.05$, FWE corrected	MNI
Chen et al. (2014)	NeuroImage: Clinical	fMRI/ALFF	17:14	17:15	41.9 ± 10.8	46.5 ± 12.6	TIN > HC HC > TIN	3 4	Siemens 3.0T	SPM8	4	$P < 0.05$, AlphaSim corrected	MNI
Yang et al. (2014)*	Journal of Otology	fMRI/ReHo	14:4	15:5	43	42	TIN > HC HC > TIN	1 1	Philips 3.0T	SPM5	NA	$P < 0.05$, FWE corrected	MNI
Ueyama et al. (2015)	Plos One	SPECT	10:7	NA	NA	NA	TIN > HC HC > TIN	6 2	FUJI FILM	SPM8	8	$P < 0.05$, AlphaSim corrected	MNI
Chen et al. (2015d)	Neural Plasticity	fMRI/ReHo	16:13	15:15	40.9 ± 10.5	46.2 ± 11.9	TIN > HC HC > TIN	4 1	Siemens 3.0T	SPM8	4	$P < 0.01$, AlphaSim corrected	MNI
Leaver et al. (2016b)	Human Brain Mapping	fMRI/ICA	10:11	9:10	47.33 ± 13.47	48.89 ± 12.49	HC > TIN	5	Siemens 3.0T	Brain Voyager	6	$P < 0.0005$, uncorrected	Tal
Chen et al. (2016)	Frontiers in Aging Neuroscience	fMRI/DC	9:15	9:13	50.8 ± 12.4	44.7 ± 15.4	TIN > HC	2	Philips 3.0T	SPM8	6	$P < 0.01$, AlphaSim corrected	MNI

*Note: TIN, tinnitus; HC, healthy control; fMRI, functional magnetic resonance imaging; PET, positron emission tomography; SPECT, single photon emission computed tomography; ALFF, amplitude of low-frequency fluctuations; ReHo, regional homogeneity; ICA, independent component analysis; DC, degree centrality; SPM, statistical parametric mapping; MNI, Montreal Neurological Institute; FDR, false discovery rate; FWE, family-wise error; NA, not available. *Only reported mean age in this study.*

TABLE 2 | The hearing and psychological status of the subjects included in all the studies.

Study	Hearing status		Psychological status
	Patients	Controls	
Maudoux et al. (2012a)	2 severe HL 7 mild/moderate HL 4 no HL	No HL	No major neurological neurosurgical or psychiatric history
Geven et al. (2014)	NA	NA	No major medical, neurological or psychiatric diagnoses
Laureano et al. (2014)	No HL	No HL	No neurologic or psychiatric disorders
Chen et al. (2014)	No HL	No HL	No depression or anxiety or other neurologic or psychiatric disorders
Yang et al. (2014)	1 profound HL 1 severe HL 4 moderate HL 9 mild HL 3 no HL	No HL	NA
Ueyama et al. (2015)	11 mild to severe HL 6 no HL	No HL	No neurologic or psychiatric disorders
Chen et al. (2015d)	No HL	No HL	No depression or anxiety or other neurologic or psychiatric disorders
Leaver et al. (2016b)	15 mild to severe HL 6 no HL	10 mild to severe HL 9 no HL	No significant symptoms of anxiety or depression
Chen et al. (2016)	No HL	No HL	No depression or anxiety or other neurologic or psychiatric disorders

Note: HL, hearing loss; NA, not available.

These non-auditory areas are parts of separable subnetworks representing multiple clinical cognitive and emotional aspects of tinnitus; resting-state disruptions in these areas may provide new insights on the neuropathological mechanisms of this disorder.

Middle Temporal Gyrus

The MTG has been suggested to be involved in cognitive processes including language, semantic memory and multimodal sensory integration (Cabeza and Nyberg, 2000). A quantitative EEG study has demonstrated higher α2-band activity in the

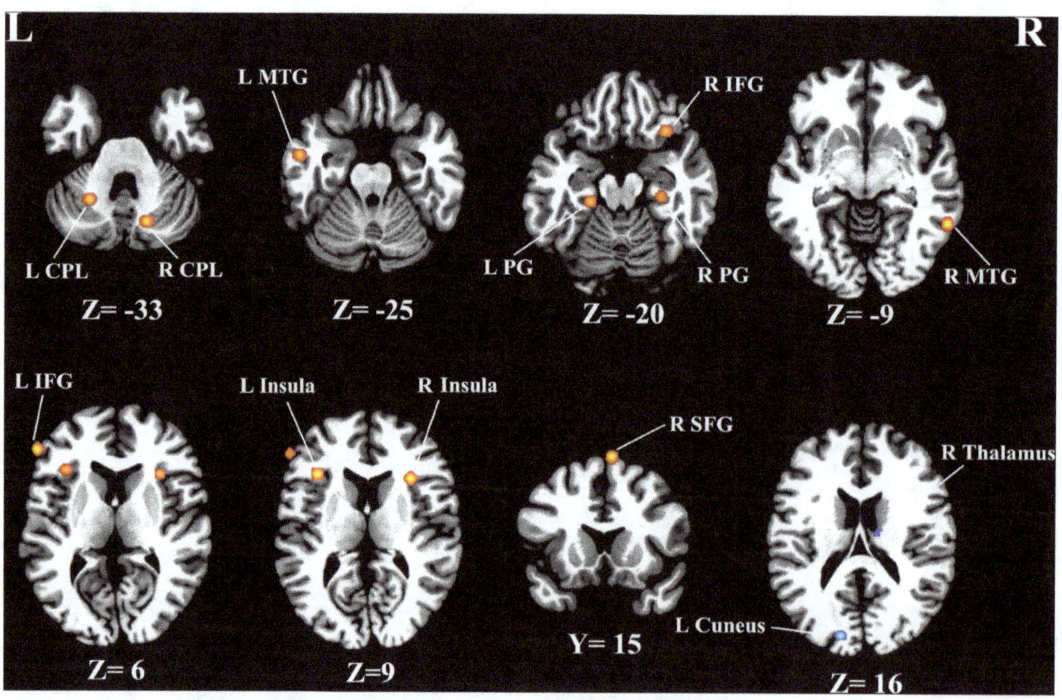

FIGURE 2 | Resting-state brain activity alterations in chronic tinnitus patients compared with healthy controls. Results are from the activation likelihood estimation (ALE) software for meta-analyses. All activations are significant at $p < 0.05$ corrected for multiple comparisons using the false-discovery rate (FDR) correction.

TABLE 3 | Regions of altered brain activity in tinnitus patients relative to healthy controls.

Brain regions	BA	MNI coordinates *x, y, z* (mm)	ALE extrema value	Cluster size (mm^3)
Tinnitus > Controls				
L Insula	13	−36, 24, 9	0.0088	880
R Cerebellar Posterior Lobe	–	17, −72, −33	0.0075	768
L Cerebellar Posterior Lobe	–	−25, −56, −33	0.0075	768
L Middle Temporal Gyrus	21	−53, −6, −25	0.0075	768
R Middle Temporal Gyrus	37	60, −51, −9	0.0086	768
R Inferior Frontal Gyrus	47	34, 22, −20	0.0072	736
R Superior Frontal Gyrus	6	6, 15, 69	0.0086	728
L Parahippocampal Gyrus	35	−22, −30, −20	0.0073	720
R Parahippocampal Gyrus	35	30, −26, −18	0.0073	720
L Inferior Frontal Gyrus	46	−57, 39, 6	0.0085	712
R Insula	13	34, 20, 10	0.0082	704
Tinnitus < Controls				
L Cuneus	17	−14, −88, 16	0.013	488
R Thalamus	–	14, −10, 14	0.0101	368

ALE, activation likelihood estimation; BA, Brodmann area; MNI, Montreal Neurological Institute; L, left; R, right. Each ALE map was thresholded using a FDR-corrected $p < 0.05$.

MTG in tinnitus patients with higher distress (Vanneste et al., 2010a). Voxel-based morphometry (VBM) analyses revealed that the gray matter increases in the MTG in tinnitus patients with hearing impairment (Boyen et al., 2013). Using resting-state fMRI, significantly increased spontaneous neural activity was observed in the right MTG in tinnitus patients (Chen et al., 2014). Moreover, Zhang et al. (2015) showed decreased functional connectivity between right MTG and left thalamus, which was negatively correlated with tinnitus severity. In addition, the MTG has been regarded as a key region of the DMN (Raichle et al., 2001). The DMN, consisting of nodes in the MTG, posterior cingulate/precuneus, angular gyrus and medial frontal gyrus, is most active at rest and shows reduced activity when a subject enters a task-based state involving attention or goal-directed behavior (Raichle et al., 2001; Mantini et al., 2007). As a condition involving the perception of a phantom auditory sensation, tinnitus might lead to dysfunction of the DMN. Previous fMRI studies found abnormal functional connectivity within the DMN associated with tinnitus distress (Burton et al., 2012; Maudoux et al., 2012b; Schmidt et al., 2013). Nevertheless, the source or type of aberrant neural activity within DMN regions in tinnitus remains unclear. Our results indicate that increased neuronal activity in the MTG may be responsible for disrupting the DMN in tinnitus patients.

Frontal Cortex

The frontal cortex, including the SFG and IFG, exhibited increased neural activity in tinnitus patients in the current study. Rauschecker et al. (2010) developed a model to demonstrate structural and functional differences in ventromedial prefrontal cortex that were associated with tinnitus subjective loudness, indicating that frontal cortex may contribute to certain perceptual features of tinnitus. Resting-state fMRI studies have pointed out that the abnormalities of the frontal cortex could act as a direct mechanism of tinnitus chronification (Burton et al., 2012; Schmidt et al., 2013; Chen et al., 2014, 2015c,d, 2016), which are confirmed by the current meta-analysis. Based on the previous fMRI studies, the SFG has been regarded as a major integrative hub of the tinnitus network architecture (Chen et al., 2016), which can receive and integrate all kinds of information from different parts of the brain from inside and outside the body. Besides, it can also timely organize efferent impulses to ensure the coordination of the central nervous system as a whole (Mathiak et al., 2007; Melloni et al., 2007). A possible explanation for our result was that the increased activity of the SFG might be due to feedback inhibition of an over active auditory network (Downar et al., 2000). Furthermore, the IFG serves as the core region of response inhibition and IFG activity might mirror the attempt to control the bottom-up attention allocation to the tinnitus percept in a top-down manner (Aron et al., 2014). In one hypothetical model, the fronto-insular cortex is part of a salience network that drives switching by a central executive control network important to maintaining and adjusting attention (Sridharan et al., 2008). In another model, the IFG and the insula act as executive control components in the attention system that regulates dorsal and VANs, which lack direct interconnections (Shulman et al., 2009). Taken together, we suggest that tinnitus distress, salience, or attentional focus is associated with increased resting-state activity in these brain subnetworks.

Parahippocampus

The parahippocampal area has been hypothesized to play a central role in memory recollection and transferring information from the hippocampus to the association areas, which might explain its involvement in the generation of simple auditory phantom percepts such as tinnitus (De Ridder et al., 2014a; Vanneste and De Ridder, 2016). EEG study suggested that tinnitus patients differed from healthy controls by increased delta and theta activity in the parahippocampus (Moazami-Goudarzi et al., 2010). Prior resting-state fMRI studies also provided further support linking tinnitus physiopathology with parahippocampal region involved in mnemonic network (Maudoux et al., 2012a; Chen et al., 2015b; Leaver et al., 2016b).

Insula

The increased response in the insula, mainly the anterior part, may be an indication of successful adaption to the tinnitus perception (van der Loo et al., 2011). On the basis of resting-state quantitative EEG, the insula has been implicated in tinnitus and specific tinnitus characteristics (van der Loo et al., 2011; Vanneste et al., 2011a,b). Greater synchrony of alpha activity was observed bilaterally in the anterior insula of patients with more severe tinnitus-related distress (Vanneste et al., 2010a). In addition, chronic tinnitus patients showed enhanced spontaneous neuronal activity and functional connectivity in bilateral anterior insula were revealed by resting-state fMRI (Burton et al., 2012; Chen et al., 2015d).

Furthermore, the insula is one of key nodes in the common brain circuit of both tinnitus and chronic pain (Rauschecker et al., 2015). Although there also exist important differences between the two disorders, the striking similarities and associations indicate that tinnitus and chronic pain share common neuropathological mechanisms. Now advances in neuroimaging have demonstrated that similar structures and functional systems are involved and probably play a central role in both disorders (Rauschecker et al., 2015). Significant loss of gray matter and compromised circuit function are detected in several specific regions, such as the ventromedial prefrontal cortex, nucleus accumbens and insula (De Ridder et al., 2011; Rauschecker et al., 2015). These areas act as a central gatekeeping system for perceptual sensations, which determines the affective value of sensory stimuli and modulates information flow in the brain (Rauschecker et al., 2015). Tinnitus and chronic pain occur when this system is compromised.

Although the EEG has been used to determine resting-state long-range functional coupling in tinnitus, it has many differences from the resting-state fMRI (Vanneste et al., 2010a,b). EEG does not offer the spatial resolution of fMRI, but offer the advantage of being quiet and not influencing the resting-state network of tinnitus. Thus these two techniques may measure different aspects of spontaneous neuronal activity (Tagliazucchi et al., 2012). Britz et al. (2010) extracted four resting-state networks from the EEG data that were the equivalent of stereotypical fMRI networks dedicated to auditory, attetional, visual and self-referential processing, but DMN was not detected by EEG in Britz's study. Other studies have correlated the DMN with beta-2 (Laufs et al., 2003) or with delta (Mantini et al., 2007) spectral bands of EEG. Therefore, a direct comparison of EEG and resting-state fMRI is complicated by the fact that similar EEG power bands may be correlated with varying fMRI-generated spatial maps and a single resting-state network may be linked with different EEG spectral patterns (Laufs et al., 2008; Musso et al., 2010).

Cerebellum

Furthermore, although the cerebellum is primarily involved in motor actions and control, several cerebellar regions such as the paraflocculus and vermis receive inputs from auditory centers (Petacchi et al., 2005). Brozoski et al. (2007) observed increased activity in the parafloccular lobe of the cerebellum in animals with tinnitus confirmed and suggested that the cerebellum acts as a gating control mechanism comparing the afferent input from the cochlea with descending signals from the auditory cortex (Bauer et al., 2013; Chen et al., 2015b). Consistent with this view, hyperactivity in the auditory cortex and increased functional connectivity between the auditory cortex and cerebellum were observed in rats with salicylate-induced tinnitus (Chen et al., 2015a). If this cerebellar-tinnitus gating hypothesis is correct, then inactivating the cerebellum could possibly suppress the sound perception of tinnitus. Based on these findings, we suggest that cerebellum may play a pivotal role of gating control in tinnitus. Furthermore, using resting-state fMRI, chronic tinnitus patients exhibited enhanced functional connectivity in the cerebellar hemisphere that was associated with tinnitus distress (Maudoux et al., 2012a; Ueyama et al., 2013), indicating the involvement of cerebellum in auditory system.

Cuneus

Our meta-analysis found decreased brain activity in the cuneus of tinnitus patients. We speculate that the connections between auditory and visual regions make it possible to alter the brain activity in the visual areas (Kaltenbach et al., 2004; Cate et al., 2009). This is consistent with prior fMRI studies showing negative correlations of functional connectivity between auditory and visual resting-state subnetworks in tinnitus patients (Burton et al., 2012; Maudoux et al., 2012b). One possibility is that the phantom sounds might act to decrease spontaneous activity in visual areas because of the salience of the tinnitus perception (Chen et al., 2014, 2015d). Thus, tinnitus may be regarded as the consequence of multisensory interactions between auditory and visual regions.

Thalamus

The thalamus, which regulates the flow of sensory information to and from the auditory cortex, has been thought to play a key role in tinnitus (Richardson et al., 2012). Llinás et al. (1999) hypothesized that tinnitus results from thalamocortical dysrhythmias triggered by peripheral damage. Prior MRI studies have identified structural and functional abnormalities involved in thalamocortical network of tinnitus (Mühlau et al., 2006; Rauschecker et al., 2010; Benson et al., 2014; Chen et al., 2014; Lanting et al., 2014; Zhang et al., 2015). Consistent with our results, Zhang et al. (2015) showed decreased functional connectivity between the thalamus and auditory cortical areas in tinnitus, which may be a reflection of disrupted thalamic gating mechanism (Rauschecker et al., 2010). The thalamus is regarded as the center of ascending noise canceling system, and thus if it is dysfunctional, noise canceling is no longer possible and the subject may perceive tinnitus (Rauschecker et al., 2010). However, the mechanisms responsible for these functional changes are unknown, but could involve aberrant inhibition (Richardson et al., 2012).

Limitations

Several inevitable limitations should be noted in our study. First, the heterogeneity of the included studies could affect the current results. In particular, hearing loss is always a complicating factor in structural and functional studies of tinnitus. Melcher et al. (2013) compared tinnitus patients with controls who were matched for hearing thresholds in the standard clinical frequencies and found that gray matter changes were not related to tinnitus but instead negatively correlated with hearing thresholds at frequencies above 8 kHz. Therefore, a more complete characterization of hearing loss is desirable. Moreover, tinnitus can become a significant psychological problem and comorbid symptoms such as depression and anxiety are potential confounds on the observed brain activity in tinnitus patients (Leaver et al., 2016a). It is necessary to characterize the psychological health problems as covariates in the analyses. The problems of differential tinnitus variables on structural and functional changes in neural activity can be solved using correlational analyses of large samples (Schecklmann et al., 2013) and comparisons of different tinnitus subtypes (Vanneste and De Ridder, 2012). Second, voxel-wise meta-analytic approach like ALE provides excellent control of false positive results, but it is more difficult to avoid false negatives (Radua et al., 2012). Voxel-wise meta-analysis is based on the pooling of peak stereotactic coordinates rather than on raw statistical brain maps from the original studies, which could give rise to less accurate results (Radua et al., 2012). Furthermore, fMRI produces aversive scanner noise which has been shown to interfere with auditory processing in the human brain at the physiological and psychological level (Perrachione and Ghosh, 2013). The concept of resting state is somewhat problematic in tinnitus studies because the auditory pathway is likely to be activated by scanner noise which is nearly impossible to completely eliminate even with ear plugs or active noise reduction (Logothetis et al., 2009). Therefore, this limitation should be taken into consideration when interpreting the resting-state fMRI data in auditory system-related researches. Finally, the number of included neuroimaging studies is relatively small. Further explorations are needed to perform the subgroup analyses or meta-regression analyses for the control of confounding factors that might influence resting-state brain function in tinnitus, such as the imaging methodology and data analysis method. Most importantly, we should establish standard protocols for resting-state fMRI researches to minimize heterogeneity on the experimental side.

CONCLUSION

Using the ALE-based meta-analysis, our study demonstrated abnormal resting-state neural activity mainly in the non-auditory brain areas, including the MTG, frontal cortex, parahippocampus, insula, cerebellum, cuneus and thalamus. In accordance to the hypothesis, these results show that there exist several important brain hubs in specific tinnitus network encompassing DMN, attentional, mnemonic, salience, visual and thalamocortical subnetworks. Aberrant resting-state brain patterns in tinnitus-related networks may help enhance our understanding of the neuropathological mechanisms underlying chronic subjective tinnitus. Nonetheless, a theoretical pathophysiological framework capable of explaining all these aspects in one model is still highly required. There is thus hope that a single cure can be found that would target a common mechanism.

AUTHOR CONTRIBUTIONS

Y-CC and FW designed the experiment, reviewed the literatures, performed the analysis and wrote the manuscript. JW, FB and WX reviewed the literatures. J-PG and XY contributed to the discussion and manuscript revision.

ACKNOWLEDGMENTS

The authors thank Prof. Richard Salvi, Center for Hearing and Deafness, University at Buffalo, Buffalo, NY, USA, for his contributions to the revision of the manuscript. This work was supported by a grant from the Natural Science Foundation of Jiangsu Higher Education Institutions (No. 16KJB320001) and National Natural Science Foundation of China (Nos. 81601477, 81600638).

REFERENCES

Aron, A. R., Robbins, T. W., and Poldrack, R. A. (2014). Inhibition and the right inferior frontal cortex: one decade on. *Trends Cogn. Sci.* 18, 177–185. doi: 10.1016/j.tics.2013.12.003

Bauer, C. A., Kurt, W., Sybert, L. T., and Brozoski, T. J. (2013). The cerebellum as a novel tinnitus generator. *Hear. Res.* 295, 130–139. doi: 10.1016/j.heares.2012.03.009

Benson, R. R., Gattu, R., and Cacace, A. T. (2014). Left hemisphere fractional anisotropy increase in noise-induced tinnitus: a diffusion tensor imaging (DTI) study of white matter tracts in the brain. *Hear. Res.* 309, 8–16. doi: 10.1016/j.heares.2013.10.005

Boyen, K., Langers, D. R., de Kleine, E., and van Dijk, P. (2013). Gray matter in the brain: differences associated with tinnitus and hearing loss. *Hear. Res.* 295, 67–78. doi: 10.1016/j.heares.2012.02.010

Britz, J., Van De Ville, D., and Michel, C. M. (2010). BOLD correlates of EEG topography reveal rapid resting-state network dynamics. *Neuroimage* 52, 1162–1170. doi: 10.1016/j.neuroimage.2010.02.052

Brozoski, T. J., Ciobanu, L., and Bauer, C. A. (2007). Central neural activity in rats with tinnitus evaluated with manganese-enhanced magnetic resonance imaging (MEMRI). *Hear. Res.* 228, 168–179. doi: 10.1016/j.heares.2007.02.003

Burton, H., Wineland, A., Bhattacharya, M., Nicklaus, J., Garcia, K. S., and Piccirillo, J. F. (2012). Altered networks in bothersome tinnitus: a functional connectivity study. *BMC Neurosci.* 13:3. doi: 10.1186/1471-2202-13-3

Cabeza, R., and Nyberg, L. (2000). Imaging cognition II: an empirical review of 275 PET and fMRI studies. *J. Cogn. Neurosci.* 12, 1–47. doi: 10.1162/08989290051137585

Cate, A. D., Herron, T. J., Yund, E. W., Stecker, G. C., Rinne, T., Kang, X., et al. (2009). Auditory attention activates peripheral visual cortex. *PLoS One* 4:e4645. doi: 10.1371/journal.pone.0004645

Chen, Y.-C., Feng, Y., Xu, J.-J., Mao, C.-N., Xia, W., Ren, J., et al. (2016). Disrupted brain functional network architecture in chronic tinnitus patients. *Front. Aging Neurosci.* 8:174. doi: 10.3389/fnagi.2016.00174

Chen, Y.-C., Li, X., Liu, L., Wang, J., Lu, C.-Q., Yang, M., et al. (2015a). Tinnitus and hyperacusis involve hyperactivity and enhanced connectivity in auditory-limbic-arousal-cerebellar network. *Elife* 4:e06576. doi: 10.7554/eLife.06576

Chen, Y.-C., Xia, W., Feng, Y., Li, X., Zhang, J., Feng, X., et al. (2015b). Altered interhemispheric functional coordination in chronic tinnitus patients. *Biomed Res. Int.* 2015:345647. doi: 10.1155/2015/345647

Chen, Y.-C., Xia, W., Luo, B., Muthaiah, V. P., Xiong, Z., Zhang, J., et al. (2015c). Frequency-specific alternations in the amplitude of low-frequency fluctuations in chronic tinnitus. *Front. Neural Circuits* 9:67. doi: 10.3389/fncir.2015.00067

Chen, Y.-C., Zhang, J., Li, X.-W., Xia, W., Feng, X., Qian, C., et al. (2015d). Altered intra-and interregional synchronization in resting-state cerebral networks associated with chronic tinnitus. *Neural Plast.* 2015:475382. doi: 10.1155/2015/475382

Chen, Y.-C., Zhang, J., Li, X.-W., Xia, W., Feng, X., Gao, B., et al. (2014). Aberrant spontaneous brain activity in chronic tinnitus patients revealed by resting-state functional MRI. *Neuroimage Clin.* 6, 222–228. doi: 10.1016/j.nicl.2014.09.011

Davies, J., Gander, P., Andrews, M., and Hall, D. (2014). Auditory network connectivity in tinnitus patients: a resting-state fMRI study. *Int. J. Audiol.* 53, 192–198. doi: 10.3109/14992027.2013.846482

Downar, J., Crawley, A. P., Mikulis, D. J., and Davis, K. D. (2000). A multimodal cortical network for the detection of changes in the sensory environment. *Nat. Neurosci.* 3, 277–283. doi: 10.1038/72991

Eickhoff, S. B., Laird, A. R., Grefkes, C., Wang, L. E., Zilles, K., and Fox, P. T. (2009). Coordinate-based activation likelihood estimation meta-analysis of neuroimaging data: a random-effects approach based on empirical estimates of spatial uncertainty. *Hum. Brain Mapp.* 30, 2907–2926. doi: 10.1002/hbm.20718

Eickhoff, S. B., Stephan, K. E., Mohlberg, H., Grefkes, C., Fink, G. R., Amunts, K., et al. (2005). A new SPM toolbox for combining probabilistic cytoarchitectonic maps and functional imaging data. *Neuroimage* 25, 1325–1335. doi: 10.1016/j.neuroimage.2004.12.034

Ellison-Wright, I., and Bullmore, E. (2010). Anatomy of bipolar disorder and schizophrenia: a meta-analysis. *Schizophr. Res.* 117, 1–12. doi: 10.1016/j.schres.2009.12.022

Genovese, C. R., Lazar, N. A., and Nichols, T. (2002). Thresholding of statistical maps in functional neuroimaging using the false discovery rate. *Neuroimage* 15, 870–878. doi: 10.1006/nimg.2001.1037

Geven, L., de Kleine, E., Willemsen, A., and van Dijk, P. (2014). Asymmetry in primary auditory cortex activity in tinnitus patients and controls. *Neuroscience* 256, 117–125. doi: 10.1016/j.neuroscience.2013.10.015

Henry, J. A., Roberts, L. E., Caspary, D. M., Theodoroff, S. M., and Salvi, R. J. (2014). Underlying mechanisms of tinnitus: review and clinical implications. *J. Am. Acad. Audiol.* 25, 5–22; quiz 126. doi: 10.3766/jaaa.25.1.2

Hinkley, L. B., Mizuiri, D., Hong, O., Nagarajan, S. S., and Cheung, S. W. (2015). Increased striatal functional connectivity with auditory cortex in tinnitus. *Front. Hum. Neurosci.* 9:568. doi: 10.3389/fnhum.2015.00568

Husain, F. T., and Schmidt, S. A. (2014). Using resting state functional connectivity to unravel networks of tinnitus. *Hear. Res.* 307, 153–162. doi: 10.1016/j.heares.2013.07.010

Jastreboff, P. J. (1990). Phantom auditory perception (tinnitus): mechanisms of generation and perception. *Neurosci. Res.* 8, 221–254. doi: 10.1016/0168-0102(90)90031-9

Jastreboff, P. J., Hazell, J. W., and Graham, R. L. (1994). Neurophysiological model of tinnitus: dependence of the minimal masking level on treatment outcome. *Hear. Res.* 80, 216–232. doi: 10.1016/0378-5955(94)90113-9

Kaltenbach, J. A., Zacharek, M. A., Zhang, J., and Frederick, S. (2004). Activity in the dorsal cochlear nucleus of hamsters previously tested for tinnitus following intense tone exposure. *Neurosci. Lett.* 355, 121–125. doi: 10.1016/j.neulet.2003.10.038

Kaltenbach, J. A., Zhang, J., and Finlayson, P. (2005). Tinnitus as a plastic phenomenon and its possible neural underpinnings in the dorsal cochlear nucleus. *Hear. Res.* 206, 200–226. doi: 10.1016/j.heares.2005.02.013

Kim, J.-Y., Kim, Y.-H., Lee, S., Seo, J.-H., Song, H.-J., Cho, J. H., et al. (2012). Alteration of functional connectivity in tinnitus brain revealed by resting-state fMRI?: a pilot study. *Int. J. Audiol.* 51, 413–417. doi: 10.3109/14992027.2011.652677

Kühn, S., and Gallinat, J. (2013). Resting-state brain activity in schizophrenia and major depression: a quantitative meta-analysis. *Schizophr. Bull.* 39, 358–365. doi: 10.1093/schbul/sbr151

Laird, A. R., Fox, P. M., Price, C. J., Glahn, D. C., Uecker, A. M., Lancaster, J. L., et al. (2005a). ALE meta-analysis: controlling the false discovery rate and performing statistical contrasts. *Hum. Brain Mapp.* 25, 155–164. doi: 10.1002/hbm.20136

Laird, A. R., McMillan, K. M., Lancaster, J. L., Kochunov, P., Turkeltaub, P. E., Pardo, J. V., et al. (2005b). A comparison of label-based review and ALE meta-analysis in the Stroop task. *Hum. Brain Mapp.* 25, 6–21. doi: 10.1002/hbm.20129

Lancaster, J. L., Tordesillas-Gutiérrez, D., Martinez, M., Salinas, F., Evans, A., Zilles, K., et al. (2007). Bias between MNI and Talairach coordinates analyzed using the ICBM-152 brain template. *Hum. Brain Mapp.* 28, 1194–1205. doi: 10.1002/hbm.20345

Landgrebe, M., Azevedo, A., Baguley, D., Bauer, C., Cacace, A., Coelho, C., et al. (2012). Methodological aspects of clinical trials in tinnitus: a proposal for an international standard. *J. Psychosom. Res.* 73, 112–121. doi: 10.1016/j.jpsychores.2012.05.002

Lanting, C. P., de Kleine, E., Langers, D. R., and van Dijk, P. (2014). Unilateral tinnitus: changes in connectivity and response lateralization measured with FMRI. *PLoS One* 9:e110704. doi: 10.1371/journal.pone.0110704

Laufs, H., Daunizeau, J., Carmichael, D. W., and Kleinschmidt, A. (2008). Recent advances in recording electrophysiological data simultaneously with magnetic resonance imaging. *Neuroimage* 40, 515–528. doi: 10.1016/j.neuroimage.2007.11.039

Laufs, H., Krakow, K., Sterzer, P., Eger, E., Beyerle, A., Salek-Haddadi, A., et al. (2003). Electroencephalographic signatures of attentional and cognitive default modes in spontaneous brain activity fluctuations at rest. *Proc. Natl. Acad. Sci. U S A* 100, 11053–11058. doi: 10.1073/pnas.1831638100

Laureano, M. R., Onishi, E. T., Bressan, R. A., Castiglioni, M. L. V., Batista, I. R., Reis, M. A., et al. (2014). Memory networks in tinnitus: a functional brain image study. *PLoS One* 9:e87839. doi: 10.1371/journal.pone.0087839

Leaver, A. M., Renier, L., Chevillet, M. A., Morgan, S., Kim, H. J., and Rauschecker, J. P. (2011). Dysregulation of limbic and auditory networks in tinnitus. *Neuron* 69, 33–43. doi: 10.1016/j.neuron.2010.12.002

Leaver, A. M., Seydell-Greenwald, A., and Rauschecker, J. P. (2016a). Auditory-limbic interactions in chronic tinnitus: challenges for neuroimaging research. *Hear. Res.* 334, 49–57. doi: 10.1016/j.heares.2015.08.005

Leaver, A. M., Turesky, T. K., Seydell-Greenwald, A., Morgan, S., Kim, H. J., and Rauschecker, J. P. (2016b). Intrinsic network activity in tinnitus investigated using functional MRI. *Hum. Brain Mapp.* 37, 2717–2735. doi: 10.1002/hbm.23204

Li, H., Chan, R. C., McAlonan, G. M., and Gong, Q. Y. (2010). Facial emotion processing in schizophrenia: a meta-analysis of functional neuroimaging data. *Schizophr. Bull.* 36, 1029–1039. doi: 10.1093/schbul/sbn190

Li, J., Zhang, Z., and Shang, H. (2012). A meta-analysis of voxel-based morphometry studies on unilateral refractory temporal lobe epilepsy. *Epilepsy Res.* 98, 97–103. doi: 10.1016/j.eplepsyres.2011.10.002

Llinás, R. R., Ribary, U., Jeanmonod, D., Kronberg, E., and Mitra, P. P. (1999). Thalamocortical dysrhythmia: a neurological and neuropsychiatric syndrome characterized by magnetoencephalography. *Proc. Natl. Acad. Sci. U S A* 96, 15222–15227. doi: 10.1073/pnas.96.26.15222

Lockwood, A. H., Salvi, R. J., Coad, M. L., Towsley, M. L., Wack, D. S., and Murphy, B. W. (1998). The functional neuroanatomy of tinnitus: evidence for limbic system links and neural plasticity. *Neurology* 50, 114–120. doi: 10.1212/WNL.50.1.114

Logothetis, N. K., Murayama, Y., Augath, M., Steffen, T., Werner, J., and Oeltermann, A. (2009). How not to study spontaneous activity. *Neuroimage* 45, 1080–1089. doi: 10.1016/j.neuroimage.2009.01.010

van der Loo, E., Congedo, M., Vanneste, S., Van De Heyning, P., and De Ridder, D. (2011). Insular lateralization in tinnitus distress. *Auton. Neurosci.* 165, 191–194. doi: 10.1016/j.autneu.2011.06.007

Mantini, D., Perrucci, M. G., Del Gratta, C., Romani, G. L., and Corbetta, M. (2007). Electrophysiological signatures of resting state networks in the human brain. *Proc. Natl. Acad. Sci. U S A* 104, 13170–13175. doi: 10.1073/pnas.0700668104

Mathiak, K., Menning, H., Hertrich, I., Mathiak, K. A., Zvyagintsev, M., and Ackermann, H. (2007). Who is telling what from where? A functional magnetic resonance imaging study. *Neuroreport* 18, 405–409. doi: 10.1097/WNR.0b013e328013cec4

Maudoux, A., Lefebvre, P., Cabay, J.-E., Demertzi, A., Vanhaudenhuyse, A., Laureys, S., et al. (2012a). Auditory resting-state network connectivity in tinnitus: a functional MRI study. *PLoS One* 7:e36222. doi: 10.1371/journal.pone.0036222

Maudoux, A., Lefebvre, P., Cabay, J. E., Demertzi, A., Vanhaudenhuyse, A., Laureys, S., et al. (2012b). Connectivity graph analysis of the auditory resting state network in tinnitus. *Brain Res.* 1485, 10–21. doi: 10.1016/j.brainres.2012.05.006

Melcher, J. R., Knudson, I. M., and Levine, R. A. (2013). Subcallosal brain structure: correlation with hearing threshold at supra-clinical frequencies (>8 kHz), but not with tinnitus. *Hear. Res.* 295, 79–86. doi: 10.1016/j.heares.2012.03.013

Melloni, L., Molina, C., Pena, M., Torres, D., Singer, W., and Rodriguez, E. (2007). Synchronization of neural activity across cortical areas correlates with conscious perception. *J. Neurosci.* 27, 2858–2865. doi: 10.1523/JNEUROSCI.4623-06.2007

Minami, S. B., Oishi, N., Watabe, T., Uno, K., Kaga, K., and Ogawa, K. (2015). Auditory resting-state functional connectivity in tinnitus and modulation with transcranial direct current stimulation. *Acta Otolaryngol.* 135, 1286–1292. doi: 10.3109/00016489.2015.1068952

Mirz, F., Gjedde, A., Ishizu, K., and Pedersen, C. B. (2000). Cortical networks subserving the perception of tinnitus–a PET study. *Acta Otolaryngol. Suppl.* 543, 241–243. doi: 10.1080/000164800454503

Moazami-Goudarzi, M., Michels, L., Weisz, N., and Jeanmonod, D. (2010). Temporo-insular enhancement of EEG low and high frequencies in patients with chronic tinnitus. QEEG study of chronic tinnitus patients. *BMC Neurosci.* 11:40. doi: 10.1186/1471-2202-11-40

Mühlau, M., Rauschecker, J. P., Oestreicher, E., Gaser, C., Röttinger, M., Wohlschlager, A. M., et al. (2006). Structural brain changes in tinnitus. *Cereb. Cortex* 16, 1283–1288. doi: 10.1093/cercor/bhj070

Musso, F., Brinkmeyer, J., Mobascher, A., Warbrick, T., and Winterer, G. (2010). Spontaneous brain activity and EEG microstates. A novel EEG/fMRI analysis approach to explore resting-state networks. *Neuroimage* 52, 1149–1161. doi: 10.1016/j.neuroimage.2010.01.093

Perrachione, T. K., and Ghosh, S. S. (2013). Optimized design and analysis of sparse-sampling FMRI experiments. *Front. Neurosci.* 7:55. doi: 10.3389/fnins.2013.00055

Petacchi, A., Laird, A. R., Fox, P. T., and Bower, J. M. (2005). Cerebellum and auditory function: an ALE meta-analysis of functional neuroimaging studies. *Hum. Brain Mapp.* 25, 118–128. doi: 10.1002/hbm.20137

Radua, J., Mataix-Cols, D., Phillips, M., El-Hage, W., Kronhaus, D., Cardoner, N., et al. (2012). A new meta-analytic method for neuroimaging studies that combines reported peak coordinates and statistical parametric maps. *Eur. Psychiatry* 27, 605–611. doi: 10.1016/j.eurpsy.2011.04.001

Raichle, M. E., MacLeod, A. M., Snyder, A. Z., Powers, W. J., Gusnard, D. A., and Shulman, G. L. (2001). A default mode of brain function. *Proc. Natl. Acad. Sci. U S A* 98, 676–682. doi: 10.1073/pnas.98.2.676

Rauschecker, J. P., Leaver, A. M., and Mühlau, M. (2010). Tuning out the noise: limbic-auditory interactions in tinnitus. *Neuron* 66, 819–826. doi: 10.1016/j.neuron.2010.04.032

Rauschecker, J. P., May, E. S., Maudoux, A., and Ploner, M. (2015). Frontostriatal gating of tinnitus and chronic pain. *Trends Cogn. Sci.* 19, 567–578. doi: 10.1016/j.tics.2015.08.002

Richardson, B. D., Brozoski, T. J., Ling, L. L., and Caspary, D. M. (2012). Targeting inhibitory neurotransmission in tinnitus. *Brain Res.* 1485, 77–87. doi: 10.1016/j.brainres.2012.02.014

De Ridder, D., Elgoyhen, A. B., Romo, R., and Langguth, B. (2011). Phantom percepts: tinnitus and pain as persisting aversive memory networks. *Proc. Natl. Acad. Sci. U S A* 108, 8075–8080. doi: 10.1073/pnas.1018466108

De Ridder, D., Vanneste, S., and Freeman, W. (2014a). The Bayesian brain: phantom percepts resolve sensory uncertainty. *Neurosci. Biobehav. Rev.* 44, 4–15. doi: 10.1016/j.neubiorev.2012.04.001

De Ridder, D., Vanneste, S., Weisz, N., Londero, A., Schlee, W., Elgoyhen, A. B., et al. (2014b). An integrative model of auditory phantom perception: tinnitus as a unified percept of interacting separable subnetworks. *Neurosci. Biobehav. Rev.* 44, 16–32. doi: 10.1016/j.neubiorev.2013.03.021

Schaette, R., and McAlpine, D. (2011). Tinnitus with a normal audiogram: physiological evidence for hidden hearing loss and computational model. *J. Neurosci.* 31, 13452–13457. doi: 10.1523/JNEUROSCI.2156-11.2011

Schecklmann, M., Landgrebe, M., Langguth, B., and TRI Database Study Group. (2014). Phenotypic characteristics of hyperacusis in tinnitus. *PLoS One* 9:e86944. doi: 10.1371/journal.pone.0086944

Schecklmann, M., Landgrebe, M., Poeppl, T. B., Kreuzer, P., Männer, P., Marienhagen, J., et al. (2013). Neural correlates of tinnitus duration and distress: a positron emission tomography study. *Hum. Brain Mapp.* 34, 233–240. doi: 10.1002/hbm.21426

Schmidt, S. A., Akrofi, K., Carpenter-Thompson, J. R., and Husain, F. T. (2013). Default mode, dorsal attention and auditory resting state networks exhibit differential functional connectivity in tinnitus and hearing loss. *PLoS One* 8:e76488. doi: 10.1371/journal.pone.0076488

Sedley, W., Friston, K. J., Gander, P. E., Kumar, S., and Griffiths, T. D. (2016). An integrative tinnitus model based on sensory precision. *Trends Neurosci.* 39, 799–812. doi: 10.1016/j.tins.2016.10.004

Seki, S., and Eggermont, J. J. (2003). Changes in spontaneous firing rate and neural synchrony in cat primary auditory cortex after localized tone-induced hearing loss. *Hear. Res.* 180, 28–38. doi: 10.1016/s0378-5955(03)00074-1

Shao, N., Yang, J., and Shang, H. (2015). Voxelwise meta-analysis of gray matter anomalies in Parkinson variant of multiple system atrophy and Parkinson's disease using anatomic likelihood estimation. *Neurosci. Lett.* 587, 79–86. doi: 10.1016/j.neulet.2014.12.007

Shargorodsky, J., Curhan, G. C., and Farwell, W. R. (2010). Prevalence and characteristics of tinnitus among US adults. *Am. J. Med.* 123, 711–718. doi: 10.1016/j.amjmed.2010.02.015

Shulman, G. L., Astafiev, S. V., Franke, D., Pope, D. L., Snyder, A. Z., McAvoy, M. P., et al. (2009). Interaction of stimulus-driven reorienting and expectation in ventral and dorsal frontoparietal and basal ganglia-cortical networks. *J. Neurosci.* 29, 4392–4407. doi: 10.1523/JNEUROSCI.5609-08.2009

Song, J. J., De Ridder, D., Van de Heyning, P., and Vanneste, S. (2012). Mapping tinnitus-related brain activation: an activation-likelihood estimation metaanalysis of PET studies. *J. Nucl. Med.* 53, 1550–1557. doi: 10.2967/jnumed.112.102939

Sridharan, D., Levitin, D. J., and Menon, V. (2008). A critical role for the right fronto-insular cortex in switching between central-executive and default-mode networks. *Proc. Natl. Acad. Sci. U S A* 105, 12569–12574. doi: 10.1073/pnas.0800005105

Stroup, D. F., Berlin, J. A., Morton, S. C., Olkin, I., Williamson, G. D., Rennie, D., et al. (2000). Meta-analysis of observational studies in epidemiology: a proposal for reporting. *JAMA* 283, 2008–2012. doi: 10.1001/jama.283.15.2008

Tagliazucchi, E., von Wegner, F., Morzelewski, A., Brodbeck, V., and Laufs, H. (2012). Dynamic BOLD functional connectivity in humans and its electrophysiological correlates. *Front. Hum. Neurosci.* 6:339. doi: 10.3389/fnhum.2012.00339

Turkeltaub, P. E., Eden, G. F., Jones, K. M., and Zeffiro, T. A. (2002). Meta-analysis of the functional neuroanatomy of single-word reading: method and validation. *Neuroimage* 16, 765–780. doi: 10.1006/nimg.2002.1131

Turkeltaub, P. E., Eickhoff, S. B., Laird, A. R., Fox, M., Wiener, M., and Fox, P. (2012). Minimizing within-experiment and within-group effects in Activation Likelihood Estimation meta-analyses. *Hum. Brain Mapp.* 33, 1–13. doi: 10.1002/hbm.21186

Ueyama, T., Donishi, T., Ukai, S., Ikeda, Y., Hotomi, M., Yamanaka, N., et al. (2013). Brain regions responsible for tinnitus distress and loudness: a resting-state fMRI study. *PLoS One* 8:e67778. doi: 10.1371/journal.pone.0067778

Ueyama, T., Donishi, T., Ukai, S., Yamamoto, Y., Ishida, T., Tamagawa, S., et al. (2015). Alterations of regional cerebral blood flow in tinnitus patients as assessed using single-photon emission computed tomography. *PLoS One* 10:e0137291. doi: 10.1371/journal.pone.0137291

Vanneste, S., and De Ridder, D. (2012). The auditory and non-auditory brain areas involved in tinnitus. An emergent property of multiple parallel overlapping subnetworks. *Front. Syst. Neurosci.* 6:31. doi: 10.3389/fnsys.2012.00031

Vanneste, S., and De Ridder, D. (2016). Deafferentation-based pathophysiological differences in phantom sound: tinnitus with and without hearing loss. *Neuroimage* 129, 80–94. doi: 10.1016/j.neuroimage.2015.12.002

Vanneste, S., Plazier, M., der Loo, E., de Heyning, P. V., Congedo, M., and De Ridder, D. (2010a). The neural correlates of tinnitus-related distress. *Neuroimage* 52, 470–480. doi: 10.1016/j.neuroimage.2010.04.029

Vanneste, S., Plazier, M., van der Loo, E., Van de Heyning, P., and De Ridder, D. (2010b). The differences in brain activity between narrow band noise and pure tone tinnitus. *PLoS One* 5:e13618. doi: 10.1371/journal.pone.0013618

Vanneste, S., Plazier, M., van der Loo, E., Van de Heyning, P., and De Ridder, D. (2011a). The difference between uni- and bilateral auditory phantom percept. *Clin. Neurophysiol.* 122, 578–587. doi: 10.1016/j.clinph.2010.07.022

Vanneste, S., van de Heyning, P., and De Ridder, D. (2011b). The neural network of phantom sound changes over time: a comparison between recent-onset and chronic tinnitus patients. *Eur. J. Neurosci.* 34, 718–731. doi: 10.1111/j.1460-9568.2011.07793.x

Wager, T. D., Jonides, J., and Reading, S. (2004). Neuroimaging studies of shifting attention: a meta-analysis. *Neuroimage* 22, 1679–1693. doi: 10.1016/j.neuroimage.2004.03.052

Weng, H.-H., Chen, C.-F., Tsai, Y.-H., Wu, C.-Y., Lee, M., Lin, Y.-C., et al. (2015). Gray matter atrophy in narcolepsy: an activation likelihood estimation meta-analysis. *Neurosci. Biobehav. Rev.* 59, 53–63. doi: 10.1016/j.neubiorev.2015.03.009

Wineland, A. M., Burton, H., and Piccirillo, J. (2012). Functional connectivity networks in nonbothersome tinnitus. *Otolaryngol. Head Neck Surg.* 147, 900–906. doi: 10.1177/0194599812451414

Yang, H., Zheng, Y., Ou, Y., and Huang, X. (2014). Regional homogeneity on resting state fMRI in patients with tinnitus. *J. Otol.* 9, 173–178. doi: 10.1016/j.joto.2014.10.001

Zhang, J., Chen, Y. C., Feng, X., Yang, M., Liu, B., Qian, C., et al. (2015). Impairments of thalamic resting-state functional connectivity in patients with chronic tinnitus. *Eur. J. Radiol.* 84, 1277–1284. doi: 10.1016/j.ejrad.2015.04.006

17

Different Teams, Same Conclusions? A Systematic Review of Existing Clinical Guidelines for the Assessment and Treatment of Tinnitus in Adults

Thomas E. Fuller[1,2*†], Haula F. Haider[3†], Dimitris Kikidis[4], Alec Lapira[5], Birgit Mazurek[6], Arnaud Norena[7], Sarah Rabau[8], Rachelle Lardinois[2], Christopher R. Cederroth[9], Niklas K. Edvall[9], Petra G. Brueggemann[6], Susanne N. Rosing[10], Anestis Kapandais[11], Dorte Lungaard[10], Derek J. Hoare[12] and Rilana F. F Cima[1,2]

[1] Clinical Psychological Science, Faculty of Psychology and Neuroscience, Maastricht University, Maastricht, Netherlands, [2] Adelante, Centre of Expertise in Rehabilitation and Audiology, Hoensbroek, Netherlands, [3] ENT Department of Hospital, Cuf Infante Santo - Nova Medical School, Lisbon, Portugal, [4] Department of Otorhinolaryngology, Head and Neck Surgery, National and Kapodistrian University of Athens, Hippocrateion General Hospital, Athens, Greece, [5] ENT Specialist, Institute of Health Care, Mater Dei Hospital, Malta, Malta, [6] Tinnitus Center, Charite University Hospital, Berlin, Germany, [7] Laboratory of Adaptive and Integrative Neuroscience, Centre National de la Recherche Scientifique, Fédération de Recherche, Aix-Marseille Université, Marseille, France, [8] Faculty of Medicine and Health Sciences, Campus Drie Eiken, University of Antwerp, Antwerp, Belgium, [9] Department of Physiology and Pharmacology, Karolinska Institutet, Stockholm, Sweden, [10] Department of Clinical Research, Faculty of Health Sciences, University of Southern Denmark, Odense, Denmark, [11] Department of Nordic Studies and Linguistics, Copenhagen University, Denmark, [12] NIHR Nottingham Hearing Biomedical Research Unit, Division of Clinical Neuroscience, School of Medicine, University of Nottingham, Nottingham, UK

Correspondence:
Thomas E. Fuller
thomas.fuller@maastrichtuniversity.nl

† These authors have contributed equally to this work.

Background: Though clinical guidelines for assessment and treatment of chronic subjective tinnitus do exist, a comprehensive review of those guidelines has not been performed. The objective of this review was to identify current clinical guidelines, and compare their recommendations for the assessment and treatment of subjective tinnitus in adults.

Method: We systematically searched a range of sources for clinical guidelines (as defined by the Institute of Medicine, United States) for the assessment and/or treatment of subjective tinnitus in adults. No restrictions on language or year of publication were applied to guidelines.

Results: Clinical guidelines from Denmark, Germany, Sweden, The Netherlands, and the United States were included in the review. There was a high level of consistency across the guidelines with regard to recommendations for audiometric assessment, physical examination, use of a validated questionnaire(s) to assess tinnitus related distress, and referral to a psychologist when required. Cognitive behavioral treatment for tinnitus related distress, use of hearing aids in instances of hearing loss and recommendations against the use of medicines were consistent across the included guidelines. Differences between the guidelines centered on the use of imaging in assessment procedures and sound therapy as a form of treatment for tinnitus distress respectively.

Conclusion: Given the level of commonality across tinnitus guidelines from different countries the development of a European guideline for the assessment and treatment of subjective tinnitus in adults seems feasible. This guideline would have the potential to benefit the large number of clinicians in countries where clinical guidelines do not yet exist, and would support standardization of treatment for patients across Europe.

Keywords: tinnitus, clinical guidelines, assessment, treatment, systematic review

INTRODUCTION

Tinnitus is essentially made up of two components, the phantom perception of a sound in the ears or head, and the degree of emotional reaction to that percept. Tinnitus can co-occur with several medical-otological disorders such as presbycusis, though etiology is unknown for the majority of tinnitus patients (Baguley et al., 2013b). In rare cases tinnitus indicates a serious underlying pathology such as vascular troubles, vestibular schwannoma (VS), or otosclerosis (Baguley et al., 2013a). In most cases however subjective tinnitus is a benign symptom. In many patients co-morbidities exist such as anxiety, depression, insomnia, and concentration problems, all of which severely impair quality of life (Langguth et al., 2011). In 1–3% of cases tinnitus causes severe health problems, with a wide range of effects on daily life functioning (Davis and Refaie, 2000; Fujii et al., 2011; Kim et al., 2015). Evidence corroborates that the aversive psychological reactions, such as cognitive problems, negative emotions, and dysfunctional attentional processes are of main importance in leading to a severe tinnitus condition (Erlandsson and Hallberg, 2000; Andersson et al., 2006; Cima et al., 2011; Kleinstauber et al., 2013; McKenna et al., 2014; Handscomb et al., 2017).

During the last decades, efforts have been made to better understand tinnitus pathophysiology and provide specialized treatments to patients (Kamalski et al., 2010; Cima et al., 2012; Langguth et al., 2013; Hoekstra et al., 2014). A large number of management strategies including various assessment and treatment procedures exist and have evolved but lack empirical support. For example, there is no evidenced treatment or licensed pharmacological therapy to eliminate the tinnitus percept (Langguth and Elgoyhen, 2012). The Cochrane Library lists 10 completed systematic reviews on different tinnitus treatments, all of which reported small numbers of studies of variable quality (e.g., Martinez-Devesa et al., 2010). These facts combined makes it difficult for healthcare professionals to decide what is best for which tinnitus patient. This is evidenced by the discrepancy between scientific and clinical perspectives on the management of tinnitus and the *actual* day-to-day practice in European healthcare settings (Hoare et al., 2012); tinnitus patient care is fragmented and *ad hoc* (Hoare and Hall, 2011; Hoare et al., 2012). To date there has been no overview of the number of existing clinical practice guidelines for tinnitus, the details included, their comparability, or their purpose. Clinical practice guidelines are defined as systematically developed statements to assist practitioner and patient decisions about appropriate health care for specific clinical circumstances (Field and Lohr, 1990). They have the benefit of simplifying and standardizing assessment and treatment options for clinicians and patients. A European Union guideline would extend this benefit to 28 countries. This systematic review aims to identify, review, and examine the clinical guidelines which do exist for tinnitus. The tinnitus assessments (diagnostics and measures), processes, and treatment options recommended by the respective guidelines will be compared and summarized.

METHODS

The aims, the work plan, and the protocol for this systematic review were developed by TINNET Working Group 1, a COST Action BM1306 (2014–2018) to create a pan-European tinnitus research network (http://tinnet.tinnitusresearch.net/). This review was registered with PROSPERO, the international register of systematic reviews (protocol number: CRD42016038588) prior to commencing the literature search. The review was exempt from human ethics procedures as there were no human participants and only secondary sources of data (the clinical guidelines) were used.

Eligibility Criteria

Records were considered eligible for inclusion if they fit the definition of a guideline by describing and making recommendations on the assessment, diagnosis, and or treatment of subjective tinnitus for adults (i.e., people aged 16 years or older). Those records were required to identify or describe themselves as guidelines, and be the most recent guideline form the country of origin. No publication date or language restrictions were imposed on the eligibility of the guidelines.

Guidelines were excluded if they were for objective tinnitus, pediatrics, referred only to the triage or referral pathways for assessing and treating tinnitus, or if they were a guide for only one specific type of assessment or treatment procedure for tinnitus.

Literature Search

The literature search for clinical guidelines included the Medline, PubMed, and the Cumulative Index to Nursing and Allied Health Literature (CINAHL), and EMBASE databases. In addition to these the National Guideline Clearinghouse (www.guideline.gov), National Institute for Health and Clinical Excellence (NICE; https://www.nice.org.uk/), Guideline International Network (GIN; http://www.g-i-n.net/), Google, and hand-search of reference lists of any included guidelines was undertaken. International experts were also contacted to ask if they were aware of any guidelines that had not already been identified from the search results. The date that the search for guidelines was first conducted was 2 May 2016 and was undertaken by TEF and HH using "tinnitus" and "guideline" as the two key terms. The final search was conducted on 24 June 2016.

Study Selection

Two reviewers independently screened search results by title and abstract, and then by full text if required. The first 20 pages of search results from Google, and all search results from GIN, NICE, and the National Guideline Clearinghouse were screened. In the event of disagreements, a third reviewer (BM) acted as an arbiter. As an additional check and in line with other systemic review searches using internet search engines, a *post-hoc* rule of stopping searching after three consecutive pages without new search results was applied. In this case, no new search results were identified after the first eight pages.

Data Extraction

Data extraction was undertaken using a tailored form that had been pilot tested and was emailed to reviewers in the form of an Excel spreadsheet. A document with guidance on the extraction of information for each of the items was provided to each of the reviewers to improve consistency of data extraction. Data extraction from each guideline was undertaken by at least two reviewers who were native speakers of or fluent in the language in which the guideline was published. Reviewers extracted information from the guidelines regarding items about the: country and year of publication, availability, author details, sponsor/funder involved, scope, target audience, developers and process related to the guideline, recommendations for assessment and treatment procedures, the level of evidence and type of rating system used (e.g., Oxford) related to the recommendations, and items related to the implementation and revision of the guideline.

Data Management

HH and TEF were responsible for data management and maintained editorial rights. All identified records were saved into a Microsoft word master file and then saved in pdf-copy.

Quality Assessment and Risk of Bias

All reviewers of the guidelines also completed the AGREE II tool (Brouwers et al., 2010) to assess the quality of the guidelines. AGREE II is an international tool to assess the quality and reporting of practice guidelines (www.agreetrust.org). It contains 23 items grouped under six guideline domains. Each item is scored on a 1–7 scale where 1 = "Strongly disagree" and 7 = "Strongly agree." Scores are standardized to provide an overall percentage score. Previous reviews have used a 60% marker to distinguish high and low quality guidelines (Sanclemente et al., 2014; Ruszczynski et al., 2016).

Details relating to the sources of funding, professional affiliations, and editorial independence of the guideline developers were extracted as indicative of risk of bias.

Data Synthesis

Data extracted by the reviewers were collated and integrated into summary tables and a narrative synthesis describing the similarities and differences between the clinical practice guidelines was completed.

RESULTS

Five clinical guidelines for tinnitus were ultimately included in this review (see **Figure 1** for details of the search and selection process). They were guidelines from Denmark (Jørgensen et al., 2007), Germany (The Association of the Scientific Medical Societies, 2015), The Netherlands (Dutch Association for Ear Nose Throat and Head surgery [Nederlandse Vereniging voor Keel – Neus – Oor heel kunde en Heelkunde van het Hoofd – Halsgebied], in press), Sweden (Idrizbegovic et al., 2011), and United States (Tunkel et al., 2014). Several documents were excluded as by definition not providing a guideline. For example, the Australian audiology clinical practice standards (Audiology Australia, 2013) underwent full-text screening but was not included as it only related to audiological management and had a brief section on tinnitus assessment. The UK Good Practice Guide (Department of Health, 2009) also was excluded as it explicitly states: "This Good Practice Guide to the delivery of services is not, and does not aim to be, an evidence-based guideline for clinical practice with individual patients" (p. 5). The Tinnitus Research Initiative (TRI) algorithm (Biesinger et al., 2010), after some debate within the review team, was also excluded because it was judged not to be a "clinical guideline." A list of full text documents considered but excluded is in Appendix 1.

Although there was not a restricting time period for the guidelines, no guidelines older than 10 years were identified. With exception of the Danish guideline (published in 2007) all were developed during the last 5 years.

Details about Development of the Clinical Guidelines

Table 1 provides detailed information about the stakeholder involvement, rigor of development, and the editorial independence associated with the respective clinical guidelines.

All the guidelines included information on the professional backgrounds of the participants in the respective development groups and in three out of the five cases (American, Dutch, and German), provided information on how views of funding bodies and competing interests were addressed. Although patient groups and the public were consulted in the development of three guidelines (American, Dutch, and German), the actual expected users of the guidelines were health professionals.

Details were provided in all guidelines (with the exception of those from Sweden which did not provide methodological information) about how literature was located and used to inform the respective recommendations. That is, details of search strategies using MeSH and other search terms and databases such as Medline and PsychInfo were included. Tools and criteria used to assess the evidence included the: Oxford Centre for Evidence Based Medicine (U.S. and German guidelines) and American Academy of Paediatrics' (American guideline) evidence criteria respectively, the AMSTAR checklist (Dutch guideline), and

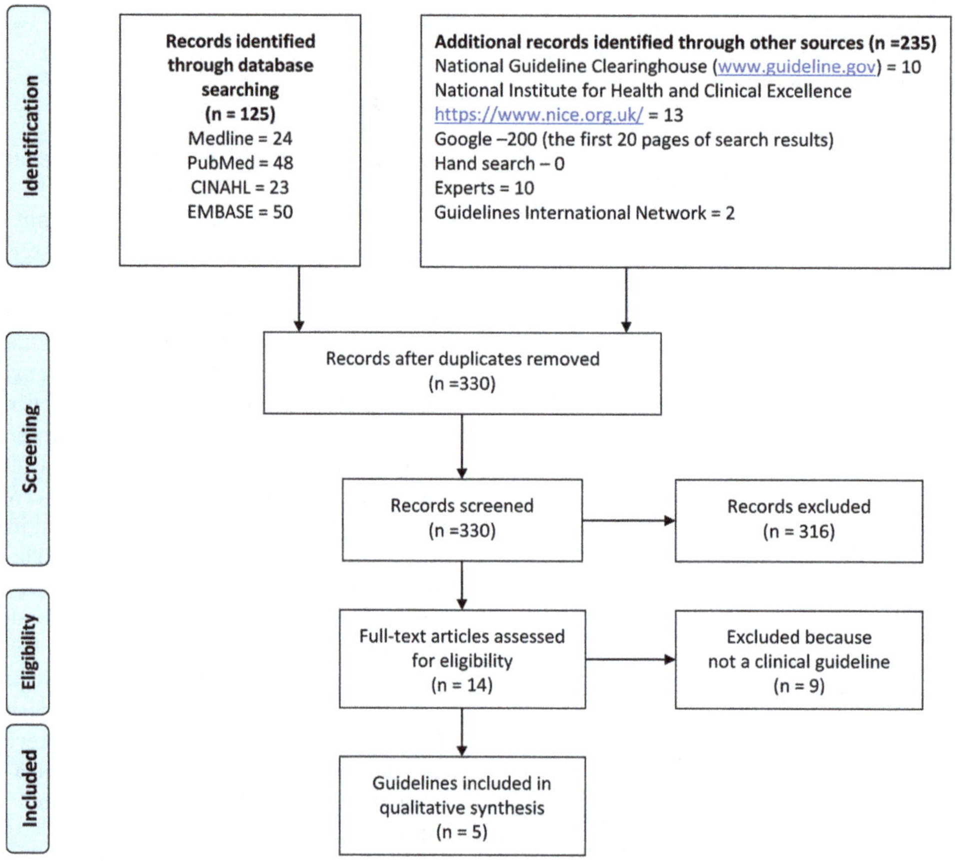

FIGURE 1 | PRISMA flowchart showing the stages of guideline search, screening and inclusion.

the GRADE ranking system of trust in conclusions of the literature (Dutch guideline). American, Danish, Dutch and German guidelines all provided information and referred to the research literature associated with each recommendation as well as describing their methods for reaching consensus on each recommendation. The Dutch, German and U.S. guidelines consider the strengths and limitations of the research literature and were reviewed externally prior to publication. Similarly, those three guidelines also state a year by and/or describe conditions under which they would be revised.

Assessment Recommendations in the Clinical Guidelines

Table 2 compares assessment recommendations between the respective national tinnitus guidelines. All guidelines, except the Danish, recommend a clinical history (anamnesis/targeted history/special tinnitus anamnesis) be taken.

All guidelines describe the need for physical examination by an ENT doctor, although physical examination is not explicitly referred to in the Swedish guideline. The American guideline recommends examination to exclude objective tinnitus, cardiovascular disease and vascular lesions, neurologic diseases, middle or outer ear infection/disease, vertigo, head-neck masses, or other treatable conditions. The German guideline additionally mentions cervical, dental, and temporomandibular joint functional exploration in a silent environment to evaluate tinnitus modulation.

Audiological assessment was recommended in all the included guidelines. The majority refers to audiometry as a general category, but the German guideline provides most detail. For example, it specifies details relating to the assessment of oto-acoustic measurements, brainstem auditory evoked responses, caloric tests, determination of tinnitus loudness and frequency using narrow-band noise and pure tones, residual inhibition, Feldmann masking curves (Feldmann, 1984), and loudness discomfort level. None of the other guidelines included in this review recommend psychoacoustic measurements of tinnitus frequency or intensity.

The German guideline does not refer to specific psychological assessments though the other guidelines do in varying terms. For example, when tinnitus is severe or accompanied by psychological factors, the Swedish guideline recommends psychological assessment while the Danish guideline recommends a structured interview. The American guideline on the other hand recommends that clinicians distinguish between patients with or without bothersome tinnitus for subsequent referral (when necessary) to a psychologist or psychiatrist.

TABLE 1 | Summary of guideline development by country.

Country	Professionals involved	Views of patients considered	Target users	Views of funding body	Competing interests
Germany	Audiologists, psychiatrist, psychologists, otolaryngologists, dentists, pediatricians, neurologists, and patient representative groups	Patient representative groups were included in the guideline development group; contributed to external review on draft documents, and patient related information was also considered from the results of a literature review	Physicians (especially ENT), phoniatry and pediatric audiology, psychiatry, psychosomatic, neurology, mouth, jaw, and facial surgeons and dentists, psychologists, general practitioners	A statement concerning financial and other interests and editorial independence is included.	Competing interests are declared and when relevant, stakeholders with competing interests were excluded
Denmark	Speech Pathologist and hearing therapists	NS	Hearing therapists	NS	NS
Netherlands	Details provided. ENT-doctors, psychologist, clinical physicist-audiologist	Dutch Association of the Hearing Impaired consulted. A literature review regarding patient preferences was also conducted	ENT doctors, audiology centers, GP's, psychologists, psychiatrists	A statement of independence was signed by professionals involved	Competing interests are declared
USA	Paediatric and adult otolaryngologists, otologists/neurotologists, geriatrician, behavioral neuroscientist, neurologist, audiologist, family physician, radiologist, psychiatrist, psycho-acoustician, nurse, physician, and consumer advocates	Yes: also included a draft of the guideline being made available for public comment	Any clinician, health care provider, specialty physicians, and non-physician providers such as audiologists and mental health professionals	Funded by American Academy of Otolaryngology—Head and Neck Surgery Foundation but no statement of independence from the process	Competing interests are declared
Sweden	Partial details provided—included medical doctors, and professional representatives from the tinnitus teams for diagnostics and rehabilitation	NS	Staff at the audiology and balance clinic at Karolinska University Hospital and professionals that might refer to the clinic (GPs, ENTs or audiologist)	NS	NS

(Continued)

TABLE 1 | Continued

Country	Methods used	Evidence criteria	Category of evidence*	Strengths and limitations	Methods for reaching consensus	Consequences of the recommendations	Link between evidence and recommendations	Peer review?	Update of the guidelines?
Germany	Systematic methods used, details provided in the guideline	Classified according to Oxford Centre of Evidence-based Medicine criteria	1a	Strengths and limitations of the body of evidence are clearly described	Formal consensus technique	The guideline includes health benefits, side effects and risks formulating the recommendations	There is an clear link between the recommendations and the supporting evidence	External review	Due in 2020.
Denmark	Systematic methods used, details provided in the guideline	NS	The guidelines are based on literature, and articles based on the consensus of leading professionals in the field of audiology (evidence level IV)	NS	Informal consensus. All recommendations are based on the ICF model	NS	Each recommendation is provided with an argument based on relevant literature	Not peer reviewed	NS
Netherlands	Systematic methods used, details provided in the guideline	Based on AMSTAR checklist	1a, 1b, IV	The strength of the evidence is specified according to GRADE. Evidence tables describe limitations and strengths of the included studies	Recommendations were evidence based and the importance the workgroup gave to them conforms to GRADE	Recommendations were made considering the scientific value, preferences of the patient, costs, and availability of the organization	There is a clear link between the recommendations and the supporting evidence	External review	Update due in 2020 or sooner if new compelling evidence warrants earlier consideration
USA	Systematic methods used, details provided in the guideline	Based on criteria from the Oxford Centre for Evidence-Based Medicine	American Academy of Pediatrics Categories of evidence (A, B, C, D, and X) updated to be in accordance with Oxford Centre for Evidence-Based Medicine	Strengths and limitations of the body of evidence are clearly described	This guideline was developed using an explicit and transparent a priori protocol for creating actionable statements based on supporting evidence and the associated balance of benefit and harm	The benefits and harms of the recommendations have been considered for each recommendation.	There is an clear link between the recommendations and the supporting evidence	External review	Update due in 2018/9 or sooner if new compelling evidence warrants earlier consideration
Sweden	No method reported	No evidence criteria	No evidence provided	None provided.	NS	NS	NS	NS	NS

**Unless stated, the level of evidence refers to/uses the Oxford Centre for Evidence Based Medicine criteria (GRADE system consists of 4 grades of degree of trust in conclusions of the literature: high, moderate, low, and very low) NS, not specified; ENT, Ear Nose Throat; GP, General Practitioner.*

TABLE 2 | Clinical guideline recommendations regarding assessment of patients with tinnitus.

Guideline	Physical examination	Hearing and audiology tests	Psychological assessment	Assessment tools/questionnaires recommended	Other assessment procedures	Procedures not recommended
Germany	Orientating neurological assessment of cervical spine, vestibular is with examination of denture (including TMJ) in silence to screen modulation of tinnitus • Orientating examination of functioning of N. facialis • ENT examination including tympanic membrane microscopy, asopharyngoscopy and eustachian respectively • stethoscopic examination of the ear and of the carotid artery, particularly in pulsatile tinnitus	• Pure tone audiometry • discomfort, possibly with categorical loudness scaling • determining of tinnitus loudness and frequency using narrow-band noise and pure tones • residual inhibition • determining the minimum masking level by white noise and pure tones; masking curves according to Feldmann • tympanometry and acoustic reflex including recording possible changes due to breathing or heart rate • TEOAE and/or DPOAE • brainstem auditory evoked response (BAER) • preliminary vestibular examination possibly including caloric testing • Brainstem audiometry (BERA) when medically justified, economically viable and likely to be useful in informing counseling might be of potential benefit	NS	• Goebel-Hiller Tinnitus Questionnaire, • VAS or other validated scales	• Special tinnitus anamnesis (see Structured Tinnitus Interview (Goebel and Hiller, 2001) • X-rays of the cervical spine, if further indicated also functional images	• Acoustic examination with more than 84 dB 1 week after acute tinnitus or tinnitus exacerbation
Denmark	NS	• Audiometry (performed by ENTs) • LDL/UCL • If necessary also: ABR	• Structured interview	• THI-DK • VAS-scale for hyperacusis • Tværfaglig Tinnitus Screening (Danish tool assessing signs of anxiety)	If necessary also: • ABR, • CT/MRI, • blood samples, • other neurological tests	NS
Netherlands	• Anamnesis, • ENT-assessment inclusive otoscopy and tuning fork tests, • Blood pressure measurement, • Flexible nasofaryngoscopy, • Palpation of neck and area around ear	• Audiometry (Air and bone conduction) • Speech audiometry	• Detailed assessment regarding the nature how tinnitus impacts on daily life and functioning, comorbid symptoms	• TQ, mini-TQ • THI • TFI • THQ • HADS	• MRI/MRA, • CT, • DSA (angiography)	• Not to use MRI with every patient with non-pulsatile, unilateral tinnitus.

(Continued)

TABLE 2 | Continued

Guideline	Physical examination	Hearing and audiology tests	Psychological assessment	Assessment tools/questionnaires recommended	Other assessment procedures	Procedures not recommended
USA	• Targeted history and physical examination of the head and neck including otoscopy and neurologic examination. • When pulsatile tinnitus is reported, the examination should focus on identification of cardiovascular disease and vascular lesions	• Prompt, comprehensive audiological examination (Tonal and Speech audiometry and Immittance) in patients with tinnitus that is unilateral, persistent ($\geq$6 months), or associated with hearing difficulties (Strong recommendation); • Initial comprehensive audiological examination (including ear specific masked air and bone conduction) in patients who present with tinnitus regardless of laterality, duration, or perceived hearing status (Option)	• Distinction between patients with bothersome tinnitus from patients with non-bothersome tinnitus. • Assess degree of tinnitus related disability (including baseline measurement for the purpose to establish effects of treatment). • Assess if further psychological treatment required	• TQ, • TEQ, • THQ, • TRQ, • THI, • TFI	NS	• Imaging studies unless patients have one or more of the following: tinnitus that localises to one ear, pulsatile tinnitus, focal neurological abnormalities, or asymmetric hearing loss
Sweden	NS	• Audiometry (including LDL when necessary) • Speech and speech in noise test and impedance audiometry • ABR and MRI when necessary	• In case of severe tinnitus: the first encounter with the psychologist/ psychiatrist is investigative and informative. (1) symptoms tinnitus, (2) individual's mental status, (3) the overall life situation	• BAS (basic own questionnaire), • THI • HADS (when necessary)	• Anamnesis focused on tinnitus onset, laterality, character and patients' problems. • Consideration of psychological factors and somatosensory factors	NS

ABR, Auditory brainstem response; BAER, Brainstem auditory evoked response; CT, Computer tomography; DSA, Digital subtraction angiography; DPOAE, Distortion product optoacoustic emission; ENT, Ear nose throat; GP, General Practitioner; HADS, Hospital Anxiety and Depression Scale; LDL, Loudness discomfort level; MRA, Magnetic resonance angiography; MRI, Magnetic resonance imaging; TEOAE, Transient evoked optoacoustic emission; TEQ, Tinnitus evaluation questionnaire; TFI, Tinnitus functional index; THI, Tinnitus handicap inventory; THQ, Tinnitus handicap questionnaire; TMJ, Temporomandibular joint; TQ, Tinnitus questionnaire; TRQ, Tinnitus reaction questionnaire; UCL, Uncomfortable listening level; VAS, Visual analog scale.

The Tinnitus Handicap Inventory (THI; Newman et al., 1996, 1998) is the most frequently referred to assessment questionnaire followed by Tinnitus Questionnaire (TQ; Goebel and Hiller, 1994). Visual Analog Scales (VAS; e.g., Germany, Denmark) and the Hospital Anxiety and Depression Scale (HADS; Zigmond and Snaith, 1983, e.g., The Netherlands, Sweden) were referred to by at least two guidelines. The American guideline referred to a large number of questionnaires including the: TQ (Goebel and Hiller, 1994), THI (Newman et al., 1996, 1998), Tinnitus Effects Questionnaire (TEQ; Hallam et al., 1988), Tinnitus Handicap Questionnaire (THQ; Kuk et al., 1990), Tinnitus Reaction Questionnaire (TRQ; Wilson et al., 1991), and Tinnitus Functional Index (TFI; Meikle et al., 2012).

Several guidelines make recommendations for or against the use of other assessment related procedures. For example, the German guideline refers to X-rays of the cervical spine. Although three guidelines recommend magnetic resonance imaging (MRI) as an assessment of tinnitus, The American and the Dutch guideline recommend against it, unless patients have one or more of: tinnitus that localizes to one ear, pulsatile tinnitus, focal neurological abnormalities, or asymmetric hearing loss. The German guideline also recommends against acoustic examination using sound pressure levels more than 84 dB 1 week after acute tinnitus or tinnitus exacerbation.

Summary of Recommendations Regarding the Assessment of Subjective Tinnitus

- Conduct a thorough physical examination to exclude possible (physical) causes of tinnitus (three of five guidelines; not stated in Danish and Swedish).
- Complete a thorough audiological assessment (all guidelines).
- Establish the degree to which a patient experiences subjective tinnitus as bothersome or distressing using a validated and reliable multi-item questionnaire such as the TQ, THI, TFI, or HADS (all guidelines).
- In situations where patients appear to be experiencing a degree of distress or difficulties related to living with tinnitus, consider making a referral for an assessment by a psychologist or psychiatrist (four of five guidelines; not stated in German guideline).
- Variation exist in recommendations regarding the use of imaging studies (e.g., MRI).

Treatment Recommendations across the Guidelines

Table 3 compares therapeutic recommendations for the treatment of subjective tinnitus between the respective national tinnitus guidelines; note the Danish guideline is not included in this table as it provides only recommendations regarding assessment procedures. Across the guidelines there is generally a high degree of consistency in the recommendations for or against: the use of medicines (prescribed drugs and herbal supplements); audiological and psychological interventions; and, transcranial magnetic stimulation. Greatest variation occurs in the recommendations concerning the use of therapies involving sound such as Tinnitus Retraining Therapy (TRT).

There is a consensus that medicines should not be prescribed for the treatment of subjective tinnitus, though some variation in the level of specificity that each guideline has. For example, the German guideline lists specific medicines that should not be prescribed for the treatment of tinnitus. The German and Swedish do however note that medicines such as antidepressants might be prescribed to treat comorbid conditions. Herbal supplements such as Gingko biloba are also specifically recommended against being used in all guidelines except for Sweden which does not make recommendations for or against their use.

The use of hearing aids is recommended by all guidelines but only when clinically meaningful hearing loss is also present in people suffering from tinnitus. The use of a cochlear implant is mentioned in the Dutch and German guidelines and only recommended when there is profound hearing loss or deafness in addition to tinnitus. The Dutch guideline is the only one to provide scores on tinnitus questionnaires (e.g., TQ, THI) for when such interventions should be considered (e.g., it recommends referral to specialized stepped-care CBT for tinnitus in cases where TQ score is greater than 30, in combination with a clinically relevant request for healthcare by the patient, as is judged by the referring party).

Psychological interventions for tinnitus can potentially include a wide range of components but there is general consensus on the use of two of them. In particular, the provision of information and education about tinnitus and treatment options is consistently recommended across the guidelines although there is some variation in the specificity of the content that each provides. Second, specialized CBT for tinnitus is specifically recommended by all the guidelines except for Sweden which mentions it only in relation to the presence of stress, anxiety, or depression.

Least consistency exists across the guidelines in relation to TRT. Specifically, the Dutch guideline recommends that TRT can only be contemplated if tinnitus is very mild (TQ < 30) and the patients specifically asks for TRT, the American guideline indicates that sound therapies "may" be recommended to patients with tinnitus, while the Swedish guideline recommends that sound stimulation be used as part of TRT for people without hearing loss. The German guideline recommends the use of notched music therapy, but recommends against the use of TRT.

In relation to other less commonly used treatments (such as acupuncture or hyperbaric oxygen), the guidelines mostly indicate that there is an insufficient body of evidence to be able to make recommendations for or against their use.

Lastly, three guidelines (Germany, The Netherlands, and U.S.) either caution that there is insufficient evidence, or make additional recommendations against the use of transcranial magnetic stimulation (rTMS), transcranial direct current stimulation (tDCS), dietary supplements, neuromodulation treatments, and hearing aids for tinnitus patients without hearing loss.

Summary of Therapeutic Recommendations regarding the Treatment of Subjective Tinnitus

- Provide information about tinnitus and treatment options (all guidelines).
- Use hearing aids only when patients also experience hearing loss (all guidelines).

TABLE 3 | Tinnitus guideline recommendations regarding treatments for tinnitus.

Country	Medicine	Audiological	Psychological	Sound therapies	Other	Treatments recommended against using
Germany	• None for tinnitus but refers to, for example, some for co-morbid depression, e.g., glutamate-antagonists.	• Hearing aids for patients with hearing loss; Cochlear Implants for patients with deafness.	• General counseling (including information provision). • Tinnitus specific CBT (aimed at reducing attention focusing toward the ear noise, reappraisal of the tinnitus and its consequences) individual or group-settings, also treatment for comorbidities. • Hospital treatment for decompensated tinnitus and/or with severe psychiatric comorbidity. • An absence of conclusive evidence of effectiveness for self-help groups.	• Audio therapy including "notched music," "coordinated reset" or music therapy.	• Absence of evidence of effectiveness for: acupuncture, cervical vertebral spine therapy/ physiotherapy, hyperbaric oxygen; and, electric stimulation (e.g., transcutaneous electric stimulation, ear and cervical spine; vagus stimulation); Acoustic Coordinated-Reset Neuromodulation. • Uncertain recommendation for rTMS.	• Sound therapy including Noiser and TRT. • Hearing aids for patients with only tinnitus. • Medicines (including: steroids, melatonin, antidepressants, Sulpirid, Apraxolam, Sertraline, Botox A, Pramiprexol, Nortriptyline, Piribedil, Vardenafil, Trazodone, Atorvastatin, Gabapentin, anticonvulsants, Paroxetine, Lamotrigine, Cyclandelat, Baclofen, Nicotinamide, Tocainid, Misoprostol, Egb 761, Amitriptyline, Misoprostol, Pramipexole Dopamine. • Herbal medicines and vitamins (including Ginkgo biloba zinc).
Netherlands	None	• Consider a trial of hearing aids. • In patients with high TQ (>60) or THI (>78) scores, and have severe hearing loss or deafness and have not responded to CBT, consider Cochlear Implant.	• Educational material about tinnitus and treatment options considered essential. • Specialised CBT for patients with TQ > 30 or THI >36.	• TRT can only be contemplated in case tinnitus is very mild (TQ<30) and the patients specifically asks for TRT.	None	• rTMS. • TDCS. • Gingko biloba. • Acupuncture. • Auditive perceptual training. • Hyperbaric oxygen.
Sweden	• None for tinnitus specifically but does state that if necessary, sleeping pills or antidepressants, can be used to treat sleep disorders or depression (no drug types, names, or dosage provided).	• For people with tinnitus and hearing loss hearing aids are fitted.	• Individual or group tinnitus information meetings. For patients without hearing loss, this is based on a modified version of TRT protocol. • There is reference to CBT in case of stress/ anxiety/ depression, but no clear recommendation.	• Sound stimulation as part of TRT for people without hearing loss.	• For middle ear dysfunctions such as otosclerosis, surgery is possible – no clear recommendation is provided. • For tensions or pain in the jaw, neck, shoulders or back, referral to "bite" therapist, or physiotherapist.	None

(Continued)

TABLE 3 | Continued

Country	Medicine	Audiological	Psychological	Sound therapies	Other	Treatments recommended against using
USA	None	• Clinicians *should* recommend a hearing aid evaluation for patients with hearing loss and persistent, bothersome tinnitus.	• Clinicians *should* educate patients with persistent, bothersome tinnitus about management strategies. • Clinicians *should* recommend cognitive behavior therapy to patients with persistent, bothersome tinnitus.	• Clinicians *may* recommend sound therapy (e.g., TMT, TRT) to patients with persistent, bothersome tinnitus but patients must be informed of potential outcomes as well as costs associated with sound therapy.	• *No recommendation* can be made regarding the effect of acupuncture in patients with persistent bothersome tinnitus based on the poor quality of trials, no benefit, and minimal harm.	Clinicians *should not* routinely recommend: • Medicine (including antidepressants, anticonvulsants, anxiolytics, or intratympanic medications for a primary indication of treating persistent, bothersome tinnitus. • Dietary supplements and herbal medicines (e.g., Ginkgo biloba, melatonin, zinc). • TMS.

CBT, Cognitive behavioral therapy; NS, not specified; rTMS, repetitive Transcranial magnetic stimulation; TCDS, Transcranial direct stimulation; THI, Tinnitus handicap inventory; TMS, Transcranial magnetic stimulation; TMT, Tinnitus management therapy; TQ, Tinnitus questionnaire; TRT, Tinnitus retraining therapy.

- Specialised CBT for tinnitus should be offered to patients (three of four guidelines; Sweden refers to use of CBT in context of co-morbid anxiety or depression).
- There is a lack of consensus on the use of TRT for tinnitus.
- Prescribed medicines and herbal supplements should not be used for the treatment of tinnitus (all guidelines).
- Treatment with TMS is recommended against by Dutch and U.S. guidelines, and German guidelines give an "uncertain" recommendation.

Quality Assessment of the Guidelines

The AGREE II tool was used by the authors who undertook data extraction of the respective guidelines and the summarized results are shown in **Table 4**. In general the domains of "stakeholder involvement" and "clarity of presentation" respectively by guideline developers were rated high (good quality). Conversely, ratings on the domain of "applicability" which refers to how the guidelines might be disseminated, implemented and evaluated were low. For the domains addressing the scope and purpose of the guidelines, rigor of development and editorial independence, a pattern emerged whereby the American, Dutch and German guidelines were rated considerably higher (AGREE II scores >60% on all domains) than the Danish and Swedish guidelines (AGREE II scores <60% on all domains).

DISCUSSION

This systematic review aims to compare existing clinical guidelines for the assessment and treatment of subjective tinnitus in adults. Five guidelines, developed in the last 10 years within Europe, Scandinavia, and North America were included in the review. Although there are differences in some specific recommendations for assessment and treatment procedures across the guidelines, in general, commonalities across guidelines were high. The fact that there are differences in some of the recommendations is not surprising and appears to reflect the relatively young state of the field and the evolving nature of assessment and treatments for subjective tinnitus—a symptom with a high level of heterogeneity. On the other hand, the level of agreement, for example, in the recommendation of specialized cognitive behavioral therapy reflects the growing evidence base for the effectiveness of this treatment to alleviate patients' distress and impairment, even though significant changes in the tinnitus percept itself as a result of CBT have been proposed, though not yet assessed across studies.

When the methods of the development of guidelines were reported, it was clear that the respective groups were making efforts to be transparent, systematic, and using the best available evidence base, and frequently linking recommendations to specific research literature. For example, systematic reviews and meta-analyses were referred to whenever available to inform recommendations. It should be noted though that there is a lack of high quality studies or powered randomized trials of some treatments either for practical or methodological reasons. Regardless, the strengths and limitations of the evidence for particular recommendations were included for the majority

TABLE 4 | Summary of AGREE II domain scores (%) by country.

	Scope & Purpose	Stakeholder involvement	Rigour of development	Clarity of presentation	Applicability	Editorial independence
Germany	61	94	83	89	71	67
Denmark	52	44	24	59	2	17
Netherlands	81	100	97	100	9	100
USA	86	97	93	100	71	88
Sweden	42	42	1	33	2	13
Median	61	94	83	89	9	67
Average	64	75	60	76	31	57

of the guidelines and thus enable the user/reader to make informed decisions about following the recommended actions. Furthermore, target users were generally clearly defined and the development groups were comprised of a range of the health professionals often involved in the assessment and treatment of tinnitus. These two factors are important not only for providing expert input into the guideline, but also for garnering "buy-in" from potential users of the guidelines and focussing the content.

Differences between the Guidelines

Differences in recommended assessment procedures tend to relate to specific techniques (questionnaires, diagnostic tests, types of scanning techniques) rather than general principles [e.g., trying to establish tinnitus severity, hearing loss, psycho-social problem(s)], or the presence or absence of severe physical pathology that might be causing the tinnitus. Differences related to, for example, the recommended questionnaires for assessing tinnitus related interference and distress. While all the guidelines referred to the THI (the German guideline indirectly refers to this), only the American, Dutch and German guidelines referred to the TQ. Recommendations for specific questionnaires to measure psychological distress (especially symptoms of anxiety and depression) also varied with some guidelines not mentioning any (e.g., United States) and others such as the Dutch and Swedish guidelines which referred to the HADS. Differences also existed between the recommendations to assess loudness discomfort levels with the American and Dutch guidelines not recommending the use of such tests while the other guidelines did.

With regard to treatments, differences are found primarily regarding recommendations for the use of sound therapies. TRT specifically is not recommended by the German guideline, conditionally by the Dutch guideline and the American guideline indicates that clinicians "may" recommend it; TRT is currently being tested in a large multicenter trial in the U.S. (clinical trials ID: NCT01177137). A lack of evidences about other treatments such as acupuncture, hyperbaric oxygen and some herbal supplements leads most groups to recommend against them. The American guideline though is more cautious and simply states that because there is a lack of evidence they can neither recommend for or against the use of such treatments.

Differences in the recommendations of assessment and treatment procedures could be explained by a combination of factors including the time of the development of the guideline and availability of translated versions of the questionnaires (e.g., the TFI was published in 2012 which was after that of the Danish and Swedish guidelines), the known psychometric properties of the questionnaires themselves [e.g., concerns have been raised about the cross-cultural use of the HADS (Maters et al., 2013)], and the different methods used to reach consensus by the different guideline groups.

Consistencies across the Guidelines

Across the guidelines consensus appears to exist on a number of important general features of assessment relating to subjective tinnitus. Specifically, there is consensus about the initial need for excluding a physical cause of the tinnitus, conducting an audiometric assessment of the patient, using standardized questionnaires to measure degrees of tinnitus related distress, and when relevant, making referrals for further psychological assessment.

Regarding the therapeutic recommendations for the treatment of subjective tinnitus, all guidelines recommend against the use of medicines for the treatment of the tinnitus specifically but note that medicines are appropriate for treating co-morbid conditions. There is also agreement in the recommendations to use hearing aids for patients experiencing hearing loss and CBT to facilitate adjustment to the symptom, alleviate distress and tinnitus-related interference in daily life.

As a group of tinnitus researchers and clinicians, we endorse the specific principles and practices of assessment and treatment that are consistently found across the guidelines. Further, while a treatment for removing the tinnitus percept does not exist, we reiterate the importance of providing patients with bothersome tinnitus, evidence based cost-effective treatment(s) in a way (such as stepped care) that is minimally burdensome to the patient. That is patients who are assessed as having relatively little tinnitus related distress and interference should receive less intensive treatment in the first instance, than someone who is assessed as having severe levels of distress and interference in activities of daily living.

Strengths and Limitations of the Review

There are two critical factors that affect the conclusions that can be drawn from the included guidelines. Firstly, and as with all systematic reviews, the search strategy and inclusion criteria used determine what is located and subsequently included. In this review, we used the search terms "tinnitus" and "guideline" to conduct the search in a wide range of databases, repositories of clinical guidelines, and search engines, with the intention of being focussed enough to identify the most relevant documents within a manageable number of search results. Only including the term "guideline" though might have resulted in relevant documents, albeit not called "guidelines," being omitted from search results. Similarly, our use of inclusion/exclusion criteria that led to the decision to exclude documents such as the TRI flowchart could be problematic as it (the TRI flowchart) is a comprehensive document potentially used in many situations to inform assessment and treatment decisions.

To minimize the risk of omitting relevant search results we contacted a range of international experts and members of guideline development groups. In addition to this, we conducted hand searches of the references lists of included guidelines for relevant sources. We also recruited native speakers to extract data from the respective guidelines in an effort to ensure that data collection was as accurate as possible. It is possible, that different search and inclusion criteria might have led to different documents being included. However, given the large range of assessment and treatment options and the limited evidence base around many treatments in particular, it is unlikely that our conclusions would differ significantly if further guidelines had been identified at this time. Future systematic reviews though will be able to use this as a reference point.

IMPLICATIONS AND CONCLUSIONS

As researchers from around the world are collecting and making efforts to better understand the heterogeneity of subjective tinnitus in adults and systematically evaluate assessment and treatment options, we have, for the first time, described the major similarities and differences between existing clinical guidelines for subjective tinnitus in adults. The results reveal true guidelines from only five countries and thus highlight a need to develop guidelines that are endorsed by the range of professionals involved in assessing and treating tinnitus. Although we do not place a great deal of weight on the quality assessment ratings of the guidelines, they do suggest that there is room for improvement particularly with regard to implementation and evaluation. The absence of guidelines contributes to the variations that exist in assessment and treatment of tinnitus internationally.

While it would be tempting to do so, it is beyond the scope of this paper to formulate a new or composite guideline based on the results that we have obtained. Instead, the results of this review in conjunction with those from a survey of European tinnitus healthcare providers and researchers (Cima et al., 2016) will form the basis of further work on the development of a set of European clinical guidelines for the assessment and treatment of tinnitus being undertaken by the COST-action TINNET: Working Group I "*Clinical.*" As with existing clinical guidelines, attention will need to be given to how the future European guideline is disseminated, subsequently evaluated, and the implications for resource management considered. We expect it to be challenging task but one that will hopefully result in a more reliable and equitable assessment and treatment of tinnitus patients across Europe.

AUTHOR CONTRIBUTIONS

TF, HH, DK, AL, BM, AN, SR and RC, conceived and designed the study. TF and HH wrote and revised the protocol and manuscripts, conducted the literature search, data extraction, and data synthesis. SR, RL, CC, NE, PB, SNR, AK, DL, and BM extracted data. DH, AN, DK, and RC reviewed and edited manuscripts and contributed intellectually to the content of the manuscript. All authors approved the manuscript for submission.

FUNDING

This research was supported by funding from SWOL Limburgs Fonds voor Revalidatie and Adelante, Centre for expertise in Rehabilitation and Audiology. A COST Action grant (BM1306) supported the collaboration between the authors and the formation of the COST Action BM1306 (2014–2018) TINNET Working Group I.

REFERENCES

American Academy of Audiology (2000). *Audiologic Guidelines for the Diagnosis and Management of Tinnitus Patients.* Available online at: http://www.audiology.org/publications-resources/document-library/audiologic-guidelines-diagnosis-management-tinnitus-patients [Accessed 22 November 2016].

American Speach Language Hearing Association (2016). *Tinnitus Triage Guidelines.* Available online at: http://www.asha.org/aud/Articles/Tinnitus-Triage-Guidelines/ [Accessed 22 November 2016].

Andersson, G., Juris, L., Classon, E., Fredrikson, M., and Furmark, T. (2006). Consequences of suppressing thoughts about tinnitus and the effects of cognitive distraction on brain activity in tinnitus patients. *Audiol. Neurotol.* 11, 301–309. doi: 10.1159/000094460

Audiology Australia (2013). *Audiology Australia Professional Practice Standards - Part B Clinical Standards.* Melbourne, VCA: Audiology Australia.

Baguley, D., Andersson, G., McFerran, D., and McKenna, L. (eds.). (2013a). *Tinnitus: A Multidisciplinary Approach.* West Sussex: John Wiley & Sons, Ltd.

Baguley, D., McFerran, D., and Hall, D. (2013b). Tinnitus. *Lancet* 382, 1600–1607. doi: 10.1016/S0140-6736(13)60142-7

Biesinger, E., Del Bo, L., De Ridder, D., Goodey, R., Herraiz, C., Kleinjung, T., et al. (2010). *Algorithm for the Diagnostic and Therapeutic Management of Tinnitus.* Available online at: http://www.tinnitusresearch.org/en/documents/downloads/TRI_Tinnitus_Flowchart.pdf [Accessed 30 Jan 2015].

Brouwers, M. C., Kho, M. E., Browman, G. P., Burgers, J. S., Cluzeau, F., Feder, G., et al. (2010). AGREE II: advancing guideline development, reporting and evaluation in health care. *CMAJ* 182, E839–E842. doi: 10.1503/cmaj.090449

Cima, R. F., Crombez, G., and Vlaeyen, J. W. (2011). Catastrophizing and fear of tinnitus predict quality of life in patients with chronic tinnitus. *Ear Hear.* 32, 634–641. doi: 10.1097/AUD.0b013e31821106dd

Cima, R. F., Haider, H., Mazurek, B., Cederroth, C. R., Lapira, A., Kikidis, D., et al. (2016). "TINNET COST Action BM1306 - clinical WG1: establishment of a standard for Tinnitus; patient assessment, characterization, and treatment options," in *10th International Tinnitus Research Initiative Conference* (Nottingham: Tinnitus Research Initiative).

Cima, R. F., Maes, I. H., Joore, M. A., Scheyen, D. J., El Refaie, A., Baguley, D. M., et al. (2012). Specialised treatment based on cognitive behaviour therapy versus usual care for tinnitus: a randomised controlled trial. *Lancet* 379, 1951–1959. doi: 10.1016/S0140-6736(12)60469-3

Davis, A., and Refaie, A. E. (2000). "Epidemiology of tinnitus," in *Handbook of Tinnitus*, ed R. S. Tyler (San Diego: Singular thompson Learning), 1–24.

Department of Health (2009). *Provision of Services for Adults with Tinnitus: A Good Practice Guide*. London: Department of Health.

Dutch Association for Ear Nose Throat and Head surgery [Nederlandse Vereniging voor Keel - Neus - Oor heel kunde en Heelkunde van het Hoofd - Halsgebied] (in press). *Guideline Tinnitus [Richtlijn Tinnitus]*. Utrecht.

Erlandsson, S. I., and Hallberg, L. R. (2000). Prediction of quality of life in patients with tinnitus. *Br. J. Audiol.* 34, 11–20. doi: 10.3109/03005364000000114

Feldmann, H. (1984). Tinnitus masking curves (updates and review). *J. Laryngol. Otol.* 98, 157–160. doi: 10.1017/S1755146300090375

Field, M. J., and Lohr, K. N. (eds.). (1990). *Clinical Practice Guidelines: Directions for a New Program*. Washington, DC: National Academy of Sciences.

Fujii, K., Nagata, C., Nakamura, K., Kawachi, T., Takatsuka, N., Oba, S., et al. (2011). Prevalence of tinnitus in community-dwelling Japanese adults. *J. Epidemiol.* 21, 299–304. doi: 10.2188/jea.JE20100124

Goebel, G., and Hiller, W. (1994). The tinnitus questionnaire. A standard instrument for grading the degree of tinnitus. Results of a multicenter study with the tinnitus questionnaire. *HNO* 42, 166–172.

Goebel, G., and Hiller, W. (2001). *Verhaltensmedizinische Tinnitus-Diagnostik. Eine Praktische Anleitung zur Erfassung Medizinischer und Psychologischer Merkmale Mittels des Strukturierten Tinnitus-Interviews (STI)*. Göttingen: Hogrefe.

Hallam, R. S., Jakes, S. C., and Hinchcliffe, R. (1988). Cognitive variables in tinnitus annoyance. *Br. J. Clin. Psychol.* 27(Pt 3), 213–222. doi: 10.1111/j.2044-8260.1988.tb00778.x

Handscomb, L. E., Hall, D. A., Shorter, G. W., and Hoare, D. J. (2017). Positive and negative thinking in tinnitus: factor structure of the tinnitus cognitions questionnaire. *Ear Hear.* 38, 126–132. doi: 10.1097/AUD.0000000000000365

Henry, J. A., Zaugg, T. L., Myers, P. J., Schmidt, C. J., Ribbe, C., Edmonds, K., et al. (2015). *Adult Tinnitus Management Clinical Practice Recommendation*. Portland, OR: Department of Veterans Affairs.

Henry, J. A., Zaugg, T. L., and Schechter, M. A. (2005a). Clinical guide for audiologic tinnitus management I: assessment. *Am. J. Audiol.* 14, 21–48. doi: 10.1044/1059-0889(2005/004)

Henry, J. A., Zaugg, T. L., and Schechter, M. A. (2005b). Clinical guide for audiologic tinnitus management II: treatment. *Am. J. Audiol.* 14, 49–70. doi: 10.1044/1059-0889(2005/005)

Hoare, D. J., Gander, P. E., Collins, L., Smith, S., and Hall, D. A. (2012). Management of tinnitus in English NHS audiology departments: an evaluation of current practice. *J. Eval. Clin. Pract.* 18, 326–334. doi: 10.1111/j.1365-2753.2010.01566.x

Hoare, D. J., and Hall, D. (2011). Clinical guidelines and practice: a commentary on the complexity of tinnitus management. *Eval. Health Prof.* 34, 413–420. doi: 10.1177/0163278710390355

Hoekstra, C. E., Wesdorp, F. M., and van Zanten, G. A. (2014). Socio-demographic, health, and tinnitus related variables affecting tinnitus severity. *Ear Hear.* 35, 544–554. doi: 10.1097/AUD.0000000000000045

Idrizbegovic, E., Kjerulf, E., and Team for Diagnostics Hearing Habilitation Children and Youth and Hearing Rehabilitation for Adults (2011). *Tinnitus Care Program [Tinnitus Vårdprogram]*. Stockholm: Karolinska Institute.

Jørgensen, H. S., Amt, F., Nemholt, S. S., Kristensen, R., and Ellesøe, H. (2007). "Guidance for Diagnosing Tinnitus and Hyperacusis [Vejledning for udredning af tinnitus og hyperakusis]," in *Vejledninger i Udredning* (Denmark: S.l. Danske Tale-Høre-Synsinstitutioner: eksp. Center for Hjælpemidler og Kommunikation).

Kamalski, D. M., Hoekstra, C. E., van Zanten, B. G., Grolman, W., and Rovers, M. M. (2010). Measuring disease-specific health-related quality of life to evaluate treatment outcomes in tinnitus patients: a systematic review. *Otolaryngol. Head Neck Surg.* 143, 181–185. doi: 10.1016/j.otohns.2010.03.026

Kim, H. J., Lee, H. J., An, S. Y., Sim, S., Park, B., Kim, S. W., et al. (2015). Analysis of the prevalence and associated risk factors of tinnitus in adults. *PLoS ONE* 10:e0127578. doi: 10.1371/journal.pone.0127578

Kleinstauber, M., Jasper, K., Schweda, I., Hiller, W., Andersson, G., and Weise, C. (2013). The role of fear-avoidance cognitions and behaviors in patients with chronic tinnitus. *Cogn. Behav. Ther.* 42, 84–99. doi: 10.1080/16506073.2012.717301

Kuk, F. K., Tyler, R. S., Russell, D., and Jordan, H. (1990). The psychometric properties of a tinnitus handicap questionnaire. *Ear Hear.* 11, 434–445. doi: 10.1097/00003446-199012000-00005

Langguth, B., and Elgoyhen, A. B. (2012). Current pharmacological treatments for tinnitus. *Expert Opin. Pharmacother.* 13, 2495–2509. doi: 10.1517/14656566.2012.739608

Langguth, B., Kleinjung, T., and Landgrebe, M. (2011). Severe tinnitus and depressive symptoms: a complex interaction. *Otolaryngol. Head Neck Surg.* 145, 519; author reply 520. doi: 10.1177/0194599811411851

Langguth, B., Kreuzer, P. M., Kleinjung, T., and De Ridder, D. (2013). Tinnitus: causes and clinical management. *Lancet Neurol.* 12, 920–930. doi: 10.1016/S1474-4422(13)70160-1

Martinez-Devesa, P., Perera, R., Theodoulou, M., and Waddell, A. (2010). Cognitive behavioural therapy for tinnitus. *Cochrane Database Syst. Rev.* CD005233. doi: 10.1002/14651858.CD005233.pub3

Maters, G. A., Sanderman, R., Kim, A. Y., and Coyne, J. C. (2013). Problems in cross-cultural use of the hospital anxiety and depression scale: "no butterflies in the desert". *PLoS ONE* 8:e70975. doi: 10.1371/journal.pone.0070975

McKenna, L., Handscomb, L., Hoare, D. J., and Hall, D. A. (2014). A scientific cognitive-behavioral model of tinnitus: novel conceptualizations of tinnitus distress. *Front. Neurol.* 5:196. doi: 10.3389/fneur.2014.00196

Meikle, M. B., Henry, J. A., Griest, S. E., Stewart, B. J., Abrams, H. B., McArdle, R., et al. (2012). The tinnitus functional index: development of a new clinical measure for chronic, intrusive tinnitus. *Ear Hear.* 33, 153–176. doi: 10.1097/AUD.0b013e31822f67c0

Newman, C. W., Jacobson, G. P., and Spitzer, J. B. (1996). Development of the tinnitus handicap inventory. *Arch. Otolaryngol. Head Neck Surg.* 122, 143–148. doi: 10.1001/archotol.1996.01890140029007

Newman, C. W., Sandridge, S. A., and Jacobson, G. P. (1998). Psychometric adequacy of the Tinnitus Handicap Inventory (THI) for evaluating treatment outcome. *J. Am. Acad. Audiol.* 9, 153–160.

NHS Scotland (2006). *Best Practice Statement - Ear Care*. Healthcare Improvement Scotland.

Ruszczynski, M., Horvath, A., Dziechciarz, P., and Szajewska, H. (2016). Cow's milk allergy guidelines: a quality appraisal with the AGREE II instrument. *Clin. Exp. Allergy* 46, 1236–1241. doi: 10.1111/cea.12784

Sanclemente, G., Acosta, J. L., Tamayo, M. E., Bonfill, X., and Alonso-Coello, P. (2014). Clinical practice guidelines for treatment of acne vulgaris: a critical appraisal using the AGREE II instrument. *Arch. Dermatol. Res.* 306, 269–277. doi: 10.1007/s00403-013-1394-x

The Association of the Scientific Medical Societies (2015). *German S3 Guideline 017/064: Chronic Tinnitus [AWMF-Register Nr. 017/064 Klasse: S3 Chronischer Tinnitus]*. AWMF online.

Tunkel, D. E., Bauer, C. A., Sun, G. H., Rosenfeld, R. M., Chandrasekhar, S. S., Cunningham, E. R., et al. (2014). Clinical practice guideline: tinnitus. *Otolaryngol. Head Neck Surg.* 151, S1–S40. doi: 10.1177/0194599814547475

Wilson, P. H., Henry, J., Bowen, M., and Haralambous, G. (1991). Tinnitus reaction questionnaire psychometric properties of a measure of distress associated with tinnitus. *J. Speech Hear. Res.* 34, 197–201. doi: 10.1044/jshr.3401.197

Zigmond, A. S., and Snaith, R. P. (1983). The hospital anxiety and depression scale. *Acta Psychiatr. Scand.* 67, 361–370. doi: 10.1111/j.1600-0447.1983.tb09716.x

18

Does Tinnitus Depend on Time-of-Day? An Ecological Momentary Assessment Study with the "TrackYourTinnitus" Application

Thomas Probst[1,2], Rüdiger C. Pryss[2], Berthold Langguth[3], Josef P. Rauschecker[4,5], Johannes Schobel[2], Manfred Reichert[2], Myra Spiliopoulou[6], Winfried Schlee[3†] and Johannes Zimmermann[7†]*

[1] Georg-Elias-Müller-Institute for Psychology, Georg-August-University Göttingen, Göttingen, Germany, [2] Department for Psychotherapy and Biopsychosocial Health, Danube University Krems, Krems an der Donau, Austria, [3] Department of Psychiatry and Psychotherapy of the University of Regensburg at Bezirksklinikum Regensburg, Regensburg, Germany, [4] Program in Cognitive and Computational Systems, Georgetown University Washington, Washington, DC, United States, [5] Institute for Advanced Study, Technical University Munich, Munich, Germany, [6] Department of Technical and Business Information Systems, Otto-von-Guericke-University Magdeburg, Magdeburg, Germany, [7] Psychologische Hochschule Berlin, Berlin, Germany

***Correspondence:**
Thomas Probst
thomas.probst@donau-uni.ac.at

Only few previous studies used ecological momentary assessments to explore the time-of-day-dependence of tinnitus. The present study used data from the mobile application "TrackYourTinnitus" to explore whether tinnitus loudness and tinnitus distress fluctuate within a 24-h interval. Multilevel models were performed to account for the nested structure of assessments (level 1: 17,209 daily life assessments) nested within days (level 2: 3,570 days with at least three completed assessments), and days nested within participants (level 3: 350 participants). Results revealed a time-of-day-dependence of tinnitus. In particular, tinnitus was perceived as louder and more distressing during the night and early morning hours (from 12 a.m. to 8 a.m.) than during the upcoming day. Since previous studies suggested that stress (and stress-associated hormones) show a circadian rhythm and this might influence the time-of-day-dependence of tinnitus, we evaluated whether the described results change when statistically controlling for subjectively reported stress-levels. Correcting for subjective stress-levels, however, did not change the result that tinnitus (loudness and distress) was most severe at night and early morning. These results show that time-of-day contributes to the level of both tinnitus loudness and tinnitus distress. Possible implications of our results for the clinical management of tinnitus are that tailoring the timing of therapeutic interventions to the circadian rhythm of individual patients (chronotherapy) might be promising.

Keywords: tinnitus, stress, circadian fluctuation, time-of-day, ecological momentary assessment

INTRODUCTION

Tinnitus, the phantom perception of sound (Baguley et al., 2013; Langguth et al., 2013), is perceived by 5.1% up to 42.7% of the population according to a recent review including 39 studies from 16 countries (McCormack et al., 2016). These percentages depend on age (with older persons showing higher prevalence), gender (with male persons showing higher prevalence), and the definition of tinnitus used in the epidemiological study (McCormack et al., 2016). Prevalence rates of tinnitus also have increased over the years (Nondahl et al., 2012; Martinez et al., 2015), and one can speculate about the reasons for this apparent increase. On a neuronal basis, auditory-limbic interactions play a central role in the development of (chronic) tinnitus (Rauschecker et al., 2010; Leaver et al., 2011). In many cases, tinnitus is associated with psychological distress and incapacity for work (Bhatt et al., 2016) resulting in high socio-economic costs (Maes et al., 2013). Cognitive-behavioral therapy (CBT) has proven to have the potential to reduce the burden of tinnitus for the individual (Hesser et al., 2011) as well as the society/economy (Maes et al., 2014). But not all tinnitus patients reach clinically relevant improvements with CBT (e.g., Jasper et al., 2014). Other therapeutic approaches, including pharmacological therapy (Langguth and Elgoyhen, 2012), auditory stimulation (Hobson et al., 2012) or brain stimulation (Langguth and De Ridder, 2013), have only revealed small and inconsistent effects in subgroups of patients. It is assumed that an important reason for the poor treatment response in clinical trials is the heterogeneity of tinnitus (Landgrebe et al., 2012; Baguley et al., 2013), both across patients (inter-individual heterogeneity) as well as within patients over time (intra-individual heterogeneity, see Dauman et al., 2015).

Therefore, it is important to understand the factors that contribute to the heterogeneity of tinnitus. Psychological variables, such as fear-related cognition (e.g., Cima et al., 2011; Kleinstäuber et al., 2013), an accepting stance toward tinnitus (e.g., Weise et al., 2013; Riedl et al., 2015), emotions (e.g., Probst et al., 2016a,b), and avoidance/safety behaviors (e.g., Hesser and Andersson, 2009; Kleinstäuber et al., 2013), have been demonstrated to account for the heterogeneity of tinnitus in several studies (see also the "scientific cognitive-behavioral model of tinnitus"; McKenna et al., 2014). Moreover, recent neuroscience studies imply that the moment-to-moment variability of tinnitus is related to brain oscillatory patterns like the alpha power in temporal regions (Schlee et al., 2014) and time-of-day (Basinou et al., 2017); circadian fluctuations have been shown, for example, in auditory pathway structures related to tinnitus like the cochlea (Meltser et al., 2014) and the inferior colliculus (Park et al., 2016). Another hint for a link between tinnitus and circadian rhythms is provided by findings of reduced tinnitus severity after intake of melatonin (e.g., Pirodda et al., 2010; Ajayi et al., 2014; Miroddi et al., 2015). Furthermore, pain, which shares many similarities with tinnitus (De Ridder et al., 2011; Rauschecker et al., 2015), has been found to underlie circadian variations (e.g., Strian et al., 1989; Gilron and Ghasemlou, 2014; Buttgereit et al., 2015). Furthermore, depression, which overlaps in its pathophysiology with tinnitus (Langguth et al., 2011), is characterized by changes in circadian rhythm (e.g., Germain and Kupfer, 2008; Wirz-Justice, 2008).

The question of whether tinnitus varies systematically over the course of the day, however, has not yet been studied systematically. The limited possibilities of traditional assessment methods to routinely track symptoms in the daily routine have made it rather difficult to validly study whether tinnitus shows time-of-day-dependence. To overcome these limitations of traditional assessment methods, newer technological developments can be used to electronically gather valid daily life data (ecological momentary assessments, EMA; Trull and Ebner-Priemer, 2013, 2014; Adams et al., 2017). Henry et al. (2012), for example, used personal digital assistants (PDA) in a 2-week pilot study with 24 participants to obtain EMA during a 12-h interval (8 a.m.–8 p.m.) and showed that the scores of the 10-item screening version of the Tinnitus Handicap Inventory (THI-S; Newman et al., 2008) were not significantly different between 3-h time blocks (8 a.m.–11 a.m., 11 a.m.–2 p.m., 2 p.m.–5 p.m., and 5 p.m.–8 p.m.). Although Henry et al. (2012) failed to demonstrate time-of-day-dependence of tinnitus, a 2-week pilot smartphone-based study with 20 participants on fluctuations of tinnitus within an 11-h interval (9 a.m.–8 p.m.) suggested that tinnitus does vary within a single day (Wilson et al., 2015). But Wilson et al. (2015) did not report at which time-of-day the participants rated their tinnitus as more or less severe. In another diary study, Flor et al. (2004) reported tinnitus being worst at the beginning of a day, thus supporting the time-of-day-dependence of tinnitus. To our knowledge there are only these three studies with ambivalent results that addressed the time-of-day-dependence of tinnitus in daily life with EMA (Flor et al., 2004; Henry et al., 2012; Wilson et al., 2015).

The current study used EMA from the "TrackYourTinnitus" (TYT) mobile application (Pryss et al., 2015a,b; Schlee et al., 2016) to explore whether tinnitus fluctuates within a 24-h interval (night and upcoming day). Tinnitus is operationalized by two questions in TYT, one question is on tinnitus loudness and the other question on tinnitus distress. Prior research suggested that an assessment of both tinnitus loudness and tinnitus distress is necessary for a comprehensive assessment, since tinnitus loudness and tinnitus distress are only moderately correlated (e.g., Hiller and Goebel, 2007; Wallhäusser-Franke et al., 2012) and processed in different but interconnected brain areas (e.g., Leaver et al., 2012; Ueyama et al., 2013; De Ridder et al., 2014; Vanneste et al., 2014). Therefore, it appears possible that tinnitus loudness and tinnitus distress show either similar or different ups and downs within a 24-h interval. Accordingly, the present study investigated the time-of-day-dependence of tinnitus loudness as well as of tinnitus distress. Moreover, stress is known to be associated with tinnitus (e.g., Hébert et al., 2004; Hébert and Lupien, 2007, 2009; Alsalman et al., 2016) and stress-related hormones like cortisol and adrenocorticotropic hormone (ACTH) underlie circadian rhythms (e.g., Dickmeis, 2009; Lightman and Conway-Campbell, 2010; Conway-Campbell et al., 2012), which could influence the potential time-of-day-dependence of tinnitus (loudness and distress). Thus, we also explored whether the stress-level as assessed with TYT depends on time-of-day and whether the 24-h fluctuations of tinnitus loudness and tinnitus distress change when taking the stress-level into account.

MATERIALS AND METHODS

The material and the methods were approved by the Ethics Committee of the University Clinic of Regensburg and were carried out in accordance with the approved guidelines. Information that the TYT data will be used for scientific analyses is included in the mobile applications of "TrackYourTinnitus" as well as on the "TrackYourTinnitus" website and, therefore, the TYT users were informed that the data will be used for scientific purposes. Written consent, however, was not possible to obtain given the nature of the study. The study participants were anonymized.

"TrackYourTinnitus" Platform

The TYT platform (www.trackyourtinnitus.org, Pryss et al., 2015a,b) consists of a website for registration, two mobile applications (for iOS and Android), and a MySQL database as a central repository for the data collected. Users can either use TYT whenever they want or they can set a user-defined schedule to receive random notifications. For the study at hand, only these notification-triggered assessments were investigated. At each of these notifications, the users are asked to rate their tinnitus and other tinnitus-related variables (e.g., subjective stress-level). Although the attention might be directed toward the tinnitus by such notifications, Henry et al. (2012) and Schlee et al. (2016) found that repeatedly rating tinnitus and associated variables in daily life does not have detrimental effects. The present study investigated the following variables the users were asked to rate at each notification: "Current tinnitus loudness" (subjective rating of current tinnitus loudness on a visual analog scale [VAS], including a zero value for moments without loudness: min: 0; max: 1), "current tinnitus distress" (subjective rating of current tinnitus distress on a VAS including a zero value for moments without distress: min: 0; max: 1), and "current stress-level" (subjective rating of current stress-level on a VAS: min: 0; max: 1). Moreover, the timestamps of the assessments were used to explore the time-of-day-dependence of tinnitus. In TYT, the timestamps represent the local time of the time zone a given user is in when providing the assessments.

The data set used for the current study was exported in June 2016. After excluding the self-initiated assessments and the assessments given within the 15 min after the last assessment (for the inter-assessment interval of 15 min see also Pryss et al., 2015b), we had access to 25,863 notification-triggered assessments. For the present study, we only included the 25,092 assessments without missing values in any of the three target variables. Furthermore, as we were interested in within-day variations, we only considered data from days with at least three completed assessments, resulting in a total number of 17,209 assessments.

Sample

The final sample consisted of 350 participants. Two-hundred and fifty three participants (72.2%) were male, 94 (26.9%) were female, and 3 did not indicate their gender. On average, participants were 45.4 ($SD = 12.1$) years old (17 participants did not report their age). The median number of years since onset of tinnitus was 5.4, ranging from 0 to 61.8 years. According to participants, onset of tinnitus was related to loud blast of sound ($n = 48$), whiplash ($n = 9$), change in hearing ($n = 38$), stress ($n = 99$), head trauma ($n = 12$), and other causes ($n = 141$) (3 participants did not report events related to onset of tinnitus). The median number of days per participant (with at least three assessments) was 11, ranging from 1 to 415 days. This corresponds to a total number of 3,570 days. The median number of assessments per day was 4, ranging from 3 (the minimum requirement to be included in this study) to 18 assessments.

Statistical Analyses

To test our hypotheses, we used multilevel modeling (MLM; Raudenbush and Bryk, 2002; Singer and Willett, 2003). MLM is ideally suited to address the nested structure of our data, with assessments (Level 1) nested in days (Level 2), and days nested in participants (Level 3). First, we estimated two MLMs predicting tinnitus loudness and tinnitus distress from time-of-day, respectively. Time-of-day was dummy-coded using five binary variables indicating whether the assessment was in the early morning (T1, from 4 a.m. to 8 a.m.), in the late morning (T2, from 8 a.m. to 12 p.m.), in the afternoon (T3, from 12 p.m. to 4 p.m.), in the early evening (T4, from 4 p.m. to 8 p.m.), or in the late evening (T5, from 8 p.m. to 12 a.m.). Assessments during the night (from 12 a.m. to 4 a.m.) were defined as the reference group. The full three-level MLM with random intercepts at Level 2 and 3 and random slopes at Level 3 (Model I) is summarized below:

$$
\begin{aligned}
\text{Level 1:}\quad & y_{ijk} = \pi_{0jk} + \pi_{1jk}(T1) + \pi_{2jk}(T2) + \pi_{3jk}(T3) \\
& \qquad + \pi_{4jk}(T4) + \pi_{5jk}(T5) + e_{ijk} \\
\text{Level 2:}\quad & \pi_{0jk} = \beta_{00k} + r_{0jk} \\
& \pi_{1jk} = \beta_{10k} \\
& \pi_{2jk} = \beta_{20k} \\
& \pi_{3jk} = \beta_{30k} \\
& \pi_{4jk} = \beta_{40k} \\
& \pi_{5jk} = \beta_{50k} \\
\text{Level 3:}\quad & \beta_{00k} = \gamma_{000} + u_{00k} \\
& \beta_{10k} = \gamma_{100} + u_{10k} \\
& \beta_{20k} = \gamma_{200} + u_{20k} \\
& \beta_{30k} = \gamma_{300} + u_{30k} \\
& \beta_{40k} = \gamma_{400} + u_{40k} \\
& \beta_{50k} = \gamma_{500} + u_{50k}
\end{aligned}
$$

The model decomposes the amount of tinnitus loudness/distress (y) of participant k on day j at assessment i into a series of fixed and random effects. The fixed effect γ_{000} represents the expected (population) tinnitus loudness/distress during the night before an average day of an average participant. The fixed effects γ_{100}, γ_{200}, γ_{300}, γ_{400}, and γ_{500} represent the expected change in tinnitus loudness/distress from night to early and late morning, afternoon and early and late evening, respectively. The random effects at Level 3, u_{00k}, u_{10k}, u_{20k}, u_{30k}, u_{40k}, and u_{50k}, indicate that the level of tinnitus loudness/distress at night as well as its later change during the day may differ between participants. The random intercept at Level 2, r_{0jk}, indicates that the baseline level of tinnitus loudness/distress may differ between days within participants. We assumed random effects to be multivariate normally distributed within levels, and residuals to be independent and identically distributed across levels.

Second, we estimated the same MLM for stress-level as the dependent variable (y). Moreover, we estimated two further MLMs predicting tinnitus loudness and tinnitus distress from time-of-day, this time including stress-level as an additional predictor. As stress-level varied across all three levels, we decomposed its variance into three separate mean-centered variables capturing variation of stress within days (S1), variation of stress within participants across days (S2), and variation of stress across participants (S3) prior to estimating the MLMs. The full three-level MLM with random intercepts at Level 2 and 3 and random slopes at Level 3 (Model II) is summarized below:

$$\begin{aligned}
\text{Level 1:}\quad & y_{ijk} = \pi_{0jk} + \pi_{1jk}(T1) + \pi_{2jk}(T2) + \pi_{3jk}(T3) \\
& \qquad + \pi_{4jk}(T4) + \pi_{5jk}(T5) + \pi_{6jk}(S1) + e_{ijk} \\
\text{Level 2:}\quad & \pi_{0jk} = \beta_{00k} + \beta_{01k}(S2) + r_{0jk} \\
& \pi_{1jk} = \beta_{10k} \\
& \pi_{2jk} = \beta_{20k} \\
& \pi_{3jk} = \beta_{30k} \\
& \pi_{4jk} = \beta_{40k} \\
& \pi_{5jk} = \beta_{50k} \\
& \pi_{6jk} = \beta_{60k} \\
\text{Level 3:}\quad & \beta_{00k} = \gamma_{000} + \gamma_{001}(S3) + u_{00k} \\
& \beta_{01k} = \gamma_{010} + u_{01k} \\
& \beta_{10k} = \gamma_{100} + u_{10k} \\
& \beta_{20k} = \gamma_{200} + u_{20k} \\
& \beta_{30k} = \gamma_{300} + u_{30k} \\
& \beta_{40k} = \gamma_{400} + u_{40k} \\
& \beta_{50k} = \gamma_{500} + u_{50k} \\
& \beta_{60k} = \gamma_{600} + u_{60k}
\end{aligned}$$

The newly defined fixed effects, γ_{001}, γ_{010}, and γ_{600}, represent the expected between-participant, between-day, and within-day effect of stress on tinnitus loudness/distress after controlling for time-of-day. The remaining fixed effects, γ_{000}, γ_{100}, γ_{200}, γ_{300}, γ_{400}, and γ_{500}, represent the expected level of tinnitus loudness/distress at night as well as its later change during the day after controlling for the influence of stress. The newly defined random effects, u_{01k} and u_{60k}, indicate that the between- and within-day effects of stress may differ between participants. Due to model identification issues, we restricted the covariances between random effects of stress and the remaining random effects in the model to be zero.

All models were estimated using full maximum likelihood estimation. Analyses were conducted with the package "lme4" (Bates et al., 2015) of the statistical platform R (R Core Team, 2015). We used Satterthwaite's approximations to derive p-values for fixed effects. Pairwise comparisons between the six distinct timeframes were explored using the Tukey Honest Significant Difference method as implemented in the package "multcomp" (Hothorn et al., 2008). Finally, we quantified the effect size of time-of-day on tinnitus loudness/distress by means of a pseudo R^2 statistic. This statistic can be computed by subtracting the residual variance $Var(e_{ijk})$ of Model I from the residual variance of an intercept-only model without any predictors, divided by this latter residual variance. It represents the relative amount of variance in tinnitus loudness/distress within days that is explained by time-of-day (i.e., by the five variables T1–T5).

RESULTS

In total, 186 assessments (1.1%) were completed at night, 460 (2.7%) were completed in the early morning, 4,200 (24.4%) were completed in the late morning, 4,941 (28.7%) in the afternoon, 4,724 (27.5%) in the early evening, and 2,698 (15.7%) were completed in the late evening (see **Figure 1**). **Table 1** summarizes the estimated fixed effects of all MLMs (standard deviations and correlations of random effects can be found in the Supplementary Material). Results suggest that tinnitus was louder and more distressing during the night and early morning hours than during all other timeframes of the day (see Models I in the first and third columns of **Table 1**). Tukey's post-hoc tests revealed that differences between late morning, afternoon, and early evening were non-significant (see **Table 2**). However, tinnitus was significantly louder in the late evening compared to the afternoon and early evening. This pattern of results is visualized in **Figures 2A,B**. The pseudo R^2 statistics revealed that time-of-day explained 20.6% of the within-day variance of tinnitus loudness, and 13.0% of the within-day variance of tinnitus distress.

Next, we tested whether time-of-day influences the subjective stress-level (see Model I in the right hand column of **Table 1** and **Figure 2C**). Tukey's post-hoc tests suggested that stress-level increased from morning to afternoon, decreased from afternoon to evening, and did not differ compared to the night (see **Table 2**). Time-of-day explained 7.8% of the within-day variance of stress.

Finally, the models predicting tinnitus loudness and tinnitus distress from time-of-day and stress-level revealed that the stress-level had incremental effects across all three levels (see Models II in **Table 1**): Tinnitus was louder and more distressing when the level of stress was higher at a specific time-of-day compared to other times-of-day, when it was higher during a whole day compared to other days, and when it was higher during the whole assessment period for a given participant (compared to other participants). Nevertheless, the effects of time-of-day on tinnitus loudness and tinnitus distress

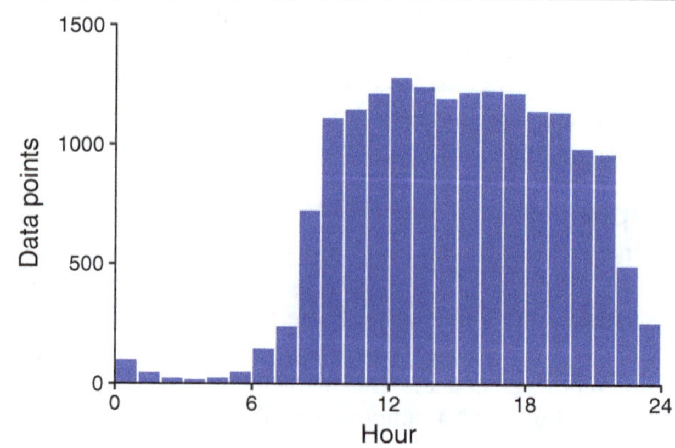

FIGURE 1 | Number of data points per hour.

TABLE 1 | Estimated fixed effects (and their standard errors) for five MLMs.

		Tinnitus loudness		Tinnitus distress		Stress-level
		Model I	Model II	Model I	Model II	Model I
Intercept (night)	γ_{000}	0.529*** (0.021)	0.521*** (0.018)	0.435*** (0.021)	0.423*** (0.016)	0.303*** (0.020)
Early morning (vs. night) effect	γ_{100}	−0.017 (0.021)	−0.015 (0.019)	−0.015 (0.022)	−0.014 (0.018)	−0.015 (0.020)
Late morning (vs. night) effect	γ_{200}	−0.089*** (0.019)	−0.086*** (0.017)	−0.083*** (0.020)	−0.077*** (0.016)	0.009 (0.019)
Afternoon (vs. night) effect	γ_{300}	−0.098*** (0.019)	−0.099*** (0.017)	−0.083*** (0.019)	−0.083*** (0.016)	0.023 (0.018)
Early evening (vs. night) effect	γ_{400}	−0.093*** (0.019)	−0.092*** (0.017)	−0.080*** (0.020)	−0.074*** (0.015)	0.006 (0.018)
Late evening (vs. night) effect	γ_{500}	−0.071*** (0.019)	−0.062*** (0.016)	−0.066*** (0.019)	−0.052*** (0.014)	−0.023 (0.018)
Within-day effect of stress	γ_{600}		0.287*** (0.020)		0.370*** (0.022)	
Between-day effect of stress	γ_{010}		0.470*** (0.037)		0.585*** (0.035)	
Between-person effect of stress	γ_{001}		0.651*** (0.051)		0.810*** (0.041)	

*Total number of assessments was 17,209. p-values were based on Satterthwaite's approximations. ***p < 0.001. night = 12 a.m.–4 a.m. early morning = 4 a.m.–8 a.m. late morning = 8 a.m.–12 p.m. afternoon = 12 p.m.–4 p.m. early evening = 4 p.m.–8 p.m. late evening = 8 p.m.–12 a.m.*

TABLE 2 | Tukey's *post-hoc* tests for five MLMs.

	Tinnitus loudness		Tinnitus distress		Stress-level
	Model I	Model II	Model I	Model II	Model I
Early_morning–night	−0.017 (0.021)	−0.015 (0.019)	−0.015 (0.022)	−0.014 (0.018)	−0.015 (0.020)
Late_morning–night	−0.089*** (0.019)	−0.086*** (0.017)	−0.083*** (0.020)	−0.077*** (0.016)	0.009 (0.019)
Afternoon–night	−0.098*** (0.019)	−0.099*** (0.017)	−0.083*** (0.019)	−0.083*** (0.016)	0.023 (0.018)
Early_evening–night	−0.093*** (0.019)	−0.092*** (0.017)	−0.080*** (0.020)	−0.074*** (0.015)	0.006 (0.018)
Late_evening–night	−0.071** (0.019)	−0.062** (0.016)	−0.066** (0.019)	−0.052** (0.014)	−0.023 (0.018)
Late_morning–early_morning	−0.072*** (0.014)	−0.071*** (0.013)	−0.068*** (0.015)	−0.063*** (0.013)	0.023 (0.012)
Afternoon–early_morning	−0.080*** (0.016)	−0.084*** (0.015)	−0.068*** (0.016)	−0.069*** (0.014)	0.038* (0.012)
Early_evening–early_morning	−0.076*** (0.016)	−0.077*** (0.015)	−0.064*** (0.016)	−0.060*** (0.014)	0.021 (0.013)
Late_evening–early_morning	−0.053** (0.016)	−0.047* (0.015)	−0.050* (0.017)	−0.038* (0.014)	−0.009 (0.012)
Afternoon–late_morning	−0.008 (0.005)	−0.013# (0.005)	−0.000 (0.005)	−0.006 (0.004)	0.014** (0.004)
Early_evening–late_morning	−0.004 (0.007)	−0.005 (0.006)	0.004 (0.006)	0.003 (0.004)	−0.003 (0.006)
Late_evening–late_morning	0.019 (0.009)	0.025* (0.008)	0.017 (0.008)	0.025** (0.007)	−0.032*** (0.006)
Early_evening–afternoon	0.004 (0.003)	0.007 (0.003)	0.004 (0.004)	0.009* (0.003)	−0.017*** (0.004)
Late_evening–afternoon	0.027** (0.007)	0.037*** (0.007)	0.017 (0.007)	0.031*** (0.006)	−0.046*** (0.005)
Late_evening–early_evening	0.023** (0.006)	0.030*** (0.006)	0.014 (0.006)	0.022*** (0.005)	−0.029*** (0.004)

*Total number of assessments was 17,209. The table presents estimated differences (and their standard errors) for all comparisons between timeframes. p-values were adjusted using the Tukey Honest Significant Difference method. #p < 0.10. *p < 0.05. **p < 0.01. ***p < 0.001. night = 12 a.m.–4 a.m. early morning = 4 a.m.–8 a.m. late morning = 8 a.m.–12 p.m. afternoon = 12 p.m.–4 p.m. early evening = 4 p.m.–8 p.m. late evening = 8 p.m.–12 a.m.*

were still significant (i.e., after controlling for the effects of stress).

DISCUSSION

This study evaluated whether subjective tinnitus loudness and subjective tinnitus distress depend on time-of-day with EMA from the "TrackYourTinnitus" (TYT) mobile application (Pryss et al., 2015a,b; Schlee et al., 2016). Strengths of the present study are that a mobile application was used to obtain EMA of high ecological validity (Trull and Ebner-Priemer, 2013, 2014; Adams et al., 2017), a much higher sampling frequency was applied than in typical clinical studies, and the sample size was much larger than in previous EMA studies on the time-of-day-dependence of tinnitus (Flor et al., 2004; Henry et al., 2012; Wilson et al., 2015).

The main result was that tinnitus (loudness and distress) was rated as more severe during the night and the early morning (from 12 a.m. to 8 a.m.) than during the upcoming day. Interestingly, tinnitus loudness and tinnitus distress showed a very similar time pattern although the neurobiological correlates of loudness and distress differ to a certain degree (e.g., De Ridder et al., 2011; Leaver et al., 2012; Ueyama et al., 2013; Vanneste et al., 2014).

Contrary to the EMA study by Henry et al. (2012), the present investigation found a time-of-day-dependence of tinnitus. The most obvious reason for this discrepancy is that Henry et al. (2012) assessed tinnitus only from 8 a.m. to 8 p.m. and could, therefore, not evaluate tinnitus during the time interval that was related to most severe tinnitus in our study (12 a.m.–8 a.m.). During a time interval (8 a.m.–12 a.m.) that included the 12-h

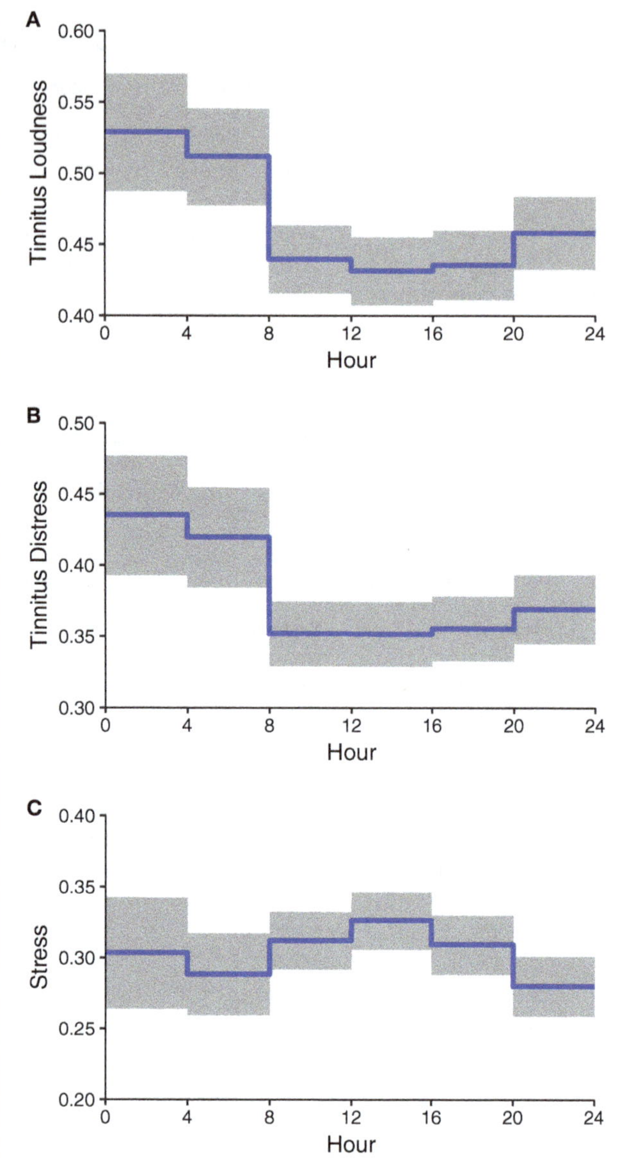

FIGURE 2 | Expected tinnitus loudness **(A)**, tinnitus distress **(B)**, and level of stress **(C)** as a function of time-of-day. The blue lines represent expected values for the average participant on an average day, the gray bands represent 95% confidence intervals.

interval analyzed by Henry et al. (2012) tinnitus did not vary much in our study either (see **Figures 2A,B**). The result that tinnitus was more severe in the early morning hours is in line with a previous diary study (Flor et al., 2004) and fits to the clinical impression of a "morning roar" as it is often anecdotally reported by tinnitus patients. Yet, our result that tinnitus was more severe during the night was not found by Flor et al. (2004). More severe tinnitus (loudness and distress) during the night could at least partially result from the possibility that several assessments at night were given by participants while having sleep disturbances. Sleep disturbances are common among tinnitus patients and their severity correlates positively with measures of tinnitus severity (e.g., Crönlein et al., 2007; Schecklmann et al., 2015; Crönlein et al., 2016). Although we aimed to control for this potential confounder by excluding data from spontaneous ratings and restricting the data analysis to the ratings provided at notifications, the fact that sleep disturbances were not assessed on a daily basis in the present study and, hence, were not available for analysis is a limitation of our study. Future research could explore whether the effect of time-of-day on tinnitus is different between days with and without sleep disturbances. Besides sleep, several other variables are time-of-day dependent and should be considered as potential confounding variables: For example, the environmental sound level depends on time-of-day and tinnitus might be more severe during the night and the early morning, because the environmental sound level in these time intervals cannot mask the tinnitus. Furthermore, a trigger of tinnitus might be (even slight) tension of specific muscles of the craniocervical connection (Bechter et al., 2016), whereby the tension depends mainly from posture, which is influenced by different aspects during the night (e.g., sleeping posture, bed pillow) and during the day. Moreover, the release of stress-related hormones is controlled by a circadian clock (Dickmeis, 2009; Lightman and Conway-Campbell, 2010; Conway-Campbell et al., 2012) and future studies could explore the relationship between circadian tinnitus variability and such stress-related hormones. In the present study, we could only analyze subjective stress-levels with the result that the 24-h course of the subjective stress-level was not parallel to the course of tinnitus (loudness and distress): While tinnitus (loudness and distress) showed their maximum between 12 a.m. and 8 a.m., the maximum of the subjective stress-level was found between 12 p.m. and 4 p.m. The discrepant time curves of tinnitus and subjective stress-level raise further questions, which need to be addressed in future longitudinal studies regarding the tinnitus-stress link. For example, it appears possible that tinnitus and subjective stress interact more in a time-lagged than in an instant manner. Thus, it should be clarified whether increases of subjective stress lead to more severe tinnitus and whether increases of tinnitus severity also lead to more subsequent subjective stress (which again might affect tinnitus severity resulting in a vicious circle). Feedback loops have been described already in research on the pituitary-adrenal system: "positive, delayed, feedforward connection between the pituitary and the adrenals" and "negative feedback of glucocorticoids on ACTH release" (Lightman and Conway-Campbell, 2010, p. 712). It should also be noted in this context that the peaks of our self-reported stress-levels (12 p.m.–4 p.m.) did not correspond to the peaks of cortisol and ACTH releases (4 a.m.–8 a.m.) as illustrated by Lightman and Conway-Campbell (2010). Therefore, the longitudinal associations between tinnitus and self-reported stress might be different from the ones between tinnitus and stress-hormones.

Regarding the observed circadian variability of tinnitus loudness, it is tempting to speculate relations to circadian variations in neuronal sensitivity of peripheral and central auditory structures, which have been identified in recent studies (Park et al., 2016; Basinou et al., 2017). However, tinnitus loudness does not directly reflect neuronal activity in auditory pathways, but also depends on other factors such as attention and emotions. For example, a previous study found that tinnitus becomes louder over time when participants experience more qualitatively different feelings (Probst et al., 2016b). Therefore, more research is needed to replicate the observed circadian rhythm of tinnitus in large samples, to identify the specific contribution of different factors (e.g., neuronal activity in auditory pathways, attention, and emotion), and to explore whether different persons show a different time-of-day dependence of tinnitus. Moderating variables might, for example, be gender, age (e.g., the time-of-day dependence of tinnitus might be different between men and women or within women before/after the menopause), and the etiology of tinnitus (e.g., the time of time-of-day dependence might be different between noise trauma as etiology and stress as etiology). Future translational and clinical studies with samples large enough to analyze such subgroups are required to explore potential moderators of the time-of-day dependence of tinnitus. These further studies could also measure tinnitus by different assessment methods, because the study at hand only analyzed self-reported tinnitus. For example, by the "gap-in-noise" paradigm (Lowe and Walton, 2015) or psychophysiological measurements such as tinnitus matching. Yet, the reliability and validity of tinnitus matching is an ongoing matter of debate (Hoare et al., 2014; De Ridder et al., 2015). For mobile applications such as TYT, portable methods to assess tinnitus more objectively (see for example, Hébert and Fournier, 2017) that can be integrated in the mobile application are needed. It is necessary to evaluate whether a similar time-of-day dependence of tinnitus can be shown for self-reported tinnitus as well as for more objectively measured tinnitus. Future studies could also compare different statistical approaches and identify the approach most suited to investigate time-of-day dependencies. For example, harmonic regression was performed in an animal study on circadian rhythm (Atger et al., 2015), and an R package for nonparametric circular methods (NPCirc) is available to analyze circular data (Oliveira et al., 2014). These approaches were not performed in the present study due to the nested structure of the data (assessments within days and days within participants).

In summary, the results of our study have implications for both tinnitus research and tinnitus management. Taking time-of-day into account in the study design might be necessary in clinical studies. Yet, the results of our study rely solely on TYT users (who are not representative for clinical tinnitus patients, see Probst et al., 2017) and on one-item questions on tinnitus distress and tinnitus loudness making it difficult to conclude whether the observed differences between night/early morning and the upcoming day are clinically relevant. Future studies using assessment instruments appropriate to distinguish between clinically relevant and clinically irrelevant change (for example the Tinnitus Handicap Inventory (THI), see Zeman et al., 2011) with clinical tinnitus samples are necessary to address this point. Chronobiological aspects should not only be considered in tinnitus research but also in tinnitus treatment. Tailoring the timing of therapeutic interventions to the circadian rhythm of individual tinnitus patients (chronotherapy) might be promising. Further translational and clinical studies are necessary to evaluate the potential of chronotherapy for tinnitus. However, this is a challenging task since "research in the topic is underfunded when compared with other diseases for which the prevalence and cost to society is relatively similar" (Cederroth et al., 2013, p. 972). Nevertheless, the current study might motivate individuals with tinnitus to observe their tinnitus fluctuations and to identify time-intervals during which the access to and the use of tinnitus coping strategies are most crucial.

AUTHOR CONTRIBUTIONS

TP substantially contributed to the design of the study and data preparation, drafted and revised the manuscript. RP substantially contributed to the design of the study, data preparation, conception, implementation and maintenance of the "TrackYourTinnitus" application, and revised the manuscript. BL substantially contributed to the design of the study and revised the manuscript. JR substantially contributed to the design of the study and revised the manuscript. JS substantially contributed to the conception, implementation and maintenance of the "TrackYourTinnitus" application, and revised the manuscript. MR substantially contributed to the conception, implementation and maintenance of the "TrackYourTinnitus" application, and revised the manuscript. MS substantially contributed to the design of the study and revised the manuscript. WS substantially contributed to the design of the study, data preparation, conception and implementation of the "TrackYourTinnitus" application, drafted and revised the manuscript. JZ substantially contributed to the design of the study and performed the statistical analysis, drafted and revised the manuscript.

ACKNOWLEDGMENTS

This work was supported by the German Research Foundation (DFG) and the Georg-August-University Göttingen (Germany) within the funding programme Open Access Publishing.

REFERENCES

Adams, W. Z., McClure, E. A., Gray, K. M., Danielson, C. K., Treiber, F. A., and Ruggiero, K. J. (2017). Mobile devices for the remote acquisition of physiological and behavioral biomarkers in psychiatric clinical research. *J. Psychiatr. Res.* 85, 1–14. doi: 10.1016/j.jpsychires.2016.10.019

Ajayi, O. V., Phillips, J. S., Laopaiboon, M., and McFerran, D. (2014). Melatonin for tinnitus. *Cochrane Database Syst. Rev.* 12:CD011435. doi: 10.1002/14651858.CD011435

Alsalman, O. A., Tucker, D., and Vanneste, S. (2016). Salivary stress-related responses in tinnitus: a preliminary study in young male subjects with tinnitus. *Front. Neurosci.* 10:338. doi: 10.3389/fnins.2016.00338

Atger, F., Gobet, C., Marquis, J., Martin, E., Wang, J., Weger, B., et al. (2015). Circadian and feeding rhythms differentially affect rhythmic mRNA transcription and translation in mouse liver. *Proc. Natl. Acad. Sci. U.S.A.* 112, E6579–E6588. doi: 10.1073/pnas.1515308112

Baguley, D., McFerran, D., and Hall, D. (2013). Tinnitus. *Lancet* 382, 1600–1607. doi: 10.1016/S0140-6736(13)60142-7

Basinou, V., Park, J.- S., Cederroth, C. R., and Canlon, B: (2017). Circadian regulation of auditory function. *Hear. Res.* 347, 47–55. doi: 10.1016/j.heares.2016.08.018

Bates, D., Maechler, M., Bolker, B, and Walker, S. (2015). Fitting linear mixed-effects models using lme4. *J. Stat. Softw.* 67, 1–48. doi: 10.18637/jss.v067.i01

Bechter, K., Wieland, M., and Hamann, G. F. (2016). Chronic cervicogenic tinnitus rapidly resolved by intermittent use of cervical collar. *Front. Psychiatry* 7:43. doi: 10.3389/fpsyt.2016.00043

Bhatt, J. M., Bhattacharyya, N., and Lin, H. W. (2016). Relationships between tinnitus and the prevalence of anxiety and depression. *Laryngoscope* 127, 466–469. doi: 10.1002/lary.26107

Buttgereit, F., Smolen, J. S., Coogan, A. N., and Cajochen, C. (2015). Clocking in: chronobiology in rheumatoid arthritis. *Nat. Rev. Rheumatol.* 11, 349–356. doi: 10.1038/nrrheum.2015.31

Cederroth, C. R., Canlon, B., and Langguth, B. (2013). Hearing loss and tinnitus-are funders and industry listening? *Nat. Biotechnol.* 31, 972–974. doi: 10.1038/nbt.2736

Cima, R. F., Crombez, G., and Vlaeyen, J. W. (2011). Catastrophizing and fear of tinnitus predict quality of life in patients with chronic tinnitus. *Ear. Hear.* 32, 634–641. doi: 10.1097/AUD.0b013e31821106dd

Conway-Campbell, B. L., Pooley, J. R., Hager, G. L., and Lightman, S. L. (2012). Molecular dynamics of ultradian glucocorticoid receptor action. *Mol. Cell. Endocrinol.* 348, 383–393. doi: 10.1016/j.mce.2011.08.014

Crönlein, T., Langguth, B., Geisler, P., and Hajak, G. (2007). Tinnitus and insomnia. *Prog. Brain. Res.* 166, 227–233. doi: 10.1016/S0079-6123(07)66021-X

Crönlein, T., Langguth, B., Pregler, M., Kreuzer, P. M., Wetter, T. C., and Schecklmann, M. (2016). Insomnia in patients with chronic tinnitus: cognitive and emotional distress as moderator variables. *J. Psychosom. Res.* 83, 65–68. doi: 10.1016/j.jpsychores.2016.03.001

Dauman, N., Erlandsson, S., Lundlin, L., and Dauman, R. (2015). Intra-individual variability in tinnitus patients: current thoughts and perspectives. *HNO.* 63, 302–306. doi: 10.1007/s00106-014-2978-2

De Ridder, D., Congedo, M., and Vanneste, S. (2015). The neural correlates of subjectively perceived and passively matched loudness perception in auditory phantom perception. *Brain Behav.* 5: e00331. doi: 10.1002/brb3.331

De Ridder, D., Elgoyhen, A. B., Romo, R., and Langguth, B. (2011). Phantom percepts: tinnitus and pain as persisting aversive memory networks. *Proc. Natl. Acad. Sci. U.S.A.* 108, 8075–8080. doi: 10.1073/pnas.1018466108

De Ridder, D., Vanneste, S., Weisz, N., Londero, A., Schlee, W., Elgoyhen, A. B., et al. (2014). An integrative model of auditory phantom perception: tinnitus as a unified percept of interacting separable subnetworks. *Neurosci. Biobehav. Rev.* 44, 16–32. doi: 10.1016/j.neubiorev.2013.03.021

Dickmeis, T. (2009). Glucocorticoids and the circadian clock. *J. Endocrinol.* 200, 3–22. doi: 10.1677/JOE-08-0415

Flor, H., Hoffmann, D., Struve, M., and Diesch, E. (2004). Auditory discrimination training for the treatment of tinnitus. *Appl. Psychophysiol. Biofeedback* 29, 113–120. doi: 10.1023/B:APBI.0000026637.77671.f4

Germain, A., and Kupfer, D. J. (2008). Circadian rhythm disturbances in depression. *Hum. Psychopharmacol.* 23, 571–585. doi: 10.1002/hup.964

Gilron, I., and Ghasemlou, N. (2014). Chronobiology of chronic pain: focus on diurnal rhythmicity of neuropathic pain. *Curr. Opin. Support. Palliat. Care* 8, 429–436. doi: 10.1097/SPC.0000000000000085

Hébert, S., and Fournier, P. (2017). Clinical validation of a new tinnitus assessment technology. *Front. Neurol.* 8:38. doi: 10.3389/fneur.2017.00038

Hébert, S., and Lupien, S. J. (2007). The sound of stress: blunted cortisol reactivity to psychosocial stress in tinnitus sufferers. *Neurosci. Lett.* 411, 138–142. doi: 10.1016/j.neulet.2006.10.028

Hébert, S., and Lupien, S. J. (2009). Salivary cortisol levels, subjective stress, and tinnitus intensity in tinnitus sufferers during noise exposure in the laboratory. *Int. J. Hyg. Environ. Health* 212, 37–44. doi: 10.1016/j.ijheh.2007.11.005

Hébert, S., Paiement, P., and Lupien, S. J. (2004). A physiological correlate for the intolerance to both internal and external sounds. *Hear. Res.* 190, 1–9. doi: 10.1016/S0378-5955(04)00021-8

Henry, J. A., Galvez, G., Turbin, M. B., Thielman, E. J., McMillan, G. P., and Istvan, J. A. (2012). Pilot study to evaluate ecological momentary assessment of tinnitus. *Ear. Hear.* 33, 179–290. doi: 10.1097/AUD.0b013e31822f6740

Hesser, H., and Andersson, G. (2009). The role of anxiety sensitivity and behavioral avoidance in tinnitus disability. *Int. J. Audiol.* 48, 295–299. doi: 10.1080/14992020802635325

Hesser, H., Weise, C., Westin, V. Z., and Andersson, G. (2011). A systematic review and meta-analysis of randomized controlled trials of cognitive-behavioral therapy for tinnitus distress. *Clin. Psychol. Rev.* 31, 545–553. doi: 10.1016/j.cpr.2010.12.006

Hiller, W., and Goebel, G. (2007). When tinnitus loudness and annoyance are discrepant: audiological characteristics and psychological profile. *Audiol. Neurootol.* 12, 391–400. doi: 10.1159/000106482

Hoare, D. J., Edmondson-Jones, M., Gander, P. E., and Hall, D. A. (2014). Agreement and reliability of tinnitus loudness matching and pitch likeness rating. *PLoS ONE* 9:e114553. doi: 10.1371/journal.pone.0114553

Hobson, J., Chisholm, E., and El Refaie, A. (2012). Sound therapy (masking) in the management of tinnitus in adults. *Cochrane Database Syst. Rev.* 11:CD006371. doi: 10.1002/14651858.cd006371.pub3

Hothorn, T., Bretz, F., and Westfall, P. (2008). Simultaneous inference in general parametric models. *Biom. J.* 50, 346–363. doi: 10.1002/bimj.200810425

Jasper, K., Weise, C., Conrad, I., Andersson, G., Hiller, W., and Kleinstäuber, M. (2014). Internet-based guided self-help versus group cognitive behavioral therapy for chronic tinnitus: a randomized controlled trial. *Psychother. Psychosom.* 83, 234–246. doi: 10.1159/000360705

Kleinstäuber, M., Jasper, K., Schweda, I., Hiller, W., Andersson, G., and Weise, C. (2013). The role of fear-avoidance cognitions and behaviors in patients with chronic tinnitus. *Cogn. Beh. Ther.* 42, 84–99. doi: 10.1080/16506073.2012.717301

Landgrebe, M., Azevedo, A., Baguley, D., Bauer, C., Cacace, A., Coelho, C., et al. (2012). Methodological aspects of clinical trials in tinnitus: a proposal for an international standard. *J. Psychosom. Res.* 73, 112–121. doi: 10.1016/j.jpsychores.2012.05.002

Langguth, B., and De Ridder, D. (2013). Tinnitus: therapeutic use of superficial brain stimulation. *Handb. Clin. Neurol.* 116, 441–467. doi: 10.1016/B978-0-444-53497-2.00036-X

Langguth, B., and Elgoyhen, A. B. (2012). Current pharmacological treatments for tinnitus. *Expert Opin. Pharmacother.* 13, 2495–2509. doi: 10.1517/14656566.2012.739608

Langguth, B., Kreuzer, P. M., Kleinjung, T., and De Ridder, D. (2013). Tinnitus: causes and clinical management. *Lancet Neurol.* 12, 920–930. doi: 10.1016/S1474-4422(13)70160-1

Langguth, B., Landgrebe, M., Kleinjung, T., Sand, G. P., and Hajak, G. (2011). Tinnitus and depression. *World J. Biol. Psychiatry* 12, 489–500. doi: 10.3109/15622975.2011.575178

Leaver, A. M., Renier, L., Chevillet, M. A., Morgan, S., Kim, H. J., and Rauschecker, J. P. (2011). Dysregulation of limbic and auditory networks in tinnitus. *Neuron* 69, 33–43. doi: 10.1016/j.neuron.2010.12.002

Leaver, A. M., Seydell-Greenwald, A., Turesky, T. K., Morgan, S., Kim, H. J., and Rauschecker, J. P. (2012). Cortico-limbic morphology separates tinnitus from tinnitus distress. *Front. Syst. Neurosci.* 6:21. doi: 10.3389/fnsys.2012.00021

Lightman, S. L., and Conway-Campbell, B. L. (2010). The crucial role of pulsatile activity of the HPA axis for continuous dynamic equilibration. *Nat. Rev. Neurosci.* 11, 710–718. doi: 10.1038/nrn2914

Lowe, A. S., and Walton, J. P. (2015). Alterations in peripheral and central components of the auditory brainstem response: a neural assay of tinnitus. *PLoS ONE* 10:e0117228. doi: 10.1371/journal.pone.0117228

Maes, I. H., Cima, R. F., Anteunis, L. J., Scheijen, D. J., Baguley, D. M., El Refaie, A., et al. (2014). Cost-effectiveness of specialized treatment based on cognitive behavioral therapy versus usual care for tinnitus. *Otol. Neurotol.* 35, 787–795. doi: 10.1097/MAO.0000000000000331

Maes, I. H., Cima, R. F., Vlaeyen, J. W., Anteunis, L. J., and Joore, M. A. (2013). Tinnitus: a cost study. *Ear. Hear.* 34, 508–514. doi: 10.1097/AUD.0b013e31827d113a

Martinez, C., Wallenhorst, C., McFerran, D., and Hall, D. A. (2015). Incidence rates of clinically significant tinnitus: 10-year trend from a cohort study in England. *Ear. Hear.* 36, e69–75. doi: 10.1097/aud.0000000000000121

McCormack, A., Edmondson-Jones, M., Somerset, S, and Hall, D. (2016). A systematic review of the reporting of tinnitus prevalence and severity. *Hear. Res.* 337, 70–79. doi: 10.1016/j.heares.2016.05.009

McKenna, L., Handscomb, L., Hoare, D. J., and Hall, D. A. (2014). A scientific cognitive-behavioral model of tinnitus: novel conceptualizations of tinnitus distress. *Front. Neurol.* 5:196. doi: 10.3389/fneur.2014.00196

Meltser, I., Cederroth, C. R., Basinou, V., Savelyev, S., Lundkvist, G. S., and Canlon, B. (2014). TrkB-mediated protection against circadian sensitivity to noise trauma in the murine cochlea. *Curr. Biol.* 24, 658–663. doi: 10.1016/j.cub.2014.01.047

Miroddi, M., Bruno, R., Galletti, F., Calapai, F., Navarra, M., Gangemi, S., et al. (2015). Clinical pharmacology of melatonin in the treatment of tinnitus: a review. *Eur. J. Clin. Pharmacol.* 71, 263–270. doi: 10.1007/s00228-015-1805-3

Newman, C. W., Sandridge, S. A., and Bolek, L. (2008). Development and psychometric adequacy of the screening version of the tinnitus handicap inventory. *Otol. Neurotol.* 29, 276–281. doi: 10.1097/MAO.0b013e31816569c4

Nondahl, D. M., Cruickshanks, K. J., Huang, G. H., Klein, B. E., Klein, R., Tweed, T. S., et al. (2012). Generational differences in the reporting of tinnitus. *Ear. Hear.* 33, 640–644. doi: 10.1097/AUD.0b013e31825069e8

Oliveira, M., Crujeiras, R. M., and Rodríguez-Casal, A. (2014). NPCirc: an R package for nonpara-metric circular methods. *J. Stat. Soft.* 61, 1–26. doi: 10.18637/jss.v061.i09

Park, J., S., Cederroth, C. R., Basinou, V., Meltser, I., Lundkvist, G., and Canlon, B. (2016). Identification of a circadian clock in the inferior colliculus and its dysregulation by noise exposure. *J. Neurosci.* 36, 5509–5519. doi: 10.1523/JNEUROSCI.3616-15.2016

Pirodda, A., Raimondi, M. C., and Ferri, G. G. (2010). Exploring the reasons why melatonin can improve tinnitus. *Med. Hypotheses* 75, 190–191. doi: 10.1016/j.mehy.2010.02.018

Probst, T., Pryss, R., Langguth, B., and Schlee, W. (2016a). Emotional states as mediators between tinnitus loudness and tinnitus distress in daily life: results from the "TrackYourTinnitus" application. *Sci. Rep.* 6:20382. doi: 10.1038/srep20382

Probst, T., Pryss, R., Langguth, B., and Schlee, W. (2016b). Emotion dynamics and tinnitus: daily life data from the "TrackYourTinnitus" application. *Sci. Rep.* 6:31166. doi: 10.1038/srep31166

Probst, T., Pryss, R. C., Langguth, B., Spiliopoulou, M., Landgrebe, M., Vesala, M., et al. (2017). Outpatient tinnitus clinic, self-help web platform, or mobile application to recruit tinnitus study samples? *Front. Aging Neurosci.* 9:113. doi: 10.3389/fnagi.2017.00113

Pryss, R., Reichert, M., Herrmann, J., Langguth, B., Schlee, W. (2015a). "Mobile crowd sensing in clinical and psychological trials - a case study," in *28th IEEE Int'l Symposium on Computer-Based Medical Systems, 22–25 June 2015* (Sao Carlos: IEEE Computer Society Press), 23–24. Available online at: http://dbis.eprints.uni-ulm.de/1144/1/PCBMS_2015.pdf (Accessed July 15, 2017)

Pryss, R., Reichert, M., Langguth, B., and Schlee, W. (2015b). "Mobile crowd sensing services for tinnitus assessment, therapy and research," in *IEEE 4th International Conference on Mobile Services (MS 2015), June 27–July 2, 2015* (New York, NY: IEEE Computer Society Press), 352–359. Available online at: http://dbis.eprints.uni-ulm.de/1152/1/ms2015rpmrblws.pdf (Accessed: July 15, 2017).

Raudenbush, S. W., and Bryk, A. S. (2002). *Hierarchical Linear Models: Applications and Data Analysis Methods.* Newbury Park, CA: Sage Publications.

Rauschecker, J. P., Leaver, A. M., and Mühlau, M. (2010). Tuning out the noise: limbic-auditory interactions in tinnitus. *Neuron* 66, 819–826. doi: 10.1016/j.neuron.2010.04.032

Rauschecker, J. P., May, E. S., Maudoux, A., and Ploner, M. (2015). Frontostriatal gating of tinnitus and chronic pain. *Trends Cogn. Sci.* 19, 567–578. doi: 10.1016/j.tics.2015.08.002

R Core Team, A. (2015). *R: A Language and Environment for Statistical Computing.* Vienna: R foundation for statistical computing. Available online at: https://www.R-project.org/ (Accessed: November 25, 2016).

Riedl, D., Rumpold, G., Schmidt, A., Zorowka, P. G., Bliem, H. R., and Moschen, R. (2015). The influence of tinnitus acceptance on the quality of life and psychological distress in patients with chronic tinnitus. *Noise Health* 17, 374–381. doi: 10.4103/1463-1741.165068

Schecklmann, M., Pregler, M., Kreuzer, P. M., Poeppl, T. B., Lehner, A., Crönlein, T., et al. (2015). Psychophysiological associations between chronic tinnitus and sleep: a cross validation of tinnitus and insomnia questionnaires. *BioMed. Res. Int.* 2015:461090. doi: 10.1155/2015/461090

Schlee, W., Pryss, R. C., Probst, T., Schobel, J., Bachmeier, A., Reichert, M., et al. (2016). Measuring the moment-to-moment variability of tinnitus: the TrackYourTinnitus smart phone app. *Front. Aging Neurosci.* 8:294. doi: 10.3389/fnagi.2016.00294

Schlee, W., Schecklmann, M., Lehner, A., Kreuzer, P. M., Vielsmeier, V., Poeppl, T. B., et al. (2014). Reduced variability of auditory alpha activity in chronic tinnitus. *Neural. Plast.* 2014:436146. doi: 10.1155/2014/436146

Singer, J. D., and Willett, J. B. (2003). *Applied Longitudinal Data Analysis: Modeling Change and Event Occurence.* New York, NY: Oxford University Press. doi: 10.1093/acprof:oso/9780195152968.001.0001

Strian, F., Lautenbacher, S., Galfe, G., and Hölzl, R. (1989). Diurnal variations in pain perception and thermal sensitivity. *Pain* 36, 125–131. doi: 10.1016/0304-3959(89)90120-6

Trull, T. J., and Ebner-Priemer, U. (2013). Ambulatory assessment. *Annu. Rev. Clin. Psychol.* 9, 151–176. doi: 10.1146/annurev-clinpsy-050212-185510

Trull, T. J., and Ebner-Priemer, U. (2014). The role of ambulatory assessment in psychological science. *Curr. Dir. Psychol. Sci.* 23, 466–470. doi: 10.1177/0963721414550706

Ueyama, T., Donishi, T., Ukai, S., Ikeda, Y., Hotomi, M., Yamanaka, N., et al. (2013). Brain regions responsible for tinnitus distress and loudness: a resting-state FMRI study. *PLoS ONE* 8:e67778. doi: 10.1371/journal.pone.0067778

Vanneste, S., Congedo, M., and De Ridder, D. (2014). Pinpointing a highly specific pathological functional connection that turns phantom sound into distress. *Cereb. Cortex* 24, 2268–2282. doi: 10.1093/cercor/bht068

Wallhäusser-Franke, E., Brade, J., Balkenhol, T., D'Amelio, R., Seegmüller, A., and Delb, W. (2012). Tinnitus: distinguishing between subjectively perceived loudness and tinnitus-related distress. *PLoS ONE* 7:e34583. doi: 10.1371/journal.pone.0034583

Weise, C., Kleinstäuber, M., Hesser, H., Westin, V. Z., and Andersson, G. (2013). Acceptance of tinnitus: validation of the tinnitus acceptance questionnaire. *Cogn. Behav. Ther.* 42, 100–115. doi: 10.1080/16506073.2013.781670

Wilson, M. B., Kallogjeri, D., Joplin, C. N., Gorman, M. D., Krings, J. G., Lenze, E. J., et al. (2015). Ecological momentary assessment of tinnitus using smartphone technology: a pilot study. *Otolaryngol. Head. Neck. Surg.* 152, 897–903. doi: 10.1177/0194599815569692

Wirz-Justice, A. (2008). Diurnal variation of depressive symptoms. *Dialogues Clin. Neurosci.* 10, 337–343.

Zeman, F., Koller, M., Figueiredo, R., Aazevedo, A., Rates, M., Coelho, C., et al. (2011). Tinnitus handicap inventory for evaluating treatment effects: which changes are clinically relevant? *Otolaryngol. Head Neck Surg.* 145, 282–287. doi: 10.1177/0194599811403882

19

Validation of Online Versions of Tinnitus Questionnaires Translated into Swedish

*Karolina Müller[1], Niklas K. Edvall[2], Esma Idrizbegovic[3], Robert Huhn[3], Rilana Cima[4,5], Viktor Persson[6], Constanze Leineweber[6], Hugo Westerlund[6], Berthold Langguth[7], Winfried Schlee[7], Barbara Canlon[2] and Christopher R. Cederroth[2]**

[1] Center for Clinical Studies, University Medical Center Regensburg, Regensburg, Germany, [2] Experimental Audiology, Department of Physiology and Pharmacology, Karolinska Institutet, Stockholm, Sweden, [3] Hörsel-och Balanskliniken, Karolinska Universitetssjukhuset, Stockholm, Sweden, [4] Clinical Psychological Science, Faculty of Psychology and Neuroscience, Maastricht University, Maastricht, Netherlands, [5] Center of Expertise in Rehabilitation and Audiology, Adelante Rehabilitation, Hoensbroek, Netherlands, [6] Stress Research Institute, Stockholm University, Stockholm, Sweden, [7] Department of Psychiatry and Psychotherapy, University Medical Center Regensburg, Regensburg, Germany

***Correspondence:**
Christopher R. Cederroth
christopher.cederroth@ki.se

Background: Due to the lack of objective measures for assessing tinnitus, its clinical evaluation largely relies on the use of questionnaires and psychoacoustic tests. A global assessment of tinnitus burden would largely benefit from holistic approaches that not only incorporate measures of tinnitus but also take into account associated fears, emotional aspects (stress, anxiety, and depression), and quality of life. In Sweden, only a few instruments are available for assessing tinnitus, and the existing tools lack validation. Therefore, we translated a set of questionnaires into Swedish and evaluated their reliability and validity in a group of tinnitus subjects.

Methods: We translated the English versions of the Tinnitus Functional Index (TFI), the Fear of Tinnitus Questionnaire (FTQ), the Tinnitus Catastrophizing Scale (TCS), the Perceived Stress Questionnaire (PSQ-30), and the Tinnitus Sample Case History Questionnaire (TSCHQ) into Swedish. These translations were delivered via the internet with the already existing Swedish versions of the Tinnitus Handicap Inventory (THI), the Hospital Anxiety and Depression Scale (HADS), the Hyperacusis Questionnaire (HQ), and the World Health Organization Quality of Life questionnaire (WHOQoL-BREF). Psychometric properties were evaluated by means of internal consistency [Cronbach's alpha (α)] and test–retest reliability across a 9-week interval [Intraclass Correlation Coefficient (ICC), Cohen's kappa] in order to establish construct as well as clinical validity using a sample of 260 subjects from a population-based cohort.

Results: Internal consistency was acceptable for all questionnaires ($\alpha > 0.7$) with the exception of the "social relationships" subscale of the WHOQoL-BREF. Test–retest reliability was generally acceptable (ICC > 0.70, Cohens kappa > 0.60) for the tinnitus-related questionnaires, except for the TFI "sense of control" subscale and 15 items of the TSCHQ. Spearmen rank correlations showed that almost all questionnaires on tinnitus are significantly related, indicating that these questionnaires measure different aspects of the same construct. The data supported good clinical validity of the tinnitus-related questionnaires.

Conclusion: Our results suggest that most Swedish adaptations of the questionnaires are suitable for clinical and research settings and should facilitate the assessment of treatment outcomes using a more holistic approach by including measures of tinnitus fears, emotional burden, and quality of life.

Keywords: tinnitus, questionnaires, anxiety, depression, stress, hyperacusis, quality of life, TFI

INTRODUCTION

Tinnitus is the perception of one or more sounds despite the physical absence of such sound(s) (Chan, 2009). This condition is chronically experienced by a large portion of the population (>15%) and severely debilitating for about 1–2% of the population, affecting sleep, concentration, and productivity at work (Dobie, 2003; Heller, 2003). Tinnitus is associated with a higher risk of receiving disability pension (Friberg et al., 2012) and perceived as an enormous socioeconomic burden (Cederroth et al., 2013). In the Netherlands, tinnitus-related costs have been estimated to be € 6.8 billion per year (Maes et al., 2013). The prevalence of tinnitus is age-dependent, peaking in the seventh decade of life (Nondahl et al., 2002; Gopinath et al., 2010a,b; Shargorodsky et al., 2010; Park B. et al., 2014; Park K. H. et al., 2014). Tinnitus remains a clinical enigma because of the lack of effective treatments for stopping phantom tinnitus perception (Chan, 2009). Presently, tinnitus assessment relies on self-report questionnaires and subjective psychoacoustic measures (Langguth et al., 2007). Tinnitus heterogeneity varies in its phenotypes and may be objective (emitted by the ear itself and perceivable by an external observer) or subjective (only perceived by the patient), chronic or occasional, pulsatile or non-pulsatile, noise or tonal, constant or intermittent, and unilateral or bilateral (Langguth et al., 2013). Tinnitus may present with a high number of etiologies (e.g., noise exposure, stress, or physical trauma) and a multitude of co-morbidities (e.g., hypertension or diabetes; Langguth et al., 2013). The large variety in tinnitus profiles is thought to partly responsible for the lack of success in clinical treatment trials (Tunkel et al., 2014). Thus, tools need to be urgently identified for reliably assessing tinnitus and enabling the classification of patient subgroups according to a defined set of characteristics.

Several efforts have been made to establish a consensus for patient assessment and outcome measurement (Langguth et al., 2007; Landgrebe et al., 2012; Zeman et al., 2012, 2014). Nevertheless, a recent systematic review has shown that more than 100 instruments are used for primary outcome measures in clinical trials (Hall et al., 2016), evincing that there is still no agreement on how to assess tinnitus. For this reason, a working group of the Cooperation in Science and Technology (COST) action TINNET, a European Tinnitus research Network (www.tinnet.tinnitusresearch.net), is currently standardizing assessment methods and defining a core set of domains and instruments (Hall et al., 2015).

In Sweden, national guidelines on the management and treatment of tinnitus are lacking, and clinics in the different counties rely on local recommendations. The only questionnaires recommended are the Tinnitus Handicap Inventory (THI) and the Hospital Anxiety and Depression Scale (HADS). However, the Swedish versions of these questionnaires lack validity. Thus, the number of patients with tinnitus in Sweden receiving appropriate care is rather small when compared to the large capacities of other European clinics (Karolinska Hospital in Stockholm Sweden, $n = 70$ patients per year vs. the Tinnitus Clinic at the Charité in Berlin, $n = 3000$ new patients per year; or in the Adelante Tinnitus Expert Center in Maastricht, Netherlands, $n = 700$ newly referred patients per year), even when considering the population size of the respective cities. We selected a number of additional questionnaires (for instance, the Tinnitus Sample Case History Questionnaire (TSCHQ), Tinnitus Functional Index (TFI), Fear of Tinnitus Questionnaire (FTQ), Tinnitus Catastrophizing Scale (TCS), and Perceived Stress Questionnaire (PSQ-30) according to recommendations given in a consensus meeting (Langguth et al., 2007) or because of their successful application in clinical trials on tinnitus (Cima et al., 2012). Each of the questionnaires was translated into Swedish. A set of validated questionnaires would not only enable Swedish clinics to assess the burden of tinnitus in a wider context but also other aspects such as measures of tinnitus fears, emotional burden, and quality of life.

MATERIALS AND METHODS

Subjects

Patients with tinnitus were identified in the fifth wave of the Swedish Longitudinal Occupational Survey of Health (SLOSH). All patients aged between 18 and 85 years who had previously agreed to be contacted ($n = 620$) were invited to join STOP and participate in an online survey. Additionally, 319 participants were recruited through flyers. Two hundred and seventy one subjects registered with STOP (http://stop.ki.se) gave their written informed consent to participate in the survey. After excluding participants without tinnitus and incomplete test–retest data, a total sample size of 260 subjects was achieved. The project was approved by the local ethics committee "*Regionala etikprövningsnämnden*" in Stockholm (2014/1998-31/4). The database project and the server were coordinated and located at the Department of Physiology and Pharmacology of the Karolinska Institutet, Sweden.

Selection of Questionnaires

Based on a consensus meeting in 2006, Langguth et al. (2007) recommended the use of several questionnaires such as the TSCHQ (Landgrebe et al., 2010), the THI (Newman et al., 1996, 1998), the Tinnitus-Beeinträchtigungs-Fragebogen (TBF-12; Greimel et al., 1999), the Major Depression Inventory (MDI; Bech and Wermuth, 1998), and the World Health

Organization-Quality of life questionnaire (WHO, 1998). These questionnaires have been used in a large number of studies, albeit preferentially in Europe (Hall et al., 2016).

The TSCHQ was designed to assess the most important tinnitus characteristics and the tinnitus history of patients (Landgrebe et al., 2010). Tinnitus-related impairment in daily life is typically assessed with the THI (Newman et al., 1996, 1998). The TFI (Meikle et al., 2012; Henry et al., 2016) has been proposed as a more recent questionnaire with very high internal consistency of 0.97 and test–retest reliability of 0.78. We favored the TFI over the TBF-12 because of its high responsiveness to treatment-related changes.

In a randomized controlled trial on cognitive behavioral therapy (CBT) that included 245 patients with tinnitus, Cima et al. (2012) reported the successful and valid use of various questionnaires developed for assessing tinnitus-related emotional affects. Tinnitus-specific emotional reactivity and cognitions were evaluated with the TCS and the FTQ (Cima et al., 2011). The TCS is used for assessing cognitive misinterpretations of tinnitus sounds and the FTQ for measuring tinnitus-related fears (Cima et al., 2011). Both questionnaires showed excellent internal consistency values (TCS: Cronbach's alpha = ·0.94; FTQ: Cronbach's alpha = 0.82). Moreover, Cima et al. (2011) evaluated negative emotional affects with the HADS that also showed good reliability (Cronbach's alpha = 0.71–0.90; Spinhoven et al., 1997). The HADS is used for evaluating both depression and anxiety and has been previously tested on the Swedish tinnitus population (Andersson et al., 2003). Therefore, we decided to replace the MDI recommended in the 2006 consensus meeting (Langguth et al., 2007) that only evaluates depression and used the HADS instead. Stress is widely evaluated with the PSQ-30 showing an internal consistency of $0.80 < \alpha < 0.86$ (Levenstein et al., 1993). The combination of HADS and PSQ-30 allows the distinct evaluation of stress, anxiety and depression.

No Hyperacusis Questionnaire (HQ) was suggested in the initial recommendation (Langguth et al., 2007). However, because about 40–55% of patients with tinnitus experience this condition (Baguley, 2003; Schecklmann et al., 2014), we also considered the HQ (Khalfa et al., 2002), which had been validated in a group of tinnitus patients showing an internal consistency of $\alpha = 0.88$ (Fackrell et al., 2015). A Swedish version was developed with an internal consistency of $\alpha = 0.92$, albeit tested on people with Williams Syndrome (Blomberg et al., 2006).

The Health Utilities Index (HUI)—validated for assessing quality of life of patients with tinnitus (Maes et al., 2011)—was used as a primary outcome measure to evaluate the efficacy of specialized CBT on quality of life (Cima et al., 2012). However, a quality of life questionnaire developed by the WHO has also been shown to be suitable for patients with tinnitus (Zeman et al., 2014). The World Health Organization Quality of Life Scale (WHOQoL-BREF), which is a shorter version of the long questionnaire (WHO, 1998), is already available in many different languages and appears to be more appropriate for world-wide use than the HUI.

Permission to translate the questionnaires into Swedish was obtained from all developers of source language questionnaires: B. Langguth and W. Schlee (TSCHQ), J. A. Henry (TFI), R. R. L. Cima (FTQ and TCS), S. Levenstein (PSQ-30). For the TFI translation, as the reproduction in whole or in part is prohibited without the written consent of Oregon Health & Science University (OHSU), a license was obtained from OHSU, who agreed on the above procedure and authorized the validation of the translated TFI questionnaire. For further use in the clinics in Sweden, additional agreements will be needed.

Translation

No clear guidelines exist on how to translate questionnaires (Epstein et al., 2015), in particular when cultural adaptations are required as in the case of translations from English into Swedish. Since the objective of our translations was to find a functional equivalent but not a literal formulation of the original versions, we relied on a procedure called TRAPD (translation, review, adjudication, pre-testing, and documentation) developed by Harkness (2003). This procedure includes translators as well as a team reviewing the translations and presenting the final version (Harkness, 2003). The original English versions of the questionnaires were thus translated into Swedish by three native Swedish speakers (whose mother tongue was the target language, who were fluent in English and country residents with experience in the target culture). All translators were briefed on the background of the project before the translation. First, all translators worked independently and then in a team to produce one single reconciled forward translation. This forward translation was then reviewed and discussed by a multidisciplinary committee from our clinic that included a doctor, an ENT specialist, an audiologist, a psychologist, two researchers, and a statistician to provide an additional level of quality control. All members of the reviewing committee agreed on the final version. Some of the questions and responses were slightly modified in order to produce fully comprehensible items in the Swedish language. Backward translation was conducted by a blinded native Swedish and fluent English speaker, with no knowledge of the original questionnaire. The backward-translated version was evaluated by the project leader and the translator and used as a tool to ensure that the meaning of the items was not altered (conceptual accuracy), rather than as a measure of translation accuracy. The Swedish versions of the questionnaires are available upon request.

Online Survey

Before field-testing from October 2015 to January 2016, we carried out a pilot test of these online surveys on a small group of respondents ($n = 6$) in order to detect any flaws in routing, layout, comprehension, length, software use (different browsers and mobile devices), and data transfer to the server. After giving written consent, patients were invited to participate in a secure online survey that included sociodemographic variables as well as the following questionnaires: the TSCHQ (Landgrebe et al., 2010), THI (Newman et al., 1996, 1998), TFI (Henry et al., 2016), FTQ (Cima et al., 2011), TCS (Cima et al., 2011), HQ (Khalfa et al., 2002), PSQ-30 (Levenstein et al., 1993), HADS

(Andersson et al., 2003), and WHOQoL-BREF (1998). **Table 1** presents an overview of the questionnaires: number of items as well as total and subscale scores. Scores were based on the scoring guideline of each questionnaire. Participants had to complete the questionnaires twice. The median time interval between initial and subsequent assessment was 70 days (Q1 = 66, Q3 = 71, range = 16–94 days). We performed no interventions between the test and re-test sessions.

Statistical Analyses

The sample and the questionnaire values underwent descriptive analysis [frequencies (*n*), percentages (%), means (*m*), standard

TABLE 1 | Questionnaire overview.

Questionnaire	Number of items	Total score	Subscale scores	
TSCHQ	35	–	–	
THI[a]	25	Range = 0–100; categories: 1. 0–16: Negligible 2. 18–36: Light weight 3. 38–56: Moderate weight 4. 58–76: Severe weight 5. 78–100: Catastrophic	–	
TFI[a]	25	Range = 0–100; Categories: 1. 0–17: Not a problem 2. 18–31: Small problem 3. 32–53: Moderate problem 4. 54–72: Big problem 5. 73–100: Very big problem	Range = 0–100 1. Intrusive 2. Sense of control 3. Cognitive 4. Sleep	5. Auditory 6. Relaxation 7. Quality of life 8. Emotional
FTQ[a]	17	Range = 0–17	–	
TCS[a]	13	Range = 0–52	–	
HQ[a]	14	Range = 0–42; Categories: 1. ≤28 = No hyperacusis 2. >28 = Hyperacusis	3. Attentional (range = 0–12) 4. Emotional (range = 0–18) 5. Social (range = 0–12)	
PSQ-30[a]	30	Range = 0–1; Categories: 1. <0.34 = Low stress level 2. 0.34–0.46 = Moderate stress level 3. >0.46 = High stress level	–	
HADS[a]	14	–	Range = 0–21 1. Anxiety 2. Depression Categories: 1. 0–7 = Normal 2. 8–10 = Borderline 3. 11–21 = Abnormal	
WHOQoL-BREF[b]	26	–	Range = 4–20 1. Physical health 2. Psychological 3. Social relationships 4. Environment	Range: 1–5 single items 5. Overall quality of life 6. Overall health

TSCHQ, Tinnitus Sample Case History Questionnaire; THI, Tinnitus Handicap Inventory; TFI, Tinnitus Functional Index; FTQ, Fear of Tinnitus Questionnaire; TCS, Tinnitus Catastrophizing Scale; HQ, Hyperacusis Questionnaire; PSQ-30, Perceived Stress Questionnaire; HADS, Hospital Anxiety and Depression Scale; WHOQoL-BREF, World Health Organization Quality of Life Scale (short version).

[a] *Higher score, higher impairment.*

[b] *Higher score, higher quality of life.*

deviations (*SD*), medians (med), and percentiles (Q1, first quartile/25th percentile; Q3, third quartile/75th percentile)]. Mann-Whitney *U*-tests were used to examine gender differences in tinnitus-related questionnaire values and Spearman's rank correlations to assess the relation between age and tinnitus-related questionnaire values.

A range of standardly-used analyses were carried out to assess the psychometric properties of tinnitus-related questionnaires. Cronbach's alpha coefficient was used to assess the internal consistency of multi-item scales based on correlations between items on the same test or subscale and to show the extent to which several items proposed to measure the same construct result in similar scores. Coefficients >0.70 are considered acceptable (Cohen, 1960; Grouven et al., 2007; see also, http://www.rehabmeasures.org/rehabweb/rhstats.aspx). Test–retest reliability is used to evaluate how stable patients respond over time. The consistency of tinnitus-related data was assessed by Cohen's kappa coefficient for categorical variables and Intraclass Correlation Coefficient (ICC) for metric variables. ICCs > 0.70 and Cohen's kappa > 0.60 are considered acceptable (Cohen, 1960; Grouven et al., 2007; see also, http://www.rehabmeasures.org/rehabweb/rhstats.aspx). Because construct validity indicates whether instruments measure the same theoretical concept, it was used to assess inter-scale correlations [Spearman's rank correlation coefficient (ρ)] within and between tinnitus-related questionnaires. Correlation coefficients ≥0.40 indicate that questionnaires or subscales measure the same aspects of tinnitus (convergent validity), whereas correlation coefficients between <0.40 indicate that questionnaires or subscales measure different aspects (discriminant validity; algebraic signs are omitted; Hays and Hayashi, 1990). Known-group comparisons were used to evaluate the clinical validity of the tinnitus-related questionnaires. The statistical significance of group differences in tinnitus occurrence, onset, and manifestation was tested with Mann-Whitney *U*-tests.

The significance level was set at $p \leq 0.050$. The software package SPSS for Windows, Version 23, was used for all statistical analyses.

RESULTS

Subject Characteristics

Sociodemographic Data

Two hundred and sixty Swedish subjects (52.3% men) were included in the study. The median age was 62.40 years (Q1 = 56.00, Q3 = 68.00, ranging from 21 to 87 years).

Tinnitus-Related Data

The majority of participants reported experiencing continuous tinnitus (86.9%). 64.6% of subjects perceived a gradual onset of tinnitus, and 65.8% described tinnitus of (very) high frequency. Most subjects reported constant tinnitus manifestation over time (73.8%) and that they had consulted with a clinician because of the condition (61.5%). The median time since the onset of tinnitus was 15.00 years (Q1 = 6.00, Q3 = 25.00, ranging from 0 to 55 years, missing information: $n = 30$). Subjects related the initial onset to the following reasons: loud blast of sound ($n = 41$, 15.8%), stress ($n = 37$, 14.2%), change in hearing ($n = 30$, 11.5%), head trauma ($n = 2$, 0.9%), whiplash ($n = 5$, 1.9%), and others ($n = 51$, 19.6%). 36.2% ($n = 94$) could not specify any specific reason. Tinnitus was reduced by music or environmental sounds in 53.5% of subjects and intensified by loud noise in 51.2% and by stress in 53.8%. Medication had no influence on tinnitus in 91.9% of subjects. On a scale from 0 to 100, the median loudness of tinnitus was 60.00 (Q1 = 35.00, Q3 = 75.00, $n = 259$), the median percentage of total awake time being aware of tinnitus was 60.00 (Q1 = 25.00, Q3 = 100.00, $n = 225$), and the median percentage of total awake time being annoyed or distressed of tinnitus was 20.00 (Q1 = 10.00, Q3 = 50.00, $n = 226$). **Table 2** presents both tinnitus-related and additional clinical data (TSCHQ).

Questionnaire Data

The median scores and quartiles of the test and re-test sessions are presented in **Table 3**. At the initial assessment, the THI was 24.00 (Q1 = 14.00, Q3 = 38.00), and 10.8% of subjects described their tinnitus as *severe* to *catastrophic*. The average TFI score was 24.0 (Q1 = 14.00, Q3 = 38.00), and 16.9% of subjects described to have a big or a very big problem. Stress was evaluated by means of the PSQ (median = 0.27, Q1 = 0.16, Q3 = 0.39), and 16.2% of subjects scored high stress levels. Anxiety was measured with the HADS (median = 2.0, Q1 = 1.0, Q3 = 5.0), in which 10% of subjects showed abnormally high scores. Depression, also evaluated with the HADS (median = 4.0, Q1 = 2.0, Q3 = 8.0), showed abnormally high scores in 4.6% of subjects. The median TCS-value was 11.5 (Q1 = 5.0, Q3 = 20.0), and that of the FTQ was 4.0 (Q1 = 3.0, Q3 = 6.0); however, no subscale is available for determining severity levels. The HQ showed that 17.7% of subjects had hyperacusis according to a >28 cut-off value. Quality of life was measured with the WHOQoL subscales for physical (median = 16.0, Q1 = 13.7, Q3 = 17.7), psychological (median = 16.0, Q1 = 14.0, Q3 = 17.3), social (median = 14.7, Q1 = 13.3, Q3 = 16.0), and environmental (median = 16.5, Q1 = 15.0, Q3 = 8.0) relationships. Age was significantly associated with tinnitus-related questionnaire scores, with exception of the THI "intrusive" subscale score, the HQ "emotional" subscale score, and the TCS total score (**Table 4**). Correlation coefficients were small to moderate in size. In general, the older the subjects, the fewer were the impairments and the better the quality of life reported. Women tended to have more impairments and less quality of life than men (**Table 4**). Significant differences were found for 17 out of 25 values.

Psychometric Properties

Internal Consistency

Cronbach's alpha for multi-item scales ranged from 0.69 to 0.97 (see **Table 4**). Thus, internal consistency was acceptable, except for the WHOQoL-BREF subscale "social relationships" that fell short of reaching the conventional cut-off value of $\alpha \leq 0.70$.

Test–Retest Reliability

ICC ranged between 0.68 and 0.90 (**Table 4**) and Cohen's kappa from 0.34 to 0.93 (**Table 2**). Test–retest reliability was acceptable, except for the subscale "sense of control" of the TFI and for 15 items of the TSCHQ. Critical items of the TSCHQ were: 3b

TABLE 2 | Tinnitus-related data and test–retest reliability assessed with the Tinnitus Sample Case History Questionnaire (TSCHQ).

	Initial assessment		Test–retest reliability
	n	%	Cohen's kappa/Intra-class correlation coefficient
Onset of tinnitus (exact date)	–	–	0.34
Relation of initial onset of tinnitus (etiology)			0.51
Loud blast of sound	41	15.8	
Stress	37	14.2	
Change in hearing	30	11.5	
Head trauma	2	0.8	
Whiplash	5	1.9	
Other	51	19.6	
Do not know	94	36.2	
Tinnitus occurrence			0.73
Occasionally	34	13.1	
Permanently	226	86.9	
Time of day of tinnitus emergence			0.50
When awakening	20	7.7	
In the morning	8	3.1	
Around noon	24	9.2	
In the afternoon	16	6.2	
In the evening	39	15.0	
Before sleeping	21	8.1	
Do not know	132	50.8	
Perceiving the onset of tinnitus			0.78
Gradual	168	64.6	
Abrupt	92	35.4	
Pulsation of tinnitus			0.69
Yes, with heartbeat	33	12.7	
Yes, different from heartbeat	12	4.6	
No	215	82.7	
Location of tinnitus			0.62
Right ear	25	9.6	
Left ear	35	13.5	
Both ears, worse in right ear	37	14.2	
Both ears, worse in left ear	38	14.6	
Both ears equally	79	30.4	
Inside the head	43	16.5	
Elsewhere	3	1.2	
Tinnitus manifestation over time			0.55
Intermittent	68	26.2	
Constant	192	73.8	
Loudness of tinnitus (median, Q1/Q3)	60	35/75	0.83
Tinnitus loudness variation from day to day			0.58
Yes	173	66.5	
No	87	33.5	

(Continued)

TABLE 2 | Continued

	Initial assessment		Test–retest reliability
	n	%	Cohen's kappa/Intra-class correlation coefficient
Percentage of total awake time of tinnitus awareness (median, Q1/Q3)	60	25/100	0.71
Percentage of total awake time being distressed by tinnitus (median, Q1/Q3)	20	10/50	0.78
Sound of tinnitus			0.56
Tone	102	39.2	
Noise	108	41.5	
Crickets	36	13.8	
Other	14	5.4	
Pitch of tinnitus			0.47
Low frequency	15	5.8	
Medium frequency	74	28.5	
High frequency	120	46.2	
Very high frequency	51	19.6	
Reduction of tinnitus by music or environmental sounds			0.44
Yes	139	53.5	
No	65	25.0	
Do not know	56	21.5	
Worsening of tinnitus by loud noise			0.54
Yes	133	51.2	
No	82	31.5	
Don't know	45	17.3	
Tinnitus affected by head movement or touch			0.66
Yes	54	20.8	
No	206	79.2	
Tinnitus affected by nap			0.60
Yes, worsening of tinnitus	7	2.7	
Yes, reducing of tinnitus	34	13.1	
No, no effect	219	84.2	
Tinnitus affected by sleep at night			0.35
Yes	49	18.8	
No	103	39.6	
Do not know	108	41.5	
Tinnitus affected by stress			0.70
Yes, worsening of tinnitus	139	53.5	
Yes, reducing of tinnitus	2	0.8	
No, no effect	119	45.8	
Tinnitus affected by medication			0.67
Yes	21	8.1	
No	239	91.9	
Contacted a clinician due to tinnitus			0.69
Yes	160	61.5	

(Continued)

TABLE 2 | Continued

	Initial assessment		Test–retest reliability
	n	%	Cohen's kappa/Intra-class correlation coefficient
No	100	38.5	
Number of different tinnitus treatments			0.61
0	196	75.4	
1	18	63.9	
2–4	28	10.8	
5 or more	18	6.9	
Tinnitus occurrence in family			0.74
Yes	187	71.9	
No	73	28.1	
Comorbidity			0.83
Yes	129	49.6	
No	131	50.4	
Medication			0.87
Yes	166	63.8	
No	94	36.2	
Currently under treatment for psychiatric problems			0.73
Yes	16	6.2	
No	244	93.8	
Hearing problem			0.74
Yes	220	84.6	
No	40	15.4	
Hearing aids			0.93
Yes, on both ears	74	28.5	
Yes, on the right ear	8	3.1	
Yes, on the left ear	9	3.5	
No	169	65.0	
Problems tolerating sounds			0.41
Never	41	15.8	
Rarely	44	16.9	
Sometimes	100	38.5	
Usually	49	18.8	
Always	26	10.0	
Sounds cause pain or physical discomfort			0.46
Yes	115	44.2	
No	124	47.2	
Do not know	21	8.1	
Headache			0.77
Yes	56	21.5	
No	204	78.5	
Vertigo or dizziness			0.56
Yes	72	27.7	
No	188	72.3	
Temporomandibular disorder			0.67
Yes	29	11.2	

(Continued)

TABLE 2 | Continued

	Initial assessment		Test–retest reliability
	n	%	Cohen's kappa/Intra-class correlation coefficient
No	231	88.8	
Neck pain			0.82
Yes	72	27.7	
No	188	72.3	
Other pain syndromes			0.65
Yes	71	27.3	
No	189	72.7	

Test–retest reliability was assessed by Cohen's kappa coefficient for categorical variables and intra-class correlation coefficient for metric variables. ICCs > 0.70 and Cohen's kappa > 0.60 are considered acceptable. Descriptive data of Tinnitus Sample Case History Questionnaire is presented at initial assessment.

(the time of day tinnitus starts), 5 (initial onset), 7 (etiology), 10 (intermittent or constant), 11 (varying loudness), 14 (sound of tinnitus), 15 (pitch of tinnitus), 18 (different treatments), 19 (reduction by ambient sounds), 20 (tinnitus worse by noise), 22 (nap effects), 23 (tinnitus affected by night sleep), 28 (problems tolerating sounds), 29 (pain induced by noise), and 31 (vertigo or dizziness).

Construct Validity

Spearmen's rank correlations showed that almost all tinnitus-related questionnaires were significantly related (mainly $p < 0.001$), with the exception of the correlation between the "auditory" subscale of the TFI and the "social relationships" subscale of WHOQoL-BREF ($\rho = -0.12$, $p = 0.053$). 55% ($n = 165$) of 300 correlations yielded coefficients of $\geq$0.40, and 10.3% ($n = 31$) substantial coefficients of $\geq$0.70. These findings indicated that the questionnaires measured different aspects of the same construct. In general, higher correlation coefficients were observed between total and subscale scores of the THI, TFI, HQ, and HADS. WHOQoL-BREF showed correlation coefficients of $\geq$0.40 mainly within its subscales but not with other tinnitus-related questionnaires. **Table 5** summarizes the correlation coefficients.

Clinical Validity

Subjects with a more severe clinical condition (permanent tinnitus, abrupt onset, and constant manifestation of tinnitus) tended to report more tinnitus-related impairments than subjects with a less severe clinical condition (occasional tinnitus, gradual onset, and intermittent manifestation of tinnitus). **Table 6** summarizes the results of the Mann-Whitney *U*-tests.

DISCUSSION

Overall, the Swedish versions of the tinnitus-specific questionnaires showed good internal consistency, test–retest reliability, construct, as well as clinical validity. Internal consistency was excellent ($\alpha > 0.90$) for the THI, TFI, TCS,

TABLE 3 | Descriptive analyses of tinnitus-related questionnaires.

N = 260		Initial assessment		Subsequent assessment	
Questionnaire		**med (Q1, Q3)**	**Range**	**med (Q1, Q3)**	**Range**
THI[b,c]					
Sum score		24.0 (14.0, 38.0)	0–90	22.0 (12.0, 36.0)	0–94
		n	%	*n*	%
Categories	Negligible	82	31.5	97	37.5
	Light weight	110	42.3	99	38.2
	Moderate weight	40	15.4	42	16.2
	Severe weight	20	7.7	14	5.4
	Catastrophic	8	3.1	7	2.7
TFI[b,c]					
Sum score		24.0 (14.0, 38.0)	0–90	22.0 (12.0, 36.0)	0–94
		n	%	*n*	%
Categories	No problem	78	30.0	84	32.4
	Small problem	57	21.9	63	24.3
	Moderate problem	81	31.2	69	26.6
	Big problem	34	13.1	28	10.8
	Very big problem	10	3.8	15	5.8
Subscales	Intrusive	43.3 (23.3, 63.3)	0–100	43.3 (23.3, 60.0)	0–100
	Sense of control	43.3 (16.7, 66.7)	0–100	43.3 (20.0, 66.7)	0–100
	Cognitive	20.0 (6.7, 43.3)	0–93	16.7 (3.3, 40.0)	0–100
	Sleep	13.3 (0.0, 43.3)	0–100	13.3 (0.0, 40.0)	0–100
	Auditory	43.3 (16.7, 69.2)	0–100	36.7 (20.0, 66.7)	0–100
	Relaxation	23.3 (10.0, 50.0)	0–100	20.0 (6.7, 50.0)	0–100
	Quality of life	20.0 (2.5, 42.5)	0–93	17.5 (2.5, 40.0)	0–100
	Emotional	6.7 (0.0, 16.7)	0–67	6.7 (0.0, 16.7)	0–67
FTQ[b]					
Sum score		4.0 (3.0, 6.0)	1–14	4.0 (3.0, 6.0)	1–17
TCS[b,c]					
Sum score		11.5 (5.0, 20.0)	0–45	10.0 (4.0, 19.0)	0–52
PSQ-30[b,c]					
PSQ index		0.27 (0.16, 0.39)	0.00–0.82	0.24 (0.13–0.39)	0.00–0.81
		n	%	*n*	%
Categories	Low stress level	163	62.7	171	65.8
	Moderate stress level	55	21.2	45	17.3
	High stress level	42	16.2	43	16.5
HQ[b,c]					
Sum score		17.0 (10.0, 25.0)	0–39	17.0 (10.0, 25.0)	0–39
		n	%	*n*	%
Categories	No hyperacusis	214	82.3	214	82.3
	Hyperacusis	46	17.7	46	17.7
Subscales	Attentional	5.0 (2.0, 7.0)	0–12	5.0 (2.0, 7.0)	0–12
	Emotional	7.0 (4.0, 11.0)	0–18	7.0 (4.0, 77.0)	0–18
	Social	5.0 (2.0, 8.0)	0–12	5.0 (2.0, 8.0)	0–12
HADS[b]					
Subscales	Anxiety	4.0 (2.0, 8.0)	0–17	4.0 (2.0, 7.0)	0–18
	Depression	2.0 (1.0, 5.0)	0–15	2.0 (1.0, 5.0)	0–18

(Continued)

TABLE 3 | Continued

N = 260		Initial assessment		Subsequent assessment	
Questionnaire		**med (Q1, Q3)**	**Range**	**med (Q1, Q3)**	**Range**
		n	%	*n*	%
THI[b,c]					
Sum score		24.0 (14.0, 38.0)	0–90	22.0 (12.0, 36.0)	0–94
		n	%	*n*	%
Categories anxiety	Normal	193	74.2	199	76.5
	Borderline	41	15.8	37	14.2
	Abnormal	26	10.0	24	9.2
Categories depression	Normal	227	87.3	226	86.9
	Borderline	21	8.1	23	8.8
	Abnormal	12	4.6	11	4.2
WHOQoL-BREF[a]					
Subscales	Physical health[c]	16.0 (13.7, 17.7)	5–20	16.0 (13.7, 17.7)	6–20
	Psychological	16.0 (14.0, 17.3)	7–20	16.0 (14.0, 17.3)	7–20
	Social relationships	14.7 (13.3, 16.0)	5–20	14.7 (13.3, 16.0)	5–20
	Environment	16.5 (15.0, 18.0)	10–20	16.5 (15.0, 18.0)	10–20
	Overall quality of life	4.0 (4.0, 5.0)	1–5	4.0 (4.0, 5.0)	1–5
	Overall health	4.0 (3.0, 4.0)	1–5	4.0 (3.0, 4.0)	1–5

THI, Tinnitus Handicap Inventory; TFI, Tinnitus Functional Index; FTQ, Fear of Tinnitus Questionnaire; TCS, Tinnitus Catastrophizing Scale; PSQ-30, Perceived Stress Questionnaire; HQ, Hyperacusis Questionnaire; HADS, Hospital Anxiety and Depression Scale; WHOQoL-BREF, World Health Organization Quality of Life Scale (short version).

[a] *Higher score, higher quality of life.*

[b] *Higher score, higher impairment.*

[c] *n = 259 at subsequent assessment.*

HQ, and PSQ-30, good for the HADS ($0.80 \leq \alpha \leq 0.90$), and acceptable for the FTQ ($0.70 \leq \alpha \leq 0.80$). However, the subscale "social relationships" of the WHOQoL-BREF showed low internal consistency that fell short of reaching the conventional cut-off value of $\alpha \leq 0.70$.

Test–retest reliability was acceptable, except for the subscale sense of control of the TFI (ICC = 0.68) and for 15 items of the TSCHQ that includes descriptive data about tinnitus. The comparison of TSCHQ scores with previously published descriptive analyses by the Tinnitus Research Initiative (Schecklmann et al., 2014) showed very similar prevalence for specific items. For instance, gradual perception of tinnitus at its onset was reported by 64.6% of subjects in STOP vs. 50% in the TRI. Similarly, high-frequency perceptions were reported by 65.8% of subjects in STOP vs. 72% in the TRI. 73.8% of subjects in the STOP reported constant tinnitus in comparison to 84% in the TRI. Cohen's kappa coefficients of several TSCHQ items (e.g., first tinnitus experience, manifestation of tinnitus over time, or suffering from headaches) were below the cut-off value of $k > 0.60$. However, this result does not mean that the questionnaire is not reliable *per-se*. The low kappa values may reflect (a) variables that differ in time or are fluctuating, (b) variables that are not accurately remembered, (c) that subjects did not understand the item, and (d) how reliably or conscientiously subjects respond to questionnaires. Nonetheless, this finding suggests that caution should be taken in the interpretation of some items of the TSCHQ. The test–retest reliability of the TSCHQ should also be investigated in a different sample in order to find out whether the phrasing of specific questions should be modified—this could also apply to the original English version of the TSCHQ.

Backward translation is often conducted to ensure the reliability of the forward translation, however, we found no guideline on how to score the reliability of a backward translation. We considered one-word change in the translated version, as a meaningful difference when comparing to the original version. Using this criterion, we found that in the case of English-Swedish translations, near 60% of backward-translated items from the TSCHQ and the TFI differed from the original version. With shorter sentences, as those found in the PSQ-30, this number went down to 40%. Importantly, of all backward-translated items in which a change from the original version was observed, only 6% of them had potentially altered meaning. Verification of the Swedish items helped confirming that they were culturally adapted and thus appropriate for testing. The low score for the subscale sense of control of the TFI (ICC = 0.68) could potentially derive from translation failures. The verb "*to cope*" in English has the equivalent "*att hantera*" in Swedish, but which has additional meanings such as "*to handle*" or "*to manage.*" Such differences, when evaluating the "sense of control" could alter the test–retest reliability. Potentially, this variability in the test–retest sessions might not necessarily occur in a more severe group of individuals such as those recruited in clinics, which is not the case with the STOP cohort (population based).

TABLE 4 | Internal consistency and test–retest reliability of tinnitus-related questionnaires and relations with age and sex.

N = 260	Internal consistency	Test–retest reliability		Age	Sex		
Questionnaire	**Cronbach's α**	**ICC (95% CI)**	***F (df)***	**Spearmen's rank correlation**	**Men med (Q1, Q3)**	**Women med (Q1, Q3)**	***U*-test**
THI total[b,c]	**0.93**	**0.90 (0.87, 0.92)**	**18.665 (258)****	**−0.26****	**22.0 (12.0, 37.5)**	**26.0 (16.0, 39.5)**	**7165.0***
TFI total[b,c]	**0.97**	**0.88 (0.85, 0.90)**	**15.314 (258)****	**−0.22****	**24.6 (12.4, 40.0)**	**34.8 (14.9, 20.1)**	**7066.0***
Intrusive	0.84	0.82 (0.78, 0.86)	10.097 (258)**	−0.09	41.7 (23.3, 63.3)	43.3 (24.2, 63.3)	7912.5
Sense of control	0.81	0.68 (0.61, 0.74)	5.256 (258)**	−0.12*	43.3 (16.7, 66.7)	41.7 (16.7, 65.8)	8322.0
Cognitive	0.95	0.81 (0.76, 0.85)	9.494 (258)**	−0.23**	16.7 (6.7, 36.7)	25.0 (6.7, 55.8)	7003.0*
Sleep	0.95	0.79 (0.74, 0.83)	8.510 (258)**	−0.13*	10.0 (0.0, 35.8)	20 (0.0, 50.0)	7000.0*
Auditory	0.95	0.76 (0.70, 0.81)	7.255 (258)**	−0.15*	33.3 (16.7, 63.3)	46.7 (20.0, 75.8)	7451.0
Relaxation	0.94	0.79 (0.74, 0.83)	8.493 (258)**	−0.24**	20.0 (6.7, 40.0)	30.0 (10.0, 60.0)	6962.5*
Quality of life	0.91	0.87 (0.84, 0.90)	14.569 (258)**	−0.21**	12.5 (2.5, 35.0)	23.8 (5.0, 46.9)	6919.0*
Emotional	0.88	0.81 (0.77, 0.85)	9.581 (258)**	−0.24**	3.3 (0.0, 13.3)	6.7 (0.0, 20.0)	7534.0
FTQ total[b]	**0.71**	**0.74 (0.68, 0.79)**	**6.638 (259)****	**−0.23****	**4.0 (3.0, 6.0)**	**4.0 (3.0, 6.0)**	**8136.0**
TCS total[b,c]	**0.93**	**0.82 (0.77, 0.86)**	**10.315 (258)****	**−0.07**	**11.0 (5.0, 19.0)**	**13.0 (5.0, 21.8)**	**7857.5**
PSQ-30 total[b,c]	**0.94**	**0.88 (0.85, 0.91)**	**16.624 (258)****	**−0.41****	**23 (0.13, .34)**	**0.3 (0.2, 0.4)**	**6358.5****
HQ total[b,c]	**0.90**	**0.88 (0.85, 0.91)**	**16.141 (258)****	**−0.18***	**13.0 (8.0, 20.0)**	**22.0 (14.0, 28.8)**	**5165.5****
Attentional	0.75	0.73 (0.67, 0.78)	6.388 (258)**	−0.22**	4.0 (1.0, 6.0)	6.0 (3.0, 9.0)	5337.0**
Emotional	0.83	0.86 (0.82, 0.89)	13.199 (258)**	−0.11	6.0 (3.3, 10.0)	9.0 (5.0, 13.0)	6313.5**
Social	0.82	0.83 (0.78, 0.86)	10.426 (258)**	−0.18*	4.0 (2.0, 6.0)	7.0 (4.0, 9.0)	5046.5**
HADS[b]							
Anxiety	0.85	0.85 (0.81, 0.88)	12.278 (259)**	−0.21**	4.0 (2.0, 6.0)	5.0 (3.0, 9.0)	6860.5*
Depression	0.83	0.85 (0.81, 0.88)	12.505 (259)**	−0.32**	2.0 (1.0, 4.8)	2.5 (1.0, 6.0)	7457.0
WHOQoL-BREF[a]							
Physical health[c]	0.84	0.88 (0.85, 0.91)	15.628 (258)**	0.18*	16.0 (14.1, 17.7)	15.4 (12.6, 17.1)	6900.5*
Psychological	0.84	0.87 (0.84, 0.90)	14.721 (259)**	0.27**	16.7 (14.7, 17.3)	15.3 (13.3, 16.7)	6261.0**
Social relationships	0.69[d]	0.78 (0.73, 0.83)	8.192 (259)**	0.21**	14.7 (12.3, 16.0)	14.7 (13.3, 16.0)	8414.5
Environment	0.78	0.80 (0.75, 0.84)	9.020 (259)**	0.26**	16.5 (15.5, 18.0)	16.0 (15.0, 17.5)	6733.0*
Overall quality of life	–	0.74 (0.69, 0.80)	6.876 (259)**	0.25**	4.0 (4.0, 5.0)	4.0 (4.0, 5.0)	7091.0*
Overall health	–	0.71 (0.65, 0.77)	5.920 (259)**	0.21**	4.0 (3.0, 4.0)	3.0 (2.0, 4.0)	6849.5*

THI, Tinnitus Handicap Inventory; TFI, Tinnitus Functional Index; FTQ, Fear of Tinnitus Questionnaire; TCS, Tinnitus Catastrophizing Scale; PSQ-30, Perceived Stress Questionnaire; HQ, Hyperacusis Questionnaire; HADS, Hospital Anxiety and Depression Scale; WHOQoL-BREF, World Health Organization Quality of Life Scale (short version).
***Correlation is significant at the 0.001 level. *Correlation is significant at the 0.05 level.*
[a] *higher score, higher quality of life.*
[b] *higher score, higher impairment.*
[c] *$n = 259$ at subsequent assessment.*
[d] *Internal consistency of domain social relationship (WHOQoL-BREF) increases to $\alpha = 0.73$ without item number 21. However, the item-total correlation between item 21 and its subscale is $r = 0.42$, which is acceptable.*

Indeed, it is possible that the low values obtained for some of the items of the TSCHQ are due to the fact that the population tested within the STOP includes participants from the general population and not clinical (outpatient) individuals. When comparing the scores of STOP participants with the scores obtained in other studies, we observed that the scores of the different questionnaires were lower than normal. Because most studies failed to report median values, we compared the mean values. Our average THI score was 28.34 in comparison to the range of 40–55 found in the literature (Kaldo et al., 2007; Westin et al., 2011; Albu and Chirtes, 2014; Jasper et al., 2014). The TFI average was 31.74 vs. 40.6 (Fackrell et al., 2016), so that the overall score was lower than that typically found in the literature. Similarly, the anxiety level of 5.12 measured with the HADS was lower than that reported in other studies (6.2–8.7; Kaldo et al., 2007; Westin et al., 2011; Albu and Chirtes, 2014; Jasper et al., 2014). The average of 3.44 for depression in the STOP cohort was also lower than the range of 4.05–6.5 described in the literature (Kaldo et al., 2007; Westin et al., 2011; Albu and Chirtes, 2014; Jasper et al., 2014). The average values of 13.86 of tinnitus-specific cognitions measured with the TCS were almost two times less than the baseline score of 21.11 in the study by Cima et al. (2012). Fear-reactivity as measured by the FTQ was 4.57 in the STOP cohort vs. 7.25 (Cima et al., 2012) at baseline. This finding may be due to the fact that all patients in the Cima trial had severely irritating tinnitus at baseline with an average THI score of 38.96 (*SD* 22.88; Cima et al., 2012) in contrast to our study sample who had significantly less severe tinnitus with an average score of 28.34. The STOP values were more comparable with the values

TABLE 5 | Convergent validity: spearmen's rank correlations between tinnitus-related questionnaires.

	THI total	TFI total	TFI intrusive	TFI sense of control	TFI cognitive	TFI sleep	TFI auditory	TFI relaxation	TFI quality of life	TFI emotional	FTQ total	TCS total	HQ total	HQ attentional	HQ emotional	HQ social	PSQ-30 total	HADS anxiety	HADS depression	WHOQoL physical health	WHOQoL psychological	WHOQoL social relationships	WHOQoL environment	WHOQoL overall quality of life	WHOQoL overall health
THI total	–																								
TFI total	0.85**	–																							
TFI intrusive	0.70**	0.85**	–																						
TFI sense of control	0.67**	0.77**	0.68**	–																					
TFI cognitive	0.78**	0.89**	0.71**	0.66**	–																				
TFI sleep	0.60**	0.73**	0.58**	0.48**	0.67**	–																			
TFI auditory	0.61**	0.73**	0.61**	0.45**	0.55**	0.39**	–																		
TFI relaxation	0.71**	0.86**	0.71**	0.65**	0.81**	0.67**	0.48**	–																	
TFI quality of life	0.79**	0.89**	0.66**	0.59**	0.77**	0.56**	0.74**	0.71**	–																
TFI emotional	0.75**	0.79**	0.65**	0.58**	0.71**	0.57**	0.50**	0.69**	0.72**	–															
FTQ total	0.55**	0.57**	0.47**	0.46**	0.52**	0.39**	0.39**	0.51**	0.49**	0.54**	–														
TCS total	0.68**	0.66**	0.59**	0.61**	0.62**	0.52**	0.37**	0.63**	0.54**	0.63**	0.65**	–													
HQ total	0.57**	0.56**	0.38**	0.32**	0.56**	0.42**	0.43**	0.52**	0.59**	0.50**	0.31**	0.37**	–												
HQ attentional	0.40**	0.43**	0.27**	0.23**	0.47**	0.31**	0.28**	0.44**	0.44**	0.38**	0.22**	0.29**	0.87**	–											
HQ emotional	0.55**	0.55**	0.39**	0.33**	0.47**	0.37**	0.51**	0.44**	0.61**	0.46**	0.32**	0.33**	0.87**	0.61**	–										
HQ social	0.52**	0.49**	0.32**	0.29**	0.55**	0.42**	0.30**	0.48**	0.46**	0.47**	0.26**	0.36**	0.87**	0.70**	0.61**	–									
PSQ-30 total	0.47**	0.44**	0.23**	0.33**	0.48**	0.33**	0.25**	0.47**	0.43**	0.43**	0.26**	0.34**	0.49**	0.46**	0.32**	0.52**	–								
HADS anxiety	0.40**	0.35**	0.19**	0.22**	0.42**	0.30**	0.20**	0.40**	0.33**	0.39**	0.28**	0.39**	0.45**	0.40**	0.31**	0.48**	0.75**	–							
HADS depression	0.42**	0.40**	0.19**	0.29**	0.44**	0.29**	0.23**	0.39**	0.43**	0.39**	0.22**	0.27**	0.43**	0.37**	0.36**	0.41**	0.71**	0.65**	–						
WHOQoL physical health	–0.41**	–0.45**	–0.27**	–0.32**	–0.46**	–0.41**	–0.22**	–0.44**	–0.43**	–0.43**	–0.22**	–0.30**	–0.44**	–0.38**	–0.34**	–0.45**	–0.64**	–0.53**	–0.60**	–					
WHOQoL psychological	–0.37**	–0.34**	–0.16*	–0.24**	–0.41**	–0.26**	–0.13*	–0.37**	–0.33**	–0.35**	–0.25**	–0.30**	–0.37**	–0.35**	–0.26**	–0.38**	–0.70**	–0.68**	–0.71**	0.66**	–				
WHOQoL social relationships	–0.30**	–0.28**	–0.15*	–0.22**	–0.27**	–0.20**	–0.12	–0.32**	–0.30**	–0.29**	–0.12	–0.23**	–0.27**	–0.26**	–0.20**	–0.27**	–0.50**	–0.42**	–0.50**	0.46**	0.57**	–			
WHOQoL environment	–0.31**	–0.33**	–0.15*	–0.23**	–0.36**	–0.26**	–0.18**	–0.34**	–0.37**	–0.28**	–0.18**	–0.20**	–0.34**	–0.28**	–0.31**	–0.31**	–0.55**	–0.49**	–0.53**	0.64**	0.61**	0.43**	–		
WHOQoL overall quality of life	–0.38**	–0.38**	–0.23**	–0.25**	–0.39**	–0.35**	–0.16**	–0.40**	–0.39**	–0.41**	–0.24**	–0.28**	–0.41**	–0.39**	–0.34**	–0.35**	–0.63**	–0.57**	–0.60**	0.64**	0.65**	0.50**	0.61**	–	
WHOQoL overall health	–0.34**	–0.33**	–0.22**	–0.23**	–0.32**	–0.31**	–0.13*	–0.34**	–0.30**	–0.34**	–0.14*	–0.23**	–0.37**	–0.30**	–0.30**	–0.37**	–0.51**	–0.43**	–0.48**	0.72**	0.55**	0.37**	0.47**	0.56**	–

THI, Tinnitus Handicap Inventory; TFI, Tinnitus Functional Index; FTQ, Fear of Tinnitus Questionnaire; TCS, Tinnitus Catastrophizing Scale; PSQ-30, Perceived Stress Questionnaire, HQ, Hyperacusis Questionnaire; HADS, Hospital Anxiety and Depression Scale; WHOQoL-BRE, World Health Organization Quality of Life Scale (short version).

***Correlation is significant at the 0.01 level (2-tailed). *Correlation is significant at the 0.05 level (2-tailed).*

TABLE 6 | Clinical validity of tinnitus-related questionnaires.

$N = 260$	Tinnitus occurrence			Tinnitus onset			Tinnitus manifestation		
Questionnaire	**Occasionally $n = 34$ med (Q1, Q3)**	**Permanently $n = 226$ med (Q1, Q3)**	***U*-test**	**Gradual $n = 168$ med (Q1, Q3)**	**Abrupt $n = 92$ med (Q1, Q3)**	**U-Test**	**Intermittent $n = 68$ med (Q1, Q3)**	**Constant $n = 192$ med (Q1, Q3)**	**U-test**
THI total[b]	**17.0 (6.0, 26.0)**	**26.0 (16.0, 42.0)**	**2239.5****	**23.0 (12.0, 36.0)**	**28.0 (16.0, 46.0)**	**6691.0**	**20.0 (10.0, 31.5)**	**26.0 (16.0, 42.0)**	**5256.0***
TFI total[b]	**11.0 (4.7, 25.4)**	**32.4 (16.3, 46.4)**	**1948.0****	**29.2 (12.1, 42.6)**	**34.4 (14.0, 50.3)**	**6738.0**	**18.2 (9.8, 38.9)**	**32.6 (17.7, 46.7)**	**4883.0***
Intrusive	20.0 (12.5, 37.5)	46.7 (26.7, 66.7)	1757.5**	43.3 (23.3, 63.3)	46.7 (23.3, 65.8)	7367.5	26.7 (14.2, 56.7)	46.7(26.7, 66.7)	4476.0**
Sense of control	11.7 (3.3, 40.8)	46.7 (20.0, 66.7)	2233.5**	40.0 (13.3, 63.3)	48.3 (24.2, 70.0)	6506.5*	36.7 (10.0, 62.5)	46.7 (20.0, 66.7)	5576.5
Cognitive	6.7 (0.0, 26.7)	20.0 (6.7, 43.3)	2708.0*	16.7 (6.7, 39.2)	23.3 (10.0, 55.8)	6671.0	10.0 (6.7, 30.0)	23.3 (6.7, 46.7)	5476.0*
Sleep	6.7 (0.0, 21.7)	16.7 (0.0, 44.2)	2970.5*	10.0 (0.0, 40.0)	16.7 (0.8, 50.0)	6741.0	8.3 (0.0, 39.2)	16.7 (0.0, 43.3)	5801.0
Auditory	10.0 (3.3, 36.7)	46.7 (22.5, 73.3)	1878.5**	46.7 (20.0, 66.7)	35.0 (10.8, 70.0)	7214.0	30.0 (10.0, 55.8)	50.0 (20.0, 73.3)	4746.5**
Relaxation	10.0 (0.0, 23.3)	26.7 (10.0, 53.3)	2426.0**	20.0 (4.2, 46.7)	33.3 (10.0, 60.0)	6370.5*	18.3 (3.3, 32.5)	26.7 (10.0, 56.7)	5278.0*
Quality of life	2.5 (0.0, 20.6)	22.5 (5.0, 47.5)	2197.0**	20.0 (2.5, 42.5)	22.5 (3.1, 47.5)	7245.0	11.3 (2.5, 26.9)	22.5 (5.0, 47.5)	5205.0*
Emotional	1.7 (0.0, 4.2)	6.7 (0.0, 16.7)	2415.5**	6.7 (0.0, 13.3)	6.7 (0.8, 26.7)	6412.0*	3.3 (0.0, 10.0)	6.7 (0.0, 20.0)	5314.5*
FTQ total[b]	**4.0 (2.8, 4.0)**	**4.0 (3.0, 6.0)**	**2921.0***	**4.0 (3.0, 6.0)**	**4.0 (3.0, 6.0)**	**7036.0**	**4.0 (3.0, 6.0)**	**4.0 (3.0, 6.0)**	**5913.5**
TCS total[b]	**8.0 (2.0, 16.0)**	**12.0 (6.0, 21.0)**	**2860.5***	**11.0 (6.0, 19.0)**	**13.5 (5.0, 22.0)**	**7184.5**	**10.0 (4.0, 16.0)**	**12.5 (6.0, 21.0)**	**5344.5***
PSQ-30 total[b]	**0.2 (0.2,0.4)**	**0.3 (0.2,0.4)**	**3735.0**	**0.3 (0.2,0.4)**	**0.3 (0.1,0.4)**	**6874.0**	**0.3 (0.2,0.4)**	**0.3 (0.2,0.4)**	**6370.5**
HQ total[b]	**14.5 (8.0, 22.5)**	**17.0 (10.0, 25.0)**	**3422.0**	**15.0 (8.3, 24.0)**	**20.0 (12.0, 27.8)**	**6204.5***	**15.0 (9.3, 21.8)**	**17.5 (10.0, 26.0)**	**5681.5**
Attentional	4.5 (2.8, 7.0)	5.0 (2.0, 8.0)	3817.0	4.0 (2.0, 6.8)	6.0 (3.0, 8.0)	6154.5*	4.0 (2.0, 6.0)	5.0 (2.0, 8.0)	5458.5*
Emotional	5.0 (3.0, 9.3)	7.0 (4.0, 11.0)	3084.0	6.0 (4.0, 10.0)	8.0 (5.0, 12.0)	6522.0*	6.0 (4.0, 10.0)	7.0 (4.0, 11.8)	5738.5
Social	5.0 (2.0, 7.5)	5.0 (2.0, 8.0)	3641.5	4.0 (2.0, 7.8)	6.0 (3.0, 9.0)	6409.5*	5.0 (2.0, 7.0)	5.0 (2.0, 8.8)	6204.5
HADS[b]									
Anxiety	4.0 (2.0, 8.0)	4.0 (2.0, 8.0)	3766.0	4.0 (2.0, 7.0)	5.0 (2.0, 8.0)	6486.5*	4.0 (2.0, 7.0)	5.0 (2.0, 8.0)	6085.5
Depression	1.0 (1.0, 4.0)	2.0 (1.0, 5.0)	3223.5	2.0 (1.0, 4.0)	3.0 (1.0, 6.8)	6501.0*	2.0 (1.0, 5.0)	2.0 (1.0, 5.0)	6475.5
WHOQoL-BREF[a]									
Physical health	17.1 (14.1, 18.3)	15.4 (13.7, 17.7)	3284.5	16.6 (13.7, 17.7)	14.9 (13.1, 17.1)	6326.5*	16.0 (13.3, 17.7)	15.4 (13.7, 17.7)	6277.0
Psychological	16.0 (14.0, 17.3)	16.0 (14.0, 17.3)	3734.5	16.0 (14.7, 17.3)	15.3 (13.3, 16.7)	6169.5*	16.0 (13.5, 17.3)	16.0 (14.0, 17.3)	6468.5
Social relationships	14.7 (12.0, 16.0)	14.7 (13.3, 16.0)	3820.0	14.7 (13.3, 16.0)	14.7 (12.3, 16.0)	7113.5	14.7 (12.0, 16.0)	14.7 (13.3, 16.0)	6034.5
Environment	16.5 (15.5, 17.1)	16.5 (15.0, 18.0)	3834.5	16.5 (15.1, 18.0)	16.0 (15.0, 17.5)	7009.0	16.5 (15.0, 18.0)	16.5 (15.0, 18.0)	6247.0
Overall quality of life	4.0 (4.0, 5.0)	4.0 (4.0, 5.0)	3638.0	4.0 (4.0, 5.0)	4.0 (3.0, 5.0)	5965.0*	4.0 (4.0, 5.0)	4.0 (4.0, 5.0)	6338.5
Overall health	4.0 (3.0, 4.0)	4.0 (3.0, 4.0)	3763.5	4.0 (3.0, 4.0)	3.0 (2.0, 4.0)	6606.5*	4.0 (3.0, 4.0)	4.0 (3.0, 4.0)	6436.0

THI, Tinnitus Handicap Inventory; TFI, Tinnitus Functional Index; FTQ, Fear of Tinnitus Questionnaire; TCS, Tinnitus Catastrophizing Scale; PSQ-30, Perceived Stress Questionnaire; HQ, Hyperacusis Questionnaire; HADS, Hospital Anxiety and Depression Scale; WHOQoL-BREF, World Health Organization Quality of Life Scale (short version).

***Correlation is significant at the 0.001 level. *Correlation is significant at the 0.05 level.*

[a]Higher score, higher quality of life.

[b]Higher score, higher impairment.

Summary of Mann-Whitney U-Tests in relation to occurrence (occasional vs. permanent), onset (gradual vs. abrupt), and manifestation (intermittent vs. constant).

for the 12 month follow-up trial by Cima et al. (2012) that were 11.73 for the TCS and 4.20 for the FTQ. Our study participants only seemed to be mildly affected by tinnitus compared to the RCT population. The average scores for quality of life were very similar to those reported in the literature (Abbott et al., 2009; Kreuzer et al., 2014; Schecklmann et al., 2014). Most published studies involved patients with tinnitus recruited in clinical centers or from medical registries, whereas the subjects recruited in the initial phase of the STOP were representative of the general population that may include individuals diagnosed and not diagnosed with tinnitus. As a consequence, this difference may potentially result in lower severity scores for all questionnaires. These findings emphasize the need of testing these questionnaires in a group of outpatients from clinics in Sweden.

Interestingly, the hyperacusis scores of the HQ were very similar to those found in the literature (Fackrell et al., 2015). However, using the criterion of >28 of Khalfa et al. (2002), we would obtain a proportion of 17.7% of subjects with hyperacusis, but this percentage is well below the reported 40–55% typically found in the tinnitus population (Baguley, 2003; Schecklmann et al., 2014). Indeed, reevaluation of the cut-off threshold has recently been recommended (Fackrell et al., 2015).

The potential to distribute questionnaires online has large benefits over paper versions, both in research and in clinical settings, because large data sets can be created with minimal administrative efforts. Moreover, the use of online questionnaires may precede anamnesis and audiological assessment to allow a more focused discussion at the clinic. Distributing the HADS and HQ questionnaires over the internet has proved successful and validated against pen and paper (Andersson et al., 2002, 2003; Thorén et al., 2012). The internal consistency and reliability of the online questionnaires tested here suggests that they could be used in paper versions in clinics that do not yet have the IT infrastructure to implement web-based versions.

CONCLUSIONS

This study shows the likely suitability of the Swedish versions of the THI, the TFI, the TCS, the FTQ, the HQ, the PSQ-30, the HADS, and the WHOQoL-BREF for measuring outcome in a clinical and research setting. The reliability and validity of these questionnaires translated into Swedish are comparable with that of the original English language versions. Some items of the TSCHQ may have to be removed or rewritten to further improve the reliability of this questionnaire. Additional research may be required to evaluate the sensitivity of each questionnaire in longitudinal studies and their usefulness for measuring treatment outcomes.

AUTHOR CONTRIBUTIONS

BL, WS, BC, RC, and CC designed the study. EI, RH, VP, CL, NE, and CC provided a consensus agreement on the final translated questionnaires. NE and CC developed the web-survey, coordinated the recruitment of subjects, and collected the data. KM and CC analyzed the data. CC, WS, and KM drafted the initial version of the manuscript. All authors contributed to the final version of the manuscript.

ACKNOWLEDGMENTS

We thank the four persons who performed the forward and backward translations of all questionnaires. We also thank Monika Schöll for proof-reading services on the final manuscript. CC and BC have received funding from Vetenskapsrådet, Tysta Skolan, and Karolinska Institutet. CC has received funding from Lars Hiertas Minne, Magnus Bergvalls Stiftelserna, and Loo och Hans Ostermans. The work was supported by an independent research program funded under the Biomedicine and Molecular Biosciences European Cooperation in Science and Technology (COST) Action framework (TINNET BM1306).

REFERENCES

Abbott, J. A., Kaldo, V., Klein, B., Austin, D., Hamilton, C., Piterman, L., et al. (2009). A cluster randomised trial of an internet-based intervention program for tinnitus distress in an industrial setting. *Cogn. Behav. Ther.* 38, 162–173. doi: 10.1080/16506070902763174

Albu, S., and Chirtes, F. (2014). Intratympanic dexamethasone plus melatonin versus melatonin only in the treatment of unilateral acute idiopathic tinnitus. *Am. J. Otolaryngol.* 35, 617–622. doi: 10.1016/j.amjoto.2014.06.009

Andersson, G., Kaldo-Sandström, V., Ström, L., and Strömgren, T. (2003). Internet administration of the Hospital Anxiety and Depression Scale in a sample of tinnitus patients. *J. Psychosom. Res.* 55, 259–262. doi: 10.1016/S0022-3999(02)00575-5

Andersson, G., Lindvall, N., Hursti, T., and Carlbring, P. (2002). Hypersensitivity to sound (hyperacusis): a prevalence study conducted via the Internet and post. *Int. J. Audiol.* 41, 545–554. doi: 10.3109/14992020209056075

Baguley, D. M. (2003). Hyperacusis. *J. R. Soc. Med.* 96, 582–585. doi: 10.1258/jrsm.96.12.582

Bech, P., and Wermuth, L. (1998). Applicability and validity of the Major Depression Inventory in patients with Parkinson's Disease. *Nord. J. Psychiatry* 52, 305–309. doi: 10.1080/08039489850149741

Blomberg, S., Rosander, M., and Andersson, G. (2006). Fears, hyperacusis and musicality in Williams syndrome. *Res. Dev. Disabil.* 27, 668–680. doi: 10.1016/j.ridd.2005.09.002

Cederroth, C. R., Canlon, B., and Langguth, B. (2013). Hearing loss and tinnitus–are funders and industry listening? *Nat. Biotechnol.* 31, 972–974. doi: 10.1038/nbt.2736

Chan, Y. (2009). Tinnitus: etiology, classification, characteristics, and treatment. *Discov. Med.* 8, 133–136.

Cima, R. F., Crombez, G., and Vlaeyen, J. W. (2011). Catastrophizing and fear of tinnitus predict quality of life in patients with chronic tinnitus. *Ear Hear.* 32, 634–641. doi: 10.1097/AUD.0b013e31821106dd

Cima, R. F., Maes, I. H., Joore, M. A., Scheyen, D. J., El Refaie, A., Baguley, D. M., et al. (2012). Specialised treatment based on cognitive behaviour therapy versus usual care for tinnitus: a randomised controlled trial. *Lancet* 379, 1951–1959. doi: 10.1016/S0140-6736(12)60469-3

Cohen, J. (1960). A coefficient of agreement for nominal scales. *Educ. Psychol. Meas.* 20, 37–46. doi: 10.1177/001316446002000104

Dobie, R. A. (2003). Depression and tinnitus. *Otolaryngol. Clin. North Am.* 36, 383–388. doi: 10.1016/S0030-6665(02)00168-8

Epstein, J., Santo, R. M., and Guillemin, F. (2015). A review of guidelines for cross-cultural adaptation of questionnaires could not bring out a consensus. *J. Clin. Epidemiol.* 68, 435–441. doi: 10.1016/j.jclinepi.2014.11.021

Fackrell, K., Fearnley, C., Hoare, D. J., and Sereda, M. (2015). Hyperacusis Questionnaire as a tool for measuring hypersensitivity to sound in a tinnitus research population. *Biomed Res. Int.* 2015:290425. doi: 10.1155/2015/290425

Fackrell, K., Hall, D. A., Barry, J. G., and Hoare, D. J. (2016). Psychometric properties of the Tinnitus Functional Index (TFI): assessment in a UK research volunteer population. *Hear. Res.* 335, 220–235. doi: 10.1016/j.heares.2015.09.009

Friberg, E., Jansson, C., Mittendorfer-Rutz, E., Rosenhall, U., and Alexanderson, K. (2012). Sickness absence due to otoaudiological diagnoses and risk of disability pension: a nationwide Swedish prospective cohort study. *PLoS ONE* 7:e29966. doi: 10.1371/journal.pone.0029966

Gopinath, B., McMahon, C. M., Rochtchina, E., Karpa, M. J., and Mitchell, P. (2010a). Incidence, persistence, and progression of tinnitus symptoms in older adults: the Blue Mountains Hearing Study. *Ear Hear.* 31, 407–412. doi: 10.1097/AUD.0b013e3181cdb2a2

Gopinath, B., McMahon, C. M., Rochtchina, E., Karpa, M. J., and Mitchell, P. (2010b). Risk factors and impacts of incident tinnitus in older adults. *Ann. Epidemiol.* 20, 129–135. doi: 10.1016/j.annepidem.2009.09.002

Greimel, K. V., Leibetseder, M., Unterrainer, J., and Albegger, K. (1999). [Can tinnitus be measured? Methods for assessment of tinnitus-specific disability and presentation of the Tinnitus Disability Questionnaire]. *HNO* 47, 196–201. doi: 10.1007/s001060050382

Grouven, U., Bender, R., Ziegler, A., and Lange, S. (2007). [The kappa coefficient]. *Dtsch. Med. Wochenschr.* 132(Suppl. 1), e65–e68. doi: 10.1055/s-2007-959046

Hall, D. A., Haider, H., Kikidis, D., Mielczarek, M., Mazurek, B., Szczepek, A. J., et al. (2015). Toward a global consensus on outcome measures for clinical trials in tinnitus: report from the First International Meeting of the COMiT Initiative, November 14, 2014, Amsterdam, The Netherlands. *Trends Hear.* 19, 270–289. doi: 10.1177/2331216515580272

Hall, D., Haider, H., Szczepek, A. J., Lau, P., Rabau, S., Jones-Diette, J., et al. (2016). Systematic review of outcome domains and instruments used in clinical trials of tinnitus treatments in adults. *Trials* 17, 1–19. doi: 10.1186/s13063-016-1399-9

Harkness, J. A. (2003). "Questionnaire translation," in *Cross-Cultural Survey Methods*, eds F. van de Vijver and P. Mohler (Hoboken, NJ: John Wiley & Sons).

Hays, R. D., and Hayashi, T. (1990). Beyond internal consistency reliability: rationale and user's guide for Multitrait Analysis Program on the microcomputer. *Behav. Res. Methods Instrum. Comput.* 22, 167–175. doi: 10.3758/BF03203140

Heller, A. J. (2003). Classification and epidemiology of tinnitus. *Otolaryngol. Clin. North Am.* 36, 239–248. doi: 10.1016/S0030-6665(02)00160-3

Henry, J. A., Griest, S., Thielman, E., McMillan, G., Kaelin, C., and Carlson, K. F. (2016). Tinnitus functional index: development, validation, outcomes research, and clinical application. *Hear. Res.* 334, 58–64. doi: 10.1016/j.heares.2015.06.004

Jasper, K., Weise, C., Conrad, I., Andersson, G., Hiller, W., and Kleinstäuber, M. (2014). Internet-based guided self-help versus group cognitive behavioral therapy for chronic tinnitus: a randomized controlled trial. *Psychother. Psychosom.* 83, 234–246. doi: 10.1159/000360705

Kaldo, V., Cars, S., Rahnert, M., Larsen, H. C., and Andersson, G. (2007). Use of a self-help book with weekly therapist contact to reduce tinnitus distress: a randomized controlled trial. *J. Psychosom. Res.* 63, 195–202. doi: 10.1016/j.jpsychores.2007.04.007

Khalfa, S., Dubal, S., Veuillet, E., Perez-Diaz, F., Jouvent, R., and Collet, L. (2002). Psychometric normalization of a Hyperacusis Questionnaire. *J. Otorhinolaryngol. Relat. Spec.* 64, 436–442. doi: 10.1159/000067570

Kreuzer, P. M., Landgrebe, M., Resch, M., Husser, O., Schecklmann, M., Geisreiter, F., et al. (2014). Feasibility, safety and efficacy of transcutaneous vagus nerve stimulation in chronic tinnitus: an open pilot study. *Brain Stimul.* 7, 740–747. doi: 10.1016/j.brs.2014.05.003

Landgrebe, M., Azevedo, A., Baguley, D., Bauer, C., Cacace, A., Coelho, C., et al. (2012). Methodological aspects of clinical trials in tinnitus: a proposal for an international standard. *J. Psychosom. Res.* 73, 112–121. doi: 10.1016/j.jpsychores.2012.05.002

Landgrebe, M., Zeman, F., Koller, M., Eberl, Y., Mohr, M., Reiter, J., et al. (2010). The Tinnitus Research Initiative (TRI) database: a new approach for delineation of tinnitus subtypes and generation of predictors for treatment outcome. *BMC Med. Inform. Decis. Mak.* 10:42. doi: 10.1186/1472-6947-10-42

Langguth, B., Goodey, R., Azevedo, A., Bjorne, A., Cacace, A., Crocetti, A., et al. (2007). Consensus for tinnitus patient assessment and treatment outcome measurement: Tinnitus Research Initiative meeting, Regensburg, July 2006. *Prog. Brain Res.* 166, 525–536. doi: 10.1016/S0079-6123(07)66050-6

Langguth, B., Kreuzer, P. M., Kleinjung, T., and De Ridder, D. (2013). Tinnitus: causes and clinical management. *Lancet Neurol.* 12, 920–930. doi: 10.1016/S1474-4422(13)70160-1

Levenstein, S., Prantera, C., Varvo, V., Scribano, M. L., Berto, E., Luzi, C., et al. (1993). Development of the perceived stress questionnaire: a new tool for psychosomatic research. *J. Psychosom. Res.* 37, 19–32. doi: 10.1016/0022-3999(93)90120-5

Maes, I. H., Cima, R. F., Vlaeyen, J. W., Anteunis, L. J., and Joore, M. A. (2013). Tinnitus: a cost study. *Ear Hear.* 34, 508–514. doi: 10.1097/AUD.0b013e31827d113a

Maes, I. H., Joore, M. A., Cima, R. F., Vlaeyen, J. W., and Anteunis, L. J. (2011). Assessment of health state in patients with tinnitus: a comparison of the EQ-5D and HUI mark III. *Ear Hear.* 32, 428–435. doi: 10.1097/AUD.0b013e3181fdf09f

Meikle, M. B., Henry, J. A., Griest, S. E., Stewart, B. J., Abrams, H. B., McArdle, R., et al. (2012). The tinnitus functional index: development of a new clinical measure for chronic, intrusive tinnitus. *Ear Hear.* 33, 153–176. doi: 10.1097/AUD.0b013e31822f67c0

Newman, C. W., Jacobson, G. P., and Spitzer, J. B. (1996). Development of the Tinnitus Handicap Inventory. *Arch. Otolaryngol. Head Neck Surg.* 122, 143–148. doi: 10.1001/archotol.1996.01890140029007

Newman, C. W., Sandridge, S. A., and Jacobson, G. P. (1998). Psychometric adequacy of the Tinnitus Handicap Inventory (THI) for evaluating treatment outcome. *J. Am. Acad. Audiol.* 9, 153–160.

Nondahl, D. M., Cruickshanks, K. J., Wiley, T. L., Klein, R., Klein, B. E., and Tweed, T. S. (2002). Prevalence and 5-year incidence of tinnitus among older adults: the epidemiology of hearing loss study. *J. Am. Acad. Audiol.* 13, 323–331.

Park, B., Choi, H. G., Lee, H. J., An, S. Y., Kim, S. W., Lee, J. S., et al. (2014). Analysis of the prevalence of and risk factors for tinnitus in a young population. *Otol. Neurotol.* 35, 1218–1222. doi: 10.1097/mao.0000000000000472

Park, K. H., Lee, S. H., Koo, J. W., Park, H. Y., Lee, K. Y., Choi, Y. S., et al. (2014). Prevalence and associated factors of tinnitus: data from the Korean National Health and Nutrition Examination Survey 2009–2011. *J. Epidemiol.* 24, 417–426. doi: 10.2188/jea.JE20140024

Schecklmann, M., Landgrebe, M., Langguth, B., and TRI Database Study Group. (2014). Phenotypic characteristics of hyperacusis in tinnitus. *PLoS ONE* 9:e86944. doi: 10.1371/journal.pone.0086944

Shargorodsky, J., Curhan, G. C., and Farwell, W. R. (2010). Prevalence and characteristics of tinnitus among US adults. *Am. J. Med.* 123, 711–718. doi: 10.1016/j.amjmed.2010.02.015

Spinhoven, P., Ormel, J., Sloekers, P. P., Kempen, G. I., Speckens, A. E., and Van Hemert, A. M. (1997). A validation study of the Hospital Anxiety and Depression Scale (HADS) in different groups of Dutch subjects. *Psychol. Med.* 27, 363–370. doi: 10.1017/S0033291796004382

Thorén, E. S., Andersson, G., and Lunner, T. (2012). The use of research questionnaires with hearing impaired adults: online vs. paper-and-pencil administration. *BMC Ear Nose Throat Disord.* 12:12. doi: 10.1186/1472-6815-12-12

Tunkel, D. E., Bauer, C. A., Sun, G. H., Rosenfeld, R. M., Chandrasekhar, S. S., Cunningham, E. R. Jr., et al. (2014). Clinical practice guideline: tinnitus. *Otolaryngol. Head Neck Surg.* 151, S1–S40. doi: 10.1177/0194599814547475

Westin, V. Z., Schulin, M., Hesser, H., Karlsson, M., Noe, R. Z., Olofsson, U., et al. (2011). Acceptance and commitment therapy versus tinnitus retraining therapy in the treatment of tinnitus: a randomised controlled trial. *Behav. Res. Ther.* 49, 737–747. doi: 10.1016/j.brat.2011.08.001

WHO (1998). Development of the World Health Organization WHOQOL-BREF quality of life assessment. The WHOQOL Group. *Psychol. Med.* 28, 551–558. doi: 10.1017/S0033291798006667

Zeman, F., Koller, M., Langguth, B., Landgrebe, M., and Tinnitus Research Initiative database study. (2014). Which tinnitus-related aspects are relevant for quality of life and depression: results from a large international multicentre sample. *Health Qual. Life Outcomes* 12:7. doi: 10.1186/1477-7525-12-7

Zeman, F., Koller, M., Schecklmann, M., Langguth, B., Landgrebe, M., and TRI database study group. (2012). Tinnitus assessment by means of standardized self-report questionnaires: psychometric properties of the Tinnitus Questionnaire (TQ), the Tinnitus Handicap Inventory (THI), and their short versions in an international and multi-lingual sample. *Health Qual. Life Outcomes* 10:128. doi: 10.1186/1477-7525-10-128

20

Disrupted Brain Functional Network Architecture in Chronic Tinnitus Patients

Yu-Chen Chen[1†], Yuan Feng[1†], Jin-Jing Xu[2], Cun-Nan Mao[1], Wenqing Xia[3], Jun Ren[1] and Xindao Yin[1*]*

[1] Department of Radiology, Nanjing First Hospital, Nanjing Medical University, Nanjing, China, [2] Department of Otolaryngology, Nanjing First Hospital, Nanjing Medical University, Nanjing, China, [3] Department of Endocrinology, Nanjing First Hospital, Nanjing Medical University, Nanjing, China

***Correspondence:**
Yu-Chen Chen
chenyuchen1989@126.com
Xindao Yin
y.163yy@163.com

Purpose: Resting-state functional magnetic resonance imaging (fMRI) studies have demonstrated the disruptions of multiple brain networks in tinnitus patients. Nonetheless, several studies found no differences in network processing between tinnitus patients and healthy controls (HCs). Its neural bases are poorly understood. To identify aberrant brain network architecture involved in chronic tinnitus, we compared the resting-state fMRI (rs-fMRI) patterns of tinnitus patients and HCs.

Materials and Methods: Chronic tinnitus patients (n = 24) with normal hearing thresholds and age-, sex-, education- and hearing threshold-matched HCs (n = 22) participated in the current study and underwent the rs-fMRI scanning. We used degree centrality (DC) to investigate functional connectivity (FC) strength of the whole-brain network and Granger causality to analyze effective connectivity in order to explore directional aspects involved in tinnitus.

Results: Compared to HCs, we found significantly increased network centrality in bilateral superior frontal gyrus (SFG). Unidirectionally, the left SFG revealed increased effective connectivity to the left middle orbitofrontal cortex (OFC), left posterior lobe of cerebellum (PLC), left postcentral gyrus, and right middle occipital gyrus (MOG) while the right SFG exhibited enhanced effective connectivity to the right supplementary motor area (SMA). In addition, the effective connectivity from the bilateral SFG to the OFC and SMA showed positive correlations with tinnitus distress.

Conclusions: Rs-fMRI provides a new and novel method for identifying aberrant brain network architecture. Chronic tinnitus patients have disrupted FC strength and causal connectivity mostly in non-auditory regions, especially the prefrontal cortex (PFC). The current findings will provide a new perspective for understanding the neuropathophysiological mechanisms in chronic tinnitus.

Keywords: chronic tinnitus, degree centrality, effective connectivity, resting-state fMRI

INTRODUCTION

Tinnitus is the perception of a sound in the absence of an external sound source. Roughly 12% of adults experience tinnitus, but the prevalence skyrockets to 50% in combat personnel (McFadden, 1982; Meikle, 1997). Chronic tinnitus usually leads to problems ranging from mild discomfort such as sleep disturbance to strong anxiety and depression

(Leske, 1981; Lockwood et al., 2002). Although most tinnitus patients localize tinnitus to one or both ears, the severity of the phantom sound could not be eliminated after sectioning the auditory nerve (Berliner et al., 1992; Jackler and Whinney, 2001). Tinnitus patients show various pathophysiological changes, such as increased spontaneous activity, enhanced neural synchrony, tonotopic map reorganization, abnormal consciousness gating mechanisms and coupling of networks involving auditory and non-auditory structures (Lenarz et al., 1993; Lockwood et al., 1998; Kaltenbach et al., 2005; Adjamian et al., 2009; Henry et al., 2014). Nonetheless, the mechanisms that maintain the disorder remain poorly understood.

Previous neuroimaging studies using electroencephalography (EEG), magnetoencephalography (MEG), positron emission tomography (PET), and functional magnetic resonance imaging (fMRI), have investigated the neuropathophysiological mechanisms implicated in chronic tinnitus (Shulman and Strashun, 1998; Mirz et al., 1999; Adjamian et al., 2009; Schlee et al., 2009; Roberts et al., 2010; Vanneste and De Ridder, 2012). Resting-state fMRI (rs-fMRI) is a promising noninvasive technique that could reflect the brain functional architecture in low frequency fluctuations (0.01–0.1 Hz) of blood oxygenation level-dependent (BOLD; Biswal et al., 1995; Fox and Raichle, 2007). Using rs-fMRI, multiple brain networks relevant to neural mechanisms of tinnitus have been demonstrated, such as the auditory network (Burton et al., 2012; Kim et al., 2012; Maudoux et al., 2012a,b; Schmidt et al., 2013; Hinkley et al., 2015; Minami et al., 2015; Leaver et al., 2016), dorsal attention network (DAN; Burton et al., 2012; Schmidt et al., 2013), ventral attention network (VAN; Burton et al., 2012), default mode network (DMN; Schmidt et al., 2013; Chen et al., 2014, 2015d; Leaver et al., 2016), and visual network (Burton et al., 2012; Chen et al., 2014). However, these results have been variable due to applied analytic methods. Burton et al. (2012) implied that there is dissociation between activity in auditory cortex and visual, attention and control networks using seed-based functional connectivity (FC) analysis. Through independent component analysis (ICA), Kim et al. (2012) found enhanced FC between the attention network and auditory network, suggesting that this network might contribute to the perception or salience of tinnitus. Schmidt et al. (2013) identified specific alterations in the connectivity of the DMN, DAN, and auditory networks due to tinnitus. Similarly, Maudoux et al. (2012a,b) provided fMRI evidence for a distributed network of auditory and non-auditory cortical and sub-cortical regions associated with chronic tinnitus pathology using ICA approach. Using the algorithms of amplitude of low-frequency fluctuations (ALFF) and regional homogeneity (ReHo), Chen et al. (2014, 2015c,d) found abnormal spontaneous neural activity within multiple cerebral networks, such as the DMN and the attention network. Nonetheless, other studies have failed to detect any differences in network processing between tinnitus patients and controls (Wineland et al., 2012; Davies et al., 2014). Heterogeneity among tinnitus cohorts may contribute to network state variations. According to these recent theories and observations, we speculated that abnormal brain FC and network might underlie the pathophysiology in chronic tinnitus.

The prefrontal cortex (PFC) exerts early inhibitory modulation of input to primary auditory cortex in humans and has been found to be associated with auditory attention (Lewis et al., 2000; Voisin et al., 2006). The vital role for the PFC in subserving tinnitus mechanism has been postulated (Jastreboff, 1990) and previous neuroimaging studies have confirmed the involvement of PFC for tinnitus (Vanneste et al., 2010, 2012; Vanneste and De Ridder, 2012; De Ridder et al., 2014). Furthermore, latest rs-fMRI studies identified abnormalities in the PFC associated with tinnitus (Burton et al., 2012; Kim et al., 2012; Schmidt et al., 2013; Ueyama et al., 2013; Chen et al., 2014, 2015b,c,d; Leaver et al., 2016). Among them, Ueyama et al. (2013) observed disrupted FC strength in distinct brain regions, especially in the left superior frontal gyrus (SFG), which was negatively correlated with tinnitus loudness. Taken together, the PFC is considered as a key region involved in tinnitus. Investigations exploring the role of PFC in the brain functional network architecture of tinnitus will provide valuable insight into the neural mechanisms underlying the chronic tinnitus.

Seed-based FC and ICA approaches have proved extremely useful in exploring connectivity patterns for specific components of interest. However, few studies have investigated the tinnitus-related alterations of whole-brain FC pattern or large-scale brain network. Degree centrality (DC) is a voxel-wise data-driven method that can quantify the importance of each node in brain network. This graph theory based network analysis can assess the network centrality without *a priori* selection of nodes or networks of interest (Zuo et al., 2012). This algorithm has been used to observe the alterations of resting-state functional networks in diverse diseases, such as Alzheimer's disease (AD), autism, and hepatic encephalopathy (Buckner et al., 2009; Di Martino et al., 2013; Chen et al., 2015a). Since the neural mechanisms underlying tinnitus are poorly understood and multiple brain systems are involved, we applied DC to analyze FC within the whole-brain network. To examine the directional connectivity network involved in tinnitus, we further used the granger causality analysis (GCA), which is a statistical method originally used in the field of economics to assess directional influences between simultaneously recorded time series (Granger, 1969; Zhou et al., 2011). GCA has been widely used to reveal the causal effects among brain regions in various neurological or psychiatric disorders, such as AD, schizophrenia, depression and hepatic encephalopathy (Qi et al., 2013; Zhong et al., 2014; Guo et al., 2015a,b). Thus, to unravel the details of the brain functional network architecture in tinnitus, we sought to evaluate the brain regions that show aberrant FC across the entire brain networks in tinnitus patients using DC and then use GCA to analyze effective connectivity to understand the directional aspect of these alterations. We hypothesized that the intrinsic dysconnectivity pattern of the PFC might play a crucial role in the brain functional network architecture of tinnitus patients.

MATERIALS AND METHODS

Subjects

All the subjects provided written informed consent before their participation in the study protocol, which was approved by the Research Ethics Committee of the Nanjing Medical University (Reference No. 2016067).

According to both the inclusion and exclusion criteria of this study, a final sample of 47 subjects including 25 chronic tinnitus patients and 22 healthy controls (HCs) were recruited through community health screening and newspaper advertisements. The tinnitus patients and healthy subjects were group-matched in terms of age, sex, and education. One tinnitus patient was subsequently excluded because the limits for head motion were exceeded during MR scanning. Ten patients reported a predominantly left-sided tinnitus, six a predominantly right-sided tinnitus and eight patients described their tinnitus as bilateral or originating within the head. All subjects were right-handed and completed at least 8 years of education. The severity of tinnitus and related distress were assessed by the Iowa version of the Tinnitus Handicap Questionnaires (THQ; Kuk et al., 1990). Hearing thresholds were determined by puretone audiometry (PTA). All of the participants had normal hearing (defined as thresholds <25 dB HL) at the frequencies of 0.25 kHz, 0.5 kHz, 1 kHz, 2 kHz, 4 kHz, and 8 kHz. There were no significant differences in auditory thresholds between tinnitus and control groups. In addition, none of the participants had symptoms of depression and anxiety according to the Self-Rating Depression Scale (SDS) and Self-Rating Anxiety Scale (SAS; overall scores <50, respectively; Zung, 1971, 1986). According to previous study (Khalfa et al., 2002), we used the Hyperacusis Questionnaire to exclude the participants with hyperacusis in the current study. Participants were also excluded from the study if they suffered from pulsatile tinnitus or Meniere's diseases, or if they had a past history of severe smoking, stroke, alcoholism, brain injury, Parkinson's disease, AD, epilepsy, major depression, neurological or psychiatric disorders that could affect cognitive function, major medical illness (e.g., anemia, thyroid dysfunction and cancer), MRI contraindications (e.g., cochlear implants, pacemakers, cerebral aneurysm clips, prosthetic valves, a history of intraocular metal fragments, and claustrophobia), or severe visual loss. The characteristics of the chronic tinnitus patients and healthy subjects are summarized in **Table 1**.

TABLE 1 | Characteristics of the tinnitus patients and healthy controls (HCs).

	Tinnitus patients (n = 24)	HCs (n = 22)	p value
Age (year)	50.8 ± 12.4 (26–67)	44.7 ± 15.4 (26–70)	0.144
Gender (male: female)	9:15	9:13	0.813
Education levels (years)	12.3 ± 3.1 (8–18)	13.4 ± 3.8 (8–22)	0.313
Tinnitus duration (months)	46.5 ± 39.1 (6–120)	–	–
THQ score	49.5 ± 15.5	–	–
Hearing thresholds (left)	13.0 ± 2.7	13.6 ± 2.2	0.414
Hearing thresholds (right)	14.6 ± 3.6	13.9 ± 3.4	0.470

Data are represented as Mean ± SD (range of min-max).

MRI Acquisition

MRI data were acquired at our hospital using a 3.0 T MRI scanner (Ingenia, Philips Medical Systems, Netherlands). Head motion and scanner noise were reduced using foam padding and earplugs. The earplugs (Hearos Ultimate Softness Series, USA) were used to attenuate scanner noise by approximately 32 dB. Subjects were instructed to lie quietly with their eyes closed without falling asleep, not think of anything in particular, and avoid any head motion during the scan. Functional images were obtained axially using a gradient echo-planar imaging (EPI) sequence as follows: repetition time (TR) = 2000 ms; echo time (TE) = 30 ms; slices = 36; thickness = 4 mm; gap = 0 mm; field of view (FOV) = 240 mm × 240 mm; acquisition matrix = 64 × 64; and flip angle (FA) = 90°. The fMRI sequence took 8 min and 8 s. Structural images were acquired with a three-dimensional turbo fast echo (3D-TFE) T1WI sequence with high resolution as follows: TR/TE = 8.1/3.7 ms; slices = 170; thickness = 1 mm; gap = 0 mm; FA = 8°; acquisition matrix = 256 × 256; FOV = 256 mm × 256 mm. The structural sequence took 5 min and 29 s.

Functional Data Preprocessing

Functional data analyses were conducted using Data Processing Assistant for Resting-State fMRI (DPARSF) programs (Chao-Gan and Yu-Feng, 2010) based on statistical parametric mapping (SPM8[1]) and rs-fMRI data analyses toolkits (REST[2]). A total of 240 volumes were scanned, and the first 10 volumes were discarded to allow for signal equilibrium of the initial magnetic resonance signals and adaptation of the subjects to scanner. The remaining 230 consecutive volumes were used for data analysis. Afterwards, the following procedures were carried out as follows: slice-timing adjustment, realignment for head-motion correction, spatial normalization to the Montreal Neurological Institute (MNI) template (resampling voxel size = 3 × 3 × 3 mm^3) and smoothing with an isotropic Gaussian kernel (full width at half maximum (FWHM) = 6 mm), detrending and filtering (0.01–0.08 Hz). Any subjects with a head motion >2.0 mm translation or a 2.0° rotation in any direction were excluded.

Degree Centrality Analysis

We restricted our voxel-wise centrality analyses to a predefined gray matter (GM) mask that included tissue with GM probabilities greater than 20% as previously described (Zuo et al., 2012). Within the mask, individual network centrality maps were generated in a voxel-wise fashion. First, the preprocessed functional runs were subjected to voxel-based whole-brain correlation analysis. The time course of each voxel from each participant was correlated with the time course of every other voxel, which resulted in a correlation matrix. An undirected adjacency matrix was then obtained by thresholding each correlation at $r > 0.25$ (Buckner et al., 2009; Zuo et al., 2012; Yan et al., 2013). As previously reported, the negative correlations were not included in DC calculation, given their ambiguous interpretation and detrimental effects

[1]http://www.fil.ion.ucl.ac.uk/spm
[2]http://www.restfmri.net

on test-retest reliability (Buckner et al., 2008; Vincent et al., 2008; Murphy et al., 2009). A high threshold was chosen to eliminate counting voxels that had low temporal correlation attributable to signal noise. Different threshold selections did not qualitatively change the results for cortex (Buckner et al., 2009). Then, the DC was computed as the number of significant correlations (binarized) or as the sum of the weights of the significant connections (weighted) for each voxel (Buckner et al., 2009; Zuo et al., 2012). This measure of connectivity (degree, D) for each voxel (i) with all other voxels (j) is given by the following: $D_i=\sum d_{ij}$ where, $j = 1 \ldots N$, $i \neq j$. The map of the connectivity was then standardized by converting to z scores so that maps across participants could be averaged and compared. The z score transformation is given by:

$$Z_i = \frac{D_i - \overline{D}}{\sigma_D} \; i = 1 \ldots N \tag{1}$$

The $\overline{D}$ is the mean degree across all the voxels in the whole-brain map and σ_D is the standard deviation of the map. DC has been shown to represent the most local and directly quantifiable centrality measure and has been widely used to examine node characteristics of intrinsic network connectivity (Zuo et al., 2012). The DC maps were transferred to z-values for group comparisons. Within brain network, the DC value of a node indicates its connectivity strength to all the other nodes and reflects its importance in functional integration.

We first estimated spatial distribution of mean DC in the tinnitus group and healthy group, respectively. The individual z values were entered into the SPM8 software for a random effect one-sample t-test in a voxel-wise way to show the average DC maps within each group. The significant threshold was set at $p < 0.01$, with multiple comparisons correction using the AFNI AlphaSim program[3] determined by Monte Carlo simulation (AlphaSim program with following parameters: single voxel p value of 0.01, a minimum cluster size of 40 voxels, 5000 simulations, cluster connection radius r = 5 mm, FWHM = 6 mm). This correction was confined within the aforementioned GM mask.

To find the disrupted brain hub regions, two-tailed two-sample t-test were then conducted to investigate the differences in the DC maps between tinnitus patients and HCs. Between-group comparisons of the DC maps were performed in the SPM8 software using general linear model (GLM) analysis, with age, sex and education included as nuisance covariates. A correction for multiple comparisons was performed by a Monte Carlo simulation using the AlphaSim program, resulting in a corrected threshold of $p < 0.01$ and minimum cluster size of 40 voxels (parameters were single voxel p value of 0.01, 5000 simulations, cluster connection radius r = 5 mm, FWHM = 6 mm). For between-group analysis, a mask was created by combining the significant clusters in both groups, which were obtained from one-sample t-test results.

[3] https://afni.nimh.nih.gov/pub/dist/doc/manual/AlphaSim.pdf

Effective Connectivity Analysis

Using DC approach, we were able to show that the bilateral SFG is a region of special functional importance in tinnitus patients revealing increased FC. To further investigate the influence of directionality, we applied GCA to evaluate changes in effective connectivity. Based on the results of the DC analysis we selected the seed regions, which showed significant differences between tinnitus patients and HCs (left and right SFG: MNI coordinates (x, y, z) ±18, 42, 27). Effective connectivity was analyzed using REST-GCA in the REST toolbox (Zang et al., 2012). In this study, two separate time series of the left and right SFG were defined as the seed time series x, and the time series y denotes the time series of all voxels in the brain. The linear direct influence of x on y ($F_{x \to y}$), and the linear direct influence of y on x ($F_{y \to x}$) were calculated voxel by voxel across the brain. Thus, two Granger causality maps were generated based on the influence measures for each subjects. The residual-based F was normalized (F′) and standardized to Z score for each voxel ($Z_{x \to y}$ and $Z_{y \to x}$, subtracting the global mean F′values, divided by standard deviation).

For the group analysis on the effective connectivity, mean values of $Z_{x \to y}$ and $Z_{y \to x}$ maps were computed for each group. All eight Granger causality maps were acquired, with four for each direction and four for each group (the left SFG with $Z_{x \to y}$ and $Z_{y \to x}$ and the right SFG with $Z_{x \to y}$ and $Z_{y \to x}$ for both tinnitus patient and HCs). Then these Granger causality maps were entered into SPM8 software for group comparison. A random effect two-sample t-test in a voxel-wise manner was performed to determine the differences of effective connectivity of the SFG between tinnitus patient and HCs, with age, sex and education including as nuisance covariates. A correction for multiple comparisons was also conducted by a Monte Carlo simulation using the AlphaSim program, with a corrected threshold of $p < 0.01$ and minimum cluster size of 40 voxels.

Correlation Analysis

To investigate the relationship between clinical characteristic of tinnitus patients and DC and effective connectivity measures, these regions showing significant differences in DC or effective connectivity between groups were extracted. Mean z values within these clusters were correlated against each tinnitus characteristic using the Pearson's correlation analysis by SPSS software (version 18.0; SPSS, Chicago, IL, USA). $P < 0.05$ was considered statistically significant, corrected for age, sex and education. Bonferroni correction for multiple comparisons was applied in the correlation analysis.

RESULTS

Degree Centrality Analysis

In both HC (**Figure 1A**) and tinnitus patients (**Figure 1B**), the spatial distribution of the weighted DC was highly localized in the occipital lobe, inferior parietal lobe (IPL), PFC, cingulate cortex, insula and thalamus. After two-sample t-test analysis, significantly increased DC within the bilateral SFG was found

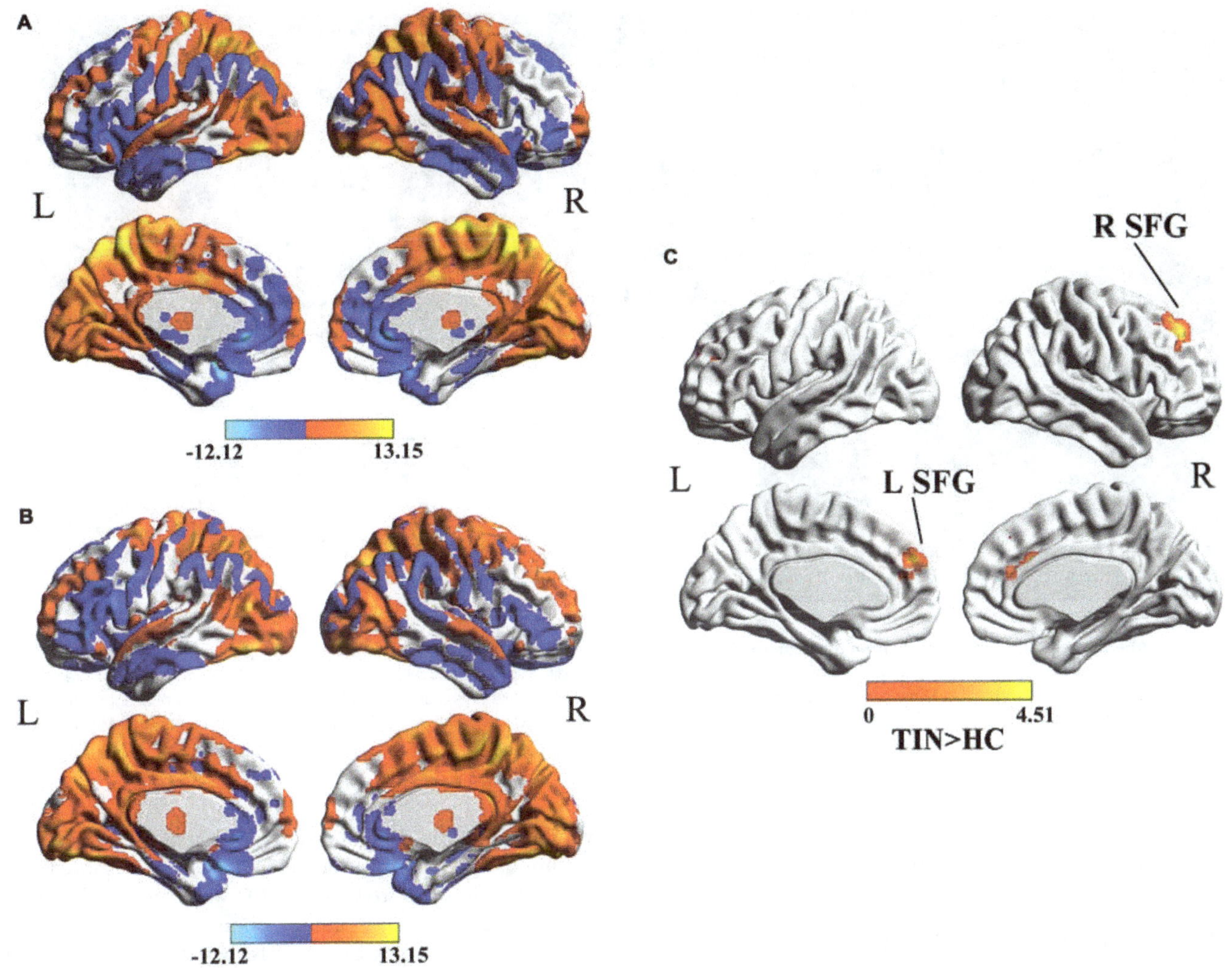

FIGURE 1 | (A) Spatial distribution of the degree centrality (DC) in the healthy controls (HCs). **(B)** Spatial distribution of the DC in the chronic tinnitus patients. **(C)** Significantly increased DC within the bilateral superior frontal gyrus (SFG) between tinnitus patients and HCs. TIN, tinnitus; HCs, healthy controls.

in tinnitus patients compared to HCs ($p < 0.01$, AlphaSim corrected; **Figure 1C**).

Effective Connectivity Analysis

Compared to HCs, patients with chronic tinnitus demonstrated significantly increased effective connectivity from the left SFG to the left middle orbitofrontal cortex (OFC), left posterior lobe of cerebellum (PLC), left postcentral gyrus (PoCG), and right middle occipital gyrus (MOG). Moreover, the right SFG exhibited enhanced effective connectivity to the right supplementary motor area (SMA; $p < 0.01$, AlphaSim corrected; **Figure 2** and **Table 2**). However, we did not find any abnormal feedback effect to the bilateral SFG in the tinnitus patients.

Correlation Results

We found no significant correlations between the DC of the bilateral SFG and the tinnitus characteristics. However, the THQ scores positively correlated with the increased effective connectivity from the left SFG to left OFC ($r = 0.504$, $p = 0.020$), and from the right SFG to right SMA ($r = 0.526$, $p = 0.014$; **Figure 3**). The other regions with enhanced effective connectivity revealed no significant correlations with tinnitus duration or THQ scores.

DISCUSSION

This is the first study to use both DC and GCA approaches to explore intrinsic functional network architecture related to tinnitus. Using DC analysis, we found significantly increased network centrality within the bilateral SFG regions in chronic tinnitus patients. Using GCA algorithm, we employed the bilateral SFG as seeds to examine their causal effect with the whole brain. Unidirectionally, bilateral SFG showed increased effective connectivity to several non-auditory regions including the prefrontal, motor, visual cortex and cerebellum. Of note,

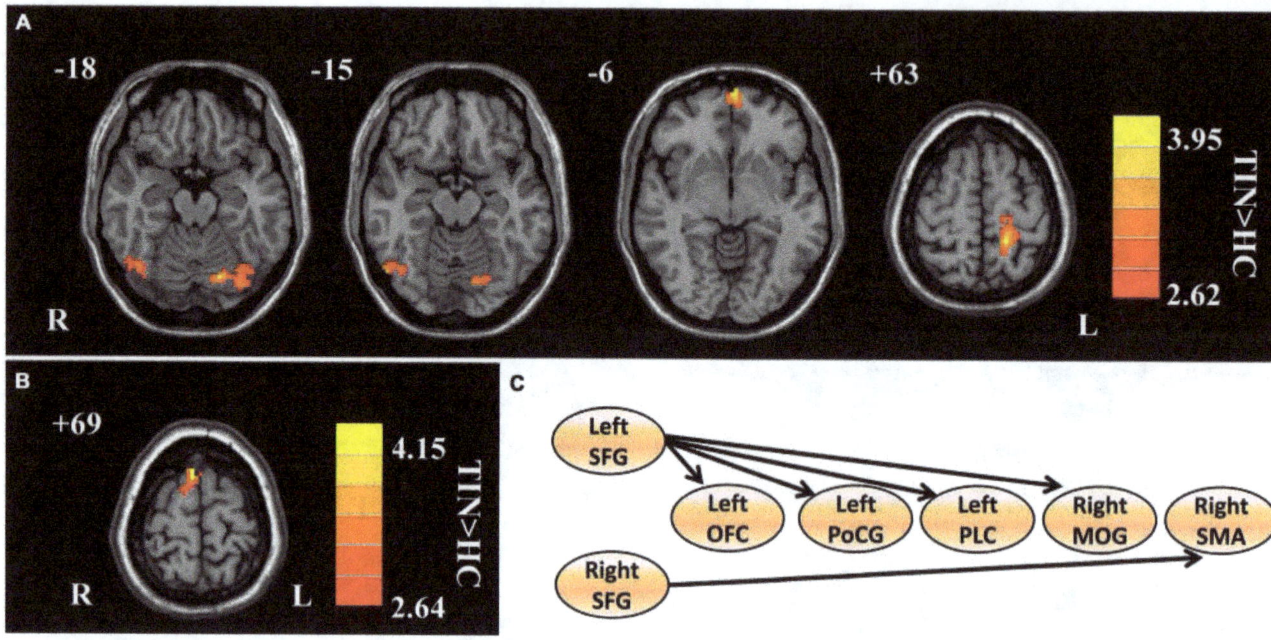

FIGURE 2 | Aberrant effective connectivity from the bilateral SFG in tinnitus patients. (A) Increased effective connectivity from the left SFG to the left orbitofrontal cortex (OFC), left PoCG, left posterior lobe of cerebellum (PLC), and right middle occipital gyrus (MOG; $p < 0.01$, AlphaSim corrected). **(B)** Increased effective connectivity from the right SFG to the right supplementary motor area (SMA; $p < 0.01$, AlphaSim corrected). **(C)** Schematic overview of changes in effective connectivity from the bilateral SFG. SFG, superior frontal gyrus; OFC, orbitofrontal cortex; PoCG, precentral gyrus; PLC, posterior lobe of cerebellum; MOG, middle occipital gyrus; SMA, supplementary motor area; TIN, tinnitus; HCs, healthy controls.

the abnormal connectivity to the OFC and the SMA revealed significant correlations with the tinnitus distress.

Increased Network Centrality in the SFG

Certain regions show strong connections with other regions within large-scale cortical networks that constitute an emerging feature of brain architecture (Sporns et al., 2007; Buckner et al., 2009; Zuo et al., 2012). Our findings show that the SFG is the main cortical hub in the brain network architecture affected by tinnitus, which is in line with the hypothesis that the dysconnectivity pattern of the PFC involved in tinnitus perception. The PFC has been regarded as a critical region by Jastreboff (1990), who suggested that the PFC integrates sensory and emotional aspects of tinnitus. Several neurophysiological models based on neuroimaging have been raised involved in tinnitus subsequently (De Ridder et al., 2014). Rauschecker et al. (2010) developed a model to demonstrate structural and functional differences in ventromedial prefrontal cortex (vmPFC) that were associated with tinnitus subjective loudness, indicating that PFC may contribute to certain perceptual features of tinnitus (Leaver et al., 2011). The current integrative model attempts to unify the different brain areas and networks associated with tinnitus in one model and propose the hypothetical neural core of conscious phantom sound perception (De Ridder et al., 2011, 2014; Vanneste and De Ridder, 2012), which is more extensive than the initially proposed auditory system (Jastreboff and Hazell, 2008).

TABLE 2 | Regions showing significant differences in effective connectivity between tinnitus patients and HCs.

Brain regions	BA	Peak MNI coordinates *x, y, z* (mm)	Peak *T* value	Voxels
Increased effective connectivity from left SFG				
Left OFC	11	−3, 66, −6	4.1302	158
Left PoCG	3	−18, −42, 63	4.0470	132
Left PLC	–	−18, −75, −18	3.7193	100
Right MOG	19	54, −69, −15	3.6185	46
Increased effective connectivity from right SFG				
Right SMA	6	6, 15, 69	4.4562	44

A corrected threshold of $p < 0.01$ was determined by Monte Carlo simulation. BA, Brodmann's area; MNI, Montreal Neurological Institute; SFG, superior frontal gyrus; OFC, orbitofrontal cortex; PoCG, precentral gyrus; PLC, posterior lobe of cerebellum; MOG, middle occipital gyrus; SMA, supplementary motor area.

Our current study suggested that the PFC, specifically the SFG, might be a major integrative hub of the model that should be involved to perceive tinnitus. However, we did not observe any abnormal neural activity in auditory system. The most parsimonious explanation for this is the absence of any hearing loss out to 8 kHz and the absence of hyperacusis in our tinnitus patients. We speculated that aberrant neural activity of the PFC may exist prior to the disruption of the auditory system in tinnitus patients with normal hearing. In addition, since our tinnitus patients showed no obvious symptoms of depression, anxiety or cognitive decline, we did not detect any abnormalities in the limbic system. Based on previous fMRI studies, the SFG is a significant part of auditory connection cortex that can receive and integrate all kinds of information from different parts of the brain from inside and outside the body. Besides, it can also timely organize efferent impulses to ensure the coordination of the central nervous system (CNS) as a whole (Mathiak et al., 2007; Melloni et al., 2007). A possible interpretation for our results was that the increased DC in bilateral SFG might be due to feedback inhibition of the over activity in auditory network.

Previous neuroimaging studies have pointed out that the abnormalities of the SFG could act as a direct mechanism of tinnitus chronification (Giraud et al., 1999; Mirz et al., 1999; Haller et al., 2010). Wunderlich et al. (2010) detected the SFG activation after acoustic stimulation in a pitch discrimination task, suggesting the perception of auditory inputs in a more emotional context due to tinnitus. Chen et al. (2014) found increased ALFF values in the right SFG in chronic tinnitus patients, which was linked with tinnitus duration and distress. The SFG was also proved to be influenced by chronic tinnitus in recent rs-fMRI studies (Maudoux et al., 2012a; Ueyama et al., 2013; Chen et al., 2015c; Zhang et al., 2015). In line with these valuable findings, our results have implications for understanding the specific role of SFG abnormalities in chronic tinnitus, suggesting the PFC may provide valuable insight into the neural mechanisms underlying tinnitus.

Increased Effective Connectivity from the SFG

Using a GCA method, the present study exhibited that the information flow is unidirectionally affected (seed to whole brain) within non-auditory areas due to tinnitus. We found increased influence from the SFG to the frontal cortex (OFC and SMA), cerebellum (PLC), visual cortex (MOG) and somatosensory cortex (PoCG). Previous neuroimaging studies have identified abnormalities in the frontal cortex which could account for tinnitus. Firstly, it has been revealed that the OFC is critical for emotional processing of sounds (Damasio et al., 1996; Blood et al., 1999). The alterations of the OFC have been found in the functional coupling of long-range cortical networks between tinnitus patients and HCs by using EEG or MEG (Schlee et al., 2009; Vanneste et al., 2012; Song et al., 2014). Moreover, recent rs-fMRI studies have also demonstrated the abnormal FC of the OFC in tinnitus patients (Maudoux et al., 2012a; Chen et al., 2015d; Zhang et al., 2015). The OFC is also regarded as part of the reward system, which might integrate the aversive information of the perceived tinnitus (Rolls, 2004; Kringelbach, 2005). The heightened effective connectivity from the SFG to the OFC might be interpreted as a dysfunctional inhibitory response directing attention away from phantom sound perception. Our finding of positive correlation between the effective connection from the SFG to the OFC and tinnitus distress also emphasized the pivotal role of the OFC in tinnitus. Furthermore, we also found positive correlation between the THQ score and increased influence from the SFG to the SMA, which is regarded as a part of the primate cerebral cortex that contributes to the control of movement (Roland et al., 1980). By using quantitative EEG (qEEG), Vanneste et al. (2011) observed aberrant neuronal activity in the SMA in unilateral or bilateral tinnitus (Vanneste and De Ridder, 2012). It was hypothesized that synchronized theta activity in the SMA might be accountable for part of the conscious perception of the phantom sound (Vanneste and De Ridder, 2012). Nevertheless, further research is needed to clarify the role of the SMA in tinnitus.

Although the cerebellum is primarily involved in motor actions and control, some cerebellar regions such as the paraflocculus and vermis receive inputs from auditory centers (Petacchi et al., 2005). Auditory sensory processing in the cerebellum has been reported. Osaki et al. (2005) revealed that the right cerebellum was involved in tinnitus and showed a decreased regional blood flow during residual inhibition. Using rs-fMRI, chronic tinnitus patients showed increased FC in the cerebellar hemisphere that was linked with tinnitus distress (Maudoux et al., 2012a; Ueyama et al., 2013), confirming the involvement of cerebellum in auditory system. Nevertheless, the association of the cerebellum with tinnitus has not been substantially elucidated. Moreover, increased effective connectivity to MOG and PoCG raised the question of whether tinnitus might be linked to phantom visual or somatosensory perceptions. Such changes seem reasonable given the multisensory interactions known to exist between auditory, visual and somatosensory regions. Possible neural correlates of visual or somatosensory modulation of tinnitus were assessed (Murray et al., 2005). One interpretation of these results is that as patients attend to their phantom auditory sensation they contemporaneously activate visual or somatosensory areas. This interpretation is consistent with previous rs-fMRI studies showing abnormal neural activity in visual network (Burton et al., 2012; Maudoux et al., 2012a; Chen et al., 2014, 2015b,c,d) or somatosensory network (Maudoux et al., 2012a; Ueyama et al., 2013) in tinnitus. Therefore, tinnitus can be regarded as the consequence of multiple brain subnetworks involved in the different aspects of tinnitus, both acoustic and affective.

Tinnitus Lateralization

Interestingly, results of effective connectivity analysis were lateralized to the left hemisphere region in tinnitus patients. Asymmetry for the tinnitus patients has been reported both structurally and functionally (Mühlau et al., 2006; Smits et al., 2007; Schecklmann et al., 2013; Chen et al., 2014). Previous PET studies have demonstrated an overactivation of the left auditory cortex independent of tinnitus laterality and anatomical hemispheric differences (Arnold et al., 1996; Langguth et al., 2006; Schecklmann et al., 2013). This lateralization may be explained as an increase in activation on the side of the perceived tinnitus, or a decrease in activation on the side contralateral to the side of perceived tinnitus. The interpretation would indicate an increased spontaneous neural activity of the affected brain area in tinnitus patients (Smits et al., 2007). However, several studies also confirmed the right-

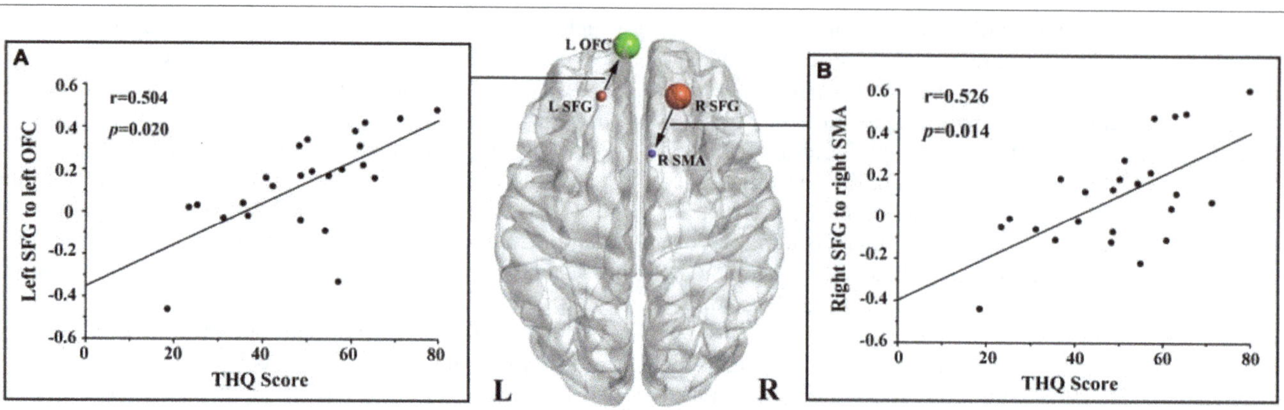

FIGURE 3 | Correlations between the increased effective connectivity of the bilateral SFG and the tinnitus handicap questionnaires (THQ) scores. **(A)** The THQ scores positively correlated with the increased effective connectivity from the left SFG to left OFC ($r = 0.504$, $p = 0.020$). **(B)** The THQ scores positively correlated with the increased effective connectivity from the right SFG to right SMA ($r = 0.526$, $p = 0.014$). L, left; R, right; THQ, tinnitus handicap questionnaires; SFG, superior frontal gyrus; OFC, orbitofrontal cortex; SMA, supplementary motor area.

lateralization in tinnitus (Chen et al., 2014; Geven et al., 2014). The inconsistencies between studies may be due to the different neuroimaging methods used to investigate tinnitus or heterogeneity of the tinnitus patients. Therefore, further studies are required to determine if the observed left hemispheric dominance is related specifically to tinnitus or some other factors.

Limitations

Study limitations must be acknowledged. First, we admit that it is difficult to make direct causal inferences regarding the relationships between the brain functional network architecture and tinnitus characteristics in tinnitus patients, considering the cross-sectional nature of our experimental design and limited sample size. Further longitudinal studies involving a greater number of subjects are required. The very nature of BOLD-fMRI makes it difficult to measure resting-state network activity given that amplitude is not measured only correlations of BOLD signals (Logothetis et al., 2001). The relationship between the measured BOLD-fMRI signal and the underlying neural activity is still largely unknown. Further studies combining fMRI with EEG may help understand the exact relationship. Second, common criticisms regarding GCA algorithm for rs-fMRI data have been raised. For example, the fallacious effects might occur because of the systematic differences across brain regions in hemodynamic delays. GCA has been confounded by the presence of vascular anatomy (Webb et al., 2013). Additionally, changes in directionality could be caused by the differences in hemodynamic coupling in different regions (Smith et al., 2011). Furthermore, we attempted to exclude subjects with hyperacusis from our study because subjects with hyperacusis exhibited robust activation in selected brain regions, such as the primary auditory cortex, thalamus, and auditory midbrain (Gu et al., 2010). However, it would be useful to include subjects with hyperacusis in future studies so as to examine if intrinsic functional network architecture is disrupted in a similar manner to that was observed in our tinnitus patients without hyperacusis. Finally, although we attempt to reduce the MR scanner noise with earplugs, the subjects cannot be completely prevented from hearing some noise that probably alters the resting-state brain networks to varying degree (Logothetis et al., 2009). This confounding factor should be taken into consideration for all rs-fMRI studies related to the auditory systems.

CONCLUSION

In this study, we show that disrupted functional network architecture within non-auditory regions revealed by DC and GCA are present in chronic tinnitus patients with normal hearing, without hyperacusis. Chronic tinnitus patients exhibited enhanced FC strength in bilateral SFG regions, which showed unidirectionally increased causal connectivity to frontal, motor, visual, somatosensory cortex and cerebellum. Furthermore, increased effective connectivity from bilateral SFG to OFC and SMA were positively correlated with tinnitus distress. Disturbance in brain functional network architecture will contribute to a better understanding of the neuropathophysiological mechanisms in tinnitus perception.

AUTHOR CONTRIBUTIONS

Y-CC and YF designed the experiment, collected the data, performed the analysis and wrote the manuscript. J-JX and C-NM collected the data. WX, JR, and XY contributed to the discussion and manuscript revision.

ACKNOWLEDGMENTS

The authors thank Prof. Richard Salvi, Center for Hearing and Deafness, University at Buffalo, Buffalo, NY, USA, for his contributions to the design of the study. This work was supported by the Collaborative Innovation Center of Suzhou Nano Science and Technology.

REFERENCES

Adjamian, P., Sereda, M., and Hall, D. A. (2009). The mechanisms of tinnitus: perspectives from human functional neuroimaging. *Hear. Res.* 253, 15–31. doi: 10.1016/j.heares.2009.04.001

Arnold, W., Bartenstein, P., Oestreicher, E., Römer, W., and Schwaiger, M. (1996). Focal metabolic activation in the predominant left auditory cortex in patients suffering from tinnitus: a PET study with [18F] deoxyglucose. *ORL J. Otorhinolaryngol. Relat. Spec.* 58, 195–199. doi: 10.1159/000276835

Berliner, K. I., Shelton, C., Hitselberger, W. E., and Luxford, W. M. (1992). Acoustic tumors: effect of surgical removal on tinnitus. *Otol. Neurotol.* 13, 13–17. doi: 10.1097/00129492-199201000-00005

Biswal, B., Zerrin Yetkin, F., Haughton, V. M., and Hyde, J. S. (1995). Functional connectivity in the motor cortex of resting human brain using echo-planar MRI. *Magn. Reson. Med.* 34, 537–541. doi: 10.1002/mrm.1910340409

Blood, A. J., Zatorre, R. J., Bermudez, P., and Evans, A. C. (1999). Emotional responses to pleasant and unpleasant music correlate with activity in paralimbic brain regions. *Nat. Neurosci.* 2, 382–387.

Buckner, R. L., Andrews-Hanna, J. R., and Schacter, D. L. (2008). The brain's default network. *Ann. N Y Acad. Sci.* 1124, 1–38. doi: 10.1196/annals.1440.011

Buckner, R. L., Sepulcre, J., Talukdar, T., Krienen, F. M., Liu, H., Hedden, T., et al. (2009). Cortical hubs revealed by intrinsic functional connectivity: mapping, assessment of stability and relation to Alzheimer's disease. *J. Neurosci.* 29, 1860–1873. doi: 10.1523/jneurosci.5062-08.2009

Burton, H., Wineland, A., Bhattacharya, M., Nicklaus, J., Garcia, K. S., and Piccirillo, J. F. (2012). Altered networks in bothersome tinnitus: a functional connectivity study. *BMC Neurosci.* 13:3. doi: 10.1186/1471-2202-13-3

Chao-Gan, Y., and Yu-Feng, Z. (2010). DPARSF: a MATLAB toolbox for "pipeline" data analysis of resting-state fMRI. *Front. Syst. Neurosci.* 4:13. doi: 10.3389/fnsys.2010.00013

Chen, H.-J., Jiang, L.-F., Sun, T., Liu, J., Chen, Q.-F., and Shi, H.-B. (2015a). Resting-state functional connectivity abnormalities correlate with psychometric hepatic encephalopathy score in cirrhosis. *Eur. J. Radiol.* 84, 2287–2295. doi: 10.1016/j.ejrad.2015.08.005

Chen, Y.-C., Xia, W., Feng, Y., Li, X., Zhang, J., Feng, X., et al. (2015b). Altered interhemispheric functional coordination in chronic tinnitus patients. *Biomed. Res. Int.* 2015:345647. doi: 10.1155/2015/345647

Chen, Y.-C., Xia, W., Luo, B., Muthaiah, V. P., Xiong, Z., Zhang, J., et al. (2015c). Frequency-specific alternations in the amplitude of low-frequency fluctuations in chronic tinnitus. *Front. Neural Circuits* 9:67. doi: 10.3389/fncir.2015.00067

Chen, Y.-C., Zhang, J., Li, X.-W., Xia, W., Feng, X., Qian, C., et al. (2015d). Altered intra-and interregional synchronization in resting-state cerebral networks associated with chronic tinnitus. *Neural Plast.* 2015:475382. doi: 10.1155/2015/475382

Chen, Y.-C., Zhang, J., Li, X.-W., Xia, W., Feng, X., Gao, B., et al. (2014). Aberrant spontaneous brain activity in chronic tinnitus patients revealed by resting-state functional MRI. *Neuroimage Clin.* 6, 222–228. doi: 10.1016/j.nicl.2014.09.011

Damasio, A. R., Everitt, B., and Bishop, D. (1996). The somatic marker hypothesis and the possible functions of the prefrontal cortex [and discussion]. *Philos. Trans. R. Soc. B Biol. Sci.* 351, 1413–1420. doi: 10.1098/rstb.1996.0125

Davies, J., Gander, P., Andrews, M., and Hall, D. (2014). Auditory network connectivity in tinnitus patients: a resting-state fMRI study. *Int. J. Audiol.* 53, 192–198. doi: 10.3109/14992027.2013.846482

De Ridder, D., Elgoyhen, A. B., Romo, R., and Langguth, B. (2011). Phantom percepts: tinnitus and pain as persisting aversive memory networks. *Proc. Natl. Acad. Sci. U S A* 108, 8075–8080. doi: 10.1073/pnas.1018466108

De Ridder, D., Vanneste, S., Weisz, N., Londero, A., Schlee, W., Elgoyhen, A. B., et al. (2014). An integrative model of auditory phantom perception: tinnitus as a unified percept of interacting separable subnetworks. *Neurosci. Biobehav. Rev.* 44, 16–32. doi: 10.1016/j.neubiorev.2013.03.021

Di Martino, A., Zuo, X.-N., Kelly, C., Grzadzinski, R., Mennes, M., Schvarcz, A., et al. (2013). Shared and distinct intrinsic functional network centrality in autism and attention-deficit/hyperactivity disorder. *Biol. Psychiatry* 74, 623–632. doi: 10.1016/j.biopsych.2013.02.011

Fox, M. D., and Raichle, M. E. (2007). Spontaneous fluctuations in brain activity observed with functional magnetic resonance imaging. *Nat. Rev. Neurosci.* 8, 700–711. doi: 10.1038/nrn2201

Geven, L. I., de Kleine, E., Willemsen, A. T., and van Dijk, P. (2014). Asymmetry in primary auditory cortex activity in tinnitus patients and controls. *Neuroscience* 256, 117–125. doi: 10.1016/j.neuroscience.2013.10.015

Giraud, A. L., Chéry-Croze, S., Fischer, G., Fischer, C., Vighetto, A., Grégoire, M.-C., et al. (1999). A selective imaging of tinnitus. *Neuroreport* 10, 1–5. doi: 10.1097/00001756-199901180-00001

Granger, C. W. (1969). Investigating causal relations by econometric models and cross-spectral methods. *Econometrica* 37, 424–438. doi: 10.2307/1912791

Gu, J. W., Halpin, C. F., Nam, E.-C., Levine, R. A., and Melcher, J. R. (2010). Tinnitus, diminished sound-level tolerance and elevated auditory activity in humans with clinically normal hearing sensitivity. *J. Neurophysiol.* 104, 3361–3370. doi: 10.1152/jn.00226.2010

Guo, W., Liu, F., Liu, J., Yu, L., Zhang, J., Zhang, Z., et al. (2015a). Abnormal causal connectivity by structural deficits in first-episode, drug-naive schizophrenia at rest. *Schizophr. Bull.* 41, 57–65. doi: 10.1093/schbul/sbu126

Guo, W., Liu, F., Zhang, Z., Liu, J., Yu, M., Zhang, J., et al. (2015b). Unidirectionally affected causal connectivity of cortico-limbic-cerebellar circuit by structural deficits in drug-naive major depressive disorder. *J. Affect. Disord.* 172, 410–416. doi: 10.1016/j.jad.2014.10.019

Haller, S., Birbaumer, N., and Veit, R. (2010). Real-time fMRI feedback training may improve chronic tinnitus. *Eur. Radiol.* 20, 696–703. doi: 10.1007/s00330-009-1595-z

Henry, J. A., Roberts, L. E., Caspary, D. M., Theodoroff, S. M., and Salvi, R. J. (2014). Underlying mechanisms of tinnitus: review and clinical implications. *J. Am. Acad. Audiol.* 25, 5–22. doi: 10.3766/jaaa.25.1.2

Hinkley, L. B., Mizuiri, D., Hong, O., Nagarajan, S. S., and Cheung, S. W. (2015). Increased striatal functional connectivity with auditory cortex in tinnitus. *Front. Hum. Neurosci.* 9:568. doi: 10.3389/fnhum.2015.00568

Jackler, R. K., and Whinney, D. (2001). A century of eighth nerve surgery. *Otol. Neurotol.* 22, 401–416. doi: 10.1097/00129492-200109000-00029

Jastreboff, P. J. (1990). Phantom auditory perception (tinnitus): mechanisms of generation and perception. *Neurosci. Res.* 8, 221–254. doi: 10.1016/0168-0102(90)90031-9

Jastreboff, P. J., and Hazell, J. W. (2008). *Tinnitus Retraining Therapy: Implementing the Neurophysiological Model.* Cambridge, UK: Cambridge University Press.

Kaltenbach, J. A., Zhang, J., and Finlayson, P. (2005). Tinnitus as a plastic phenomenon and its possible neural underpinnings in the dorsal cochlear nucleus. *Hear. Res.* 206, 200–226. doi: 10.1016/j.heares.2005.02.013

Khalfa, S., Dubal, S., Veuillet, E., Perez-Diaz, F., Jouvent, R., and Collet, L. (2002). Psychometric normalization of a hyperacusis questionnaire. *ORL J. Otorhinolaryngol. Relat. Spec.* 64, 436–442. doi: 10.1159/000067570

Kim, J.-Y., Kim, Y.-H., Lee, S., Seo, J.-H., Song, H.-J., Cho, J. H., et al. (2012). Alteration of functional connectivity in tinnitus brain revealed by resting-state fMRI? a pilot study. *Int. J. Audiol.* 51, 413–417. doi: 10.3109/14992027.2011.652677

Kringelbach, M. L. (2005). The human orbitofrontal cortex: linking reward to hedonic experience. *Nat. Rev. Neurosci.* 6, 691–702. doi: 10.1038/nrn1747

Kuk, F. K., Tyler, R. S., Russell, D., and Jordan, H. (1990). The psychometric properties of a tinnitus handicap questionnaire. *Ear Hear.* 11, 434–445. doi: 10.1097/00003446-199012000-00005

Langguth, B., Eichhammer, P., Kreutzer, A., Maenner, P., Marienhagen, J., Kleinjung, T., et al. (2006). The impact of auditory cortex activity on characterizing and treating patients with chronic tinnitus–first results from a PET study. *Acta Otolaryngol. Suppl.* 126, 84–88. doi: 10.1080/03655230600895317

Leaver, A. M., Renier, L., Chevillet, M. A., Morgan, S., Kim, H. J., and Rauschecker, J. P. (2011). Dysregulation of limbic and auditory networks in tinnitus. *Neuron* 69, 33–43. doi: 10.1016/j.neuron.2010.12.002

Leaver, A. M., Turesky, T. K., Seydell-Greenwald, A., Morgan, S., Kim, H. J., and Rauschecker, J. P. (2016). Intrinsic network activity in tinnitus investigated using functional MRI. *Hum. Brain Mapp.* doi: 10.1002/hbm.23204 [Epub ahead of print].

Lenarz, T., Schreiner, C., Snyder, R. L., and Ernst, A. (1993). Neural mechanisms of tinnitus. *Eur. Arch. Otorhinolaryngol.* 249, 441–446. doi: 10.1007/bf00168851

Leske, M. C. (1981). Prevalence estimates of communicative disorders in the US Language, hearing and vestibular disorders. *ASHA* 23, 229–237.

Lewis, J. W., Beauchamp, M. S., and DeYoe, E. A. (2000). A comparison of visual and auditory motion processing in human cerebral cortex. *Cereb. Cortex* 10, 873–888. doi: 10.1093/cercor/10.9.873

Lockwood, A. H., Salvi, R. J., and Burkard, R. F. (2002). Tinnitus. *N. Engl. J. Med.* 347, 904–910. doi: 10.1056/NEJMra013395

Lockwood, A. H., Salvi, R., Coad, M., Towsley, M., Wack, D., and Murphy, B. (1998). The functional neuroanatomy of tinnitus Evidence for limbic system links and neural plasticity. *Neurology* 50, 114–120. doi: 10.1212/wnl.50.1.114

Logothetis, N. K., Murayama, Y., Augath, M., Steffen, T., Werner, J., and Oeltermann, A. (2009). How not to study spontaneous activity. *Neuroimage* 45, 1080–1089. doi: 10.1016/j.neuroimage.2009.01.010

Logothetis, N. K., Pauls, J., Augath, M., Trinath, T., and Oeltermann, A. (2001). Neurophysiological investigation of the basis of the fMRI signal. *Nature* 412, 150–157. doi: 10.1038/35084005

Mathiak, K., Menning, H., Hertrich, I., Mathiak, K. A., Zvyagintsev, M., and Ackermann, H. (2007). Who is telling what from where? A functional magnetic resonance imaging study. *Neuroreport* 18, 405–409. doi: 10.1097/wnr.0b013e328013cec4

Maudoux, A., Lefebvre, P., Cabay, J.-E., Demertzi, A., Vanhaudenhuyse, A., Laureys, S., et al. (2012a). Auditory resting-state network connectivity in tinnitus: a functional MRI study. *PLoS One* 7:e36222. doi: 10.1371/journal.pone.0036222

Maudoux, A., Lefebvre, P., Cabay, J.-E., Demertzi, A., Vanhaudenhuyse, A., Laureys, S., et al. (2012b). Connectivity graph analysis of the auditory resting state network in tinnitus. *Brain Res.* 1485, 10–21. doi: 10.1016/j.brainres.2012.05.006

McFadden, D. (1982). *Tinnitus: Facts, Theories and Treatments.* Washington, DC: National Academies.

Meikle, M. B. (1997). Electronic access to tinnitus data: the oregon tinnitus data archive. *Otolaryngol. Head Neck Surg.* 117, 698–700. doi: 10.1016/s0194-5998(97)70055-x

Melloni, L., Molina, C., Pena, M., Torres, D., Singer, W., and Rodriguez, E. (2007). Synchronization of neural activity across cortical areas correlates with conscious perception. *J. Neurosci.* 27, 2858–2865. doi: 10.1523/jneurosci.4623-06.2007

Minami, S. B., Oishi, N., Watabe, T., Uno, K., Kaga, K., and Ogawa, K. (2015). Auditory resting-state functional connectivity in tinnitus and modulation with transcranial direct current stimulation. *Acta Otolaryngol.* 135, 1286–1292. doi: 10.3109/00016489.2015.1068952

Mirz, F., Pedersen, B., Ishizu, K., Johannsen, P., Ovesen, T., Stødkilde-Jørgensen, H., et al. (1999). Positron emission tomography of cortical centers of tinnitus. *Hear. Res.* 134, 133–144. doi: 10.1016/s0378-5955(99)00075-1

Mühlau, M., Rauschecker, J., Oestreicher, E., Gaser, C., Röttinger, M., Wohlschläger, A., et al. (2006). Structural brain changes in tinnitus. *Cereb. Cortex* 16, 1283–1288. doi: 10.1093/cercor/bhj070

Murphy, K., Birn, R. M., Handwerker, D. A., Jones, T. B., and Bandettini, P. A. (2009). The impact of global signal regression on resting state correlations: are anti-correlated networks introduced? *Neuroimage* 44, 893–905. doi: 10.1016/j.neuroimage.2008.09.036

Murray, M. M., Molholm, S., Michel, C. M., Heslenfeld, D. J., Ritter, W., Javitt, D. C., et al. (2005). Grabbing your ear: rapid auditory-somatosensory multisensory interactions in low-level sensory cortices are not constrained by stimulus alignment. *Cereb. Cortex* 15, 963–974. doi: 10.1093/cercor/bhh197

Osaki, Y., Nishimura, H., Takasawa, M., Imaizumi, M., Kawashima, T., Iwaki, T., et al. (2005). Neural mechanism of residual inhibition of tinnitus in cochlear implant users. *Neuroreport* 16, 1625–1628. doi: 10.1097/01.wnr.0000183899.85277.08

Petacchi, A., Laird, A. R., Fox, P. T., and Bower, J. M. (2005). Cerebellum and auditory function: an ALE meta-analysis of functional neuroimaging studies. *Hum. Brain Mapp.* 25, 118–128. doi: 10.1002/hbm.20137

Qi, R., Zhang, L. J., Zhong, J., Zhang, Z., Ni, L., Jiao, Q., et al. (2013). Altered effective connectivity network of the basal ganglia in low-grade hepatic encephalopathy: a resting-state fMRI study with Granger causality analysis. *PLoS One* 8:e53677. doi: 10.1371/journal.pone.0053677

Rauschecker, J. P., Leaver, A. M., and Mühlau, M. (2010). Tuning out the noise: limbic-auditory interactions in tinnitus. *Neuron* 66, 819–826. doi: 10.1016/j.neuron.2010.04.032

Roberts, L. E., Eggermont, J. J., Caspary, D. M., Shore, S. E., Melcher, J. R., and Kaltenbach, J. A. (2010). Ringing ears: the neuroscience of tinnitus. *J. Neurosci.* 30, 14972–14979. doi: 10.1523/JNEUROSCI.4028-10.2010

Roland, P. E., Larsen, B., Lassen, N., and Skinhøj, E. (1980). Supplementary motor area and other cortical areas in organization of voluntary movements in man. *J. Neurophysiol.* 43, 118–136.

Rolls, E. T. (2004). The functions of the orbitofrontal cortex. *Brain Cogn.* 55, 11–29. doi: 10.1016/S0278-2626(03)00277-X

Schecklmann, M., Landgrebe, M., Poeppl, T. B., Kreuzer, P., Männer, P., Marienhagen, J., et al. (2013). Neural correlates of tinnitus duration and distress: a positron emission tomography study. *Hum. Brain Mapp.* 34, 233–240. doi: 10.1002/hbm.21426

Schlee, W., Mueller, N., Hartmann, T., Keil, J., Lorenz, I., and Weisz, N. (2009). Mapping cortical hubs in tinnitus. *BMC Biol.* 7:80. doi: 10.1186/1741-7007-7-80

Schmidt, S. A., Akrofi, K., Carpenter-Thompson, J. R., and Husain, F. T. (2013). Default mode, dorsal attention and auditory resting state networks exhibit differential functional connectivity in tinnitus and hearing loss. *PLoS One* 8:e76488. doi: 10.1371/journal.pone.0076488

Shulman, A., and Strashun, A. (1998). Descending auditory system/cerebellum/tinnitus. *Int. Tinnitus J.* 5, 92–106.

Smith, S. M., Miller, K. L., Salimi-Khorshidi, G., Webster, M., Beckmann, C. F., Nichols, T. E., et al. (2011). Network modelling methods for FMRI. *Neuroimage* 54, 875–891. doi: 10.1016/j.neuroimage.2010.08.063

Smits, M., Kovacs, S., De Ridder, D., Peeters, R. R., Van Hecke, P., and Sunaert, S. (2007). Lateralization of functional magnetic resonance imaging (fMRI) activation in the auditory pathway of patients with lateralized tinnitus. *Neuroradiology* 49, 669–679. doi: 10.1007/s00234-007-0231-3

Song, J.-J., De Ridder, D., Weisz, N., Schlee, W., Van de Heyning, P., and Vanneste, S. (2014). Hyperacusis-associated pathological resting-state brain oscillations in the tinnitus brain: a hyperresponsiveness network with paradoxically inactive auditory cortex. *Brain Struct. Funct.* 219, 1113–1128. doi: 10.1007/s00429-013-0555-1

Sporns, O., Honey, C. J., and Kötter, R. (2007). Identification and classification of hubs in brain networks. *PLoS One* 2:e1049. doi: 10.1371/journal.pone.0001049

Ueyama, T., Donishi, T., Ukai, S., Ikeda, Y., Hotomi, M., Yamanaka, N., et al. (2013). Brain regions responsible for tinnitus distress and loudness: a resting-state fMRI study. *PLoS One* 8:e67778. doi: 10.1371/journal.pone.0067778

Vanneste, S., and De Ridder, D. (2012). The auditory and non-auditory brain areas involved in tinnitus. An emergent property of multiple parallel overlapping subnetworks. *Front. Syst. Neurosci.* 6:31. doi: 10.3389/fnsys.2012.00031

Vanneste, S., Joos, K., and De Ridder, D. (2012). Prefrontal cortex based sex differences in tinnitus perception: same tinnitus intensity, same tinnitus distress, different mood. *PLoS One* 7:e31182. doi: 10.1371/journal.pone.0031182

Vanneste, S., Plazier, M., Van der Loo, E., Van de Heyning, P., Congedo, M., and De Ridder, D. (2010). The neural correlates of tinnitus-related distress. *Neuroimage* 52, 470–480. doi: 10.1016/j.neuroimage.2010.04.029

Vanneste, S., Plazier, M., van der Loo, E., Van de Heyning, P., and De Ridder, D. (2011). The difference between uni- and bilateral auditory phantom percept. *Clin. Neurophysiol.* 122, 578–587. doi: 10.1016/j.clinph.2010.07.022

Vincent, J. L., Kahn, I., Snyder, A. Z., Raichle, M. E., and Buckner, R. L. (2008). Evidence for a frontoparietal control system revealed by intrinsic functional connectivity. *J. Neurophysiol.* 100, 3328–3342. doi: 10.1152/jn.90355.2008

Voisin, J., Bidet-Caulet, A., Bertrand, O., and Fonlupt, P. (2006). Listening in silence activates auditory areas: a functional magnetic resonance imaging study. *J. Neurosci.* 26, 273–278. doi: 10.1523/jneurosci.2967-05.2006

Webb, J. T., Ferguson, M. A., Nielsen, J. A., and Anderson, J. S. (2013). BOLD granger causality reflects vascular anatomy. *PLoS One* 8:e84279. doi: 10.1371/journal.pone.0084279

Wineland, A. M., Burton, H., and Piccirillo, J. (2012). Functional connectivity networks in nonbothersome tinnitus. *Otolaryngol. Head Neck Surg.* 147, 900–906. doi: 10.1177/0194599812451414

Wunderlich, A. P., Schönfeldt-Lecuona, C., Wolf, R. C., Dorn, K., Bachor, E., and Freund, W. (2010). Cortical activation during a pitch discrimination task in tinnitus patients and controls-an fMRI study. *Audiol. Neurootol.* 15, 137–148. doi: 10.1159/000241094

Yan, C.-G., Craddock, R. C., Zuo, X.-N., Zang, Y.-F., and Milham, M. P. (2013). Standardizing the intrinsic brain: towards robust measurement of inter-individual variation in 1000 functional connectomes. *Neuroimage* 80, 246–262. doi: 10.1016/j.neuroimage.2013.04.081

Zhang, J., Chen, Y.-C., Feng, X., Yang, M., Liu, B., Qian, C., et al. (2015). Impairments of thalamic resting-state functional connectivity in patients with chronic tinnitus. *Eur. J. Radiol.* 84, 1277–1284. doi: 10.1016/j.ejrad.2015.04.006

Zang, Z.-X., Yan, C.-G., Dong, Z.-Y., Huang, J., and Zang, Y.-F. (2012). Granger causality analysis implementation on MATLAB: a graphic user interface toolkit for fMRI data processing. *J. Neurosci. Methods* 203, 418–426. doi: 10.1016/j.jneumeth.2011.10.006

Zhong, Y., Huang, L., Cai, S., Zhang, Y., von Deneen, K. M., Ren, A., et al. (2014). Altered effective connectivity patterns of the default mode network in Alzheimer's disease: an fMRI study. *Neurosci. Lett.* 578, 171–175. doi: 10.1016/j.neulet.2014.06.043

Zhou, Z., Wang, X., Klahr, N. J., Liu, W., Arias, D., Liu, H., et al. (2011). A conditional Granger causality model approach for group analysis in functional magnetic resonance imaging. *Magn. Reson. Imaging* 29, 418–433. doi: 10.1016/j.mri.2010.10.008

Zung, W. W. (1971). A rating instrument for anxiety disorders. *Psychosomatics* 12, 371–379. doi: 10.1016/s0033-3182(71)71479-0

Zung, W. (1986). "Zung self-rating depression scale and depression status inventory," in *Assessment of Depression*, eds N. Sartorius and T. A. Ban (Berlin: Springer), 221–231.

Zuo, X.-N., Ehmke, R., Mennes, M., Imperati, D., Castellanos, F. X., Sporns, O., et al. (2012). Network centrality in the human functional connectome. *Cereb. Cortex* 22, 1862–1875. doi: 10.1093/cercor/bhr269

21

Gender-Specific Risk Factors and Comorbidities of Bothersome Tinnitus

Laura Basso[1], Benjamin Boecking[1], Petra Brueggemann[1], Nancy L. Pedersen[2], Barbara Canlon[3], Christopher R. Cederroth[3,4,5] and Birgit Mazurek[1]*

[1] Tinnitus Center, Charité – Universitätsmedizin Berlin, Berlin, Germany, [2] Department of Medical Epidemiology and Biostatistics, Karolinska Institutet, Stockholm, Sweden, [3] Laboratory of Experimental Audiology, Department of Physiology and Pharmacology, Karolinska Institutet, Stockholm, Sweden, [4] National Institute for Health Research (NIHR) Nottingham Biomedical Research Centre, Nottingham University Hospitals NHS Trust, Nottingham, United Kingdom, [5] Hearing Sciences, Division of Clinical Neuroscience, School of Medicine, University of Nottingham, Nottingham, United Kingdom

***Correspondence:**
Birgit Mazurek
birgit.mazurek@charite.de

Objective: This study aims to identify gender-specific risk factors associated with the presence of bothersome tinnitus (compared with non-bothersome tinnitus), including sociodemographic and lifestyle factors, tinnitus-associated phenomena (hearing loss, traumatic experiences, sleep disturbances), and physical as well as mental comorbidities.

Methods: We conducted a cross-sectional study using survey data from the Swedish LifeGene cohort containing information on self-reported tinnitus (N = 7615). We (1) analyzed risk factor and comorbidity frequencies, (2) computed multivariate logistic regression models to identify predictors of bothersome tinnitus within both genders, and (3) moderated logistic regression models to compare effects between genders.

Results: (1) The majority of factors that differed in frequencies between bothersome and non-bothersome tinnitus were equal for both genders. Women with bothersome tinnitus specifically reported higher rates of cardiovascular disease, thyroid disease, epilepsy, fibromyalgia, and burnout, and men with bothersome tinnitus reported higher rates of alcohol consumption, Ménière's disease, anxiety syndrome, and panic (compared with non-bothersome tinnitus, respectively).

(2) Across both genders, multivariate logistic regression analyses revealed significant associations between bothersome tinnitus and age, reduced hearing ability, hearing-related difficulties in social situations, and reduced sleep quality. In women, bothersome tinnitus was specifically associated with cardiovascular disease and epilepsy; in men, with lower education levels and anxiety syndrome.

(3) Moderated logistic regression analyses revealed that the effects of low education and anxiety syndrome were present in men, but not in women, whereas the effects of age, reduced hearing ability and related difficulties, cardiovascular disease, epilepsy, and burnout were not gender specific.

Conclusion: Irrespective of gender, bothersome tinnitus is associated with higher age, reduced hearing ability, hearing-related difficulties, cardiovascular disease, epilepsy, and burnout. Gender-specific effects comprise low levels of education and the presence of anxiety syndrome for men. These findings need to be interpreted with caution, yet they suggest the presence of gender-specific biopsychosocial influences in the emergence or maintenance of bothersome tinnitus. Future studies ought to investigate the underlying mechanisms of the observed relationships.

Keywords: tinnitus, gender difference, risk factors, cardiovascular disease, epilepsy, burnout, anxiety, education

INTRODUCTION

Tinnitus is a highly prevalent symptom with 10–15% of adults being affected (Baguley et al., 2013). Many affected individuals perceive tinnitus as harmless and not debilitating (Henry et al., 2005). However, for 1% up to 7% of the population (Nondahl et al., 2002; Gallus et al., 2015; Ramage-Morin et al., 2019), tinnitus is a highly bothersome experience. In those individuals, the sound is generally perceived as an intrusive threat, leading to emotional distress (Henry et al., 2005; Cima, 2018).

Epidemiological research on tinnitus is mixed. While most studies have cross-sectional designs with inherent limitations, a handful of longitudinal studies has contributed to identifying risk factors for tinnitus. The most clearly identified risk factor is hearing loss (Nondahl et al., 2002; Gopinath et al., 2010; Aarhus et al., 2015; Bogo et al., 2017). Symptoms of temporomandibular disorders (Bernhardt et al., 2011; Lee et al., 2016) and smoking were found to be associated with an increased risk of tinnitus (Nondahl et al., 2010), whereas higher caffeine intake (Glicksman et al., 2014) and moderate alcohol consumption were associated with a lower risk (Nondahl et al., 2010). Cross-sectional studies further suggest associations between tinnitus and increased age (Shargorodsky et al., 2010; Park et al., 2014; Gallus et al., 2015; Kim et al., 2015), sleep disturbances (Axelsson and Ringdahl, 1989; Izuhara et al., 2013), and sociodemographic factors (Unterrainer et al., 2001; Hoekstra et al., 2014; Gallus et al., 2015; Kim et al., 2015).

Tinnitus can be associated with a range of physical and mental conditions (Baguley et al., 2013), some of which appear relevant for bothersome tinnitus (Basso et al., submitted). Many of these conditions, like cardiovascular diseases (Regitz-Zagrosek and Kararigas, 2017), chronic musculoskeletal pain (Wijnhoven et al., 2006), thyroid diseases (Vanderpump et al., 1995), Ménière's disease (Smith et al., 2019), depression (Salk et al., 2017), and anxiety disorders (Bandelow and Michaelis, 2015) are marked by gender differences.

Regarding bothersome tinnitus, relationships with stress were found in cross-sectional studies (Park et al., 2014; Kim et al., 2015). Moreover, adverse life events can contribute to tinnitus aggravation (Zeng et al., 2016) and bidirectional links between symptoms of posttraumatic stress disorder (PTSD) and tinnitus severity are known (Hinton et al., 2006; Fagelson, 2007).

Whether sex or gender impacts on tinnitus severity is poorly understood. For instance, in some studies, women were found to exhibit higher levels of tinnitus-related distress or annoyance (Seydel et al., 2013; Gallus et al., 2015; Schlee et al., 2017), but opposite findings exist as well (Jalessi et al., 2013), and some studies found no severity differences between men and women (Axelsson and Ringdahl, 1989; Gopinath et al., 2010; Hoekstra et al., 2014). Moreover, a recent study found an association between tinnitus severity and suicide attempts in women only (Lugo et al., 2019), highlighting the importance to investigate gender differences in severe tinnitus. Differences in risk factors for bothersome tinnitus between men and women have not yet been investigated.

Given the paucity of research using sex as a biological variable (SABV), the aim of the present study is to investigate gender differences in risk factors for bothersome tinnitus in a large general population sample, covering sociodemographic factors, lifestyle factors, hearing loss, traumatic experiences, sleep disturbances, and physical and mental comorbidities. Logistic regression models are used to identify risk factors within both genders, and moderation models are used to assess whether the effects of the respective factors on bothersome tinnitus are moderated by gender, that is, are different for women and men.

MATERIALS AND METHODS

Data Source and Study Design

The sample of this study was drawn from the LifeGene cohort. LifeGene is a population-based study conducted in Sweden (Almqvist et al., 2011; LifeGene, 2017). Cross-sectional data of the web-based LifeGene survey collected between 2009 and 2016 were used. Participants were recruited via random selection, invitation by other participants, and self-registration (Almqvist et al., 2011; LifeGene, 2017). From the 31926 participants who completed the survey, all individuals with self-reported tinnitus [N = 7615 (23.9%)] were included in the present study. The same sample was used in Basso et al. (submitted). All participants provided informed consent (for participants under the age of 18, informed consent was provided by the participants' legal guardian/next of kin). The project has been approved by the local ethics committee "*Regionala etikprövningsnämnden*" in Stockholm (2015/2129-31/1).

Variables

The investigated risk factors were grouped into (1) sociodemographic and lifestyle factors (age, marital status, education level, employment, alcohol use, smoking status, snus and drug use), (2) tinnitus-associated phenomena (hearing ability and hearing-related difficulties in social situations, sleep quality and sleep disturbances, and traumatic/stressful experiences), and (3) physical and (4) mental comorbidities; see **Supplementary Figure S1**. Information on sociodemographic factors was selected from the "socio-demography" module of the LifeGene survey, information on lifestyle factors from the "living habits" module, information on comorbidities (past or present), sleep quality/disturbances, hearing ability and hearing-related difficulties in social situations from the "medical history" module, and information regarding traumatic/stressful life events from the "mental health" module. Participants' experience of the tinnitus ["Is there a constant ringing in the ears or do you have any other bothersome sound in the ears (tinnitus)?"] as constant and bothersome ("All the time, the sound is very bothersome") or intermittent and non-bothersome ("Sometimes, but the sound doesn't bother me") was defined as the dependent variable in all analyses.

Sociodemographic factors included age, marital status (married, cohabiting, single, separated/divorced, living apart, widowed, same-sex marriage), highest or current level of education (9-year primary school, secondary school, university, other), and employment [employed, unemployed, running an owned or part-owned company, age pension, activity or sickness benefit (early retirement) due to illness/disability, sick leave (for 2 months or longer), parental leave (for 2 months or longer), student, on leave, housewife/man, other]. Lifestyle factors included smoking status and the use of alcohol, snus, and illicit drugs. Alcohol consumption was assessed by the question: "If you consider the last 12 months, how often have you been drinking alcohol?" ("four times a week or more," "2–3 times per week," "once a week," "2–3 times per month," "once a month or less," "never"). Smoking status was categorized as "current smoker" (>100 cigarettes in life, at least 1 cigarette/day when smoking most AND currently smoking), "ex-smoker" (>100 cigarettes in life, at least 1 cigarette/day when smoking most, NOT currently smoking), and "non-smoker" (never or occasional: <100 cigarettes in life OR less than 1 cigarette/day when smoking most). The use of snus, a smokeless tobacco product (moist powder) usually placed under the upper lip, was categorized as "current snus user" (>5 boxes in life, 1 box lasting <1 week when using it most AND present use), "ex-user" (>5 boxes in life, 1 box lasting <1 week when using it most, NO present use), "non-user" (never, <5 boxes in life, OR 1 box lasting >1 week when using it most). The use of illicit drugs or unprescribed medication was categorized as "current drug user" (tried more than once AND present use), "ex-user" (tried more than once, NO present use), "non-user" (never OR not more than once) with regard to the following substances: (1) cannabis, marijuana, hash; (2) amphetamine; (3) cocaine; (4) sobril, oxascand, stesolid, diazepam, xanor, alprazolam; (5) stilnoct, zolpidem, imovane, zopiclone; (6) growth hormone; (7) anabolic steroids; (8) codeine, citodon, treo comp, panocod; (9) tramadol, tradolan, tiparol, nobligan; (10) heroin; (11) opium; (12) hallucinogens (psilocybin, psilocin); (13) LSD; (14) ecstasy; (15) GHB; (16) methylphenidate (ritalin, concerta); (17) morphine; (18) subutex, suboxone; or (19) other drug or medication.

Tinnitus-associated phenomena included hearing ability, hearing-related difficulties in social situations, sleep quality, sleep disturbances, and traumatic/stressful experiences. Hearing ability was assessed by the question "How is your hearing?" ("good," "somewhat reduced," "very reduced"). Hearing-related difficulties in social situations were assessed by combining the following questions into a mean variable: "Do you have difficulties hearing when speaking to one person in a silent room?," "Do you have difficulties hearing when speaking to multiple people at the same time?," "Do you have difficulties hearing when speaking to someone in city traffic?," "Do you have difficulties hearing where different sounds come from, e.g., cars in traffic?" and "Do you have problems with your hearing and are therefore avoiding meeting people?" (3 = "yes, very difficult," 2 = "sometimes, a little difficult," 1 = "no, not at all"). Sleep quality was assessed by the question "How do you sleep usually?" (response scale ranging from 1 = "very bad" to 5 = "very good"; for the analyses, the scale was inverted so that higher values reflect poorer sleep quality). In addition, participants were asked to rate how problematic their sleep disturbances are ("To what degree are sleep disturbances a problem in your life?"), with the response scale ranging from 1 = "no problem at all" to 5 = "a big problem." Traumatic/stressful life events were assessed by calculating the sum of reported traumatic/stressful life events experienced in childhood or adulthood, see **Supplementary Table S1** for all 32 items.

The following physical comorbidities were selected because of their proposed association with tinnitus in the literature: hypertension, hyperlipidemia, cardiovascular disease (angina, myocardial infarction, or cardiac arrhythmia), asthma, diabetes, thyroid disease, chronic shoulder pain, osteoarthritis, rheumatoid arthritis, systemic lupus erythematosus, migraine, Ménière's disease, epilepsy, multiple sclerosis, and fibromyalgia. The following mental comorbidities were included: burnout, depression, bipolar disease, (generalized) anxiety syndrome, panic, agoraphobia, social anxiety/phobia, obsessive-compulsive disorder, and PTSD. The survey questions assessing these conditions asked for their past or present occurrence.

Statistical Analysis

Statistical analyses were computed with IBM SPSS Statistics (version 25) for Windows 7. The significance level was set to $\alpha = 0.05$. In the first step, we identified risk factors for bothersome (vs. non-bothersome) tinnitus within each gender: (1) by comparing frequencies and medians of each variable between non-bothersome and bothersome tinnitus for women and men separately and (2) by further analyzing relevant variables [identified in (1)] as predictors of bothersome tinnitus in logistic regression analyses for women and men separately. Lastly, (3) for the comparison between genders, we tested whether gender moderated the effects of each risk factor [identified in (2)] across the whole sample.

(1) Pearson's X^2 tests were conducted to compare the frequencies of categorical variables between non-bothersome and bothersome tinnitus for both genders separately. Continuity correction was used for 2×2 tables, and adjusted residuals (ARs) were calculated to compare between the frequencies of categories (ARs $\geq$ 1.96 or ≤ -1.96 indicate significant differences). For continuous variables, Mann–Whitney U tests were used because of non-normally distributed data. (2) To test the unique association of relevant variables with bothersome tinnitus (identified by previous analyses), multivariate logistic

regression models were calculated for women and men separately including the following predictors: Model 1: sociodemographic and lifestyle factors, Model 2: tinnitus-associated phenomena, Model 3: physical comorbidities, Model 4: mental comorbidities, and Model 5: all significant predictors from Models 1 to 4. The assumptions of logistic regression were met (no multicollinearity was present among predictors, all variance inflation factor (VIF) values <2, and the Box-Tidwell approach showed a linear relationship between the continuous predictor age and the logit of the outcome). Regarding outliers, 150 female participants (3.5%) and 123 male participants (3.7%) had studentized residuals greater than 2 in Model 5, which were kept in the analyses; no cases had studentized residuals greater than 3. For model evaluation, Nagelkerke R^2 is reported as a measure of goodness-of-fit. (3) To test whether the relationships between the predictors included in Model 5 and bothersome tinnitus are different depending on gender, separate moderation models by gender were conducted for each predictor by using the PROCESS syntax version 3.4 by Hayes (2018). For all odds ratios (OR), 95% confidence intervals were computed.

Completeness of the data was high; in total, 1.5% of values were missing. The response rate was lowest with 83.8% on hearing-related difficulties in social situations, followed by 88.3% on employment; other response rates varied between 96.7 and 98.9% on eight variables (marital status, education, alcohol consumption, smoking status, snus use, drug use, hearing ability, traumatic experiences), and between 99.5 and 99.7% on 26 variables (sleep quality, sleep disturbances, and all comorbidities). All data was available for age and gender.

RESULTS

Sample Description

Of the 7615 participants with tinnitus, 697 reported bothersome tinnitus (9.2%). Females represented 56.5% of the sample (4301 participants): 393 with bothersome tinnitus (9.1%). In males (3314 participants), 304 reported bothersome tinnitus (9.2%). Participants were between 11 and 84 years old ($M = 35.80$ years, SD = 12.44 years); on average, female participants were 35.62 years old (SD = 12.45 years) and male participants were 36.03 years old (SD = 12.42 years); $U = 6931148$, $p = 0.040$. The composition of the sample by age and gender for non-bothersome and bothersome tinnitus is displayed in **Figure 1**. Most frequently, participants were cohabiting (33.4%), married (25.0%), or single (24.0%); education (highest or current) was mostly at university level (61.7%); and most participants were employed (53.7%) or students (15.0%).

Gender Differences Between Bothersome and Non-bothersome Tinnitus

Differences in Frequencies/Medians

Sociodemographic factors

Female participants with bothersome tinnitus were significantly older than those with non-bothersome tinnitus, $U = 598970$, $p < 0.001$; they differed in marital status, $X^2(6) = 20.82$, $p = 0.002$ (more often married, less often cohabiting, less often single, more often separated or divorced), in their highest or current level of education, $X^2(3) = 18.69$, $p < 0.001$ (less often university, more often "other"), as well as in their present employment situation, $X^2(10) = 60.60$, $p < 0.001$ (less often employed, more often unemployed, more often in age pension, and more often in early retirement due to illness/disability); see **Table 1**.

Male participants with bothersome tinnitus were significantly older than those with non-bothersome tinnitus, $U = 341380$, $p < 0.001$; they differed in marital status, $X^2(6) = 40.12$, $p < 0.001$ (more often married, less often single, and more often widowed), in their highest or current level of education, $X^2(3) = 49.05$, $p < 0.001$ (more often primary school, more often secondary school, and less often university), as well as in their present employment situation, $X^2(10) = 35.51$, $p < 0.001$ (more often running an owned or part-owned company, more often in age pension, less often student, and more often "other"); see **Table 2**.

Lifestyle factors

Compared with women with non-bothersome tinnitus, women with bothersome tinnitus were more often ex-smokers, $X^2(2) = 8.39$, $p = 0.015$. Men with bothersome tinnitus were more often ex-smokers and less often non-smokers than male participants with non-bothersome tinnitus, $X^2(2) = 12.60$, $p = 0.002$, and in addition, they reported more often drinking alcohol four times a week and never than those with non-bothersome tinnitus, $X^2(5) = 16.78$, $p = 0.005$. Other lifestyle variables did not differ; see **Table 1** for women and **Table 2** for men.

Tinnitus-associated phenomena

For both women and men, participants with bothersome tinnitus reported more often somewhat reduced or very reduced hearing ability compared with participants with non-bothersome tinnitus [women: $X^2(2) = 196.13$, $p < 0.001$; men: $X^2(2) = 189.60$, $p < 0.001$], as well as more hearing-related difficulties in social situations (women: $U = 388097$, $p < 0.001$; men: $U = 243912$, $p < 0.001$), more traumatic/stressful experiences (women: $U = 653215$, $p < 0.001$; men: $U = 391945$, $p = 0.001$), poorer sleep quality (women: $U = 649596$, $p < 0.001$; men: $U = 349794$, $p < 0.001$), and more problematic sleep disturbances (women: $U = 659704$, $p < 0.001$; men: $U = 355895$, $p < 0.001$); see **Tables 1, 2**.

Physical and mental comorbidities

Women with bothersome tinnitus reported higher rates of hypertension, $X^2(1) = 4.98$, $p = 0.026$, hyperlipidemia, $X^2(1) = 8.19$, $p = 0.004$, cardiovascular disease, $X^2(1) = 18.40$, $p < 0.001$, thyroid disease, $X^2(1) = 13.82$, $p < 0.001$, chronic shoulder pain, $X^2(1) = 21.68$, $p < 0.001$, osteoarthritis, $X^2(1) = 18.41$, $p < 0.001$, epilepsy, $X^2(1) = 6.87$, $p = 0.009$, and fibromyalgia, $X^2(1) = 16.56$, $p < 0.001$, than women with non-bothersome tinnitus, as well as higher rates of burnout, $X^2(1) = 17.62$, $p < 0.001$, depression, $X^2(1) = 7.93$, $p = 0.005$, and social anxiety, $X^2(1) = 5.06$, $p = 0.025$; see **Table 3**.

Men with bothersome tinnitus reported higher rates of hypertension, $X^2(1) = 9.41$, $p = 0.002$, hyperlipidemia, $X^2(1) = 10.58$, $p = 0.001$, chronic shoulder pain, $X^2(1) = 23.29$, $p < 0.001$, osteoarthritis, $X^2(1) = 8.05$, $p = 0.005$, and Ménière's

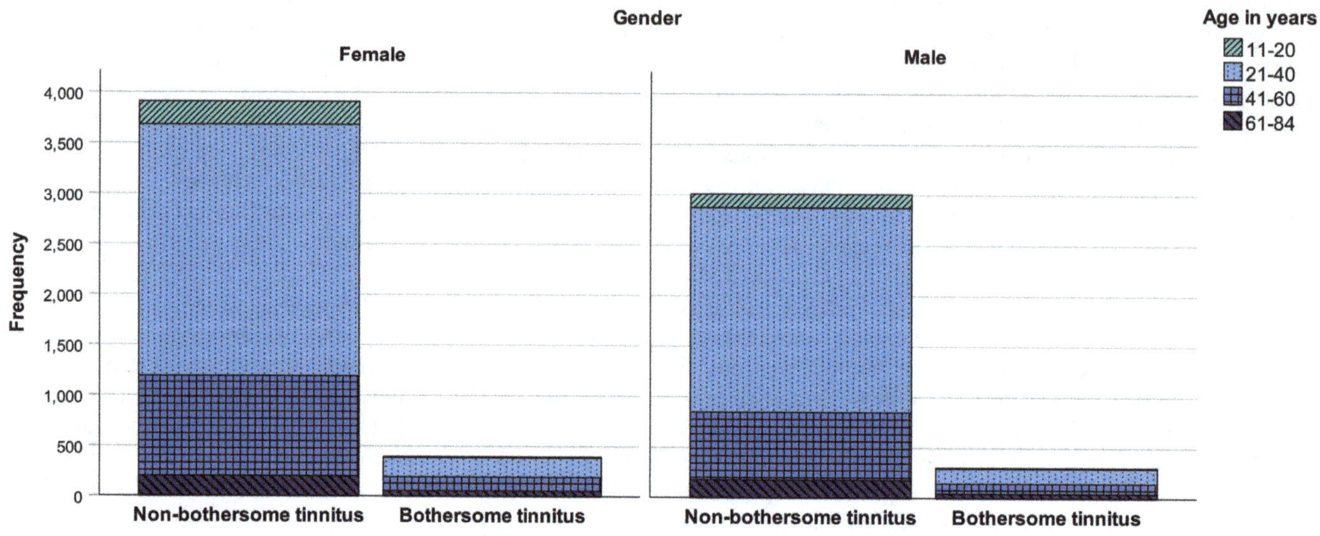

FIGURE 1 | Histogram of non-bothersome and bothersome tinnitus (count data) by age and gender.

disease, $X^2(1) = 15.39, p < 0.001$, than men with non-bothersome tinnitus, as well as higher rates of depression, $X^2(1) = 7.26$, $p = 0.007$, anxiety syndrome, $X^2(1) = 15.65$, $p < 0.001$, panic, $X^2(1) = 11.96$, $p = 0.001$, and social anxiety, $X^2(1) = 10.49$, $p = 0.001$; see **Table 3**.

Logistic Regression Analysis (Comparison Within Genders)

Female participants

Model 1: Sociodemographic and lifestyle factors. Higher age, level of education (all factor levels non-significant), and employment status (being unemployed, in early retirement due to illness/disability, and student; contrasted with being employed) significantly predicted bothersome tinnitus, Nagelkerke $R^2 = 0.050$. Marital status and smoking status showed no effect. See **Table 4**, Model 1.

Model 2: Tinnitus-associated phenomena. Hearing ability (somewhat reduced hearing ability and very reduced hearing ability; contrasted with good hearing), hearing-related difficulties in social situations, and poor sleep quality significantly predicted bothersome tinnitus, Nagelkerke $R^2 = 0.117$. Traumatic experiences and sleep disturbances showed no effect. See **Table 4**, Model 2.

Model 3: Physical comorbidities. The past or present occurrence of cardiovascular disease, thyroid disease, chronic shoulder pain, osteoarthritis, epilepsy, and fibromyalgia significantly predicted bothersome tinnitus, Nagelkerke $R^2 = 0.035$. Hypertension and hyperlipidemia showed no influence. See **Table 4**, Model 3.

Model 4: Mental comorbidities. The past or present occurrence of burnout significantly predicted bothersome tinnitus, Nagelkerke $R^2 = 0.011$. Depression and social anxiety showed no influence. See **Table 4**, Model 4.

Male participants

Model 1: Sociodemographic and lifestyle factors. Higher age and level of education (secondary school, university, and "other"; contrasted with primary school) significantly predicted bothersome tinnitus, Nagelkerke $R^2 = 0.078$. Marital status, employment, alcohol consumption, and smoking status showed no influence. See **Table 5**, Model 1.

Model 2: Tinnitus-associated phenomena. Hearing ability (somewhat reduced hearing ability and very reduced hearing ability; contrasted with good hearing), hearing-related difficulties in social situations, and poor sleep quality significantly predicted bothersome tinnitus, Nagelkerke $R^2 = 0.138$. Traumatic experiences and sleep disturbances were not associated with bothersome tinnitus. See **Table 5**, Model 2.

Model 3: Physical comorbidities. The past or present occurrence of chronic shoulder pain and Ménière's disease significantly predicted bothersome tinnitus, Nagelkerke $R^2 = 0.028$. Hypertension, hyperlipidemia, and osteoarthritis showed no effect. See **Table 5**, Model 3.

Model 4: Mental comorbidities. The past or present occurrence of anxiety syndrome significantly predicted bothersome tinnitus, Nagelkerke $R^2 = 0.014$. Depression, panic, and social anxiety showed no effect. See **Table 5**, Model 4.

Model 5: Multivariable adjusted model

In the final regression analysis, all significant predictors from Models 1 to 4 were included in the same model for multivariable adjustment (for women and men, respectively). For both genders, higher age, somewhat reduced and very reduced hearing ability, hearing-related difficulties in social situations, and poor sleep quality were significant predictors

TABLE 1 | Female participants: Differences in sociodemographic, lifestyle factors, and tinnitus-associated phenomena between bothersome and non-bothersome tinnitus.

	Non-bothersome tinnitus		Bothersome tinnitus	
Variable	**Frequency (count data)**	**Adjusted residuals**	**Frequency (count data)**	**Adjusted residuals**
Marital status**	n = 3781		n = 386	
Married	25.7% (971)	−3.0	32.6% (126)	3.0
Cohabiting	33.7% (1274)	2.0	28.8% (111)	−2.0
Single	24.3% (918)	2.4	18.9% (73)	−2.4
Separated/divorced	5.6% (210)	−2.8	9.1% (35)	2.8
Living apart	10.2% (386)	0.1	10.1% (39)	−0.1
Widowed	0.5% (20)	0.0	0.5% (2)	0.0
Same-sex marriage	0.1% (2)	0.5	0.0% (0)	−0.5
Education***	n = 3807		n = 386	
Nine-year primary school	2.2% (83)	−1.8	3.6% (14)	1.8
Secondary school	23.1% (880)	−0.8	24.9% (96)	0.8
University	66.1% (2516)	3.4	57.5% (222)	−3.4
Other	8.6% (328)	−3.5	14.0% (54)	3.5
Employment***	n = 3416		n = 356	
Employed	60.6% (2069)	2.4	53.9% (192)	−2.4
Unemployed	3.2% (108)	−3.0	6.2% (22)	3.0
Running an owned or part-owned company	6.6% (225)	0.9	5.3% (19)	−0.9
Age pension	3.0% (103)	−6.0	9.3% (33)	6.0
Activity or sickness benefit (early retirement) due to illness/disability	1.0% (34)	−3.0	2.8% (10)	3.0
Sick leave (for 2 months or longer)	1.2% (42)	0.2	1.1% (4)	−0.2
Parental leave (for 2 months or longer)	3.6% (123)	0.2	3.4% (12)	−0.2
Student	18.6% (636)	1.6	15.2% (54)	−1.6
On leave	0.1% (3)	0.6	0.0% (0)	−0.6
Housewife/man	0.3% (9)	1.0	0.0% (0)	−1.0
Other	1.9% (64)	−1.2	2.8% (10)	1.2
Smoking status*	n = 3811		n = 384	
Non-smoker	60.9% (2321)	1.4	57.3% (220)	−1.4
Ex-smoker	28.7% (1095)	−2.6	35.2% (135)	2.6
Smoker	10.4% (395)	1.7	7.6% (29)	−1.7
Hearing ability***	n = 3780		n = 377	
Good	70.4% (2663)	12.1	39.8% (150)	−12.1
Somewhat reduced	28.4% (1073)	−9.7	52.5% (198)	9.7
Very reduced	1.2% (44)	−9.2	7.7% (29)	9.2
	n	**Median**	***n***	**Median**
Age***	3908	32	393	40
Hearing-related difficulties in social situations***	3245	1.4	356	1.5
Traumatic/stressful experiences***	3843	3	388	4
Poor sleep quality***	3898	2	393	3
Problematic sleep disturbances***	3895	2	393	3

*Factors/categories in bold font indicate significant differences in frequencies (adjusted residuals ≥1.96 or ≤−1.96). ***p < 0.001, **p < 0.01, *p < 0.05.*

of bothersome tinnitus. Additionally, cardiovascular disease and epilepsy were significant predictors for women, and education and anxiety syndrome for men. Regarding the level of education, secondary school, university, and "other" were associated with a lower risk of bothersome tinnitus compared with primary school. Model summary can be found in **Table 6**; female participants: Nagelkerke R^2 = 0.153; male participants: R^2 = 0.167.

TABLE 2 | Male participants: Differences in sociodemographic, lifestyle factors, and tinnitus-associated phenomena between bothersome and non-bothersome tinnitus.

Variable	Non-bothersome tinnitus		Bothersome tinnitus	
	Frequency (count data)	Adjusted residuals	Frequency (count data)	Adjusted residuals
Marital status* **	$n = 2915$		$n = 299$	
Married	23.9% (696)	−5.0	37.1% (111)	5.0
Cohabiting	36.5% (1063)	1.5	32.1% (96)	−1.5
Single	26.6% (776)	2.8	19.1% (57)	−2.8
Separated/divorced	3.5% (102)	−0.5	4.0% (12)	0.5
Living apart	9.5% (276)	1.4	7.0% (21)	−1.4
Widowed	0.0% (1)	−3.4	0.7% (2)	3.4
Same-sex marriage	0.0% (1)	0.3	0.0% (0)	−0.3
Education* **	$n = 2944$		$n = 301$	
Nine-year primary school	2.7% (80)	−6.1	9.3% (28)	6.1
Secondary school	27.9% (820)	−2.0	33.2% (100)	2.0
University	61.7% (1815)	4.8	47.5% (143)	−4.8
Other	7.8% (229)	−1.3	10.0% (30)	1.3
Employment* **	$n = 2679$		$n = 275$	
Employed	62.4% (1671)	1.6	57.5% (158)	−1.6
Unemployed	3.2% (86)	−0.1	3.3% (9)	0.1
Running an owned or part-owned company	11.4% (305)	−2.1	15.6% (43)	2.1
Age pension	3.8% (101)	−4.7	9.8% (27)	4.7
Activity or sickness benefit (early retirement) due to illness/disability	0.4% (11)	−0.8	0.7% (2)	0.8
Sick leave (for 2 months or longer)	0.6% (15)	−0.3	0.7% (2)	0.3
Parental leave (for 2 months or longer)	1.0% (28)	0.5	0.7% (2)	−0.5
Student	15.9% (425)	3.0	9.1% (25)	−3.0
On leave	0.3% (7)	0.8	0.0% (0)	−0.8
Housewife/man	0.0% (1)	0.3	0.0% (0)	−0.3
Other	1.1% (29)	−2.1	2.5% (7)	2.1
Alcohol **	$n = 2957$		$n = 298$	
4 times a week or more	5.5% (163)	−2.5	9.1% (27)	2.5
2–3 times a week	26.4% (781)	0.3	25.5% (76)	−0.3
Once a week	21.5% (637)	1.4	18.1% (54)	−1.4
2–3 times a month	26.1% (772)	1.4	22.5% (67)	−1.4
Once a month or less	17.7% (522)	−0.6	19.1% (57)	0.6
Never	2.8% (82)	−2.8	5.7% (17)	2.8
Smoking status **	$n = 2952$		$n = 299$	
Non-smoker	64.5% (1903)	3.5	54.2% (162)	−3.5
Ex-smoker	28.5% (842)	−3.2	37.5% (112)	3.2
Smoker	7.0% (207)	−0.9	8.4% (25)	0.9
Hearing ability* **	$n = 2974$		$n = 299$	
Good	66.1% (1966)	11.8	31.4% (94)	−11.8
Somewhat reduced	32.9% (977)	−9.5	60.5% (181)	9.5
Very reduced	1.0% (31)	−9.0	8.0% (24)	9.0
	n	**Median**	***n***	**Median**
Age* **	3010	33	304	39.5
Hearing-related difficulties in social situations* **	2497	1.2	281	1.4
Traumatic/stressful experiences **	2966	3	299	3
Poor sleep quality* **	2997	2	304	3
Problematic sleep disturbances* **	2996	2	304	2

*Factors/categories in bold font indicate significant differences in frequencies (adjusted residuals ≥1.96 or ≤−1.96). ***p < 0.001, **p < 0.01, *p < 0.05.*

TABLE 3 | Differences in physical and mental comorbidities between bothersome and non-bothersome tinnitus.

Variable	Non-bothersome tinnitus		Bothersome tinnitus	
	Frequency (count data)	Adjusted residuals	Frequency (count data)	Adjusted residuals
		Female participants		
	n = 3894		n = 392	
Hypertension*	5.7% (223)	−2.3	8.7% (34)	2.3
Hyperlipidemia**	2.5% (97)	−3.0	5.1% (20)	3.0
Cardiovascular disease***	4.2% (165)	−4.4	9.2% (36)	4.4
Asthma	12.5% (485)	0.0	12.5% (49)	0.0
Diabetes	0.5% (19)	−1.4	1.0% (4)	1.4
Thyroid disease***	5.8% (226)	−3.8	10.7% (42)	3.8
	n = 3891		n = 392	
Chronic shoulder pain***	7.2% (282)	−4.8	14.0% (55)	4.8
Osteoarthritis***	5.4% (212)	−4.4	11.0% (43)	4.4
Rheumatoid arthritis	0.8% (30)	0.0	0.8% (3)	0.0
Systemic lupus erythematosus	0.1% (5)	0.7	0.0% (0)	−0.7
Migraine	19.2% (749)	−1.2	21.7% (85)	1.2
Ménière's disease	0.2% (8)	−1.2	0.5% (2)	1.2
Epilepsy**	0.7% (26)	−2.9	2.0% (8)	2.9
Multiple sclerosis	0.1% (5)	0.7	0.0% (0)	−0.7
Fibromyalgia***	1.3% (50)	−4.3	4.1% (16)	4.3
Burnout***	12.1% (470)	−4.3	19.6% (77)	4.3
Depression**	25.0% (972)	−2.9	31.6% (124)	2.9
Bipolar disease	0.7% (29)	−1.6	1.5% (6)	1.6
Anxiety syndrome	12.3% (478)	−1.6	15.1% (59)	1.6
Panic	13.9% (542)	−0.3	14.5% (57)	0.3
Agoraphobia	0.7% (28)	−1.2	1.3% (5)	1.2
Social anxiety*	3.7% (143)	−2.4	6.1% (24)	2.4
Obsessive-compulsive disorder	2.5% (97)	−0.7	3.1% (12)	0.7
Posttraumatic stress disorder	2.2% (84)	−1.8	3.6% (14)	1.8
		Male participants		
	n = 2992		n = 303	
Hypertension**	5.9% (176)	−3.2	10.6% (32)	3.2
Hyperlipidemia**	3.8% (114)	−3.4	7.9% (24)	3.4
Cardiovascular disease	3.7% (112)	−1.9	5.9% (18)	1.9
Asthma	9.7% (289)	−0.9	11.2% (34)	0.9
Diabetes	0.7% (22)	1.5	0.0% (0)	−1.5
Thyroid disease	0.8% (25)	−1.4	1.7% (5)	1.4
	n = 2991		n = 303	
Chronic shoulder pain***	2.8% (85)	−5.0	8.3% (25)	5.0
Osteoarthritis**	3.7% (111)	−3.0	7.3% (22)	3.0
Rheumatoid arthritis	0.3% (9)	−1.0	0.7% (2)	1.0
Systemic lupus erythematosus	0.0% (0)	0.0	0.0% (0)	0.0
Migraine	8.9% (267)	−0.8	10.2% (31)	0.8
Ménière's disease***	0.2% (5)	−4.5	1.7% (5)	4.5
Epilepsy	0.7% (21)	0.8	0.3% (1)	−0.8
Multiple sclerosis	0.2% (5)	0.7	0.0% (0)	−0.7
Fibromyalgia	0.1% (4)	0.6	0.0% (0)	−0.6
Burnout	7.6% (227)	−1.0	9.2% (28)	1.0
Depression**	14.5% (433)	−2.8	20.5% (62)	2.8
Bipolar disease	0.8% (23)	0.9	0.3% (1)	−0.9

(Continued)

TABLE 3 | Continued

	Non-bothersome tinnitus		Bothersome tinnitus	
Variable	**Frequency (count data)**	**Adjusted residuals**	**Frequency (count data)**	**Adjusted residuals**
Anxiety syndrome* **	7.0% (210)	−4.1	13.5% (41)	4.1
Panic**	7.4% (221)	−3.6	13.2% (40)	3.6
Agoraphobia	0.3% (10)	−0.9	0.7% (2)	0.9
Social anxiety**	2.9% (88)	−3.4	6.6% (20)	3.4
Obsessive-compulsive disorder	1.4% (43)	−1.2	2.3% (7)	1.2
Posttraumatic stress disorder	0.8% (23)	−1.6	1.7% (5)	1.6

*Factors in bold font indicate significant differences in frequencies (adjusted residuals ≥1.96 or ≤−1.96). ***$p < 0.001$, **$p < 0.01$, *$p < 0.05$.*

TABLE 4 | Female participants: Logistic regression models for sociodemographic and lifestyle factors (Model 1), tinnitus-associated phenomena (Model 2), physical comorbidities (Model 3), and mental comorbidities (Model 4).

						95% CI	
Variable	**β**	**SE β**	**Wald's X^2**	***p***	**OR**	**Lower**	**Upper**
			Model 1: sociodemographic and lifestyle factors				
Age***	0.027	0.007	17.41	<0.001	1.028	1.015	1.041
Marital status							
Education*			8.92	0.030			
Employment*			22.13	0.014			
Unemployed**	0.860	0.256	11.25	0.001	2.364	1.430	3.908
Early retirement due to illness/disability*	0.775	0.394	3.87	0.049	2.172	1.003	4.704
Student*	0.370	0.186	3.97	0.046	1.447	1.006	2.082
Smoking status							
			Model 2: tinnitus-associated phenomena				
Hearing ability***			47.52	<0.001			
Somewhat reduced***	0.853	0.133	41.38	<0.001	2.347	1.810	3.043
Very reduced***	1.438	0.304	22.43	<0.001	4.213	2.323	7.640
Hearing-related difficulties in social situations***	1.023	0.165	38.27	<0.001	2.782	2.012	3.848
Traumatic/stressful experiences							
Poor sleep quality**	0.206	0.074	7.76	0.005	1.229	1.063	1.420
Problematic sleep disturbances							
			Model 3: physical comorbidities				
Hypertension							
Hyperlipidemia							
Cardiovascular disease**	0.658	0.198	11.09	0.001	1.931	1.311	2.844
Thyroid disease**	0.536	0.182	8.70	0.003	1.708	1.197	2.439
Chronic shoulder pain**	0.506	0.167	9.15	0.002	1.659	1.195	2.304
Osteoarthritis**	0.550	0.184	8.92	0.003	1.733	1.208	2.487
Epilepsy*	1.041	0.415	6.31	0.012	2.833	1.257	6.383
Fibromyalgia*	0.759	0.312	5.94	0.015	2.137	1.160	3.937
			Model 4: mental comorbidities				
Burnout**	0.488	0.148	10.94	0.001	1.629	1.220	2.176
Depression							
Social anxiety							

*Only significant results are displayed. OR, odds ratio. The coefficients of employment are contrasted with being employed; those of self-rated hearing ability are contrasted with good hearing. ***$p < 0.001$, **$p < 0.01$, *$p < 0.05$.*

TABLE 5 | Male participants: Logistic regression models for sociodemographic and lifestyle factors (Model 1), tinnitus-associated phenomena (Model 2), physical comorbidities (Model 3), and mental comorbidities (Model 4).

Variable	β	SE β	Wald's X^2	*p*	OR	95% CI Lower	95% CI Upper
Model 1: sociodemographic and lifestyle factors							
Age***	0.032	0.007	18.57	<0.001	1.033	1.018	1.048
Marital status							
Education***			21.08	<0.001			
Secondary school**	−0.878	0.272	10.44	0.001	0.416	0.244	0.708
University***	−1.193	0.266	20.11	<0.001	0.303	0.180	0.511
Other**	−0.891	0.321	7.69	0.006	0.410	0.219	0.770
Employment							
Alcohol							
Smoking status							
Model 2: tinnitus-associated phenomena							
Hearing ability***			68.13	<0.001			
Somewhat reduced***	1.130	0.153	54.90	<0.001	3.097	2.296	4.176
Very reduced***	2.125	0.340	39.02	<0.001	8.372	4.298	16.308
Hearing-related difficulties in social situations***	0.799	0.207	14.93	<0.001	2.224	1.483	3.336
Traumatic/stressful experiences							
Poor sleep quality**	0.226	0.085	7.01	0.008	1.253	1.060	1.481
Problematic sleep disturbances							
Model 3: physical comorbidities							
Hypertension							
Hyperlipidemia							
Chronic shoulder pain***	0.992	0.243	16.71	<0.001	2.697	1.676	4.339
Osteoarthritis							
Ménière's disease**	2.084	0.658	10.02	0.002	8.037	2.211	29.211
Model 4: mental comorbidities							
Depression							
Anxiety syndrome*	0.449	0.224	4.00	0.045	1.566	1.009	2.430
Panic							
Social anxiety							

*Only significant results are displayed. OR, odds ratio. The coefficients of education are contrasted with 9-year primary school; those of self-rated hearing ability are contrasted with good hearing. ***p < 0.001, **p < 0.01, *p < 0.05.*

Gender-Moderated Logistic Regression Analysis (Comparison Between Genders)

Predictors identified by the logistic regression analysis within men and women (all predictors included in Model 5 for female and/or male participants) were further analyzed to investigate whether gender moderates their effects on bothersome tinnitus, that is, whether their effects on bothersome tinnitus are different for women and men. These analyses revealed main effects (gender-independent) of age, hearing ability, hearing-related difficulties in social situations, cardiovascular disease, epilepsy and burnout; and moderating effects of gender for education and anxiety syndrome, see **Table 7**. In female participants, the effect of education was non-significant (p = 0.826); in male participants, higher education levels were negatively related to the presence of bothersome vs. non-bothersome tinnitus: $\beta = -0.374$, SE = 0.090, OR = 0.688 [0.577, 0.821], $p < 0.001$. For anxiety syndrome, the effect was non-significant in female participants (p = 0.116); in male participants, anxiety syndrome was associated with an increase of odds of bothersome tinnitus: $\beta = 0.729$, SE = 0.183, OR = 2.072 [1.449, 2.964], $p < 0.001$. For all other variables (employment, sleep quality, thyroid disease, fibromyalgia, chronic shoulder pain, osteoarthritis, Ménière's disease) neither main effects nor moderation effects by gender were present.

DISCUSSION

The current study investigated a range of potential risk factors for bothersome tinnitus in a large Swedish sample. Our results indicate that participants with bothersome tinnitus differ from those with non-bothersome tinnitus in several aspects. Higher age, reduced hearing ability, more hearing-related difficulties in

TABLE 6 | Multivariable adjusted regression model for the prediction of bothersome tinnitus (Model 5).

Variable	β	SE β	Wald's X^2	*p*	OR	95% CI Lower	95% CI Upper
				Female participants			
Age*	0.013	0.007	3.86	0.049	1.013	1.000	1.027
Education							
Employment							
Self-rated hearing ability***			38.42	<0.001			
Somewhat reduced***	0.823	0.823	32.69	<0.001	2.277	1.717	3.018
Very reduced***	1.431	0.319	20.12	<0.001	4.182	2.238	7.815
Hearing-related difficulties in social situations***	0.834	0.177	22.15	<0.001	2.302	1.627	3.258
Poor sleep quality*	0.122	0.060	4.08	0.043	1.129	1.004	1.271
Cardiovascular disease*	0.480	0.237	4.11	0.043	1.616	1.016	2.568
Thyroid disease							
Fibromyalgia							
Chronic shoulder pain							
Osteoarthritis							
Epilepsy*	1.059	0.457	5.36	0.021	2.883	1.176	7.067
Burnout							
				Male participants			
Age**	0.017	0.005	11.20	0.001	1.017	1.007	1.027
Education**			16.20	0.001			
Secondary school**	−0.781	0.280	7.76	0.005	0.458	0.265	0.793
University***	−1.059	0.271	15.23	<0.001	0.347	0.204	0.590
Other**	−0.899	0.329	7.46	0.006	0.407	0.214	0.776
Self-rated hearing ability***			52.96	<0.001			
Somewhat reduced***	1.053	0.156	45.32	<0.001	2.865	2.109	3.893
Very reduced***	1.872	0.357	27.50	<0.001	6.499	3.229	13.082
Hearing-related difficulties in social situations**	0.635	0.211	9.06	0.003	1.887	1.248	2.852
Poor sleep quality***	0.267	0.068	15.35	<0.001	1.306	1.143	1.493
Chronic shoulder pain							
Ménière's disease							
Anxiety syndrome*	0.464	0.216	4.62	0.032	1.590	1.042	2.427

*Only significant results are displayed. OR, odds ratio. The coefficients of education are contrasted with 9-year primary school; those of self-rated hearing ability are contrasted with good hearing. ***p < 0.001, **p < 0.01, *p < 0.05.*

TABLE 7 | Moderation analysis by gender for the prediction of bothersome tinnitus.

	β	SE β	*p*	OR	95% CI Lower	95% CI Upper
		Main effects				
Age**	0.029	0.009	0.001	1.029	1.011	1.047
Self-rated hearing ability***	1.039	0.220	<0.001	2.828	1.837	4.351
Hearing-related difficulties in social situations***	1.589	0.316	<0.001	4.897	2.636	9.096
Cardiovascular disease*	1.168	0.465	0.012	3.216	1.293	7.997
Epilepsy*	3.020	1.310	0.021	20.481	1.571	267.040
Burnout**	0.938	0.344	0.007	2.554	1.301	5.013
		Moderation effects				
Education × Gender**	−0.393	0.125	0.002	0.675	0.528	0.863
Anxiety syndrome × Gender*	0.494	0.236	0.036	1.638	1.032	2.601

*Only significant results are displayed. OR, odds ratio. ***p < 0.001, **p < 0.01, *p < 0.05.*

social situations, the past or present occurrence of cardiovascular disease, epilepsy, and burnout were associated with bothersome tinnitus in both genders, whereas associations of low education and anxiety syndrome were only present in male participants.

Clear Associations With Bothersome Tinnitus

The effects of age and hearing loss on bothersome tinnitus are in accordance with the findings of Kim et al. (2015). Relationships between cardiovascular diseases and severe tinnitus have been reported previously (Nondahl et al., 2002; Stobik et al., 2005; Park et al., 2014), however, the mechanisms linking cardiovascular health and tinnitus are poorly understood. In a recent study, tinnitus was found to be twice as prevalent in patients with epilepsy than control subjects, and the authors argue that tinnitus may be related to the disease itself as well as to its long-term drug treatment (Hamed and Oseilly, 2018). Moreover, both conditions are linked to cortical hyperexcitability (Chai et al., 2019). Our study suggests an association between epilepsy and severe tinnitus, however, the nature of this association remains to be established. Burnout, a syndrome resulting from chronic occupational stress, is not a diagnostic category in itself, but can be understood as a form of depression (Bianchi et al., 2015). Our finding of a relationship between bothersome tinnitus and burnout is consistent with the results of a cross-sectional study by Hébert et al. (2012), who report that emotional exhaustion (which is part of the burnout symptomatology) is a predictor of tinnitus severity. In addition, Herr et al. (2016) found that burnout mediates the effects of work-related stress (low organizational justice) on tinnitus. However, we only found an effect of burnout in the moderation analysis, but not in the multivariable adjusted regression analysis.

Unclear Associations With Bothersome Tinnitus

Female and male participants with bothersome tinnitus differed from those with non-bothersome tinnitus regarding marital status and employment (in frequency analyses). Being separated, divorced or widowed, and being unemployed, in early retirement, or running an owned or part-owned company might constitute stress factors, which can trigger or increase adverse tinnitus effects (Henry et al., 2005). Stress and tinnitus annoyance have been linked in the literature (Park et al., 2014; Kim et al., 2015). Higher alcohol consumption frequencies in men with bothersome tinnitus (more often drinking alcohol four times a week) could reflect maladaptive coping strategies to reduce tinnitus-related distress, as drinking to cope with negative affect is a relatively common drinking motive (Cooper et al., 1995; Kuntsche et al., 2014; Mohr et al., 2018). However, these sociodemographic and lifestyle factors showed no significant influence in regression analyses. Previous studies found a higher risk of tinnitus in patients with sleep apnea (Koo and Hwang, 2017), as well as associations between sleep disturbances and severe tinnitus (Axelsson and Ringdahl, 1989; Izuhara et al., 2013). In our analyses, poor sleep quality was a significant predictor of bothersome tinnitus in regression analyses for both male and female participants (with adjustment for other relevant factors), but no main effect of sleep quality was present in the moderation analysis.

Gender-Specific Associations With Bothersome Tinnitus

Lower levels of education and past or present comorbid anxiety syndrome were specifically related to bothersome tinnitus in men. Several studies report links between low education levels and tinnitus (Fujii et al., 2011; Kim et al., 2015; House et al., 2018), as well as a relationship between lower education levels and higher tinnitus impairment (Unterrainer et al., 2001). Moreover, low education levels in individuals with tinnitus seem associated with poorer quality of life (Jung et al., 2019). Yet other studies found no relationship between tinnitus and education (Michikawa et al., 2010; Gallus et al., 2015), and one study observed higher tinnitus severity in individuals with higher education levels (Hoekstra et al., 2014). Thus, the literature is not conclusive in this regard. In addition, the relationship between low education and severe tinnitus might be confounded by socioeconomic status, occupational factors (e.g., noise exposure), or reduced openness to or accessibility of psychological treatment approaches (Unterrainer et al., 2001; Jung et al., 2019). Some of these confounding influences could potentially be stronger for men. As we did not assess these factors, we cannot exclude confounding influences. Furthermore, women generally reported higher education levels in our sample than men, which limits the generalization of this result.

Comorbidity between tinnitus and anxiety disorders is high, and they might share underlying neurobiological mechanisms (Pattyn et al., 2016; Lin et al., 2018). Anxiety can be not only a predisposing factor for severe tinnitus, but also a consequence of it, which can in turn increase tinnitus-related distress and impede habituation (Henry et al., 2005; Pattyn et al., 2016). Thus, the link between anxiety and bothersome tinnitus is not surprising. However, the prevalence of most anxiety disorders is around twice as high in women as in men (Bandelow and Michaelis, 2015). Accordingly, previous studies found higher anxiety levels in women with constant tinnitus than men (Schlee et al., 2017), and also in our sample, anxiety syndrome was more frequent in women than in men (12.5 vs. 7.6%). This result might indicate that even though men are less likely to be affected by anxiety symptoms, for them the contribution of anxiety on tinnitus annoyance is particularly strong.

Clinical Implications

The medical assessment of tinnitus patients should include screenings for comorbidities, especially cardiovascular disease and epilepsy, which must be considered in clinical management. Anxiety and burnout should also be routinely investigated, as psychological treatments that target cognitive-affective sequelae of bothersome tinnitus have great potential to improve tinnitus burden (Henry et al., 2005; Pattyn et al., 2016; Cima,

2018). Similarly, hearing loss and sleep disturbances need to be addressed in all patients. In men particularly, the use of alcohol should be considered as a possible maladaptive coping strategy. Although different factors might be important for the emergence and maintenance of tinnitus-related distress in women and men, treatment should always be tailored to the individual physical and mental situation – including stress factors, cognitive and emotional reactions, and coping behaviors – to help the individual to better accept and habituate to the tinnitus (Henry et al., 2005; Cima, 2018).

Limitations

Some limitations must be considered. As the design of this study is cross-sectional, no information on the causality of relationships can be derived. For many factors, the relationships with bothersome tinnitus are most likely complex and bidirectional; for example, anxiety can precede, be caused by, or increase tinnitus-related distress (Henry et al., 2005; Pattyn et al., 2016). The temporal relation between comorbidities and bothersome tinnitus could not be determined in our data. The aim of this study was to identify potential risk factors and comorbidities of bothersome tinnitus in women and men, yet case-control and longitudinal cohort studies are needed to investigate the mechanisms behind these associations. Furthermore, the investigated risk factors are not independent and, in some cases, moderately correlated. We conducted multivariate regression models in order to adjust for intercorrelations between variables, however, not all potentially confounding variables could be controlled for. Another limitation is the fact that all information on the investigated conditions (including tinnitus) stems from self-report data with apparent validity and reliability limitations. Furthermore, most variables were assessed with single-item questions as opposed to well-constructed and validated psychometric instruments. Regarding tinnitus specifically, no information on duration, localization or other characteristics was available. The comparatively high tinnitus rate in our sample may have been influenced by the fact that the question used to assess tinnitus did not specify a minimum duration of the experience (e.g., at least 5 min) unlike many other studies (McCormack et al., 2016), and did not specify the tinnitus onset, thus combining acute and chronic tinnitus. In addition, the question confounded continuity and annoyance of tinnitus, as "non-bothersome tinnitus" was defined as occurring sometimes, and "bothersome tinnitus" was defined as occurring constantly. Yet studies indicate that the tinnitus-associated burden and functional impact of constant tinnitus are indeed higher than those of intermittent/occasional tinnitus (Schlee et al., 2017; Koops et al., 2019).

CONCLUSION

In summary, the present study found general associations between bothersome tinnitus and higher age, reduced hearing ability, hearing-related difficulties in social situations, cardiovascular disease, epilepsy, and burnout. In men, low education levels and comorbid anxiety might exert specific influences in the emergence or maintenance of bothersome tinnitus. Yet the effects of low education, in particular, must be interpreted with caution because of possible confounding influences. These new findings obtained from a large general population sample add to the literature of gender differences in tinnitus and imply the need for medical as well as psychological screenings of affected individuals and personalization of clinical treatment pathways. Future studies should investigate the mechanisms behind these general and gender-specific associations with bothersome tinnitus.

ETHICS STATEMENT

The studies involving human participants were reviewed and approved by the Local Ethics Committee "Regionala etikprövningsnämnden" in Stockholm (2015/2129-31/1). Adult participants provided their written informed consent to participate in this study. For participants under the age of 18, written informed consent to participate in this study was provided by the participants' legal guardian/next of kin.

AUTHOR CONTRIBUTIONS

BM, CC, NP, and BC devised the project. BM, BB, PB, and LB conceived the study. NP provided the data. BB and LB devised the analysis strategy. LB performed the statistical analysis and wrote the first draft of the manuscript. BM, BB, PB, CC, NP, and BC critically reviewed the manuscript. All authors contributed to the article and approved the submitted version.

FUNDING

This project has received funding from the European Research Council (ERC) under the European Union's Horizon 2020 Research and Innovation Programme (grant agreement no. 764604) as well as the GENDER-Net Co-Plus Fund (GNP-182). We acknowledge support from the German Research Foundation (DFG) and the Open Access Publication Fund of Charité – Universitätsmedizin Berlin.

REFERENCES

Aarhus, L., Engdahl, B., Tambs, K., Kvestad, E., and Hoffman, H. J. (2015). Association between childhood hearing disorders and tinnitus in adulthood. *JAMA Otolaryngol. Head Neck Surg.* 141, 983–989. doi: 10.1001/jamaoto.2015.2378

Almqvist, C., Adami, H.-O., Franks, P. W., Groop, L., Ingelsson, E., Kere, J., et al. (2011). LifeGene—a large prospective population-based study of global relevance. *Eur. J. Epidemiol.* 26, 67–77. doi: 10.1007/s10654-010-9521-x

Axelsson, A., and Ringdahl, A. (1989). Tinnitus—a study of its prevalence and characteristics. *Br. J. Audiol.* 23, 53–62. doi: 10.3109/03005368909077819

Baguley, D., McFerran, D., and Hall, D. (2013). Tinnitus. *Lancet* 382, 1600–1607. doi: 10.1016/S0140-6736(13)60142-7

Bandelow, B., and Michaelis, S. (2015). Epidemiology of anxiety disorders in the 21st century. *Dialogues Clin. Neurosci.* 17, 327–335.

Bernhardt, O., Mundt, T., Welk, A., Köppl, N., Kocher, T., Meyer, G., et al. (2011). Signs and symptoms of temporomandibular disorders and the incidence of tinnitus. *J. Oral Rehabil.* 38, 891–901. doi: 10.1111/j.1365-2842.2011.02224.x

Bianchi, R., Schonfeld, I. S., and Laurent, E. (2015). Is it time to consider the "burnout syndrome" a distinct illness? *Front. Public Health* 3:158. doi: 10.3389/fpubh.2015.00158

Bogo, R., Farah, A., Karlsson, K. K., Pedersen, N. L., Svartengren, M., and Skjönsberg, Å (2017). Prevalence, incidence proportion, and heritability for tinnitus: a longitudinal twin study. *Ear Hear.* 38, 292–300. doi: 10.1097/AUD.0000000000000397

Chai, Z., Ma, C., and Jin, X. (2019). Cortical stimulation for treatment of neurological disorders of hyperexcitability: a role of homeostatic plasticity. *Neural. Regen. Res.* 14, 34–38. doi: 10.4103/1673-5374.243696

Cima, R. F. F. (2018). Bothersome tinnitus: cognitive behavioral perspectives. *HNO* 66, 369–374. doi: 10.1007/s00106-018-0502-9

Cooper, M. L., Frone, M. R., Russell, M., and Mudar, P. (1995). Drinking to regulate positive and negative emotions: a motivational model of alcohol use. *J. Personal. Soc. Psychol.* 69, 990–1005. doi: 10.1037/0022-3514.69.5.990

Fagelson, M. A. (2007). The association between tinnitus and posttraumatic stress disorder. *Am. J. Audiol.* 16, 107–117. doi: 10.1044/1059-0889(2007/015)

Fujii, K., Nagata, C., Nakamura, K., Kawachi, T., Takatsuka, N., Oba, S., et al. (2011). Prevalence of tinnitus in community-dwelling Japanese adults. *J. Epidemiol.* 21, 299–304. doi: 10.2188/jea.JE20100124

Gallus, S., Lugo, A., Garavello, W., Bosetti, C., Santoro, E., Colombo, P., et al. (2015). Prevalence and determinants of tinnitus in the Italian adult population. *Neuroepidemiology* 45, 12–19. doi: 10.1159/000431376

Glicksman, J. T., Curhan, S. G., and Curhan, G. C. (2014). A prospective study of caffeine intake and risk of incident tinnitus. *Am. J. Med.* 127, 739–743. doi: 10.1016/j.amjmed.2014.02.033

Gopinath, B., McMahon, C. M., Rochtchina, E., Karpa, M. J., and Mitchell, P. (2010). Incidence, persistence, and progression of tinnitus symptoms in older adults: the Blue Mountains Hearing Study. *Ear Hear.* 31, 407–412. doi: 10.1097/AUD.0b013e3181cdb2a2

Hamed, S. A., and Oseilly, A. M. (2018). Cochlear function in adults with epilepsy and treated with carbamazepine. *Audiol. Neurotol.* 23, 63–72. doi: 10.1159/000490232

Hayes, A. F. (2018). *Introduction to Mediation, Moderation, and Conditional Process Analysis: a Regression-Based Approach*, 2nd Edn. New York, NY: Guilford Press.

Hébert, S., Canlon, B., and Hasson, D. (2012). Emotional exhaustion as a predictor of tinnitus. *Psychother. Psychosom.* 81, 324–326. doi: 10.1159/000335043

Henry, J. A., Dennis, K. C., and Schechter, M. A. (2005). General review of tinnitus: prevalence, mechanisms, effects, and management. *J. Speech Lang. Hear. Res.* 48, 1204–1235. doi: 10.1044/1092-4388(2005/084)

Herr, R. M., Loerbroks, A., Bosch, J. A., Seegel, M., Schneider, M., and Schmidt, B. (2016). Associations of organizational justice with tinnitus and the mediating role of depressive symptoms and burnout—findings from a cross-sectional study. *Int. J. Behav. Med.* 23, 190–197. doi: 10.1007/s12529-015-9505-z

Hinton, D. E., Chhean, D., Pich, V., Hofmann, S. G., and Barlow, D. H. (2006). Tinnitus among Cambodian refugees: relationship to PTSD severity. *J. Traumat. Stress* 19, 541–546. doi: 10.1002/jts.20138

Hoekstra, C. E. L., Wesdorp, F. M., and van Zanten, G. A. (2014). Socio-demographic, health, and tinnitus related variables affecting tinnitus severity. *Ear Hear.* 35, 544–554. doi: 10.1097/AUD.0000000000000045

House, L., Bishop, C. E., Spankovich, C., Su, D., Valle, K., and Schweinfurth, J. (2018). Tinnitus and its risk factors in African Americans: the Jackson Heart Study. *Laryngosc.* 128, 1668–1675. doi: 10.1002/lary.26964

Izuhara, K., Wada, K., Nakamura, K., Tamai, Y., Tsuji, M., Ito, Y., et al. (2013). Association between tinnitus and sleep disorders in the general Japanese population. *Ann. Otol. Rhinol. Laryngol.* 122, 701–706. doi: 10.1177/000348941312201107

Jalessi, M., Farhadi, M., Asghari, A., Kamrava, S. K., Amintehran, E., Ghalehbaghi, S., et al. (2013). Tinnitus: an epidemiologic study in Iranian population. *Acta Med. Iran* 51, 886–891.

Jung, D. J., Yoo, M. H., Jung, Y. J., Lee, H. J., and Lee, K.-Y. (2019). The influence of education level on tinnitus and quality of life in Korean adults. *Korean J. Otorhinol. Head Neck Surg.* 62, 499–506. doi: 10.3342/kjorl-hns.2018.00773

Kim, H.-J., Lee, H.-J., An, S.-Y., Sim, S., Park, B., Kim, S. W., et al. (2015). Analysis of the prevalence and associated risk factors of tinnitus in adults. *PLoS One* 10:e0127578. doi: 10.1371/journal.pone.0127578

Koo, M., and Hwang, J.-H. (2017). Risk of tinnitus in patients with sleep apnea: a nationwide, population-based, case-control study. *Laryngosc.* 127, 2171–2175. doi: 10.1002/lary.26323

Koops, E. A., Husain, F. T., van Dijk, P., (2019). Profiling intermittent tinnitus: a retrospective review. *Int. J. of Audiol.* 58, 434–440. doi: 10.1080/14992027.2019.1600058

Kuntsche, E., Gabhainn, S. N., Roberts, C., Windlin, B., Vieno, A., Bendtsen, P., et al. (2014). Drinking motives and links to alcohol use in 13 European countries. *J. Stud. Alcohol. Drugs* 75, 428–437. doi: 10.15288/jsad.2014.75.428

Lee, C.-F., Lin, M.-C., Lin, H.-T., Lin, C.-L., Wang, T.-C., and Kao, C.-H. (2016). Increased risk of tinnitus in patients with temporomandibular disorder: a retrospective population-based cohort study. *Eur. Arch. Otorhinolaryngol.* 273, 203–208. doi: 10.1007/s00405-015-3491-2

LifeGene (2017). *Description of the LifeGene Resource*. Available online at: https://lifegene.se/wp-content/uploads/1LifeGeneresource20170203version24.pdf (accessed March 27, 2020).

Lin, C.-E., Chen, L.-F., Chou, P.-H., and Chung, C.-H. (2018). Increased prevalence and risk of anxiety disorders in adults with tinnitus: a population-based study in Taiwan. *Gen. Hosp. Psychiatry* 50, 131–136. doi: 10.1016/j.genhosppsych.2017.11.006

Lugo, A., Trpchevska, N., Liu, X., Biswas, R., Magnusson, C., Gallus, S., et al. (2019). Sex-specific association of tinnitus with suicide attempts. *JAMA Otolaryngol. Head Neck Surg.* 145, 685–687. doi: 10.1001/jamaoto.2019.0566

McCormack, A., Edmondson-Jones, M., Somerset, S., and Hall, D. (2016). A systematic review of the reporting of tinnitus prevalence and severity. *Hear. Res.* 337, 70–79. doi: 10.1016/j.heares.2016.05.009

Michikawa, T., Nishiwaki, Y., Kikuchi, Y., Saito, H., Mizutari, K., Okamoto, M., et al. (2010). Prevalence and factors associated with tinnitus: a community-based study of Japanese elders. *J. Epidemiol.* 20, 271–276. doi: 10.2188/jea.JE20090121

Mohr, C. D., McCabe, C. T., Haverly, S. N., Hammer, L. B., and Carlson, K. F. (2018). Drinking motives and alcohol use: the SERVe study of U.S. current and former service members. *J. Stud. Alcohol. Drugs* 79, 79–87. doi: 10.15288/jsad.2018.79.79

Nondahl, D. M., Cruickshanks, K. J., Wiley, T. L., Klein, B. E. K., Klein, R., Chappell, R., et al. (2010). The ten-year incidence of tinnitus among older adults. *Int. J. Audiol.* 49, 580–585. doi: 10.3109/14992021003753508

Nondahl, D. M., Cruickshanks, K. J., Wiley, T. L., Klein, R., Klein, B. E. K., and Tweed, T. S. (2002). Prevalence and 5-year incidence of tinnitus among older adults: the epidemiology of hearing loss study. *J. Am. Acad. Audiol.* 13, 323–331. doi: 10.1055/s-0040-1715975

Park, K. H., Lee, S. H., Koo, J.-W., Park, H. Y., Lee, K. Y., Choi, Y. S., et al. (2014). Prevalence and associated factors of tinnitus: data from the Korean National Health and Nutrition Examination Survey 2009–2011. *J. Epidemiol.* 24, 417–426. doi: 10.2188/jea.JE20140024

Pattyn, T., Van Den Eede, F., Vanneste, S., Cassiers, L., Veltman, D. J., Van De Heyning, P., et al. (2016). Tinnitus and anxiety disorders: a review. *Hear. Res.* 333, 255–265. doi: 10.1016/j.heares.2015.08.014

Ramage-Morin, P. L., Banks, R., Pineault, D., and Atrach, M. (2019). Tinnitus in Canada. *Health Rep.* 30, 3–11. doi: 10.25318/82-003-x201900300001-eng

Regitz-Zagrosek, V., and Kararigas, G. (2017). Mechanistic pathways of sex differences in cardiovascular disease. *Physiol. Rev.* 97, 1–37. doi: 10.1152/physrev.00021.2015

Salk, R. H., Hyde, J. S., and Abramson, L. Y. (2017). Gender differences in depression in representative national samples: meta-analyses of diagnoses and symptoms. *Psychol. Bull.* 143, 783–822. doi: 10.1037/bul0000102

Schlee, W., Hall, D. A., Edvall, N. K., Langguth, B., Canlon, B., and Cederroth, C. R. (2017). Visualization of global disease burden for the optimization of patient management and treatment. *Front. Med.* 4:86. doi: 10.3389/fmed.2017.00086

Seydel, C., Haupt, H., Olze, H., Szczepek, A. J., and Mazurek, B. (2013). Gender and chronic tinnitus: differences in tinnitus-related distress depend on age and duration of tinnitus. *Ear Hear.* 34, 661–672. doi: 10.1097/AUD.0b013e31828149f2

Shargorodsky, J., Curhan, G. C., and Farwell, W. R. (2010). Prevalence and characteristics of tinnitus among US adults. *Am. J. Med.* 123, 711–718. doi: 10.1016/j.amjmed.2010.02.015

Smith, P. F., Agrawal, Y., and Darlington, C. L. (2019). Sexual dimorphism in vestibular function and dysfunction. *J. Neurophysiol.* 121, 2379–2391. doi: 10.1152/jn.00074.2019

Stobik, C., Weber, R. K., Münte, T. F., Walter, M., and Frommer, J. (2005). Evidence of psychosomatic influences in compensated and decompensated tinnitus: evidencia de influencias psicosomáticas en acúfenos compensados y descompensados. *Int. J. Audiol.* 44, 370–378. doi: 10.1080/14992020500147557

Unterrainer, J., Greimel, K. V., and Leibetseder, M. (2001). Are demographic and socioeconomic factors predictive for perceived tinnitus impairment? *Int. Tinnitus J.* 7, 109–111.

Vanderpump, M. P. J., Tunbrldge, W. M. G., French, J. M., Appleton, D., Bates, D., Clark, F., et al. (1995). The incidence of thyroid disorders in the community: a twenty-year follow-up of the Whickham Survey. *Clin. Endocrinol.* 43, 55–68. doi: 10.1111/j.1365-2265.1995.tb01894.x

Wijnhoven, H. A. H., de Vet, H. C. W., and Picavet, S. J. H. (2006). Explaining sex differences in chronic musculoskeletal pain in a general population. *Pain* 124, 158–166. doi: 10.1016/j.pain.2006.04.012

Zeng, X., Li, P., Li, Z., Cen, J., Li, Y., and Zhang, G. (2016). Analysis of acutely exacerbated chronic tinnitus by the tinnitus handicap inventory. *J. Laryngol. Otol.* 130, 38–41. doi: 10.1017/S0022215115003060

22

Sex Differences in the Response to Different Tinnitus Treatment

Annemarie Van der Wal[1,2]†, Tine Luyten[1,3]†, Emilie Cardon[1,3]†, Laure Jacquemin[1,3], Olivier M. Vanderveken[1,3], Vedat Topsakal[1,3], Paul Van de Heyning[1,3], Willem De Hertogh[2], Nancy Van Looveren[4], Vincent Van Rompaey[1,3], Sarah Michiels[1,2,3] and Annick Gilles[1,3,5]**

[1] Department of Otorhinolaryngology – Head and Neck Surgery, Antwerp University Hospital, Edegem, Belgium, [2] Department of Rehabilitation Sciences and Physiotherapy, Antwerp University, Antwerp, Belgium, [3] Department of Translational Neurosciences, Antwerp University, Antwerp, Belgium, [4] Hoorzorg Van Looveren BVBA, Borsbeek, Belgium, [5] Department of Education, Health and Social Work, University College Ghent, Ghent, Belgium

***Correspondence:**
Sarah Michiels
sarah.michiels@uantwerpen.be
Annick Gilles
annick.gilles@uza.be

† These authors have contributed equally to this work

Introduction: Tinnitus is a complex symptom requiring a thorough multidisciplinary assessment to construct an individual's tinnitus profile. The Antwerp University Hospital hosts a tertiary tinnitus clinic providing intensive, multidisciplinary tinnitus care in the form of combinational psychological treatment with either Tinnitus Retraining Therapy (TRT)/Cognitive Behavioral Therapy (CBT) or TRT/eye movement desensitization and reprocessing therapy (EMDR), high-definition transcranial direct current stimulation (HD-tDCS), and physical therapy treatment (in cases of somatic influence of the neck or the temporomandibular area). Several factors may contribute to therapy effect of which the role of gender has recently gained more interest. As such, the current manuscript explores gender differences in the outcome of different tinnitus treatments.

Methods: Data on treatment outcome of four distinct tinnitus treatments (1. HD-tDCS; 2. orofacial physical therapy; 3. combination TRT + CBT; and 4. combination TRT + EMDR) were pooled and compared. Treatment outcome was assessed via the Tinnitus Functional Index (TFI). Participants completed the TFI at baseline, immediately after treatment and after 9 weeks (±3 weeks) follow-up. To explore the effect of gender on different treatment outcomes, a linear mixed model was designed including *Time point*, *Gender*, and *Therapy Group* as fixed factors as well as all interactions between these factors.

Results: TFI scores improved significantly over time regardless of therapy group ($p < 0.0001$). A mean TFI decrease of at least 13 points was obtained by all participants except by those in the HD-tDCS. Significant interactions between Gender and Time point were identified in all groups except for the TRT +EMDR group. Female subjects improved more extensively than males in the HD-tDCS ($p = 0.0009$) and orofacial therapy group ($p = 0.0299$). Contrarily, in the TRT +CBT group, male participants showed a significant improvement whereas the mean TFI scores of female subjects remained on baseline levels ($p = 0.0138$).

Conclusion: Our data suggest that male and female tinnitus patients seem to react differently to different therapy options. We strongly encourage further prospective studies to discern the relevance of gender in therapy outcome.

Keywords: gender, tinnitus, gender-related outcome, TRT, CBT, neuromodulation, HDtDCS, tDCS

INTRODUCTION

Tinnitus, the perception of sound in the absence of an external sound source, is a frequently experienced symptom in modern society. The prevalence of tinnitus in an adult population is around 15% (Seidman and Jacobson, 1996; Gilles et al., 2012). In 2–3% of patients, the tinnitus is sufficiently bothersome to affect the quality of life due to the association with anxiety, depression, sleep disorders, concentration difficulties, and elevated stress levels (Henry et al., 2005). As a consequence, many patients find their way to the clinic seeking for alleviating treatment. In the management of tinnitus, a multi-disciplinary approach is essential in order to tailor therapy toward the patient's requirements and needs. Thorough evaluation of the patient comprises a systematic history including tinnitus characteristics, potential tinnitus triggers, and the evaluation of coexisting symptoms such as subjective hearing loss, otalgia, decreased speech understanding (Gilles et al., 2016), vertigo, and hyperacusis (Van de Heyning et al., 2015). The presence of cervical spine dysfunction as well as bruxism or known history of temporomandibular dysfunctions should be inquired and assessed accordingly as somatosensory influences may cause tinnitus and/or increase pre-existing tinnitus loudness or alter pitch (Michiels et al., 2015a, 2018b). In addition, the comorbidity with depression or anxiety disorders should be assessed, as emotional factors typical in these disorders are strong predictors of poor adjustment to the symptom of tinnitus (Zoger et al., 2006; Pattyn et al., 2016). Following extensive anamnesis, further multidisciplinary investigations as well as imaging may be required leading toward an individual tinnitus profile guiding the patient toward the most appropriate patient-specific therapy (Van de Heyning et al., 2015).

Yearly, approximately 1500 patients consult the tertiary expertise tinnitus clinic [Tinnitus Treatment and Research Centre Antwerp (TINTRA)] at the Antwerp University Hospital, with tinnitus being their primary complaint. Through a multidisciplinary approach, patients receive treatment according to their tinnitus profile, underlying causes/mediators and psychological burden. For all patients, pre-therapeutic tinnitus burden is measured at baseline, post-therapy, and at 9 weeks (±3 weeks) follow-up moment using tinnitus questionnaires.

Several treatments provided at TINTRA are psychology-based focusing on altering the coping strategies in order to change emotional responses toward the tinnitus. Cognitive Behavioral Therapy (CBT) in particular aims to change non-constructive cognitive distortions/behaviors and develop personal coping strategies targeting the tinnitus issues. Tinnitus Retraining Therapy (TRT) on the other hand is a habituation therapy in which directive counseling aims to reclassify the tinnitus percept to a neutral signal in combination with the use of sound therapy. Both CBT and TRT have proven to be effective in the treatment of tinnitus (Jastreboff and Jastreboff, 2000; Jastreboff, 2007, 2015; Cima et al., 2014). Eye movement desensitization and reprocessing (EMDR) therapy is a form of psychotherapy in which the patient is enquired to recall distressing thoughts/images (i.e., associated with the tinnitus) after which the therapist directs the patient with bilateral sensory input (i.e., hand tapping, auditory stimuli, or side-to-side eye movements). EMDR is a widely used technique in the treatment of post-traumatic stress disorder (Guideline Development Panel for the Treatment of PTSD in Adults, and American Psychological Association, 2019). In the field of tinnitus, a first preliminary study on EMDR was recently published showing promising results as significant improvement on tinnitus burden (measured by the Tinnitus Handicap Inventory) and depressive symptoms (measured by the Beck Depression Inventory) was shown up until 6 months after EMDR treatment (Phillips et al., 2019).

Also, transcranial direct current stimulation (tDCS) has been a topic of research at TINTRA. TDCS is a form of neuromodulation delivering a constant, low direct current to the brain through electrodes positioned on the head. Up until now, a total of 31 studies evaluated the effects of tDCS on tinnitus reporting various degrees of effect, ranging from no effect to significant tinnitus reduction. A large heterogeneity in used tDCS protocols and outcomes is apparent which constrains the comparability of these studies (Lefaucheur, 2016; Lefaucheur et al., 2017). At our department tDCS trials have shown clinically significant improvement in 32% of patients with large inter-individual variability (Jacquemin et al., 2018).

For patients who experience a somatosensory influence on tinnitus originating in a dysfunction of the cervical spine or temporomandibular area (Michiels et al., 2015b, 2016b, 2018a), physiotherapy treatment is provided. Depending on the area of the dysfunction that is primarily influencing the tinnitus, the physical therapy treatment is adjusted. In case of a primary influence from the cervical spine, a multimodal manual physical therapy can be provided (Michiels et al., 2016a, 2017). This type of treatment showed a significant improvement on the global perceived effect in 53% of the patients in our clinic (Michiels et al., 2016c). In case temporomandibular dysfunctions are primarily influencing the tinnitus, orofacial physiotherapy is provided, when needed combined with occlusal splints provided by the dentist. A recent systematic review on the topic showed promising results, although differences in treatment modalities and outcome measures make it hard to draw any definitive conclusions (Michiels et al., 2019).

As the tinnitus population is highly heterogeneous, a one-therapy-fits-all approach is non-existent and many treatments may add to tinnitus alleviation depending on the patients' tinnitus profile. Due to the heterogeneity, treatment outcomes also tend to vary tremendously. Recently the role of gender on the perception of tinnitus has gathered more attention. In a study by Seydel et al. (2013), women showed more tinnitus-related distress compared to men with this effect depending on age and duration of the tinnitus. These results were partially confirmed by a recent study by Han et al. (2019) and some authors have mentioned gender difference in the amount of tinnitus-related distress as well (Hiller and Goebel, 2006), whereas others did not find any gender differences (Meric et al., 1998; Pinto et al., 2010). As a result, the role of gender remains elusive. Recently, severe tinnitus was shown to be associated with an increased risk of suicide attempts in female patients only (Lugo et al., 2019). Interestingly, those patients who had been diagnosed with tinnitus in a clinical setting were no longer at risk, highlighting the need for specialty care in the tinnitus population. If males and females perceive tinnitus differently and, as a consequence, possibly show distinct reactions toward therapeutic intervention, caregivers should take these gender differences into account. The current manuscript reports on the effects of gender on the outcomes of the distinct tinnitus therapies provided at TINTRA.

MATERIALS AND METHODS

Study Protocol

The current manuscript describes the effects of gender on tinnitus treatment outcome. Therefore, all data collected prior to treatment, post-treatment, and at a follow-up visit (9 ± 3 weeks) of patients who received tinnitus treatment, were analyzed retrospectively. All patients had chronic, non-pulsatile, subjective tinnitus for longer than 3 months. Patients with active middle ear pathology were excluded from analysis. Pure tone audiometry was performed at baseline using a two-channel Interacoustics AC-40 audiometer and headphones in a soundproof booth. Air conduction thresholds were measured at 125, 250, 500, 1000, 2000, 3000, 4000, 6000, and 8000 Hz. Bone conduction thresholds were tested at 250, 500, 1000, 2000, 3000, and 4000 Hz. Tinnitus evaluation was performed using self-administering questionnaires.

Treatment

Psychological Treatment

Two combination psychological therapies were provided with either TRT +CBT combination (five sessions TRT/five sessions CBT) or TRT+EMDR combination (five sessions TRT/five sessions EDMR). All therapies were provided by licensed TRT audiologists and CBT/EMDR psychologists. The full approach of this bimodal psychotherapy is described in Luyten et al. (2019).

High-Definition Transcranial Direct Current Stimulation

Patients received six sessions of high-definition tDCS (HD-tDCS) over 3 weeks' time (2x/week) with silver/silverchloride electrodes placed on the right dorsolateral prefrontal cortex (dLPFC). A direct current of 2 mA was applied with a 20 s fade-in/fade-out time delivered by a battery-driven 1 × 1 tDCS low-intensity stimulator and 4 × 1 multichannel stimulation adaptor (Soterix Medical Inc., New York, NY, United States) as described in the HD-tDCS stimulation guidelines (Villamar et al., 2013). During each session, the patient received 20 min of stimulation.

Conservative Temporomandibular Treatment

Patients received a maximum of 18 sessions of orofacial therapy during a fixed time window of 9 weeks. This therapy was primarily directed to the temporomandibular joint and masticatory muscles. If present, cervical spine dysfunctions were treated as well, using a combination of manual mobilizations and exercise therapy. In case of severe bruxism, an occlusal splint was provided in addition to the physiotherapy. Therapists, providing the orofacial physiotherapy, were trained to the study protocol prior to the start of the study. More details can be found in the published study protocol (Michiels et al., 2018b).

Treatment Allocation

Treatment allocation to one of the four interventions described below was based on patients' complaints and needs as discussed during an intake visit at the TINTRA tinnitus consultation. For instance, only patients with self-reported temporomandibular complaints were considered for the orofacial therapy. Different therapy options were discussed based on individual patients' tinnitus profiles, and final treatment decisions were made by the patients. Thus, a certain level of selection bias was present in the treatment allocation, but this was solely based on individual patients' needs. Demographic variables, such as gender, were never taken into account as a deciding factor for treatment choice.

Ethics

All patients filled out an informed consent in which permission was granted to use their data gathered during and prior to tinnitus treatment. Ethics Committee approval numbers involved in the current analysis are 16/41/415, 16/35/360, and 16/48/513.

Questionnaires

Tinnitus Functional Index

The Tinnitus Functional Index (TFI) (Meikle et al., 2012; Rabau et al., 2014) consists of 25 items assessing the tinnitus severity as well as the impact of tinnitus in daily life. In addition to a total score reflecting the total tinnitus burden, eight subscales define the level of inconvenience for the following aspects: intrusiveness, reduced sense of control, cognitive interference, sleep disturbance, auditory difficulties, interference with relaxation, reduced quality of life, and emotional distress. The TFI has proven to be useful in the assessment of treatment-related changes in tinnitus. As such, a reduction of 13 points on the total TFI score after tinnitus treatment is considered as a clinically relevant and subjectively perceived reduction for the patient (Meikle et al., 2012).

Visual Analog Scale

The mean tinnitus loudness throughout the day was assessed by use of a Visual Analog Scale (VAS). In this case, the patient had to indicate the mean tinnitus loudness over the last week on a scale from 0 (no tinnitus at all) to 100 (the most extreme loudness one can imagine) by use of a ruler.

Hyperacusis Questionnaire

The Hyperacusis Questionnaire (HQ) (Khalfa et al., 2002; Meeus et al., 2010) determines the presence/absence of hyperacusis. According to Khalfa's original HQ, one can speak of hyperacusis when the score on the HQ is 28 or higher (Khalfa et al., 2002).

Hospital Anxiety and Depression Scale

The Hospital Anxiety and Depression Scale (HADS) is a screening tool to detect symptoms of anxiety and/or depression (Zigmond and Snaith, 1983). The HADS consists of 14 items in total assessing increased signs of anxiety (seven items) or depression (seven items). For each of the subscales, a score between 8 and 10 is considered as "borderline" while a score of 11 and higher is considered as "case."

Statistics

A linear mixed model was designed using JMP® Pro software (JMP® Pro, Version 14.0.0, 2018 SAS Institute Inc., Cary, NC, United States, 1989–2019) to explore the effects of gender on outcomes of different tinnitus treatments. Total TFI score was chosen as the outcome variable. The model applied the following fixed factors: Time point (baseline, post-treatment, follow-up), Gender (male, female), and Therapy group (HD-tDCS, orofacial therapy, TRT combined with CBT, TRT combined with EMDR). All possible two-way interactions between these factors were added to the model, as well as the three-way interaction Time point*Gender*Therapy group. Possible confounding factors were added to the model in a stepwise additive manner. These factors were age, hearing level (pure tone averages for 1, 2, and 4 kHz), tinnitus characteristics (type, duration, and laterality of the tinnitus), scores on the HADS depression and anxiety subscales, and scores on the HQ. Considerably more men than women were in all therapy groups except for the orofacial therapy group, in which the gender distribution was more balanced. Participant was added as a random intercept. *Post hoc* analyses were performed using linear mixed models for each of the four therapy groups separately. Here, Time point and Gender were added as fixed factors with an additional two-way interaction of Time point*Gender. *P*-values of < 0.05 were considered significant.

RESULTS

Data from 316 patients were included in the analysis. An overview of patients' characteristics at baseline can be found in **Table 1**. Considerably more men than women were included in all therapy groups except for the orofacial therapy group, in which the gender distribution was more balanced. Age varied slightly between therapy groups, with mean age in the HD-tDCS group being the highest and participants in the orofacial therapy group being the youngest. Hearing levels did not differ significantly between groups, nor did tinnitus characteristics (duration, type, and laterality of the tinnitus) or TFI scores at baseline. Some group level differences were found for the

TABLE 1 | Demographic details and tinnitus characteristics at baseline.

	HD-tDCS (*n* = 117)			Orofacial therapy (*n* = 109)			TRT + CBT (*n* = 44)			TRT + EDMR (*n* = 46)		
	M	**F**	***p***	**M**	**F**	***p***	**M**	**F**	***p***	**M**	**F**	***p***
Gender (*n*)	97	20		56	53		34	10		30	16	
Age (years: mean [SD])	50.02 [12.60]	53.65 [10.81]	0.2329	42.68 [15.44]	47.68 [14.22]	0.0819	49.32 [13.46]	44.5 [12.34]	0.3165	48.33 [12.44]	46[12.13]	0.5443
Hearing level: PTA (db HL: mean [SD])	19.29 [13.48]	15.38 [11.84]	0.2309	13.85 [13.02]	16.30 [13.92]	0.3491	19.75 [15.60]	8.92 [5.93]	0.0385	17.22 [14.41]	16.09 [17.39]	0.8151
Tinnitus characteristics												
Tinnitus duration(years: mean[SD])	6.59 [7.49]	4.06 [5.63]	0.1546	5.27 [7.30]	4.98 [7.14]	0.8351	9.08 [10.56]	3.35 [1.81]	0.0978	8.23 [8.98]	3.97 [2.89]	0.0728
Tinnitus laterality(*n*: right/left/bilateral/central)	13/12/57/15	1/3/13/3	0.7066	6/9/27/13	6/5/33/7	0.2132	2/8/15/9	0/3/6/1	0.4497	3 / 6 /12 / 9	2 / 4 /6 / 4	0.9624
Tinnitus type(*n*: pure tone/noise/polyphonic)	67/22/8	12/4/4	0.3468	32/16/7	22/25/4	0.0862	25/7/2	3/4/3	0.0310	18 / 8 / 4	11 / 3 / 2	0.8126
TFI scores(mean [SD])	45.5 [18.62]	55.5 [23.44]	0.0390	50.64 [18.67]	54.02 [15.35]	0.3050	48.92 [22.10]	54.24 [22.11]	0.5068	51.37 [18.31]	58.58 [18.22]	0.2098
Questionnaire scores												
HADS anxiety(mean [SD])	7.29 [3.60]	9.2[4.82]	0.0443	8.91 [4.06]	8.43 [4.22]	0.5524	8.79 [4.42]	12.6 [4.43]	0.0212	8.53 [4.01]	11[3.92]	0.0512
HADS depression(mean [SD])	6.77 [4.05]	7.65 [5.49]	0.4106	7.09 [4.49]	5.36 [4.54]	0.0488	6.91 [4.25]	9.7[4.52]	0.0794	7.53 [4.61]	7.56 [4.07]	0.9831
HQ scores(mean [SD])	18.34 [7.74]	21.25 [9.59]	0.1448	17.22 [7.19]	17.61 [8.89]	0.8039	20.74 [9.15]	26.9 [7.72]	0.0600	20.93 [7.90]	26.81 [3.87]	0.0077

HD-tDCS: High-Definition transcranial Direct Current Stimulation; TRT: Tinnitus Retraining Therapy; CBT: Cognitive Behavioral Therapy; EMDR: eye movement desensitization and reprocessing therapy; PTA: Pure Tone Average for 1, 2, and 4 kHz; TFI: Tinnitus Functional Index; HADS: Hospital Anxiety and Depression Scale; HQ: Hyperacusis Questionnaire. Standard least squares (for continuous variables) or nominal logistic models (for dichotomous variables) were designed to test whether male and female participants in each of the four therapy groups differed significantly; resulting p-values are shown in the last column.

TABLE 2 | Results of the linear mixed model analysis.

	p-value
Fixed factors	
Time point	<0.0001
Gender	0.0496
Therapy group	0.1072
HADS depression subscale scores	<0.0001
HQ scores	0.0007
Interactions	
Time point * Gender	0.7613
Time point * Therapy group	0.0023
Gender * Therapy group	0.5761
Time point * Gender * Therapy group	0.0002

HADS: Hospital Anxiety and Depression Scale; HQ: Hyperacusis Questionnaire.

additional questionnaire scores, with participants in the HD-tDCS and orofacial therapy groups scoring lower on the anxiety subscale of the HADS and on the HQ than patients in both psychotherapeutic groups.

Results of the linear mixed model analysis are summarized in **Table 2**. Of all putative confounding factors, only the HADS depression subscale score and the HQ score were found to contribute significantly to the model. All other possible confounding factors (age, hearing level, tinnitus characteristics, and HADS anxiety subscale scores) did not have any demonstrable effect on the model and were excluded from the analysis. Thus, the final model included two additional factors (HADS depression scores and HQ scores) next to the fixed factors Time point, Gender, and Therapy group. Overall, a significant fixed effect of time point was found, with TFI scores decreasing over time for all therapy groups and for both genders ($p < 0.0001$) (**Figure 1A**). Additionally, the main effect of gender was found to be significant, with women generally having a higher TFI score than men ($p = 0.0496$) (**Figure 1B**). A significant interaction between Time point and Therapy group was identified ($p = 0.0023$), indicating that TFI scores of participants in different therapy groups evolved differently over time. Crucially, a significant three-way interaction between Time point, Gender, and Therapy group was found ($p = 0.0002$). This interaction implies that treatment response in the different therapy groups was modulated by gender (**Figure 2**).

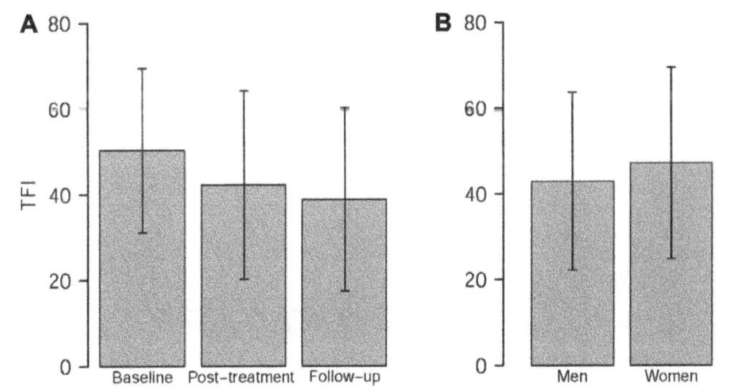

FIGURE 1 | Main effects of time point **(A)** and gender **(B)**. **(A)** TFI scores change significantly over time, independently of therapy group or gender ($p < 0.0001$). TFI scores at baseline: 50.34 ± 19.13; TFI scores at the post-treatment time point: 42.24 ± 21.99; TFI scores at follow-up: 38.84 ± 21.39; mean ± SD. **(B)** TFI scores are higher in women than in men, independently of therapy group or time point ($p = 0.0496$). TFI scores for women: 47.19 ± 22.28; TFI scores for men: 42.93 ± 20.79; mean ± SD. Error bars represent SD. TFI: Tinnitus Functional Index.

To further explore this highly significant three-way interaction, *post hoc* analyses were performed for each therapy group. Similar to the primary analysis, HADS depression subscale scores and HQ scores were added to the model as confounding factors. In three out of four therapy groups, significant interactions between *Time point* and *Gender* were found. These interactions indicate that the evolution of TFI scores depended on gender in these specific therapy groups. In the HD-tDCS (*Time point*Gender*: $p = 0.0009$) and orofacial therapy group (*Time point*Gender*: $p = 0.0299$), female participants generally had higher TFI scores at baseline, but improved more extensively than male subjects (**Figures 2A,B**). On average, TFI scores of female participants in the HD-tDCS group decreased by 15.83 ± 24.27 points from baseline to follow-up, whereas male participants' TFI scores dropped by only 2.53 ± 13.79 points. In the orofacial therapy group, female participants' TFI scores decreased by 19.02 ± 16.85 points while scores of male participants decreased by 10.53 ± 19.65 points.

Contrarily, in the TRT + CBT group, male subjects improved significantly over time whereas female participants' mean TFI scores only decreased slightly after treatment ($p = 0.327$) but did not remain stable at follow-up (**Figure 2C**) (*Time point*Gender*: $p = 0.0138$). From baseline to follow-up, male participants' TFI scores decreased by 22.42 ± 23.02 points whereas TFI scores of female subjects in this group actually increased marginally with 0.44 ± 21.26 points. Finally, in the TRT + EMDR group, the two-way interaction *Time point*Gender* was not significant ($p = 0.5240$), with men and women improving over time in a highly similar way (**Figure 2D**). The decrease in TFI scores from baseline to follow-up was 19.1 ± 18.52 and 16.46 ± 14.3 points in female and male participants, respectively.

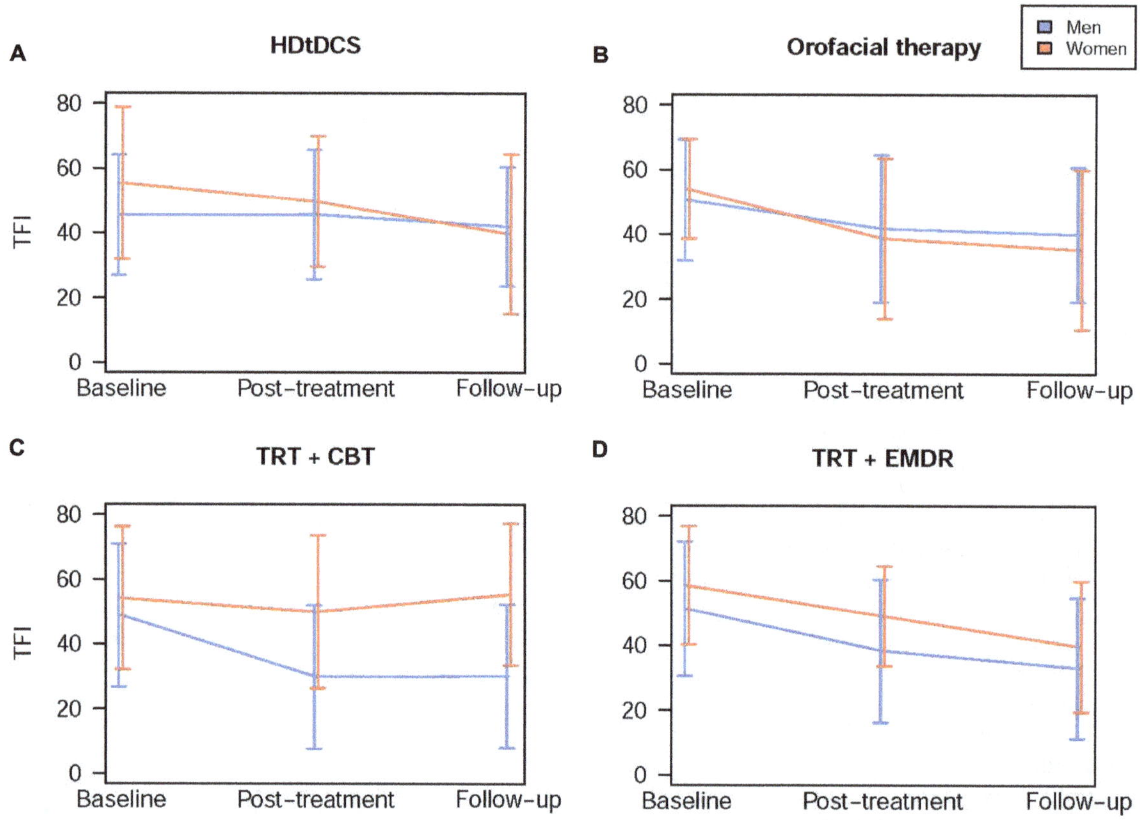

FIGURE 2 | Treatment outcome in different therapy groups differs according to gender. Blue lines represent male subjects and red lines represent female subjects. Data are presented as mean TFI scores for each time point ± SD. **(A)** Female participants benefit more from HDtDCS treatment than men. TFI scores decreased more in female participants (−15.83 ± 24.27) than male (−2.53 ± 13.79) from baseline to follow-up. **(B)** Female participants benefit more from orofacial therapy than men. TFI scores decreased more in female participants (−19.02 ± 16.85) than male (−10.53 ± 19.65) from baseline to follow-up. **(C)** Male participants benefit more from TRT combined with CBT than women. TFI scores decreased more in male participants (−22.42 ± 23.02) than female (0.44 ± 21.26) from baseline to follow-up. **(D)** Male and female participants benefit equally from TRT combined with EMDR. TFI scores decreased similarly in male (−19.1 ± 15.82) and female participants (−16.46 ± 14.3) from baseline to follow-up. TFI: Tinnitus Functional Index; HDtDCS: High-Definition transcranial Direct Current Stimulation; TRT: Tinnitus Retraining Therapy; CBT: Cognitive Behavioral Therapy; EMDR: Eye Movement Desensitization and Reprocessing.

HADS depression subscale scores and HQ scores were found to contribute significantly to the model. *Post hoc* analyses revealed that both questionnaire scores had a significant effect on tinnitus severity, with higher scores on both questionnaires equaling higher total TFI scores. These effects were not dependent on either *Time point* or *Gender*, as evidenced by the non-significance of the interactions between these questionnaire scores and *Time point* (p = 0.5914 for HADS depression scores, p = 0.1814 for HQ scores) or *Gender* (p = 0.6806 for HADS depression scores, p = 0.1868 for HQ scores).

DISCUSSION

The large variability in tinnitus treatment outcomes may be driven by differences in individual patient characteristics. The current manuscript retrospectively explored whether gender may account for any of this heterogeneity. We report remarkable gender effects on treatment outcomes of several tinnitus therapy options. Overall, our results indicate that gender might be an influential mediator of treatment outcome.

In a large group of tinnitus patients, we found that women benefited from orofacial physiotherapy to a greater extent than men. In the general population, a recent meta-analysis showed that the risk for developing temporomandibular disorders (TMD) is twice as high in women than in men (Bueno et al., 2018). Likewise, a study of Vielsmeier et al. (2011) showed that significantly more women than men had TMD in a population of patients with tinnitus, something which was also found in the general population (Edvall et al., 2019). Therefore, we hypothesize that the proportion of true TMD sufferers was higher in female than in male patients. This gender difference in baseline TMD burden may then explain the higher success ratio of conservative orofacial treatment in female tinnitus patients. Currently, no other studies reported on gender differences in orofacial treatment effect on tinnitus complaints. It must also be noted that although statistically significant, the difference in decrease in TFI score between males and females in this treatment group is small. Our results should therefore be confirmed in future research, specifically designed to investigate gender differences.

In our study population, women also demonstrated a better treatment response after receiving consecutive sessions of HD-tDCS. These results are in agreement with Frank et al. (2012), who reported larger beneficial effects of frontal tDCS in women. Both protocols comprised anodal stimulation of the right dLPFC, suggesting that this gender difference might be driven by true underlying physiological differences. Indeed, dLPFC volume has been shown to be greater in women than men (Schlaepfer et al., 1995; Luders et al., 2009), and anodal tDCS of the prefrontal cortex might have greater effects in females (Fumagalli et al., 2010). These findings cannot be explained by the amount of current intensity going through the brain as it was previously shown that females receive significantly less current compared to males when targeting parietal and frontal areas due to more dense parietal bone in females (Russell et al., 2014). A significant difference in TFI at baseline between males and females was observed with females showing higher TFI scores which may imply a greater opportunity for improvement in this population. However, even after correcting for this difference in baseline TFI score, the effect of gender over time remained significant. In addition, no equal proportion of male and female subjects was obtained in this therapy group so these results need to be interpreted with caution.

Conversely, in our study population, male patients benefited more than females from TRT combined with CBT, while both males and females experienced significant improvement through EMDR therapy. Although some evidence exists for gender differences in tinnitus perception and distress, literature on gender effects on the efficacy of psychological tinnitus treatments is scarce. To date, meta-analyses on psychotherapy outcomes report minimal to no gender differences (Bowman et al., 2001; Felmingham and Bryant, 2012; Swift et al., 2013; Tao et al., 2015; Budge and Moradi, 2019).

In a study reporting on the long-term effects of TRT combined with cognitive-behavioral elements, Seydel et al. (2010) reported subtle gender differences on treatment outcome. Male and female patients showed similar outcomes of this treatment overall, but women experiencing longer (>2 years and especially >10 years) tinnitus duration were less likely to maintain positive treatment effect at a 1-year follow-up time point. In our dataset, we did not identify any effects of tinnitus duration. However, the relatively long average tinnitus duration (7.78 years) might account for this gender difference on the outcome of a treatment combining TRT and CBT. About 70% of the female participants included in the TRT + CBT group reported a psychiatric diagnosis in the present or the past. These findings suggest that 10 sessions might not be sufficient to alleviate the complex tangle of aggravating complaints. The proportion of patients with psychiatric comorbidity was lower in the TRT + EMDR group. Given the fact that 40% of female participants did report a significant decrease of 13 points or more in the TRT + CBT group, we emphasize the identifiable influence of psychiatric comorbidity on treatment outcome. However, the cognitive behavioral approach could have influenced therapy outcome on the basis of the cognitive therapeutic techniques that were used. Some evidence can be found on women to experience more therapeutic gain through an emotion-focused treatment (Ogrodniczuk et al., 2001; Matud, 2004; Ogrodniczuk, 2006; Meléndez et al., 2012) whereas men tend to react better to a problem-focused therapy which is more integrated in the CBT approach (Samoilov and Goldfried, 2000). More empirical evidence is required to investigate whether these findings can be replicated. We interpret these results with caution, taking into account the importance of the individual characteristics of the female participants in this considerably small sample size compared to the proportion of male participants.

The results presented here are highly explorative, and large prospective trials are needed to confirm or disprove the gender effects we demonstrate. It would be especially prudent for future studies to ensure an even inclusion of men and women, as the gender balance is disturbed in many studies, as well as in several of the therapy groups discussed in this paper. Furthermore, as we identified additional effects of symptoms of depression and hyperacusis, controlling for these factors is undeniably crucial.

We have demonstrated considerable effects of gender on tinnitus treatment outcome for different therapy options. Our results suggest that women might experience greater effects of orofacial physiotherapy and transcranial direct current stimulation compared to men. Within the psychotherapeutic treatments, we identified subtle gender differences between the outcome of CBT compared to eye movement desensitization and retraining, but mainly note that individual differences and psychiatric comorbidity affect the therapeutic pathway and treatment outcome. We report remarkable gender effects on treatment outcomes of several tinnitus therapy options. Overall, our results indicate that gender might be of influence for treatment outcome. Consequently, it might be important to consider gender when estimating the chance for treatment success.

AUTHOR CONTRIBUTIONS

AV, TL, LJ, and NV contributed to data collection. AG and SM contributed to PI. VV, OV, VT, PV, and WD contributed to protocol and statistics. EC, SM, and AG contributed to analysis. AG, AV, TL, and EC contributed to manuscript writing.

REFERENCES

Bowman, D., Scogin, F., Floyd, M., and McKendree-Smith, N. (2001). Psychotherapy length of stay and outcome: a meta-analysis of the effect of therapist sex. *Psychotherapy* 38, 142–148. doi: 10.1037/0033-3204.38.2.142

Budge, S. L., and Moradi, B. (2019). Gender identity. *Psychother. Relationsh. Work* 2:133.

Bueno, C. H., Pereira, D. D., Pattussi, M. P., Grossi, P. K., and Grossi, M. L. (2018). Gender differences in temporomandibular disorders in adult populational studies: a systematic review and meta-analysis. *J. Oral Rehabil.* 45, 720–729. doi: 10.1111/joor.12661

Cima, R. F., Andersson, G., Schmidt, C. J., and Henry, J. A. (2014). Cognitive-behavioral treatments for tinnitus: a review of the literature. *J. Am. Acad. Audiol.* 25, 29–61. doi: 10.3766/jaaa.25.1.4

Edvall, N. K., Gunan, E., Genitsaridi, E., Lazar, A., Mehraei, G., Billing, M., et al. (2019). Impact of temporomandibular joint complaints on tinnitus-related distress. *Front. Neurosci.* 13:879. doi: 10.3389/fnins.2019.00879

Felmingham, K. L., and Bryant, R. A. (2012). Gender differences in the maintenance of response to cognitive behavior therapy for posttraumatic stress disorder. *J. Consult. Clin. Psychol.* 80, 196–200. doi: 10.1037/a0027156

Frank, E., Schecklmann, M., Landgrebe, M., Burger, J., Kreuzer, P., Poeppl, T. B., et al. (2012). Treatment of chronic tinnitus with repeated sessions of prefrontal transcranial direct current stimulation: outcomes from an open-label pilot study. *J. Neurol.* 259, 327–333. doi: 10.1007/s00415-011-6189-4

Fumagalli, M., Vergari, M., Pasqualetti, P., Marceglia, S., Mameli, F., Ferrucci, R., et al. (2010). Brain switches utilitarian behavior: does gender make the difference? *PLoS One* 5:e8865. doi: 10.1371/journal.pone.0008865

Gilles, A., De Ridder, D., Van Hal, G., Wouters, K., Kleine Punte, A., and Van de Heyning, P. (2012). Prevalence of leisure noise-induced tinnitus and the attitude toward noise in university students. *Otol. Neurotol.* 33, 899–906. doi: 10.1097/MAO.0b013e31825d640a

Gilles, A., Schlee, W., Rabau, S., Wouters, K., Fransen, E., and Van de Heyning, P. (2016). Decreased speech-in-noise understanding in young adults with tinnitus. *Front. Neurosci.* 10:288. doi: 10.3389/fnins.2016.00288

Guideline Development Panel for the Treatment of PTSD in Adults, and American Psychological Association (2019). Summary of the clinical practice guideline for the treatment of posttraumatic stress disorder (PTSD) in adults. *Am. Psychol.* 74, 596–607. doi: 10.1037/amp0000473

Han, T. S., Jeong, J. E., Park, S. N., and Kim, J. J. (2019). Gender differences affecting psychiatric distress and tinnitus severity. *Clin. Psychopharmacol. Neurosci.* 17, 113–120. doi: 10.9758/cpn.2019.17.1.113

Henry, J. A., Dennis, K. C., and Schechter, M. A. (2005). General review of tinnitus: prevalence, mechanisms, effects, and management. *J. Speech Lang Hear.Res.* 48, 1204–1235. doi: 10.1044/1092-4388(2005/084)

Hiller, W., and Goebel, G. (2006). Factors influencing tinnitus loudness and annoyance. *Arch. Otolaryngol. Head Neck Surg.* 132, 1323–1330. doi: 10.1001/archotol.132.12.1323

Jacquemin, L., Shekhawat, G. S., Van de Heyning, P., Mertens, G., Fransen, E., Van Rompaey, V., et al. (2018). Effects of electrical stimulation in tinnitus patients: conventional versus high-definition tDCS. *Neurorehabil. Neural Repair* 32, 714–723. doi: 10.1177/1545968318787916

Jastreboff, P. J. (2007). Tinnitus retraining therapy. *Prog. Brain Res.* 166, 415–423. doi: 10.1016/S0079-6123(07)66040-3

Jastreboff, P. J. (2015). 25 years of tinnitus retraining therapy. *HNO* 63, 307–311. doi: 10.1007/s00106-014-2979-1

Jastreboff, P. J., and Jastreboff, M. M. (2000). Tinnitus Retraining Therapy (TRT) as a method for treatment of tinnitus and hyperacusis patients. *J. Am. Acad. Audiol.* 11, 162–177.

Khalfa, S., Dubal, S., Veuillet, E., Perez-Diaz, F., Jouvent, R., and Collet, L. (2002). Psychometric normalization of a hyperacusis questionnaire. *ORL J. Otorhinolaryngol. Relat. Spec.* 64, 436–442. doi: 10.1159/000067570

Lefaucheur, J. P. (2016). A comprehensive database of published tDCS clinical trials (2005-2016). *Neurophysiol. Clin.* 46, 319–398. doi: 10.1016/j.neucli.2016.10.002

Lefaucheur, J. P., Antal, A., Ayache, S. S., Benninger, D. H., Brunelin, J., Cogiamanian, F., et al. (2017). Evidence-based guidelines on the therapeutic use of transcranial direct current stimulation (tDCS). *Clin. Neurophysiol.* 128, 56–92. doi: 10.1016/j.clinph.2016.10.087

Luders, E., Gaser, C., Narr, K. L., and Toga, A. W. (2009). Why sex matters: brain size independent differences in gray matter distributions between men and women. *J. Neurosci.* 29, 14265–14270. doi: 10.1523/JNEUROSCI.2261-09.2009

Lugo, A., Trpchevska, N., Liu, X., Biswas, R., Magnusson, C., Gallus, S., et al. (2019). Sex-specific association of tinnitus with suicide attempts. *JAMA Otolaryngol. Head Neck Surg.* 145, 685–687. doi: 10.1001/jamaoto.2019.0566

Luyten, T., Van de Heyning, P., Jacquemin, L., Van Looveren, N., Declau, F., Fransen, E., et al. (2019). The value of eye movement desensitization reprocessing in the treatment of tinnitus: study protocol for a randomized controlled trial. *Trials* 20:32. doi: 10.1186/s13063-018-3121-6

Matud, M. P. (2004). Gender differences in stress and coping styles. *Pers. Individ. Diff.* 37, 1401–1415. doi: 10.1016/j.paid.2004.01.010

Meeus, O. M., Spaepen, M., Ridder, D. D., and Heyning, P. H. (2010). Correlation between hyperacusis measurements in daily ENT practice. *Int. J. Audiol.* 49, 7–13. doi: 10.3109/14992020903160868

Meikle, M. B., Henry, J. A., Griest, S. E., Stewart, B. J., Abrams, H. B., McArdle, R., et al. (2012). The tinnitus functional index: development of a new clinical measure for chronic, intrusive tinnitus. *Ear Hear.* 33, 153–176. doi: 10.1097/AUD.0b013e31822f67c0

Meléndez, J. C., Mayordomo, T., Sancho, P., and Tomás, J. M. (2012). Coping strategies: gender differences and development throughout life span. *Span. J. Psychol.* 15, 1089–1098. doi: 10.5209/rev_sjop.2012.v15.n3.39399

Meric, C., Gartner, M., Collet, L., and Chery-Croze, S. (1998). Psychopathological profile of tinnitus sufferers: evidence concerning the relationship between tinnitus features and impact on life. *Audiol. Neurootol.* 3, 240–252. doi: 10.1159/000013796

Michiels, S., De Hertogh, W., Truijen, S., and Van de Heyning, P. (2015a). Cervical spine dysfunctions in patients with chronic subjective tinnitus. *Otol. Neurotol.* 36, 741–745. doi: 10.1097/MAO.0000000000000670

Michiels, S., Van de Heyning, P., Truijen, S., and De Hertogh, W. (2015b). Diagnostic value of clinical cervical spine tests in patients with cervicogenic somatic tinnitus. *Phys. Ther.* 95, 1529–1535. doi: 10.2522/ptj.20140457

Michiels, S., De Hertogh, W., Truijen, S., and Van De Heyning, P. (2016a). The effect of cervical physical therapy in patients with cervicogenic somatic tinnitus. *Man. Ther.* 25:e102. doi: 10.1016/j.math.2016.05.180

Michiels, S., Naessens, S., Van de Heyning, P., Braem, M., Visscher, C. M., Gilles, A., et al. (2016b). The effect of physical therapy treatment in patients with subjective tinnitus: a systematic review. *Front. Neurosci.* 10:545. doi: 10.3389/fnins.2016.00545

Michiels, S., Van de Heyning, P., Truijen, S., Hallemans, A., and De Hertogh, W. (2016c). Does multi-modal cervical physical therapy improve tinnitus in patients with cervicogenic somatic tinnitus? *Man. Ther.* 26, 125–131. doi: 10.1016/j.math.2016.08.005

Michiels, S., Ganz Sanchez, T., Oron, Y., Gilles, A., Haider, H. F., Erlandsson, S., et al. (2018a). Diagnostic criteria for somatosensory tinnitus: a delphi process and face-to-face meeting to establish consensus. *Trends Hear.* 22:2331216518796403. doi: 10.1177/2331216518796403

Michiels, S., van der Wal, A. C., Nieste, E., Van de Heyning, P., Braem, M., Visscher, C., et al. (2018b). Conservative therapy for the treatment of patients with somatic tinnitus attributed to temporomandibular dysfunction: study protocol of a randomised controlled trial. *Trials* 19:554. doi: 10.1186/s13063-018-2903-1

Michiels, S., Nieste, E., Van de Heyning, P., Braem, M., Visscher, C., Topsakal, V., et al. (2019). Does conservative temporomandibular therapy affect tinnitus complaints? A systematic review. *J. Oral Facial Pain Headache* 33, 308–317. doi: 10.11607/ofph.2055

Michiels, S., Van de Heyning, P., Truijen, S., Hallemans, A., and De Hertogh, W. (2017). Prognostic indicators for decrease in tinnitus severity after cervical physical therapy in patients with cervicogenic somatic tinnitus. *Musculoskelet. Sci. Pract.* 29, 33–37. doi: 10.1016/j.msksp.2017.02.008

Ogrodniczuk, J. S. (2006). Men, women, and their outcome in psychotherapy. *Psychother. Res.* 16, 453–462. doi: 10.1080/10503300600590702

Ogrodniczuk, J. S., Piper, W. E., Joyce, A. S., and McCallum, M. (2001). Effect of patient gender on outcome in two forms of short-term individual psychotherapy. *J. Psychother. Pract. Res.* 10:69.

Pattyn, T., Van Den Eede, F., Vanneste, S., Cassiers, L., Veltman, D. J., Van De Heyning, P., et al. (2016). Tinnitus and anxiety disorders: a review. *Hear. Res.* 333, 255–265. doi: 10.1016/j.heares.2015.08.014

Phillips, J. S., Erskine, S., Moore, T., Nunney, I., and Wright, C. (2019). Eye movement desensitization and reprocessing as a treatment for tinnitus. *Laryngoscope* 129, 2384–2390. doi: 10.1002/lary.27841

Pinto, P. C., Sanchez, T. G., and Tomita, S. (2010). The impact of gender, age and hearing loss on tinnitus severity. *Braz. J. Otorhinolaryngol.* 76, 18–24.

Rabau, S., Wouters, K., and Van de Heyning, P. (2014). Validation and translation of the Dutch tinnitus functional index. *B ENT* 10, 251–258.

Russell, M., Goodman, T., Wang, Q., Groshong, B., and Lyeth, B. G. (2014). Gender differences in current received during transcranial electrical stimulation. *Front. Psychiatry* 5:104. doi: 10.3389/fpsyt.2014.00104

Samoilov, A., and Goldfried, M. R. (2000). Role of emotion in cognitive-behavior therapy. *Clin. Psychol. Sci. Pract.* 7, 373–385. doi: 10.1093/clipsy.7.4.373

Schlaepfer, T. E., Harris, G. J., Tien, A. Y., Peng, L., Lee, S., and Pearlson, G. D. (1995). Structural differences in the cerebral cortex of healthy female and male subjects: a magnetic resonance imaging study. *Psychiatry Res.* 61, 129–135. doi: 10.1016/0925-4927(95)02634-a

Seidman, M. D., and Jacobson, G. P. (1996). Update on tinnitus. *Otolaryngol. Clin. North Am.* 29, 455–465.

Seydel, C., Haupt, H., Olze, H., Szczepek, A. J., and Mazurek, B. (2013). Gender and chronic tinnitus: differences in tinnitus-related distress depend on age and duration of tinnitus. *Ear Hear.* 34, 661–672. doi: 10.1097/AUD.0b013e31828149f2

Seydel, C., Haupt, H., Szczepek, A. J., Klapp, B. F., and Mazurek, B. (2010). Long-term improvement in tinnitus after modified tinnitus retraining therapy enhanced by a variety of psychological approaches. *Audiol. Neurootol.* 15, 69–80. doi: 10.1159/000231632

Swift, J. K., Callahan, J. L., Ivanovic, M., and Kominiak, N. (2013). Further examination of the psychotherapy preference effect: a meta-regression analysis. *J. Psychother. Integr.* 23:134. doi: 10.1037/a0031423

Tao, K. W., Owen, J., Pace, B. T., and Imel, Z. E. (2015). A meta-analysis of multicultural competencies and psychotherapy process and outcome. *J. Counsel. Psychol.* 62, 337–350. doi: 10.1037/cou0000086

Van de Heyning, P., Gilles, A., Rabau, S., and Van Rompaey, V. (2015). Subjective tinnitus assessment and treatment in clinical practice: the necessity of personalized medicine. *Curr. Opin. Otolaryngol. Head. Neck. Surg* 23, 369–375. doi: 10.1097/MOO.0000000000000183

Vielsmeier, V., Kleinjung, T., Strutz, J., Bürgers, R., Kreuzer, P. M., and Langguth, B. (2011). Tinnitus with temporomandibular joint disorders: a specific entity of tinnitus patients? *Otolaryngol. Head Neck Surg.* 145, 748–752. doi: 10.1177/0194599811413376

Villamar, M. F., Volz, M. S., Bikson, M., Datta, A., Dasilva, A. F., and Fregni, F. (2013). Technique and considerations in the use of 4x1 ring high-definition transcranial direct current stimulation (HD-tDCS). *J. Vis. Exp.* 77:e50309. doi: 10.3791/50309

Zigmond, A. S., and Snaith, R. P. (1983). The hospital anxiety and depression scale. *Acta Psychiatr. Scand.* 67, 361–370.

Zoger, S., Svedlund, J., and Holgers, K. M. (2006). Relationship between tinnitus severity and psychiatric disorders. *Psychosomatics* 47, 282–288. doi: 10.1176/appi.psy.47.4.282

Permissions

All chapters in this book were first published by Frontiers; hereby published with permission under the Creative Commons Attribution License or equivalent. Every chapter published in this book has been scrutinized by our experts. Their significance has been extensively debated. The topics covered herein carry significant findings which will fuel the growth of the discipline. They may even be implemented as practical applications or may be referred to as a beginning point for another development.

The contributors of this book come from diverse backgrounds, making this book a truly international effort. This book will bring forth new frontiers with its revolutionizing research information and detailed analysis of the nascent developments around the world.

We would like to thank all the contributing authors for lending their expertise to make the book truly unique. They have played a crucial role in the development of this book. Without their invaluable contributions this book wouldn't have been possible. They have made vital efforts to compile up to date information on the varied aspects of this subject to make this book a valuable addition to the collection of many professionals and students.

This book was conceptualized with the vision of imparting up-to-date information and advanced data in this field. To ensure the same, a matchless editorial board was set up. Every individual on the board went through rigorous rounds of assessment to prove their worth. After which they invested a large part of their time researching and compiling the most relevant data for our readers.

The editorial board has been involved in producing this book since its inception. They have spent rigorous hours researching and exploring the diverse topics which have resulted in the successful publishing of this book. They have passed on their knowledge of decades through this book. To expedite this challenging task, the publisher supported the team at every step. A small team of assistant editors was also appointed to further simplify the editing procedure and attain best results for the readers.

Apart from the editorial board, the designing team has also invested a significant amount of their time in understanding the subject and creating the most relevant covers. They scrutinized every image to scout for the most suitable representation of the subject and create an appropriate cover for the book.

The publishing team has been an ardent support to the editorial, designing and production team. Their endless efforts to recruit the best for this project, has resulted in the accomplishment of this book. They are a veteran in the field of academics and their pool of knowledge is as vast as their experience in printing. Their expertise and guidance has proved useful at every step. Their uncompromising quality standards have made this book an exceptional effort. Their encouragement from time to time has been an inspiration for everyone.

The publisher and the editorial board hope that this book will prove to be a valuable piece of knowledge for researchers, students, practitioners and scholars across the globe.

List of Contributors

Thomas W. Allan, Julien Besle, Alan R. Palmer and Peyman Adjamian
Medical Research Council Institute of Hearing Research, The University of Nottingham, Nottingham, UK

Dave R. M. Langers, Jeff Davies and Deborah A. Hall
Nottingham Hearing Biomedical Research Unit, National Institute for Health Research (NIHR), Nottingham, UK
Otology and Hearing Group, Division of Clinical Neuroscience, School of Medicine, The University of Nottingham, Nottingham, UK

Yu-Chen Chen, Fang Wang, Fan Bo, Yuan Feng, Cun-Nan Mao, Jun Ren and Xindao Yin
Department of Radiology, Nanjing First Hospital, Nanjing Medical University, Nanjing, China

Jie Wang and Jin-Jing Xu
Department of Otolaryngology, Nanjing First Hospital, Nanjing Medical University, Nanjing, China

Jian-Ping Gu
Department of Vascular and Interventional Radiology, Nanjing First Hospital, Nanjing Medical University, Nanjing, China

Wenqing Xia
Department of Endocrinology, Nanjing First Hospital, Nanjing Medical University, Nanjing, China

Jeff E. Davies
Division of Audiology, Faculty of Health and Life Sciences, School of Allied Health Sciences, De Montfort University, Leicester, UK
National Institute for Health Research, Nottingham Hearing Biomedical Research Unit, Nottingham, UK
Otology and Hearing Group, Division of Clinical Neuroscience, School of Medicine, University of Nottingham, Nottingham, UK

Phillip E. Gander
National Institute for Health Research, Nottingham Hearing Biomedical Research Unit, Nottingham, UK
Otology and Hearing Group, Division of Clinical Neuroscience, School of Medicine, University of Nottingham, Nottingham, UK

Jan Wielopolski
Department of Psychiatry and Psychotherapy, University Hospital Zurich, University of Zurich, Zurich, Switzerland

Tobias Kleinjung, Melanie Koch and Nicole Peter
Department of Otorhinolaryngology, University Hospital Zurich, University of Zurich, Zurich, Switzerland

Martin Meyer
Neuroplasticity and Learning in the Healthy Aging Brain, University of Zurich, Zurich, Switzerland

Michael Rufer and Steffi Weidt
Department of Psychiatry, Psychotherapy and Psychosomatics, Psychiatric Hospital, University of Zurich, Zurich, Switzerland

Berthold Langguth, Verena Hund and Martin Schecklmann
Department of Psychiatry and Psychotherapy, University of Regensburg, Regensburg, Germany

Michael Landgrebe
Department of Psychiatry and Psychotherapy, University of Regensburg, Regensburg, Germany
Department of Psychiatry, Psychosomatics and Psychotherapy, kbo-Lech-Mangfall-Klinik Agatharied, Hausham, Germany

Rosemarie Arnold, Emile de Kleine and Rutger Hofman
Department of Otorhinolaryngology/Head and Neck Surgery, University of Groningen, University Medical Center Groningen, Groningen, Netherlands

Minke J. C. van den Berge, Rolien H. Free and Pim van Dijk
Department of Otorhinolaryngology/Head and Neck Surgery, University of Groningen, University Medical Center Groningen, Groningen, Netherlands
Graduate School of Medical Sciences (Research School of Behavioural and Cognitive Neurosciences), University of Groningen, Groningen, Netherlands

J. Marc C. van Dijk
Graduate School of Medical Sciences (Research School of Behavioural and Cognitive Neurosciences), University of Groningen, Groningen, Netherlands
Department of Neurosurgery, University of Groningen, University Medical Center Groningen, Groningen, Netherlands

Karolina Müller
Center for Clinical Studies, University Medical Center Regensburg, Regensburg, Germany

Niklas K. Edvall, Barbara Canlon and Christopher R. Cederroth
Experimental Audiology, Department of Physiology and Pharmacology, Karolinska Institutet, Stockholm, Sweden

Esma Idrizbegovic and Robert Huhn
Hörsel-och Balanskliniken, Karolinska Universitetssjukhuset, Stockholm, Sweden

Rilana Cima
Clinical Psychological Science, Faculty of Psychology and Neuroscience, Maastricht University, Maastricht, Netherlands
Center of Expertise in Rehabilitation and Audiology, Adelante Rehabilitation, Hoensbroek, Netherlands

Viktor Persson, Constanze Leineweber and Hugo Westerlund
Stress Research Institute, Stockholm University, Stockholm, Sweden

Berthold Langguth and Winfried Schlee
Department of Psychiatry and Psychotherapy, University Medical Center Regensburg, Regensburg, Germany

Sylvie Hébert and Philippe Fournier
Faculty of Medicine, School of Speech Pathology and Audiology, Université de Montréal, Montréal, QC, Canada
BRAMS - International Laboratory for Research on Brain, Music, and Sound, Université de Montréal, Montréal, QC, Canada

Roland Moschen, Gerhard Rumpold and David Riedl
University Clinic of Medical Psychology, Medical University of Innsbruck, Innsbruck, Austria

Alessandra Fioretti and Eleonora Natalini
Tinnitus Center, European Hospital, Rome, Italy

Alberto Eibenstein
Tinnitus Center, European Hospital, Rome, Italy
Department of Applied Clinical and Biotechnological Sciences, University of Aquila, L'Aquila, Italy

Domenico Cuda
Department of Otorhinolaryngology, Guglielmo da Saliceto Hospital, Piacenza, Italy

Giuseppe Chiarella
Department of Experimental and Clinical Medicine, Unit of Audiology and Phoniatrics, Magna Græcia University, Catanzaro, Italy

Małgorzata Wrzosek
Department of Logic and Cognitive Science, Adam Mickiewicz University, Poznań, Poland

Eugeniusz Szymiec, Małgorzata Modrzyńska and Agnieszka Lang-Małecka
ENT Department, University of Medical Sciences, Poznań, Poland

Wiesława Klemens
ENT Private Practice, Gdynia, Poland

Piotr Kotyło
Audiology and Phoniatrics Clinic, Nofer Institute of Occupational Medicine in Łódź, Łódź, Poland

Winfried Schlee
Department of Psychiatry and Psychotherapy, University of Regensburg, Regensburg, Germany

Anna Preis
Institute of Acoustics, Adam Mickiewicz University, Poznań, Poland

Jan Bulla
Department of Mathematics, University of Bergen, Bergen, Norway

Isabel Diges
ACURE-Tinnitus and Hyperacusis Clinic, Madrid, Spain

Francisco Simón and Pedro Cobo
Institute of Physical and Information Technologies, Consejo Superior de Investigaciones Científicas (CSIC), Madrid, Spain

Jae-Jin Song, Woongsang Sunwoo and Sang-Youp Lee
Department of Otorhinolaryngology-Head and Neck Surgery, Seoul National University Bundang Hospital, Seongnam, South Korea

Kyungsoo Kim, Kyung-Joon Park and Ji-Woong Choi
Department of Information and Communication Engineering, Daegu Gyeongbuk Institute of Science and Technology, Daegu, South Korea

Griet Mertens and Paul Van de Heyning
Department of Otorhinolaryngology and Head and Neck Surgery, University Hospital Antwerp, Edegem, Belgium

Dirk De Ridder
Department of Surgical Sciences, Section of Neurosurgery, Dunedin School of Medicine, University of Otago, Dunedin, New Zealand

Sven Vanneste
Lab for Clinical and Integrative Neuroscience, School of Behavioral and Brain Sciences, The University of Texas at Dallas, Richardson, TX, USA

Hongsoo Choi
Department of Robotics Engineering, Daegu Gyeongbuk Institute of Science and Technology, Daegu, South Korea

Winfried Schlee and Berthold Langguth
Department for Psychiatry and Psychotherapy, University Hospital Regensburg, Regensburg, Germany

Deborah A. Hall
National Institute for Health Research (NIHR) Nottingham Biomedical Research Centre, Nottingham, United Kingdom
Otology and Hearing Group, Division of Clinical Neuroscience, School of Medicine, University of Nottingham, Nottingham, United Kingdom

Barbara Canlon, Christopher R. Cederroth and Niklas K. Edvall
Experimental Audiology, Department of Physiology and Pharmacology, Karolinska Institutet, Stockholm, Sweden

Sarah Engel, Robert Daniel Heinrich Markewitz, Berthold Langguth and Martin Schecklmann
Department of Psychiatry and Psychotherapy, University of Regensburg, Regensburg, Germany

Alain Londero
Service ORL et CCF, Hôpital Européen G. Pompidou, Paris, France

Thomas E. Fuller and Rilana F. F Cima
Clinical Psychological Science, Faculty of Psychology and Neuroscience, Maastricht University, Maastricht, Netherlands
Adelante, Centre of Expertise in Rehabilitation and Audiology, Hoensbroek, Netherlands

Rachelle Lardinois
Adelante, Centre of Expertise in Rehabilitation and Audiology, Hoensbroek, Netherlands

Haula F. Haider
ENT Department of Hospital, Cuf Infante Santo - Nova Medical School, Lisbon, Portugal

Dimitris Kikidis
Department of Otorhinolaryngology, Head and Neck Surgery, National and Kapodistrian University of Athens, Hippocrateion General Hospital, Athens, Greece

Birgit Mazurek and Petra G. Brueggemann
Tinnitus Center, Charite University Hospital, Berlin, Germany

Arnaud Norena
Laboratory of Adaptive and Integrative Neuroscience, Centre National de la Recherche Scientifique, Fédération de Recherche, Aix-Marseille Université, Marseille, France

Alec Lapira
ENT Specialist, Institute of Health Care, Mater Dei Hospital, Malta

Sarah Rabau
Faculty of Medicine and Health Sciences, Campus Drie Eiken, University of Antwerp, Antwerp, Belgium

Niklas K. Edvall and Christopher R. Cederroth
Department of Physiology and Pharmacology, Karolinska Institutet, Stockholm, Sweden

Susanne N. Rosing and Dorte Lungaard
Department of Clinical Research, Faculty of Health Sciences, University of Southern Denmark, Odense, Denmark

Anestis Kapandais
Department of Nordic Studies and Linguistics, Copenhagen University, Denmark

Derek J. Hoare
NIHR Nottingham Hearing Biomedical Research Unit, Division of Clinical Neuroscience, School of Medicine, University of Nottingham, Nottingham, UK

Grant D. Searchfield, Mithila Durai and Tania Linford
Section of Audiology, Eisdell Moore Centre, The University of Auckland, Auckland, New Zealand

Marie Wegger
Department of Clinical Medicine, Aarhus University, Aarhus, Denmark

Therese Ovesen
Department of Clinical Medicine, Aarhus University, Aarhus, Denmark
Department of Otorhinolaryngology, Holstebro Regional Hospital, Holstebro, Denmark

Dalia Gustaityte Larsen
Department of Otorhinolaryngology, Aarhus University Hospital, Aarhus, Denmark

Thomas Probst
Georg-Elias-Müller-Institute for Psychology, Georg-August-University Göttingen, Göttingen, Germany
Department for Psychotherapy and Biopsychosocial Health, Danube University Krems, Krems an der Donau, Austria

Rüdiger C. Pryss, Johannes Schobel and Manfred Reichert
Department for Psychotherapy and Biopsychosocial Health, Danube University Krems, Krems an der Donau, Austria

Berthold Langguth and Winfried Schlee
Department of Psychiatry and Psychotherapy of the University of Regensburg at Bezirksklinikum Regensburg, Regensburg, Germany

Josef P. Rauschecker
Program in Cognitive and Computational Systems, Georgetown University Washington, Washington, DC, United States
Institute for Advanced Study, Technical University Munich, Munich, Germany

Myra Spiliopoulou
Department of Technical and Business Information Systems, Otto-von-Guericke-University Magdeburg, Magdeburg, Germany

Laura Basso, Benjamin Boecking, Petra Brueggemann and Birgit Mazurek
Tinnitus Center, Charité - Universitätsmedizin Berlin, Berlin, Germany

Nancy L. Pedersen
Department of Medical Epidemiology and Biostatistics, Karolinska Institutet, Stockholm, Sweden

Barbara Canlon
Laboratory of Experimental Audiology, Department of Physiology and Pharmacology, Karolinska Institutet, Stockholm, Sweden

Christopher R. Cederroth
Laboratory of Experimental Audiology, Department of Physiology and Pharmacology, Karolinska Institutet, Stockholm, Sweden
National Institute for Health Research (NIHR) Nottingham Biomedical Research Centre, Nottingham University Hospitals NHS Trust, Nottingham, United Kingdom
Hearing Sciences, Division of Clinical Neuroscience, School of Medicine, University of Nottingham, Nottingham, United Kingdom

Johannes Zimmermann
Psychologische Hochschule Berlin, Berlin, Germany

Annemarie Van der Wal
Department of Otorhinolaryngology - Head and Neck Surgery, Antwerp University Hospital, Edegem, Belgium
Department of Rehabilitation Sciences and Physiotherapy, Antwerp University, Antwerp, Belgium

Willem De Hertogh
Department of Rehabilitation Sciences and Physiotherapy, Antwerp University, Antwerp, Belgium

Sarah Michiels
Department of Otorhinolaryngology - Head and Neck Surgery, Antwerp University Hospital, Edegem, Belgium
Department of Rehabilitation Sciences and Physiotherapy, Antwerp University, Antwerp, Belgium
Department of Translational Neurosciences, Antwerp University, Antwerp, Belgium

Tine Luyten, Emilie Cardon, Laure Jacquemin, Olivier M. Vanderveken, Vedat Topsakal, Paul Van de Heyning and Vincent Van Rompaey
Department of Otorhinolaryngology - Head and Neck Surgery, Antwerp University Hospital, Edegem, Belgium
Department of Translational Neurosciences, Antwerp University, Antwerp, Belgium

Annick Gilles
Department of Otorhinolaryngology - Head and Neck Surgery, Antwerp University Hospital, Edegem, Belgium
Department of Translational Neurosciences, Antwerp University, Antwerp, Belgium
Department of Education, Health and Social Work, University College Ghent, Ghent, Belgium

Nancy Van Looveren
Hoorzorg Van Looveren BVBA, Borsbeek, Belgium

Index

www.ingramcontent.com/pod-product-compliance
Lightning Source LLC
LaVergne TN
LVHW082202200926
848484LV00008B/2202

* 9 7 9 8 8 8 7 4 0 5 1 5 5 *